The Royal Marsden Hospital Handbook of Cancer Chemotherapy

A Guide for the Multidisciplinary Team

Edited by

David Brighton

Professional Development Facilitator (eLearning & IT), Nursing, Rehabilitation & Quality Assurance, The Royal Marsden NHS Foundation Trust, Sutton, Surrey, UK

Miriam Wood

Senior Practice Development Facilitator, The Royal Marsden NHS Foundation Trust, Sutton, Surrey, UK

Medical Editors

Stephen RD Johnston

Consultant Medical Oncologist, Department of Medicine – Breast Unit, The Royal Marsden NHS Foundation Trust, London, UK

Hugo Ford

Consultant Medical Oncologist, Addenbrooke's Hospital, Cambridge, UK

Paul J Ross

Department of Medical Oncology, Guy's & St Thomas NHS Foundation Trust, London, UK

Advisors

Jane Mallett

Head of Practice Development, Ashford & St Peter's Hospitals NHS Trust, Chertsey, Surrey, UK

Lisa Dougherty

Nurse Consultant Intravenous Therapy, The Royal Marsden NHS Foundation Trust, London, UK

Foreword

Dickon Weir-Hughes

The Chief Nurse, The Royal Marsden NHS Foundation Trust, London, UK

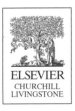

ELSEVIER
CHURCHILL
LIVINGSTONE

EDINBURGH LONDON NEW YORK OXFORD PHILADELPHIA ST LOUIS SYDNEY TORONTO 2005

ELSEVIER
CHURCHILL
LIVINGSTONE

First published 2005

ISBN 0 443 07101 2

British Library Cataloguing in Publication Data
A catalogue record for this book is available from the British Library

Library of Congress Cataloging in Publication Data
A catalog record for this book is available from the Library of Congress

Notice
Knowledge and best practice in this field are constantly changing. As new research and experience broaden our knowledge, changes in practice, treatment and drug therapy may become necessary or appropriate. Readers are advised to check the most current information provided (i) on procedures featured or (ii) by the manufacturer of each product to be administered, to verify the recommended dose or formula, the method and duration of administration, and contraindications. It is the responsibility of the practitioner, relying on their own experience and knowledge of the patient, to make diagnoses, to determine dosages and the best treatment for each individual patient, and to take all appropriate safety precautions. To the fullest extent of the law, neither the publisher nor the editors assumes any liability for any injury and/or damage.   *The Publisher*

ELSEVIER   your source for books,
            journals and multimedia
            in the health sciences
www.elsevierhealth.com

Working together to grow
libraries in developing countries

www.elsevier.com | www.bookaid.org | www.sabre.org

ELSEVIER   BOOK AID   Sabre Foundation
            International

The
publisher's
policy is to use
**paper manufactured
from sustainable forests**

Printed in China

Contents

Contributors

Caroline Archer MRCP
Consultant Medical Oncologist, Portsmouth Oncology Centre, St. Mary's Hospital, Portsmouth, Hampshire, UK

Amanda Baxter RGN RMN Onc cert BSc PG Diplom
Clinical Nurse Specialist, Pelvic Care, The Royal Marsden NHS Foundation Trust, London, UK

Maggie Breen RGN RSCN RHV Paed onc cert BSc Social Sciences MSc Palliative care
Macmillan Paediatric Clinical Nurse Specialist, Paediatric Outreach Nursing Team, The Royal Marsden NHS Foundation Trust, Sutton, Surrey, UK

David Brighton RGN BSc (Cancer Nursing)
Professional Development Facilitator (eLearning & IT), Nursing, Rehabilitation & Quality Assurance, The Royal Marsden NHS Foundation Trust, Sutton, Surrey, UK

Maria Caulfield RGN DipN BSc MSc
Research Nurse, Breast Unit, The Royal Marsden NHS Foundation Trust, Sutton, UK

Patsy Caunter RGN RSCN Onc Cert
Sister, McElwain Ward, Children's Unit, The Royal Marsden NHS Foundation Trust, Sutton, Surrey, UK

Ian Chau MBBS
Clinical Research Fellow, Department of Medicine, The Royal Marsden NHS Foundation Trust, Sutton, Surrey, UK

David Cunningham MD FRCP
Consultant, Clinical Unit Head of Gastrointestinal Unit/Lymphoma, The Royal Marsden NHS Foundation Trust, Sutton, Surrey, UK

Tom Devine RN RSCN BSc(Hons)
Previously *Paediatric Research Fellow, The Royal Marsden NHS Foundation Trust, Sutton, Surrey, UK*

Shelley Dolan RN BA (Hons) MSc
Nurse Consultant Cancer: Critical Care, Critical Care Unit, The Royal Marsden NHS Foundation Trust, London, UK

Lisa Dougherty RGN RM MSc
Nurse Consultant Intravenous Therapy, The Royal Marsden NHS Foundation Trust, London, UK

Jacqueline Edwards RGN RSCN BSc (Hon) MSC
Clinical Nurse Specialist, Paediatric Oncology Outreach (CLIC) (Lead for Neuro-oncology), The Oxford Radcliffe Hospitals NHS Trust, Oxford, Oxfordshire, UK

Timothy G Eisen PhD FRCP
Senior Lecturer/Consultant Medical Oncologist, The Royal Marsden NHS Foundation Trust, Sutton, Surrey, UK

Martin Gore PhD FRCP
Consultant: Medical Oncology, Specialties: Melanoma, Renal Cancer, Ovarian Cancer, Director: Rare Cancers Division, The Royal Marsden NHS Foundation Trust, London, UK

Douglas Guerrero MSc Clinical Neurosciences BSc(Hons) RGN NDN OncNCert NDN COD Cert Counselling Cert
Clinical Nurse Specialist, Neuro-Oncology, The Royal Marsden NHS Foundation Trust, Sutton, Surrey, UK

Karen Handscomb BSc(Hons) PGDE
Macmillan Senior Lecturer Practitioner, Cancer Care, University of Hertfordshire and Mount Vernon Cancer Centre, University of Hertfordshire, Hatfield, Hertfordshire, UK

Kevin J Harrington MBBS MRCP FRCR
Consultant: Clinical Oncologist, The Royal Marsden NHS Foundation Trust, London, UK

Sarah Hart MSc Bsc(Hons) RGN FETC Infection Control
Oncology HIV certificate
*Clinical Nurse Specialist, Infection Control and Radiation
Protection, The Royal Marsden NHS Foundation Trust,
London, UK and The Royal Marsden NHS Foundation
Trust, Sutton, Surrey, UK*

Louise Henry Bsc(Hons) Msc Cancer Care
*Senior Dietician, The Royal Marsden NHS Foundation
Trust, Sutton, Surrey, UK*

Mark Hill MBBS FRCP MD
*Consultant Medical Oncologist and Honorary Senior
Lecturer, Department of Medical Oncology, Kent
Oncology Centre, Maidstone, Kent, UK*

Hilary Hollis Bsc(Hons) Nursing Studies Msc Nursing Studies
Msc Clinical Oncology PG Dip Nursing (Education) RN RNT
ENB 237
*The School of Cancer Nursing and Rehabilitation,
The Royal Marsden NHS Foundation Trust, London, UK*

Robert A Huddart MA MB BS MRCP FRCR PhD
*Senior Lecturer, Academic Unit of Radiotherapy, Institute
of Cancer Research and The Royal Marsden NHS
Foundation Trust, Sutton, Surrey, UK*

Lorraine Hyde RGN ONC Dip Nursing Studies BSc(Hons)
Nursing Studies
*Senior Sister, Day Care Services The Royal Marsden NHS
Foundation Trust, Sutton, Surrey, UK*

Sarah Jefferies BSc MB BS MRCP FRCR
*Consultant Oncologist, Oncology Department,
Addenbrooke's Hospital, Cambridge, UK*

Stephen RD Johnston MA PhD FRCP
*Consultant Medical Oncologist, Department of Medicine –
Breast Unit, The Royal Marsden NHS Foundation Trust,
London, UK*

Ian Judson MA MB BChir MD FRCP
*Professor of Cancer Pharmacology, The Institute of Cancer
Research and Honorary Consultant Medical Oncologist,
The Royal Marsden NHS Foundation Trust, London, UK*

Stanley Kaye BSc MD FRCP FRCR FRSE FMedSci
*Professor of Medical Oncology, The Royal Marsden NHS
Foundation Trust, Sutton, Surrey, UK*

Lloyd R Kelland BPharm PhD DSc MRPharmS
*Professor Basic Medical Sciences, Antisoma Laboratories,
St George's Hospital Medical School, London, UK*

Shirley Langham RGN/RSCN MA
*Clinical Nurse Specialist, Department of Endocrinology,
Great Ormond Street Hospital for Children NHS Trust,
London, UK*

Diane Laverty RGN BSc(Hons) MSc
*Clinical Nurse Specialist, Horder Ward, The Royal
Marsden NHS Foundation Trust, London, UK*

Sally Legge RGN MSc
*Clinical Nurse Specialist, Gastrointestinal Unit,
The Royal Marsden NHS Foundation Trust, London, UK*

Andrew Lomath BSc PhD
*Quality Officer, The Royal Marsden NHS Foundation
Trust, London, UK*

Jane Mashru RGN RSCN Onc Cert
*Sister, Children's Unit, The Royal Marsden NHS
Foundation Trust, Sutton, Surrey, UK*

Rachel Merien-Bennett RN ENB 998 934 A11 BSc(Hons)
Cancer Nursing
*Oncology Nurse, Antoni van Leeuwenhoek Ziekenhuis,
Amsterdam, The Netherlands*

Rahul Kumar Mukherjee MBBS FRANZCR FAMS
*Consultant Radiation Oncologist, The Cancer Institute,
Department of Radiation Oncology, National University
Hospital, Singapore*

Tracey Murray RGN BSc(Hons) MSc
*Lymphoma Clinical Nurse Specialist, The Royal Marsden
NHS Foundation Trust, Sutton, Surrey, UK*

Wayne Naylor BSc(Hons) PG Cert (Palliative Care) RN Dip
Nursing Onc Cert
*Clinical Nurse Specialist, Wellington Cancer Centre,
Wellington Hospital, Wellington South, New Zealand*

Jillian Noble MBChB MRCP(UK)
*Clinical Research Fellow, The Institute of Cancer
Research, London, UK*

Mary ER O'Brien MD FRCP
*Consultant Medical Oncologist, Head, Lung Unit, Chair,
SWLC, Tumour Working Group, The Royal Marsden
NHS Foundation Trust, Sutton, Surrey, UK*

Ross Pinkerton MD FRCPI FRCPH
*Director of Cancer Services, Mater Hospitals, Brisbane
and Professor of Oncology, University of Queensland,
Australia*

Charlotte Rees BSc MRCP
*Consultant in Medical Oncology and Honorary Senior
Lecturer, St George's NHS Trust and St George's Medical
School, London, UK*

Alistair Ring MA MRCP
*Specialist Registrar in Medical Oncology, Department of
Medical Oncology, Guy's & St Thomas NHS Foundation
Trust, London, UK*

Timothy Root BSc Pharmacy MRPharmS
*Specialist Pharmacist, Clinical Governance & Technical
Services, London, East & South East Specialist Pharmacy
Services, Chelsea & Westminster Hospital, London, UK*

Paul Ross PhD MRCP
*Department of Medical Oncology, Guy's & St Thomas
NHS Foundation Trust, London, UK*

Corinne Diana Rowbotham RGN
*Macmillan Breast Care Specialist Nurse, Breast
Screening Unit, Royal Lancaster Infirmary,
Morecambe Bay NHS Trust, Lancaster, UK*

Mave Salter RN NDN (Cert) Onc Cert Cert Ed Dip Couns
B.Sc(Hons) MSc Research and Evaluation
*Clinical Nurse Specialist, Community Liaison,
Rehabilitation Department, The Royal Marsden NHS
Foundation Trust, Sutton, Surrey, UK*

Michelle Scurr BMed FRACP
*Clinical Research Fellow, DDU/CR-UK Centre for Cancer
Therapeutics, The Royal Marsden NHS Foundation Trust,
Sutton, Surrey, UK*

Riyaz Shah PhD MRCP
*Department of Medicine, The Royal Marsden NHS
Foundation Trust, Sutton, Surrey, UK*

Joanne Sims MBA BSc(Hons) MIOSH RSP
*Governance Manager, Clinical Governance & Risk
Management Department, Royal Bournemouth &
Christchurch Hospitals NHS Foundation Trust,
Bournemouth, Dorset, UK*

Ramani Sitamvaram MSc BSc(Hons) Onc Cert RGN
*Clinical Nurse Specialist – Gastrointestinal Cancer,
The Royal Marsden NHS Foundation Trust, Sutton,
Surrey, UK*

Sheila Small BSc RGN RGM Onc Cert MSc PGDip Ed
*Macmillan Lecturer, Macmillan Education Unit,
King's College, London, UK*

Caroline Soady RGN BSc in Cancer Nursing
*Clinical Nurse Specialist, Head & Neck, The Royal
Marsden NHS Foundation Trust, London, UK*

Louise Soanes RGN/RSCN BSc MSc
*Senior Sister for Children's Services, The Royal Marsden
NHS Foundation Trust, Sutton, Surrey, UK*

Justin Stebbing MA MRCP PhD
*MRC Clinical Training Fellow and Specialist Registrar in
Medical Oncology, Department of Oncology, Chelsea and
Westminster Hospital, London, UK*

Moira Stephens RN DPSN BSc(Hons) MSc PGC Ed Cert Onc
*Clinical Nurse Consultant, Haematology/Oncology,
Liverpool Hospital, South West Sydney Area Health
Service, New South Wales, Australia*

Anna-Marie Stevens RN RM MSc BSc(Hons) Onc Cert
*Clinical Nurse Specialist, Palliative Care, The Royal
Marsden NHS Foundation Trust, London, UK*

Jennifer Treleaven MD FRCP FRCPath
*Consultant Haematologist, Department of Haematology,
The Royal Marsden NHS Foundation Trust, Sutton,
Surrey, UK*

Sally Trent BSc MB BS MRCP FRCR
*Radiotherapy, The Royal Marsden NHS Foundation
Trust, London, UK*

Beverley van der Molen RGN MSc BSc FETC Onc Cert
*Patient Information Services Manager, The Royal
Marsden NHS Foundation Trust, Sutton, Surrey, UK*

Suzanne Vizor RGN Dip Cancer Nursing
*Clinical Nurse Specialist, Lung Cancer, St George's NHS
Trust, London, UK*

Dana Walker RGN BSc(Hons)
*Clinical Nurse Specialist, North Glamorgan NHS Trust,
Merthyr Tydfil, South Wales, UK*

Andrew Webb MRCP MD
*Consultant Medical Oncologist' Sussex Cancer Centre,
Brighton and Sussex University Hospital Trust,
Brighton, UK*

Lisa Wolf RGN BSocSc MSc
*Clinical Nurse Specialist, Breast Care, Patient Services,
The Royal Marsden NHS Foundation Trust, Sutton,
Surrey, UK*

Miriam Wood RGN BSc(Hons)
*Senior Practice Development Facilitator, The Royal
Marsden NHS Foundation Trust, Sutton, Surrey, UK*

Foreword

Chemotherapy has become one of the most significant treatment modalities in cancer care. Over the past 20 years new therapies have emerged and innovation in this area is constantly evolving. In some cases therapy is safer and more straightforward. However, when compared with many other types of drug therapy, chemotherapy remains complex, potentially high risk and difficult to manage. It must also be remembered that even when chemotherapy is branded as 'simple' the patient's needs may be complex. The complexity of the therapy is therefore not the only consideration.

The safe management of chemotherapy within a healthcare organisation requires a whole systems approach involving a wide range of clinical professionals and clinical leaders at all stages of the patient journey and the health care organisation's functions. Proper systems of education, prescriber supervision and expert pharmacy advice, integrated governance and risk management are essential. Physicians and pharmacists clearly have a key role to play in ensuring that the gap between 'bench and bedside' is reduced and that patients benefit from the latest innovation in therapy.

For the healthcare professional, chemotherapy might provide opportunities for scientific endeavour or simply a fascination with the effects of the therapy. However, for the patient, chemotherapy is much more. Within our world of science and innovation how easily we could forget that for the patient chemotherapy holds the chance of recovery from illness, or at the very least the hope of an improved quality of life. For patients and their loved ones chemotherapy often remains a frightening and unpleasant treatment modality. Nurses, physicians, pharmacists and rehabilitation therapists play a crucial part in ensuring that the latest evidence-based techniques are used when safely administering chemotherapy and when enabling patients to deal with the side-effects. Nurses have a particularly key role in getting alongside patients when they are feeling sick, fatigued, weary and vulnerable by simply being there for them, not only as a professional adviser, but as a confidante and friend.

The Royal Marsden's approach to ensuring high standards of clinical care is legendary. This impressive piece of work, which we acknowledge will require frequent updating in order to keep up with the pace of change in this area of practice, is an excellent demonstration of the commitment of cancer care professionals to the sharing of good practice. The work brings together all that which is excellent about the Royal Marsden.

This project has been an enormous undertaking for the contributors and editors. I would like to take this opportunity to express my heartfelt thanks to them for their commitment in delivering this product.

Professor Dickon Weir-Hughes
Chief Nurse/Deputy Chief Executive
The Royal Marsden NHS Foundation Trust

Preface

Cancer chemotherapy is given in a wide variety of settings with different intent to people with a range of disease classifications. There have been a number of advances in chemotherapy over recent years, but as yet there has been no 'magic bullet' and the experience of the patient undergoing chemotherapy treatment may sometimes be less than ideal. For this group of patients, good patient assessment and management are reliant upon the clinician's expertise and judgement.

This book grew from the realization that there was a need for a wide-ranging clinically based resource for the different professional groups caring for patients. For this reason, we have included as wide a range of contributors and editors as possible. To create a resource that would meet our aims we drew on the expertise available to us from the extensive range of professions at the Royal Marsden NHS Foundation Trust and our research partner, the Institute of Cancer Research. Many of our contributors' roles have changed during the development of this book; their new roles recognize and reward their expertise and provide them with further challenges. This includes

Jane Mallett, who was instrumental in helping to develop the book and was to be co-editor before she moved on.

When planning what to cover we identified how best to meet the needs of readers and have addressed the following:

- principles and practice of chemotherapy
- management of side-effects
- medical management and patient group specific information.

Because chemotherapy should not be viewed independently of other forms of treatment, there is reference to surgery and radiotherapy where appropriate in a number of the chapters to provide a better overview of the issues for the patient presenting for chemotherapy. Above all, we have tried to keep the patient at the forefront.

We hope you find this a useful resource in your professional practice.

David Brighton,
Miriam Wood

Abbreviations

5-HIAA	5-hydroxyindole acetic acid
ABMT	allogeneic bone marrow transplant
ABO	antigens (proteins) located on the surface of the erythrocyte that determine blood group
ADH	antidiuretic hormone
ADP	adenosine diphosphate
AGVHD	acute graft versus host disease
AIM HIGH	adjuvant interferon in melanoma – high risk
AJCC	American Joint Committee on Cancer
AL	amyloidosis
ALL	acute lymphoblastic leukaemia
Allo-HSCT	allogeneic haemopoietic stem cell transplant
Allo-PBT	allogeneic peripheral blood transfusion
AML	acute myeloid leukaemia
ANLL	acute non-lymphocytic leukaemia
ANP	atrial natriuretic peptide
ARF	acute renal failure
AUC	area under the curve
BASO	British Association of Surgical Oncologists
BBB	blood–brain barrier
BSA	body surface area
CA125	protein used as a marker for ovarian cancer
CAK	CDK-activating kinase, also known as CDK7/cyclinH
CALGB	cancer and leukaemia group B
CBR	clinical benefit response
CCN	childrens' community nurse

CDK	cyclin-dependent kinases
CGH	comparative genomic hybridisation
CHART	continuous hyperfractionated accelerated radiotherapy
CLL	chronic lymphocytic leukaemia
CML	chronic myeloid leukaemia
CMMoL	chronic myelomonocytic leukaemia
CMT	combined modality treatment
CMV	cytomegalovirus
C-MYC	an oncogene
CNS	central nervous system
CNST	Clinical Negligence Scheme for Trusts
CP	clinical protocol
CR	complete remission or response
CRF	case record forms
CS	clinical stage
CSF	cerebrospinal fluid
CT	computed tomography
CTC	clinical trial certificate
CTL	cytotoxic T-lymphocytes
CTX	clinical trial exemption
CVVHDF	continuous veno-venus haemodiafiltration
DCIS	ductal carcinoma in situ
DDX	doctors and dentists exemption
DFS	disease-free survival
DH or DOH	Department of Health
DLBC	diffuse large B-cell non-Hodgkin's lymphoma
DLI	donor lymphocyte infusion
DLT	dose-limiting toxicity
DNA	deoxyribonucleic acid

EBMT	European Bone Marrow Transplant group
EBV	Epstein–Barr virus
ECF	extracellular fluid
ECG	electrocardiograph
ECOG	Eastern Cooperative Oncology Group
EDTA	ethylenediaminetetraacetic acid
ELCAP	Early Lung Cancer Action Project
EOC	epithelial ovarian cancer
EORTC	European Organisation for Research and Treatment of Cancer
EPO	erythropoietin
ER	oestrogen receptor
ERCP	endoscopic retrograde cholangiopancreatography
ESPAC-1	European Study Group for Pancreatic Cancer
ESR	erythrocyte sedimentation rate
FAB	French American British cooperative group
FEV	forced expiratory volume
FIGO	International Federation of Gynaecology and Obstetrics
FISH	fluorescent in-situ hybridisation
FNA	fine needle aspiration
FSH	follicle-stimulating hormone
G-CSF	granulocyte colony-stimulating factor
GFR	glomerular filtration rate
GI	gastrointestinal
GITSG	the gastrointestinal study group
GM-CSF	granulocyte–macrophage colony-stimulating factor
GOG	gynae oncology group
GP	general practitioner (family doctor)
GvHD	graft versus host disease
HBG	health benefit groups
HCV	hepatitis C virus
HD	Hodgkin's disease
HDI	high-dose interferon
HLA	human leukocyte antigen
HNPCC	hereditary non-polyposis colorectal cancer
HPOA	hypertrophic pulmonary osteopathy
HRG	healthcare resource groups
HRT	hormone replacement therapy
HSC	haemopoietic stem cell
HSCT	haemopoietic stem cell transplant
HSR	homogeneously staining regions

IAP	inhibitors of apoptosis
ICSI	intracytoplasmic sperm injection
IFN	interferon
IGCCCG	International Germ Cell Cancer Consensus Group
IM	intramuscular injection
IPI	International Prognostic Index
IPV	inactivated polio vaccine
ISCTR	International Bone Marrow Transplant Registry
IV	intravenous
IVF	in-vitro fertilisation
LAK	lymphokine activated killer cells
LDH	lactate dehydrogenase
LDHL	lymphocyte-depleted Hodgkin's lymphoma
LH	luteinising hormone
LHRH	luteinising hormone releasing hormone
LP	lumbar puncture
LREC	local research ethics committee
LRHL	lymphocyte-rich classical Hodgkin's lymphoma
LV	leucovorin
MACH-NC	Meta Analysis of Chemotherapy on Head & Neck Cancer
MALT	mucosa-associated lymphoid tissue lymphoma
MC	mixed cellularity Hodgkin's lymphoma
MDA	Medical Devices Agency
MDS	myelodysplastic syndrome
MHC	major histocompatability complex
MIBG ^{131}I	m-iodobenzylguanidine
MMR	measles mumps & rubella vaccine
MPA	medroxyprogesterone acetate
MRC	Medical Research Council (UK)
MRD	minimal residual disease
MREC	multi-centre research ethics committee
MTD	maximum tolerated dose
MUD	matched unrelated donor
NER	nucleotide excision repair
NF2	neurofibromatosis type 2
NHL	non-Hodgkin's lymphoma
NHS	National Health Service
NICE	National Institute for Clinical Excellence (UK)
NK	natural killer cells
NLPHL	nodular lymphocyte predominant Hodgkin's lymphoma

NOS	not otherwise specified		SAML	secondary acute myeloid leukaemia
NS	nodular sclerosis Hodgkin's lymphoma		SCLC	small cell lung cancer
NSABP	National Surgical Adjuvant Breast and Bowel Project		SCT	stem cell transplant
			SD	stable disease
NSCLC	non small cell lung cancer		SIADH	syndrome of inappropriate antidiuretic hormone secretion
NSGCT	non-seminoma germ cell tumours			
			SIOP	International Society of Paediatric Oncology
OPV	oral polio vaccine			
OS	overall survival		STLI	sub total lymphoid irradiation
			SVC	superior vena cava
PBSCT	peripheral blood stem cell harvest		SVCO	superior vena cava obstruction
PBT	peripheral blood transplant		SWOG	Southwest Oncology Group
PCI	prophylactic cranial irradiation			
PET	positron emission tomography		TBI	total body irradiation
PGE$_2$	prostaglandin E$_2$		TLI	total lymphoid irradiation
PN	parenteral nutrition		TLS	tumour lysis syndrome
PNET	primitive neuroectodermal tumour		TNM	tumour node metastasis (staging system)
POC	paediatric oncology centre			
POSCU	paediatric oncology shared care unit		TRM	transplant-related mortality
PPE	personal protective equipment		TUR	trans-urethral resection
PR	partial response		TVC	true vomiting center
PS	pathological stage			
PTEN/ MMAC1	phosphatase, tensin homologue/mutated in multiple advanced cancers		UCNT	undifferentiated nasopharyngeal cancers
			UICC	Union Internationale Contre le Cancer
PVI	protracted venous infusion			
			UKCCCR	UK Coordinating Committee on Cancer Research
QOL	quality of life			
			UKCCSG	United Kingdom Children's Cancer Study Group
RA	refractory anaemia			
RAEB	refractory anaemia with excess of blasts		ULN	upper limit of normal
RARS	refractory anaemia with ringed sideroblasts		VAS	visual analogue scale
			VDRL	Venereal Disease Research Laboratory Slide Test
RBC	red blood cells			
RCC	renal cell cancer		VHL	von Hippel–Lindau gene
RCT	randomised controlled trial		VOD	venoocclusive disease
Rh-Tpa	recombinant tissue plasminogen activator			
			WBC	white blood cells
RT	radiation therapy		WHO	World Health Organisation
RTOG	Radiation Therapy Oncology Group			

SECTION 1

Cytotoxic chemotherapy principles and practice

Caring for the patient with cancer relies on an understanding of the disease and treatments, but there are also background principles that influence decisions in care. This section examines some of the principles of cancer chemotherapy and treatment (although the Management of Cancer section covers specific cancer management) and covers some of the core knowledge. The chapters are written by a range of professional groups and specialities and tap into their particular expertise and professional perspectives. Carcinogenesis, standardised protocols and ethics are some of the principles covered here, along with practice issues such as consent, self-administration and intravenous access. Chapter 8 brings many practical themes together to help the practitioner gain a better understanding of the patient's pathway and care in the health system.

Practice is not developed in isolation and the chapters in this section have links and common themes with each other. Where possible, these links and relationships are indicated to help the reader find further information or to explore a different perspective. All of these chapters provide some of the context around how treatments are decided for patients and their disease.

Chapter **1**

Cancer cell biology, drug action and resistance

Lloyd R Kelland

CANCER CELL BIOLOGY

Cancer has long been recognised as a genetic disease and where, in humans, the incidence rises exponentially in the final decades of life. Tumours may be divided into two main types: benign where the disease is limited within a well-defined capsule; malignant, where the disease invades surrounding tissue and spreads around the body. Several lines of evidence support the view that cancer formation in man is a multi-step process, probably four to seven being rate-limiting, where genetic alterations accumulate and progressively drive changes from normal cells to transformed, invasive, malignant cells (for example as described for colorectal cancer[1]). Typically, cancer cells contain numerous genomic alterations, ranging from gross changes in chromosomes (e.g. translocations or loss of regions) to more subtle point mutations within specific genes. Such genetic alterations may arise from multiple endogenous and/or exogenous factors. There are more than 100 distinct types of cancer illustrative of the complexity of these genetic changes and the wide range of organs affected.

Today, cancer at the cellular level is recognised as a state where a variety of normal regulatory processes controlling fundamental cell behaviour, such as proliferation, death and motility, are upset. In a recent review[2] the 'hallmarks of cancer' are described in terms of six basic acquired properties:

1. self-sufficiency in growth signals
2. insensitivity to antigrowth signals
3. evading cell death or apoptosis
4. limitless replicative potential
5. sustained tumour blood vessel formation (angiogenesis)
6. tumour invasion and metastasis.

Oncogenes and tumour suppressor genes

Oncogenes

It is now around 25 years since the identification of the first cellular 'cancer gene' or oncogene (c-SRC) and 20 years since the discovery of the prototype tumour suppressor genes (p53 and retinoblastoma, pRB).[3] There are now known to be at least 100 oncogenes (see Table 1.1 for major ones), which broadly can be divided into five functional categories according to their protein products: growth factors, growth factor receptors, cytoplasmic protein kinases (enzymes which add phosphate groups to specific amino acids on substrate proteins), GTP-binding proteins and transcription factors (which bind to specific DNA sequences and activate the transcription of genes).

There are various ways in which oncogenes may be activated. A common mechanism is through chromosomal translocation. An important translocation is that associated with the Philadelphia chromosome, Ph1, present in virtually all cases of chronic myeloid leukaemia (CML) and involving t(9;22)(q34;q11). This results in the fusion of the Abl proto-oncogene on chromosome 9, which encodes a tyrosine kinase, and the Bcr (breakpoint cluster region) gene on chromosome 22; the resulting fusion protein possesses enhanced constitutive tyrosine kinase activity. (See also Ch. 47 for discussion of Ph1.)

Many translocations involve the *Myc* oncogene on chromosome 8q24, resulting in constitutive activation of this transcription factor. Virtually all cases of Burkitt lymphoma, a B-cell derived, immunoglobulin-producing tumour, possess a translocation of the *Myc* gene with either the Ig heavy chain gene on chromosome 14 or the light chain genes on chromosomes 2 or 22. MYC, in association with protein partners MAX (which results in activation) and MAD and MXI1 allow MYC to act as a transcription factor.

Another important chromosomal translocation is that involving the Bcl-2 gene on chromosome 18 and various immunoglobulin genes. The translocation is observed in about 80% of cases of follicular lymphoma and 20% of diffuse B-cell lymphomas and results in activation of BCL-2, a protein involved in protecting cells from apoptosis (see below).

A second means of oncogene activation is through gene amplification. DNA amplification may be detected by the classical cytogenetic methods of double minute (DM) chromosomes or homogeneously staining regions (HSRs) or by direct DNA analyses (Southern blotting) or by fluorescence in situ hybridization (FISH) or comparative genomic hybridization (CGH). Oncogenes where gene amplification has been reported include the Myc family (e.g. N-Myc in neuroblastoma, c-Myc in small cell lung cancer) and oncogenes associated with the HER family (e.g. HER1 or EGFR in glioblastomas and many epithelial cell carcinomas and HER2/ErbB2 in breast and ovarian cancer).

Furthermore, some oncogenes, notably those of the Ras family (Harvey, Kirsten and N), are activated by point mutations. The activating mutations are usually single amino acid changes in specific positions (12, 13 and 61) which result in mutant RAS proteins with reduced intrinsic GTPase activity, thereby keeping the protein in the 'on' activated GTP-bound form rather than the 'off' GDP-bound state compared to the wild-type normal protein. As shown in Table 1.1, a number of tumours (about 25% in total) contain Ras mutations.

Tumour suppressor genes

There are also several tumour suppressor genes now known (Table 1.2). Many, such as p53 and pRB, play critical roles in the cell cycle (see below). Another important tumour suppressor is PTEN/MMAC1 (phosphatase, tensin homologue/mutated in multiple advanced cancers) on chromosome 10q23.3 which is deleted or mutated in many tumours, including brain, breast, prostate, endometrium and ovarian.[4] PTEN encodes a phosphatase (enzymes opposite in effect to kinases in that they remove phosphate groups, generally leading to inactivation), which in vivo dephosphorylates the lipid phosphatidylinositol

Table 1.1	Major oncogenes	
Oncogene	Function	Tumour examples
Ras-K	GTP/GDP binding	Pancreatic, colon
Ras-H	GTP/GDP binding	Bladder
Ras-N	GTP/GDP binding	Thyroid
Wnt1	Growth factor	–
ErbB2	Growth factor receptor	Breast, ovary
Kit	Growth factor receptor	–
Abl	Tyrosine kinase	Leukaemia
Src	Tyrosine kinase	–
Yes	Tyrosine kinase	Gastric
Lck	Tyrosine kinase	–
Akt	Serine/threonine kinase	–
Mos	Serine/threonine kinase	–
Raf	Serine/threonine kinase	–
Bcl-2	Anti-apoptosis	Follicular lymphoma
Myc	Transcription factor	Burkitt's lymphoma, neuroblastoma, leukaemia
Myb	Transcription factor	–
Fos	Transcription factor	–
Jun	Transcription factor	–
Ets	Transcription factor	Ewing's sarcoma

Table 1.2	Major tumour suppressors	
Tumour suppressors	Function	Tumour examples
RB1	Cell cycle control	Retinoblastoma
P53	Cell cycle control, apoptosis	Many types
WT1	Cell proliferation and differentiation	Wilm's
APC	Cell matrix adhesion	Colon
PTEN	Phosphatase, cell survival	Many
P16	Cell cycle control	Melanoma
BRACA1	DNA repair	Breast and ovary
MLH1	DNA mismatch repair	Colon

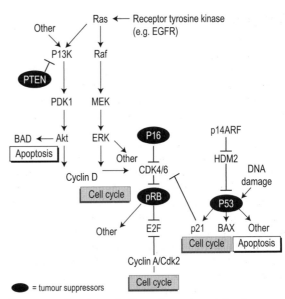

Figure 1.1   Signal transduction pathway deregulation in cancer.

3,4,5-triphosphate (PIP3). This forms part of the PI3K/Akt survival pathway (see below).

Complementary to the identification of oncogenes and tumour suppressor genes is a better understanding of the normal cell cycle and, moreover, how many oncogenes and tumour suppressor genes act to dysregulate the cell cycle. Oncogenes act in a dominant manner and may be viewed as cell cycle accelerators, whereas tumour suppressors are analogous to cell cycle brakes. A third class of cancer-causing gene is genes involved in the DNA repair processes nucleotide excision repair and mismatch repair. When such genes are mutated, cells acquire more mutations in, for example, oncogenes and tumour suppressor genes, leading to increased tumour formation. With the completion of the human genome and the ongoing cancer genome projects, all genes associated with cancer will then be known, although it will take some additional time to elucidate how the various genes/proteins function and interact with one another to cause cancer.

Pathways

Only in some cases, has the complex interaction of various proteins (some being oncogenic, others being tumour suppressors) into pathways been elucidated. Among the most well-defined are those shown in Figure 1.1, which describes the transmission of external growth signals (such as the epidermal growth factor EGF family) to protein receptors on the cell membrane (such as receptor tyrosine kinases), leading to events occurring within the nucleus. Other growth, anti-growth or survival factors include the fibroblast growth factor FGF family, the platelet-derived growth factor PDGF family, the transforming growth factor TGFβ family, insulin-like growth factors, the WNT family, scatter factor/hepatocyte growth factor, chemokines and cytokines. The various companion cell surface receptors for these growth factors are often activated in tumours by homo and hetero dimerization induced by ligand binding.

A common means of intracellular signal transduction is through protein phosphorylation either on tyrosines by non-receptor tyrosine kinases (e.g. the SRC, FPS, ABL, CSK, SYK, JAK, BTK and FAK families) or on serine or threonine amino acids by serine/threonine kinases (e.g. RAF, AKT, MOS). Often these are oncogenic (see Table 1.1). The non-receptor tyrosine kinases often possess homologous sequences or domains of amino acids, the SRC homology or SH1, 2 and 3 domains, which are important for activity, regulation and substrate recognition. One of the most well-defined signal transduction membrane to nucleus pathways is that containing the RAS protein; the RAS/RAF/MEK (MAP kinase kinase)/ERK (MAP kinase) pathway (see Fig. 1.1). Drugs designed to inhibit at various points in this pathway (see below) are already entering clinical testing. An important feature of the pathway is the observation that RAS (H-Ras in particular) is also able to activate the PI3Kinase/Akt survival pathway, thereby providing evidence of cross-talk between pathways.

The cell cycle and cancer

All proliferating cells go through a series of four carefully controlled distinct phases that comprise the cell cycle whereby DNA is duplicated and the cell divides (Fig. 1.2). At the most basic level, following cell division/mitosis (M), which generally occurs

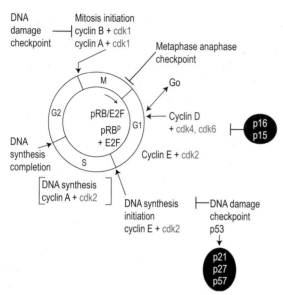

Figure 1.2 The cell cycle and its control.

within 1 hour, cells enter the first gap or G_1 phase, where cells are preparing to synthesise DNA but where synthesis of RNA and protein occurs. Then, after varying lengths of time, the S phase is entered, where there is a doubling of the DNA content; then finally the second gap G_2 phase, where the cell is preparing for cell division. Typically, cell cycle times are of the order of 16–24 hours. In addition, some cells may be out of cycle (G_0 phase). A fundamental discovery, and of great significance in cancer, is that there are various points (or checkpoints) within the cell cycle where checks are made before progressing to the next phase of the cycle (e.g. at the R/START point within G_1 and at the G_2/M border; see Fig. 1.2). Under normal conditions, these checkpoints are silent but various signals (such as DNA damage or when chromosomes are incorrectly aligned in metaphase) switch the checkpoints on and stop the cell cycle. In normal cell growth there is a finely controlled balance between growth-promoting and growth-retarding signals. Only within the past decade have the genes (originally discovered largely in yeast) involved in the cell cycle control of human cells been elucidated.

Control of the cell cycle
Progression through the cell cycle and through checkpoints is tightly regulated by a family of proteins known as cyclin-dependent kinases (CDKs) (see Fig. 1.2).[5] There are at least 9 known CDKs in human cells that act together with specific protein partners (cyclins) to form 1:1 complexes to produce the CDK holoenzyme. Cyclin expression (there at least 15 known, from A to T)

varies throughout the cell cycle and defines the start of each phase. The holoenzyme is activated by the phosphorylation of specific amino acids (tyrosines, threonines or serines) in the catalytic CDK subunit, in some cases by CAK (CDK-activating kinase also known as CDK7/cyclin H). CDKs often have specific roles within the cell cycle such as CDK1 (also known as cdc2) with cyclin B, which is involved at the G_2/M phase, while CDK4 and CDK6 (with D-cyclins) are involved within the G_1 phase (see Fig. 1.2). The first checkpoint is known as START, or the restriction (R point), and occurs late in the G_1 phase. It is at this point that cells commit themselves to a further round of DNA replication; hence loss of this checkpoint can lead to genomic instability and survival of damaged cells. The phosphorylation status of the retinoblastoma protein pRB by CDKs is a critical determinant of cell cycle progression from the G_1 phase of the cell cycle. In the G_1 phase pRB is hypophosphorylated, permitting the binding and sequestration of the E2F family of transcription factors. However, at the end of G_1 various CDKs (CDK4, 6 and 2) together with their cyclin partners, add additional phosphate groups to pRB (hyperphosphorylated state), thereby releasing E2F and allowing transcription of genes required for the S phase (including thymidylate synthase (TS) and dihydrofolate reductase). Another family of proteins known as cyclin-dependent kinase inhibitors (CDKIs) provide an additional level of control by inhibiting the activity of the various CDKs. These are divided into two groups, the INK4 (inhibitor of CDK4) family comprise $p16^{INK4a}$, $p15^{INK4b}$, $p18^{INK4c}$ and $p19^{INK4d}$ and specifically inhibit cyclin D associated kinases (CDK4 and 6). The second group the CIP CDKIs includes $p21^{WAF1}$, which is primarily activated by the important tumour suppressor gene, p53 (see below). Other members are $p27^{KIP1}$ and $p57^{KIP2}$, which inhibit cyclin E/CDK2 and cyclin A/CDK2 complexes (see Fig. 1.2).

Cell cycle deregulation in cancer
Normal cells, for proliferation and cell cycling, require growth signals which are transmitted from the cell membrane via various receptors. It is now apparent that the great majority of human cancers possess deregulation in the control of the cell cycle, in particular through loss of checkpoints. This may occur by numerous means and include inactivation of the p53 gene (see below, primarily leading to loss of a normal G_1/S checkpoint). Another important pathway that is often deregulated in cancer is the pRB/CDK4/cyclin D pathway controlling the START G_1/S checkpoint. Deregulation may occur through mutation or loss of the $p16^{INK4a}$ CDK1 on chromosome 9p21, which normally inhibits CDK4/cyclin D. For example, p16

deletion has been reported in 55% of gliomas and mesothelioma and mutation observed in 40% of pancreatic cancers. Furthermore, in some tumours there is amplification (chromosome 11q13) or over-expression of cyclin D1; for example, some head and neck, eosophageal and breast cancers show amplification while overexpression occurs in some colon cancers through chromosomal translocations. In other tumours there is amplification of CDK4 (chromosome 12q13; e.g. sarcomas, gliomas) or inactivation of pRB itself (chromosome 13q14; e.g. 100% of retinoblastomas, 90% of small cell lung cancer). Taken together, this pathway is altered in a wide range of tumours.

p53

One of the major contributors to cancer formation is the p53 protein, which plays a fundamental role in normal cell cycle progression and apoptosis but which is inacti-vated, by a variety of means, in the vast majority of tumours. The p53 protein was discovered in 1979 in studies aimed at determining the intracellular target of the protein known as large T antigen encoded by the tumour-inducing small DNA virus SV40. Mapping to the short arm of chromosome 17, the p53 gene is now the most commonly mutated gene known in human cancer.[6] Most mutations (over 10 000 have been described in a wide range of organisms) have been shown to occur within specific regions (or 'hot-spots') of the gene, especially in those involved in the bind-ing of the p53 protein to specific DNA sequences. Examples of tumours where p53 mutation is commonly found include lung, breast, colon, bladder, brain and pancreatic cancers. However, in about half of tumours where p53 is inactivated, other mechanisms not involv-ing gene mutation are involved. These include viral infection (e.g. degradation by the E6 protein encoded by the human papillomavirus (HPV) involved in the causation of cervical cancer); multiplication of the HDM2 gene, which stimulates the degradation of p53 (e.g. in sarcomas); mislocalisation of p53 to the cyto-plasm and not the nucleus where it is required to func-tion (e.g. breast cancer, neuroblastomas) and deletion of the p14[ARF] gene which results in a failure to inhibit HDM2 (e.g. some breast, lung, and brain tumours).[6]

Activation of p53   Normally, p53 is inactive but acti-vation occurs by stabilisation (through inhibition of degradation) and conformational changes following cellular stress or damage. Various stresses are known to activate p53: DNA damage, especially that leading to single strand breaks (e.g. ionising radiation); aberrant growth signals (e.g. from the activation of ras and myc oncogenes), which is dependent on the p14[ARF] protein; and chemotherapeutic agents and ultraviolet light.

Damage to DNA is recognised by checkpoint protein kinases such as ATM (ataxia telangiectasia mutated), DNA-dependent protein kinase, chk1 and chk2 which phosphorylate p53 and probably thereby reduce its degradation by HDM2. The major function of p53 is to:

- bind to particular DNA sequences, leading to the activation of adjacent genes such as those involved in cell cycle arrest (e.g. the CDKI, p21 and the 14-3-3σ protein involved in the G_1/S and G_2/M checkpoints)
- apoptosis (e.g. the bcl2 family member, bax; see below)
- DNA repair
- inhibition of the development of tumour blood vessels (angiogenesis).[6]

The end result is that p53 normally acts to mainly shut down the multiplication of stressed cells, via either inhibiting progress through the cell cycle and allowing repair of damaged DNA (hence it being termed the 'guardian of the genome') or by promoting apoptosis, thereby protecting the organism from cells containing damage.

Apoptosis/programmed cell death

The realisation that cells may die by the activation of specific death pathways (apoptosis or programmed cell death) represents a significant finding in cancer cell biology. It appears probable that an acquired resistance to apoptosis is a feature of perhaps all types of cancer. Apoptosis, discovered in the early 1970s, is an intrinsic orchestrated mechanism of cell suicide whereby aged, damaged or unnecessary cells are removed. It is a highly conserved process, being observed in organisms ranging from worms to human beings. Thus, controlled cell loss along with cell prolif-eration play opposing critical roles in organ develop-ment and maintenance of appropriate cell numbers during homeostasis.

Apoptosis was originally defined by pathologists because of its distinct morphological features in com-parison to necrosis where the cell membrane breaks down. The features of cells undergoing apoptosis include plasma membrane blebbing (although the membrane remains intact), cell shrinkage and loss of cell–cell contact (with detachment from plastic dishes in vitro) and condensation of chromatin. In vivo, apoptotic cells are rapidly phagocytosed, often by macrophages, typically within 24 hours. In cells, a commonly observed end-effect is the non-random cleavage of DNA to 50 kb fragments and, in some cells, to smaller inter-nucleosomal fragments of around 200 base pairs. This may be detected using agarose gel electrophoresis where the cleaved DNA appears

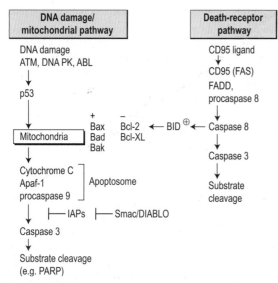

Figure 1.3 Major apoptotic pathways.

as 'DNA ladders' or by a sub-G_1 peak on DNA histograms obtained by flow cytometry.

In the past 10 years, much has been learned of the underlying genes/proteins involved in cell death pathways (Fig. 1.3).[7] The components of apoptosis may be divided into sensors, which monitor the extra-cellular and intracellular environment to check whether normal or abnormal conditions persist, and effectors, which carry out the programmed death. Essentially, there are two major apoptotic pathways in human cells. One pathway is triggered by members of the death receptor superfamily such as CD95 (Apo-1/Fas) and tumour necrosis factor receptor 1. The second is used in response to external and internal insults such as DNA damage, hypoxia and the damage caused by many anticancer drugs (see below). Most of the signals that initiate apoptosis converge on the mitochondria, where members of the BCL2 family of proteins compete and play a key role in determining whether cell death results or not. The BCL2 family may be divided into those which protect the cell from apoptosis (BCL2 itself, BCL-XL and BCL-W) and those which possess a pro-apoptotic function (BAX, BAD, BAK, BID). Exactly how the BCL-2 proteins function remains unclear, although models based on the forma-tion of channels in the outer mitochondrial membrane or the rupture of the outer mitochondrial membrane have been proposed. As described above, p53 plays an important role in the sensing of DNA damage and one of its functions is to directly increase levels of BAX. If there are more pro-apoptotic than anti-apoptotic mol-ecules a variety of molecules is released from mito-chondria, especially cytochrome c, which together

with Apaf-1 and procaspase 9, form the 'apoptosome'. The ultimate effectors of apoptosis are a family of enzymes termed caspases (cysteine proteases that are activated specifically in apoptotic cells and cleave substrate proteins after aspartic acid residues), a key member being caspase 3. Further regulation of the pathway is provided by the activity of IAP (inhibitors of apoptosis) proteins, which antagonise the action of cas-pase 3 and a recently described protein Smac/DIABLO released from mitochondria that antagonises the IAP proteins.[7]

In summary, a failure of cells to undergo apoptosis could contribute to genetically damaged (mutated) cells persisting in the organism, thereby promoting carcino-genesis. Secondly, a failure of tumours to undergo apoptosis leads to tumour resistance to radiotherapy (DNA strand breaks being the main cellular effect of radiation) and to multiple chemotherapy drugs (see below). The loss of the p53 tumour suppressor, as described above, represents the most common means by which tumours have lost a pro-apoptotic regulator. Activation of the PI3kinase-AkT anti-apoptotic survival pathway (which occurs through sequestering of pro-apoptotic BAD protein) is also commonly observed (e.g. by H-ras activation or loss of PTEN- see above).

Unlimited replicative potential of cancer cells

Another key feature of cancer cells as opposed to nor-mal cells is their ability to grow indefinitely. About 40 years ago, Hayflick showed that normal cells in cul-ture have a finite life span. Once a certain number of doublings have occurred (the Hayflick limit or mortal-ity M1), cells stop growing and enter senescence. This may be by-passed by transformation with oncogenes and/or loss of tumour suppressor genes (see above). However, these cells will divide only for a further finite time, at which point (mortality 2, M2) a state known as crisis occurs. The crisis state is characterised by mas-sive cell death, end-to-end fusion of chromosomes and the occasional emergence of a variant cell that is termed immortalised and can multiply without limit.

Control of unlimited replicative potential The under-lying control of unlimited cell growth in cancer cells has been shown in the last 10 years to involve telomeres, repetitive DNA sequences (TTAGGG in humans) and associated proteins present at the ends of chromo-somes. In normal cells some telomeric DNA is lost (around 100 base pairs) every time the cell divides due to the 'end-replication' problem, as DNA polymerases cannot completely replicate the 3' ends of chromo-somal DNA in S phase. When telomeres eventually become critically shortened, crisis occurs. Cancer cells, however, maintain telomere length and thereby are able to grow indefinitely. This occurs in 85–90% of cases by the reactivation of an enzyme termed telomerase that adds the hexanucleotide TTAGGG repeats onto telomeres with the aid of its own RNA template. In the remaining 10% of cases, telomeres are also maintained but by an alternate (ALT) mechanism involving recombinational exchanges. The structural components of telomerase (the catalytic domain hTERT and RNA component hTR) and proteins associated with telomeres have been elucidated in the past 5 years. Due to the selective expression of telomerase in cancer versus normal cells there is currently considerable interest in developing inhibitors of this enzyme as a novel therapy for cancer.[8]

Angiogenesis, invasion and metastases

A final feature of most tumours is their ability to form new blood vessels and to invade and metastasise to distant parts of the body. Angiogenesis-inducing signals appear to be generated from endothelial cells. There are also endogenous inhibitors of angiogenesis such as thrombospondin-1 and β-interferon that are downregulated, or inhibitors such as angiostatin released by proteolysis of plasmin. The ability to induce and sustain angiogenesis occurs in a discrete step in tumour development, the 'angiogenic switch'. Two major signals are vascular endothelial growth factor (VEGF) and acidic and basic fibroblast growth factors (FGF1/2). Basic FGF may be released from the extracellular matrix by proteases. VEGF and FGF each binds to transmembrane tyrosine kinase receptors present on endothelial cells. Integrins and adhesion molecules mediating cell–matrix and cell–cell association also play key roles. There is currently much interest in the discovery and study of angiogenesis inhibitors (e.g. anti-VEGF antibodies such as bevacizumab (Avastin), VEGF inhibitors, angiostatin).

Metastases are the cause of 90% of human cancer deaths. The underlying control of invasion and metastases is complex and incompletely eludicated. Several classes of proteins involved in the holding of cells together in a tissue are altered in invasive or metastatic tumour cells. These include CAMs (cell–cell adhesion molecules), members of the immunoglobulin (e.g. N-CAM) and calcium-dependent cadherin families and integrins responsible for linking cells to extracellular matrix substrates. An important protein is E-cadherin, which is normally present on epithelial cells and, through interaction with β-catenin, acts as a potent suppressor of invasion and metastasis. E-cadherin function, however, is lost in the vast majority of epithelial cancers by mechanisms that include mutation of E-cadherin or β-catenin genes. Extracellular proteases, especially those involved in

matrix degradation, are also important in invasion and metastases with protease genes upregulated and protease inhibitor genes downregulated. A family known as matrix metalloproteinases (MMPs) is of particular importance. It comprises collagenases (e.g. MMPs 1 and 8) that degrade fibrillar collagens, stromelysins (e.g. MMPs 3 and 10) that degrade proteoglycans and glycoproteins and gelatinases (e.g. MMPs 2 and 9) that degrade gelatins and some collagens. Inhibitors of MMPs are being evaluated in clinical trials.[9]

CANCER CHEMOTHERAPY

Since the origins of cancer chemotherapy, from observations of the effects of sulphur mustard gas used during World War I, there are now around 50 drugs licensed for the treatment of the disease. However, in comparison to the explosion in our knowledge of the fundamental cellular and molecular processes in cancer formation (see above), these currently available drugs may be considered to be rather blunt, crude instruments. Essentially, virtually all of these drugs (with the exception of the more specific anti-hormonal agents for the treatment of breast and prostate cancers) target rapidly proliferating cells either through effects on DNA or factors involved in mitosis. The majority of these agents were discovered during the 1950s, 1960s and 1970s through large-scale screening of natural products and synthetic molecules administered to mice bearing leukaemias. Since the 1980s, there has been a fundamental shift away from this essentially random approach to anticancer drug discovery to a more 'target-driven' strategy that exploits the recently elucidated differences between cancer and normal cells and to testing in human cancer models (tissue culture continuous cell lines and human tumours grown as xenografts on immune-suppressed or deficient mice).[10] The first members of this 'new generation' of anticancer drug which offer the potential for greater selectivity to cancer versus normal cells are now entering the clinic. Examples include antibodies directed against the products of oncogenes (e.g. Herceptin (trastuzumab) and cetuximab targeted to ERBB2/HER2 and HER1 receptors, respectively); antibodies directed against cell surface antigens (e.g. rituximab directed against the CD-20 antigen of B lymphocytes); inhibitors of tyrosine kinases (e.g. STI-571/imatinib (Gleevec) directed against the oncogenic Bcr/Abl kinase present in most chronic myeloid leukaemias – see above; Iressa (gefitinib) directed against HER1/EGFR); inhibitors of cyclindependent kinases (such as flavopiridol); and inhibitors of the enzyme farnesyltransferase involved in the membrane localisation and activation of RAS proteins. In the future, inhibitors of angiogenesis and telomerase and gene therapy to correct genetic defects may also play a role in cancer treatment.

Tumour growth

The application of chemotherapy is governed by some general concepts based on tumour growth characteristics. In tumours that are clinically detectable ($1 \, cm^3 = 10^9$ cells), growth follows a Gompertzian function; i.e. as the size of a tumour increases, its rate of growth slows. Conversely, as suggested by Norton and Simon in 1977, the rate of regrowth of a tumour may increase as it shrinks with therapy. Thus, drug levels required to initiate a regression may be insufficient to maintain the regression and induce a cure. Consequently, it is common to either increase the dose of agents for remission induction or switch to additional drugs in an aggressive schedule. Furthermore, chemotherapy studies performed by Skipper in the 1960s in mice bearing leukaemias showed that animal survival was inversely related to tumour burden. A single tumour cell was capable of multiplying and killing the animal for most drugs, increasing dose led to increasing tumour cell kill and a given dose of drug kills a constant fraction (not a constant number) of cells. This formed the basis of the cell kill hypothesis, which states that tumours are best treated when they are small in volume and that treatment must continue until the last cell is killed. (Tumour growth is also discussed in Ch 2.)

Classes of anticancer drugs

In general terms, anticancer drugs may be classified into a limited number of broad categories: alkylating agents, antimetabolites, antimicrotubule agents, topoisomerase inhibitors and anti-hormonal agents (Table 1.3).

Alkylating agents

The alkylating agents kill cells by direct interaction with DNA. Some are bifunctional (i.e. have two chemically reactive sites and produce two sites of damage or covalent adducts on DNA), whereas others are monofunctional and produce one adduct on DNA. Examples of bifunctional alkylating agents, where two R-CH$_2$ groups are added to DNA via the formation of a highly reactive cyclical immonium ion, include cyclophosphamide, ifosfamide, nitrogen mustard, melphalan, thiotepa, busulfan and chlorambucil. Cyclophosphamide is inactive as the parent drug but requires metabolic activation in the liver by cytochrome P450 enzymes to generate the active metabolite phosphoramide mustard. The elucidation of the complex

Table 1.3 Major classes of anticancer drugs

Class	Examples
Alkylating agents	Melphalan, chlorambucil, cyclophosphamide
	BCNU, CCNU
	Procarbazine, dacarbazine, temozolomide
	Cisplatin, carboplatin, oxaliplatin
Antimetabolites	Methotrexate, 5-fluorouracil, raltitrexed
	Ara-C, gemcitabine
	6-mercaptopurine, pentostatin, 6-thioguanine
	Hydroxyurea
Antimicrotubule agents	Vincristine, vinblastine, vinorelbine
	Paclitaxel, docetaxel
Topoisomerase inhibitors:	
Topo II	Doxorubicin, mitoxantrone
	Etoposide, m-AMSA
Topo I	Irinotecan, topotecan
Anti-hormonal agents:	
Breast	Tamoxifen, anastrozole
Prostate	Goserelin, cyproterone acetate

metabolism of cyclophosphamide led to the routine usage of MESNA to combat the urotoxicity caused by another metabolite, acrolein. The most susceptible region for alkylation of DNA is the N-7 position of the guanine bases. Alkylation of guanine pairs leads to crosslinked DNA strands that cannot replicate and leads to cell death (generally by apoptosis – see above). Dacarbazine, procarbazine and temozolomide act as methylating agents on DNA, dacarbazine and procarbazine requiring metabolic activation in the liver.

The platinum-containing compounds cisplatin, carboplatin and oxaliplatin also kill cells by binding to and platinating DNA. Cisplatin is essentially a prodrug where the chlorine groups on the molecule are displaced within cells by highly reactive water ions. Interestingly, cisplatin is only active when the chlorines are in the cis formation – the isomer transplatin is inactive. The formation of the positively charged aquated products of carboplatin occurs more slowly than with cisplatin and may account for its reduced nephrotoxicity. A variety of platinum-containing DNA adducts have been observed; some 90% involving crosslinks on the same strand of DNA (intrastrand crosslinks between adjacent guanines or adjacent guanine and adenine) but with a small proportion involving crosslinks on guanines on different DNA strands (interstrand crosslinks). There is still doubt as to which of these types of DNA lesion is the more biologically significant in terms of cell killing.

Antimetabolites

The antimetabolite class of anticancer drugs comprises analogues of natural compounds required for DNA or RNA synthesis. One of the earliest discovered was methotrexate, the first drug, in 1947, to cause complete remissions in children with acute lymphoblastic leukaemia (ALL). Methotrexate is a potent inhibitor of the enzyme dihydrofolate reductase (DHFR), which catalyses the reduction of dihydrofolate to tetrahydrofolate. As a consequence, levels of intracellular folate coenzymes are decreased. These coenzymes are required for thymidylate biosynthesis as well as purine biosynthesis and thus, when depleted, DNA synthesis is inhibited and cell replication stops. Methotrexate is retained inside cells by the chemical addition of, up to 5, glutamate groups onto the parent molecule, by the enzyme folylpolyglutamate synthetase (FPGS).

5-Fluorouracil (5FU) causes cell death by both being incorporated into RNA instead of uracil and by inhibition of another important enzyme involved in DNA synthesis, thymidylate synthase (TS). The drug may be activated inside cells to 5-fluorouridine monophosphate (FUMP), which may be incorporated into RNA or to the nucleotide 5-fluoro-2'-deoxyuridine 5'-phosphate (FdUMP), which inhibits TS. Recently, more specific TS inhibitors have been developed, among them, raltitrexed (Tomudex).

Another important antimetabolite drug is cytosine arabinoside (Ara-C). Inside cells, phosphate groups are added to the parent molecule by deoxycytidine kinase to produce Ara-CTP, which inhibits DNA chain elongation by being incorporated directly into DNA. The drug may also be inactivated by two intracellular enzymes, cytidine deaminase and deoxycytidylate deaminase. An important new analogue of Ara-C is gemcitabine (2',2'-difluorodeoxycytidine), which is less susceptible to inactivation by deamination than Ara-C.

Important antimetabolites based on purine DNA bases include 6-mercaptopurine (6-MP) and 6-thioguanine (6-TG). 6-MP is activated intracellularly by hypoxanthine-guanine phosphoribosyl transferase (HGPRT) to nucleotide 6-mercaptopurine ribose phosphate, which inhibits purine nucleotide synthesis. It may be inactivated by xanthine oxidase. Pentostatin (2'-deoxycoformycin) inhibits adenosine deaminase, thereby causing high levels and imbalances in pools of adenosine and deoxyadenosine nucleotides. Cladribine (2-chlorodeoxyadenosine) is phosphorylated by deoxycytidine kinase, is resistant to adenosine deaminase and becomes incorporated into DNA. Another antimetabolite class of drug is hydroxyurea, which directly inhibits the enzyme ribonucleotide reductase. The enzyme catalyses the conversion of ribonucleotides to deoxyribonucleotides and is a crucial rate-limiting enzyme in the synthesis of DNA. Hydroxyurea preferentially affects cells in the S phase of the cell cycle.

Antimicrotubule agents

The antimicrotubule agents comprise two distinct classes: the vinca alkaloids (vincristine and vinblastine isolated from the leaves of the Madagascar periwinkle plant) and the taxanes paclitaxel and docetaxel isolated from the *Taxus* or yew tree. The vinca alkaloids bind to tubulin, which is essential for forming the mitotic spindle fibres along which the chromosomes migrate during mitosis and for maintaining cell structure, and inhibit spindle assembly. In contrast, the taxanes bind to the β subunit of tubulin and stabilise the microtubule structure, thereby inhibiting depolymerisation. These drugs are cell cycle specific, acting at the G_2/M phase.

Topoisomerase inhibitors

Topoisomerase inhibitors comprise two classes of drug: those inhibiting topoisomerase II and others inhibiting topoisomerase I. These are enzymes important in maintaining DNA topology and in DNA replication and recombination as they introduce transient double- or single-stranded DNA breaks followed by strand passage and rejoining. Topoisomerase II inhibitors form a ternary complex between the enzyme and DNA, which results in the formation of DNA strand breaks. Examples include etoposide, m-AMSA and the anthracyclines, doxorubicin, daunorubicin, epirubicin and mitoxantrone. The anthracyclines may also bind (intercalate) between DNA strands and, in addition, doxorubicin may exert its killing and toxic (especially cardiotoxic) effects through the generation of free radicals. Actinomycin D is primarily a DNA intercalating drug and blocks RNA synthesis. The topoisomerase I inhibitors irinotecan and topotecan are analogues of camptothecin and act by binding to topoisomerase I, thereby resulting in DNA double-strand breaks.

Anti-hormonal drugs

The anti-hormonal group of drugs exploit the hormone dependence for the growth of some cancers, notably the common requirement for oestrogen in breast cancer and androgens in prostate cancer. One of the main anti-endocrine drugs used to treat breast cancer is the oestrogen receptor antagonist, tamoxifen. Another class of agent, inhibitors of the enzyme aromatase such as anastrozole and formestane, are used in the treatment of postmenopausal breast cancer. The main drugs used in the anti-endocrine treatment of prostate cancer are the anti-androgens (such as cyproterone acetate, flutamide and bicalutamide) and luteinising hormone releasing hormone (LHRH) analogues (such as goserelin, buserelin and leuprorelin).

Miscellaneous drugs

A final miscellaneous group of drugs includes mitomycin C and bleomycin. Mitomycin C is a prodrug which requires activation by enzymatic reduction (including under hypoxic conditions) to produce a molecule that forms crosslinks on DNA. Bleomycin causes both single- and double-strand breaks on DNA as a consequence of generating free radicals and, in some respects, resembles the biological effects of radiotherapy.

Drug effects on the cell cycle

An understanding of the cell cycle (see above) is essential for achieving the optimal use of anticancer drugs as many act at specific phases of the cell cycle whereas others act independently of the phase of the cell cycle. Phase-dependent drugs (i.e. drugs that exert their effects on cells primarily in a particular phase of the cell cycle) include the S-phase specific drugs Ara-C, methotrexate, hydroxyurea, 6-thioguanine and raltitrexed and agents which act predominantly at the G_2/M phase of the cell cycle such as etoposide, bleomycin, the vinca alkaloids vincristine and vinblastine and the taxanes paclitaxel and docetaxel. Other drugs may be classified as cell cycle independent; these include the alkylating agents, platinum agents, doxorubicin and mitomycin C.

Drug resistance

From the early days of the use of cancer drugs it was recognised in clinical practice that some patients' tumours were resistant to the effects of a particular drug (or combination), whereas other patients presenting with other tumour types or even the same tumour type by histology, responded. Furthermore, another common clinical observation was that of resistance to drugs acquired during successive courses of chemotherapy. Thus, drug resistance may be intrinsic and present at the onset of chemotherapy or acquired and represents one of the major causes of treatment failure.

Most drug resistance is considered to result from the high spontaneous mutation rate of cancer cells (i.e. genetic instability). The Goldie–Coldman random mutation hypothesis suggested that tumours may

become resistant through spontaneous mutation: the higher the number of tumour cells, the greater the probability. The model also provides a basis for the use of combination chemotherapy to help combat resistance. The main principles of combination chemotherapy are that the drugs should all be active as single agents, possess differing mechanisms of action and have minimally overlapping toxicities. Examples include cyclophosphamide, doxorubicin, vincristine and prednisone (CHOP) in the treatment of lymphoma and bleomycin, cisplatin and vinblastine (or etoposide) in the treatment of testicular cancer. (See also Ch 2.)

In the past 25 years, much has been learned of the underlying mechanisms involved in the causes of intrinsic and acquired drug resistance, predominantly through the use of laboratory cell line and animal models of cancer. In basic terms, drug resistance may be caused by 'pharmacological' factors where insufficient drug reaches the cellular target or some change in the target has occurred or through 'post-target' mechanisms where, although the drug has reached the target, the tumour cells are not killed (Fig. 1.4).

'Pharmacological' resistance mechanisms

Some genes/proteins involved in drug resistance merit special mention as these have been shown (at least in the laboratory) to confer resistance to multiple classes of anticancer drug. Foremost among these is a 170 kDa protein termed P-glycoprotein (PgP) originally discovered around 25 years ago and now known to be part of a family of membrane proteins responsible for the energy-dependent active efflux of toxins from cells.[11]

P–glycoprotein and other multidrug resistance proteins

When tumour cells in culture are repeatedly exposed to some anticancer drugs (e.g. doxorubicin, vincristine),

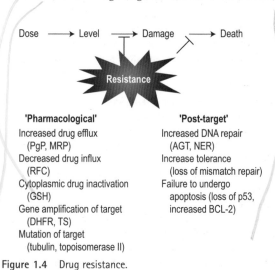

'Pharmacological'	'Post-target'
Increased drug efflux (PgP, MRP)	Increased DNA repair (AGT, NER)
Decreased drug influx (RFC)	Increase tolerance (loss of mismatch repair)
Cytoplasmic drug inactivation (GSH)	Failure to undergo apoptosis (loss of p53, increased BCL-2)
Gene amplification of target (DHFR, TS)	
Mutation of target (tubulin, topoisomerase II)	

Figure 1.4   Drug resistance.

amplification of the MDR1 gene (also known as ABCB1) encoding PgP is commonly observed. Significantly, as well as resistance being observed to the agent used to generate resistance, loss of sensitivity to a variety of additional drugs, so-called multidrug resistance (MDR), is commonly observed. The drugs involved in this MDR phenotype include the natural products vincristine, vinblastine, etoposide, paclitaxel, docetaxel, topotecan and the anthracyclines doxorubicin and daunorubicin and the synthetic drug mitoxantrone. P-glycoprotein is also normally expressed in some tissues such as the lining of the gut, the brush border of the kidney, adrenal cortical cells, pancreatic ductules and endothelial cells of capillary blood vessels in the brain, probably also to deal with environmental toxins. Evidence for a role for PgP contributing to drug resistance in clinical practice is less clear than from laboratory cell-line studies. However, there have been some reports, especially in childhood sarcoma and neuroblastoma, correlating relapse from chemotherapy to increased expression of PgP. Expression may also be increased in some recurrent leukaemias and lymphomas.

P-glycoprotein is now known to belong to a group of so-called ATP-binding cassette (ABC) superfamily of drug transporters. Another member, MDR-related protein (MRP1 also known as ABCC1; 190 kDa) also contributes to drug resistance in some cases. Another six members of the MRP family of genes have also been discovered (ABCC2 to ABCC7).[12] The MRPs appear to be organic ion transporters and are able to transport a wide variety of substances out of cells, including anionic drugs such as methotrexate, neutral drugs conjugated to glutathione, glucuronate or sulphate or together with free glutathione (such as doxorubicin, daunorubicin, vincristine, vinblastine and etoposide).[12] MRP1 may therefore act as a glutathione (GSH) S-conjugate pump (GS-X pump) and reduction in levels of GSH using a γ-glutamyl synthetase inhibitor, buthionine sulfoximine reduces its drug export properties. The range of drugs exported by MRP1 is wider than for PgP but it is not as effective as transporting paclitaxel. MRP1 is expressed in most human tissues and tumours but no strong association has yet been established between MRP1 levels and clinical drug resistance. Overexpression of MRP2 (also known as cMOAT, ABCC2), but not MRP1, may contribute to resistance to cisplatin. Another protein that has been shown to cause multidrug resistance in cancer cells and to correlate with drug resistance in patients with ovarian cancer and acute myeloid leukaemia is the lung resistance-related protein (LRP; 110 kDa). This is believed to be a vault protein involved in transport between the nucleus and cytoplasm in cells. Another

protein, breast cancer resistance protein (BCRP1), when overexpressed causes resistance to mitoxantrone, doxorubicin, daunorubicin and topotecan and SN38 (the active metabolite of irinotecan).

Changes in topoisomerase   Mutations in or changes in the phosphorylation status of topoisomerase II give rise to so-called alternate multidrug resistance (ALT-MDR), which confers resistance to the family of drugs targeting topoisomerase II (such as etoposide, m-AMSA, doxorubicin and mitoxantrone).

Other pharmacological mechanisms of drug resistance
Impaired drug transport, but not due to PgP, has also been shown to contribute to acquired resistance to some drugs; e.g. methotrexate and cisplatin. With cisplatin, membrane transport mediated resistance appears to be due mainly to a reduced drug influx rather than by increased efflux. With methotrexate and other antifolates such as raltitrexed, uptake is mediated via a specific carrier protein, the reduced folate carrier (RFC), which may be reduced in resistant tumour cells.

Increased levels of intracellular thiol-containing species, especially the tripeptide glutathione (γ-glutamylcysteinylglycine, GSH), give rise to resistance to the alkylating agents and platinum drugs and doxorubicin. GSH's conjugation with a compound, either spontaneously or catalysed by glutathione S-transferases (α, π, μ, θ isozymes), makes the compound less toxic and more hydrophilic and excretable from cells.[13] GST π has been shown to be overexpressed in some tumour types (ovarian, colorectal, ALL).

Gene amplification of the target may also contribute to resistance; e.g. overexpression of DHFR causes resistance to methotrexate, overexpression of TS causes resistance to 5-FU and raltitrexed, and overexpression of ribonucleotide reductase causes resistance to hydroxyurea. Mutation of the target tubulin is also applicable to resistance to the tubulin-interactive drugs vincristine (and vinblastine) and the taxanes paclitaxel and docetaxel. In some cases, changes in levels of activating or inactivating enzymes may contribute to drug resistance: examples include increased levels of a hydrolase that degrades bleomycin; reduced levels of deoxycytidine kinase, the activating enzyme for Ara-C; reduced levels of activity of HGPRT, which activates 6-mercaptopurine; and reduced levels of FPGS, the enzyme which adds polyglutamate groups to methotrexate and raltitrexed, thereby maintaining high intracellular drug concentrations.

Post-target mechanisms of drug resistance
As the majority of the cytotoxic class of cancer drugs target DNA, the processes by which cells repair DNA

damage may also contribute to drug resistance. At least four DNA repair processes are known in human cells. One of the simplest repair pathways is mediated through the enzyme O^6 alkyltransferase (AGT), which is responsible, through an enzyme suicide mechanism, for removing alkyl groups from the oxygen in the 6-position of the DNA base guanine. High levels of AGT cause resistance to drugs that induce lesions on this position on guanines; the methylating agents dacarbazine and temozolomide and the chloroethylating agents BCNU and CCNU.

One of the major DNA repair pathways in human cells is nucleotide excision repair (NER), which involves the complex interaction of at least 20 proteins to recognise and excise damaged DNA, then synthesise new DNA to fill the resulting gap and reseal. Enhanced NER may contribute to resistance to the alkylating agents, platinum drugs, mitomycin C and bleomycin. Another, more recently discovered, DNA repair pathway is DNA mismatch repair (MMR), which corrects for base mismatches in DNA. In contrast to NER, where an increase leads to resistance, with MMR it is a loss of this pathway that causes low-level resistance (2–3 fold) to drugs such as the methylating agents, 6-thioguanine, cisplatin and doxorubicin.

In recent years, it has become apparent that a failure to engage programmed cell death (apoptosis) – see above – may also contribute to resistance to multiple cancer drugs:[14] e.g. loss of the p53 tumour suppressor gene has been shown, particularly in cancer cell lines, to often lead to resistance to DNA-damaging drugs. In addition, there is some evidence to suggest that resistance, especially in vivo, may be caused by imbalances in the BCL-2 family of proteins: i.e. relatively high levels of anti-apoptotic members such as BCL-2 or BCL-XL relative to pro-apoptotic members.[15]

In most cases, drug resistance in clinical practice appears to be due to multiple mechanisms involving combinations of the above. For example, resistance to the platinum drugs cisplatin and carboplatin has been shown to be due to decreased drug influx, increased cytoplasmic detoxification through increased levels of glutathione and or metallothioneins, increased DNA nucleotide excision repair, increased tolerance through loss of DNA mismatch repair and decreased apoptosis through changes in the levels of pro- or anti-apoptotic proteins of the BCL2 family (Table 1.4).

Methods to overcome clinical drug resistance

As mechanisms of drug resistance have become elucidated in recent years, methods to circumvent resistance in the clinic are now an important area of study.

Table 1.4	Examples of multiple resistance mechanisms
A	**Cisplatin**
	Reduced membrane transport
	Increased GSH/metallothionein
	Increased DNA excision repair
	Loss of DNA mismatch repair
	Decreased apoptosis (e.g. loss of p53, increased BCL-2)
B	**Methotrexate**
	Defect in reduced folate carrier (RFC) protein
	Decrease in FPGS
	Gene amplification of DHFR
C	**Etoposide**
	Increased drug efflux (PgP or MRP)
	Altered topoisomerase II (mutation or phosphorylation) decreased apoptosis

A pharmacological means might be to administer higher doses of combination chemotherapy in combination with haematopoietic growth factors or stem cells (to overcome life-threatening myelosuppression). To date, such dose-intensity studies have not been particularly successful, however.

Several non-cytotoxic modulators of PgP-mediated drug resistance have been discovered, the calcium channel blocker verapamil being one of the earliest. In recent years, clinical trials of MDR modulators in combination with cytotoxic drugs such as etoposide or doxorubicin have been performed with ciclosporin A and a derivative, PSC833. As yet, there have been no clinical trials with modulators of the MRP family of MDR proteins.

Other biochemical means of overcoming resistance being evaluated in clinical practice include the co-administration of DNA repair inhibitors with cytotoxic drugs. For example, benzylguanine, an agent that depletes the enzyme AGT, is being tested in studies where it is administered prior to methylating drugs. Other studies have used an inhibitor of GSH synthesis, buthionine sulfoxime (BSO), in combination with the alkylating agent chlorambucil. Additionally, there have been efforts to design analogues of existing drugs that are less susceptible to particular mechanisms of resistance. Examples include doxorubicin analogues not exported by PgP and cisplatin analogues, such as AMD473, which are less susceptible to inactivation by thiol-containing species. There have also been efforts to design prodrugs that are selectively activated under the low oxygen (hypoxic) conditions found in many solid tumours (e.g. tirapazamine). Finally, in the future, various gene therapy approaches may be applied.

These include transfection of the normal p53 gene into tumours, which may increase tumour sensitivity to DNA-damaging agents. Alternatively, the MDR1 gene may be transfected into normal haematopoietic cells so that higher doses of drugs that cause myelosuppression may be given to patients.

References

1. Fearon ER, Vogelstein B. A genetic model for colorectal tumorigenesis. Cell 1990; 61:759–767.
2. Hanahan D, Weinberg RA. The hallmarks of cancer. Cell 2000; 100:57–70.
3. Peters G, Vousden KH (eds). Oncogenes and tumour suppressors. New York: IRL Press at Oxford University Press; 1997.
4. Ali IU, Schriml LM, Dean M. Mutational spectra of PTEN/MMAC1 gene: a tumour suppressor with lipid phosphatase activity. J Natl Cancer Inst 1999; 91:1922–1932.
5. Senderowicz AM, Sausville EA. Preclinical and clinical development of cyclin-dependent kinase modulators. J Natl Cancer Inst 2000; 92:376–387.
6. Vogelstein B, Lane D, Levine AJ. Surfing the p53 network. Nature 2000; 408:307–310.
7. Hengartner MO. The biochemistry of apoptosis. Nature 2000; 407: 770–776.
8. Kelland LR. Telomerase: biology and phase I trials. Lancet Oncol 2001; 2:95–102.
9. Chambers AF, Matrisian LM. Changing views of the role of matrix metalloproteinases in metastasis. J Natl Cancer Inst 1997; 89:1260–1270.
10. Garrett MD, Workman P. Discovering novel chemotherapeutic drugs for the third millennium. Eur J Cancer 1999; 35:2010–2030.
11. Aran JM, Pastan I, Gottesman MM. Therapeutic strategies involving the multidrug resistance phenotype: the MDR1 gene as target, chemoprotectant, and selectable marker in gene therapy. Adv Pharmacol 1999; 46: 1–42.
12. Borst P, Evers R, Kool M, Wijnholds J. A family of drug transporters: the multidrug resistance-associated proteins. J Natl Cancer Inst 2000; 92:1295–1302.
13. O'Brien ML, Tew KD. Glutathione and related enzymes in multidrug resistance. Eur J Cancer 1996; 32A:967–978.
14. Hickman JA. Apoptosis and chemotherapy resistance. Eur J Cancer 1996; 32A:921–926.
15. Fujita N, Tsuruo T. In vivo veritas: Bcl-2 and Bcl-X$_L$ mediate tumor cell resistance to chemotherapy. Drug Resist Update 2000; 3:149–154.

Chapter 2

Combination chemotherapy and chemotherapy principles

Michelle Scurr, Ian Judson and Timothy Root

INTRODUCTION

For at least the last 50 years chemotherapy has played an important role in the management of many cancers. From early on in the development of chemotherapy it was realised that the window in which the dose range is both efficacious and safe is small. This has led to much research into designing chemotherapy regimens that optimise the efficacy, and the safety and tolerability of these regimens. There has been extraordinary progress since the 1940s, as will be discussed in this chapter, but also much that is yet to be done.

It is important to recognise that methods must be in place to ensure delivery of appropriate and safe chemotherapy treatment to the patient. There is evidence to show that the use of standardised protocols is a satisfactory method of ensuring safe and appropriate delivery of chemotherapy and some of the issues surrounding good protocol design will be discussed in this chapter.

CHEMOTHERAPY REGIMENS

Single agent chemotherapy

The use of cytotoxic drugs in malignant disease was first developed from the chemical weapons programme of the USA during both World Wars. The observation that exposure to nitrogen mustard (mustard gas) caused bone marrow and lymphoid hypoplasia led to research into its use in malignant diseases, and in 1946 the first study was published showing responses to nitrogen mustard in leukaemia and Hodgkin's disease.[1] In 1948 Farber et al[2] showed that an antifolate, aminopterin, was a very active agent in leukaemia. Unfortunately, these remarkable results were quickly tempered by the fact that almost all patients rapidly relapsed and died.

It is now recognised that, with the exception of gestational choriocarcinoma, hairy cell leukaemia and Burkitt's lymphoma, single agent chemotherapy does not lead to cure and the principal reason is the presence of drug-resistant clones in the tumour population prior to commencement of treatment. Luria and Delbruck[3] observed that bacterial populations exposed to bacteriophages developed 'resistance' to the bacteriophages. They found that random mutations that occur continually in the bacterial population had led to the spontaneous development of a clone that was resistant to infection. Law[4] showed that the same mechanism was involved in the emergence of methotrexate resistance in a leukaemic cell line. Goldie and Coldman[5] proposed that tumour cells mutate to a resistant phenotype at a rate intrinsic to the genetic instability of that tumour, and that the probability of a drug-resistant cell being present in a tumour increases as tumour size increases. They predicted that this would be likely to occur, in tumours with only minimal genetic instability, at only 10^6 cells. As tumours are only clinically detectable at approximately 10^9 cells (1 cm diameter tumour), it is highly probable that detectable tumours will have a resistant cell population prior to any chemotherapy. (See also the Drug Resistance section of Ch. 1.)

Combination chemotherapy

By the mid 1950s there was preclinical evidence to suggest that combining cytotoxic drugs improved the cell kill.[6,7] The curative potential of combination chemotherapy, as evidenced by the results in the 1960s in childhood leukaemia[8] and Hodgkin's disease,[9] led to the more widespread use of combination chemotherapy in solid tumours. For a few tumours, such as testis cancer, this potential has been realised, but for the majority of tumours improvements have been modest at the most. (See also Ch. 1.)

General principles of combination chemotherapy

The aims of combination chemotherapy are:

- To circumvent existing drug resistance and prevent development of new resistant clones in a heterogeneous tumour by using different classes of drugs.
- To achieve a greater cell kill with acceptable toxicity, through the use of different classes of drugs.

To achieve these aims, certain general principles in designing a combination chemotherapeutic regimen need to be considered:

- Only drugs that have shown activity as single agents for the specific tumour type should be used.

The inclusion of drugs with little to no activity may lead to a suboptimal dose for a more active drug because of toxicity and thus compromise the efficacy of the combination.

- To ensure that adequate doses of active agents are feasible, there should be as little overlap in the toxicity profile as possible. Although exposing the patient to a potentially broader range of side effects, this approach minimises the risk of a serious or lethal toxicity.
- All drugs in the combination should be given at optimal dose and in the appropriate sequence and schedule.
- The interval between treatments needs to be consistent and as short as possible.

Models for combination chemotherapy

It was evident early on in the evolution of chemotherapy that not only was a single drug not sufficient but also that a single treatment, either of single drug or combination chemotherapy, was not sufficient. Skipper et al[10] showed that for a specific mouse leukaemia cell line, the growth of the tumour was exponential. Skipper also showed that a given dose of a drug destroyed a constant fraction, and not a constant number of cells (log kill hypothesis).[11] The fact that a constant fraction of cells are killed (Fig. 2.1) means that multiple courses (cycles) of treatment are required. Most human tumours do not follow an exponential growth pattern, but rather a Gompertzian pattern, in which the fraction of cells that are actively dividing (growth fraction) reaches its maximum at approximately one-third of the maximum tumour size and decreases thereafter (Fig. 2.2).[12] Cytotoxic agents in general require the cells to be actively cycling to be effective, and thus multiple cycles of chemotherapy are required as cell populations enter and leave the growth fraction of a tumour at differing time points.

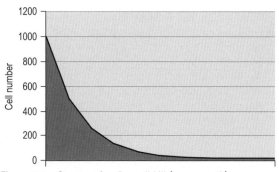

Figure 2.1 Constant fraction cell kill (no regrowth).

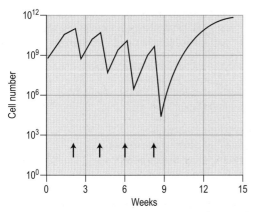

Figure 2.2 Log kill from chemotherapy showing Gompertzian growth of cancer cells.

Using their model of drug resistance, Goldie et al proposed that the optimal chemotherapy regimen would be to give all active drugs at the same time. It was readily apparent that the level of toxicity made this model unfeasible, and they therefore proposed a model in which all active drugs were given in alternating courses.[13] This model requires symmetry, with the alternating treatments being equally effective and completely non-cross resistant, two conditions that are neither easily proven nor easily achieved in clinical practice. Many clinical trials have evaluated an alternating schedule and, although some have shown superior results, in most of these studies the requirements for symmetry have not been met, and the trial design flawed. Bonadonna et al[14] compared alternating MOPP-ABVD with MOPP alone in advanced Hodgkin's disease. This study was based on the assumption that MOPP is non-cross resistant and equally efficacious to ABVD, and the result of the study was a significant survival advantage with the alternating regimen. A comparison of MOPP alone, ABVD alone and alternating MOPP/ABVD confirmed that the alternating sequence was superior to MOPP alone, but also that ABVD was as efficacious as the alternating schedule.[15] To date, the alternating schedule model has not shown true superiority over other models.

Day[16] proposed a model that relaxed the requirements for symmetry. This model again showed that in most circumstances a sequential rather than alternating treatment regimen was superior. Norton and Simon[17] proposed that increasing the dose density of chemotherapy would improve the efficacy of a regimen and that this could be achieved by shortening the interval between treatments and/or by using a sequential schedule. There have been many studies over the last 15 years evaluating sequential chemotherapy. In adjuvant breast cancer, Bonadonna et al[18] showed that sequential administration of doxorubicin followed by CMF was superior to an alternating regimen of two cycles of CMF followed by one cycle of doxorubicin repeated four times. Day[16] also devised the 'worst drug rule', in which the least active of the agents available is used first. The aim of this is to control the cells resistant to the stronger drug at an earlier stage in the treatment. A study by Colucci et al,[19] evaluating this rule in patients with non-small cell lung cancer, did not, however, support this hypothesis.

As more has become understood about the complexities of chemotherapy, models incorporating this knowledge are being designed. Iliadis and Barbolosi[20] developed a mathematical model describing the pharmacokinetics, toxicity and efficacy of a regimen. The optimal drug administration was an initial high dose of chemotherapy followed by a maintenance continuous infusion at a moderate rate. Simulations of this model provided greater cytoreduction while limiting the risks of unacceptable toxicity, compared with standard chemotherapy delivery models. The incorporation of newer agents that are cytostatic rather than cytotoxic will provide great challenges in the future design of combination regimens.

CHEMOTHERAPY PROTOCOLS

Definition of a chemotherapy protocol

A chemotherapy protocol is essentially a standard prescription for the supply and administration of anticancer drugs, either as a single drug or in a defined combination in an identified clinical situation. The prescription should not only detail the drugs administration details such as dose and sequence but also detail the requirements to ensure patient safety. These include the patient parameters that must be met, as well as the prescription of agents required to support the patient: e.g. mouthwashes, antiemetics, granulocyte colony-stimulating factor (G-CSF), and sodium bicarbonate. The two important aims of prescribing chemotherapy are to provide an efficacious treatment and to ensure patient safety. The use of validated protocols would provide a means of achieving these aims.

Evidence for the benefits of protocols

There is evidence that the use of protocols can improve patient management, both in the oncological and non-oncological setting. Drake et al[21] performed a study assessing the impact of an antiemetic protocol on postoperative nausea and vomiting in children. The introduction of the protocol resulted in a decrease in the incidence of moderate to severe postoperative nausea and vomiting and a decrease in the number of patients with repeated nausea. Mitchell et al[22] developed a standardised total parenteral nutrition protocol form that provided the prescription guidelines and compared the number of prescription errors before and after the introduction of this form. The introduction of the form was associated with a marked reduction from 93% to 11% in the numbers of prescription errors that occurred.

The clinical importance of ensuring standardisation of care through oncological protocols is demonstrated by a study by Peeters et al.[23] The authors reviewed the prescription patterns of maintenance chemotherapy (oral methotrexate and 6-mercaptopurine) in a single institution in 288 children with acute lymphoblastic leukaemia and correlated these with duration of complete response. For the overall patient group the doses received were significantly lower than that recommended, and analysis showed this to be primarily due to the dose prescribed rather than patient-related causes. Patients who received a lower than recommended dose of methotrexate were significantly more likely to relapse. Picozzi et al[24] performed an audit of the records of patients with intermediate non-Hodgkin's lymphoma over a 7-year period in a single institution to assess the delivery of chemotherapy. The results showed that 43% of the patients received suboptimal chemotherapy due either to the regimen chosen or the dose intensity delivered.

Errors in drug prescription and administration of chemotherapy are serious issues, with serious implications for both patient safety and disease outcome. This has been borne out in the well-publicised serious events and even fatalities caused by prescription or delivery errors. It would be unrealistic to expect a completely foolproof system, but methods that significantly lessen the risk of errors should be employed. A study by Pastel et al[25] compared chemotherapy prescriptions using standard prescription forms or specific chemotherapy forms. They assessed the completeness of the prescriptions for information including height, weight, dosage, dose, infusion rates, route of administration, frequency of administration and the total number of scheduled doses. The use of the specific chemotherapy form provided a significant improvement in completeness and accuracy of the prescriptions, thus lessening the risk of errors. The NIH Clinical Centre analysed all chemotherapy-related medication errors, and identified seven areas where improvements needed to be made. These included protocol development, computer system enhancements and dose verification.[26] Through the implementation of the above, there was an overall 23% decrease in prescribing errors and a 53% decrease in serious

prescribing errors. Thus, the use of standardised protocols can provide a means of improving the quality of care of patients undergoing chemotherapy.

Basic requirements of a chemotherapy protocol

The general principles that should be met in any protocol include:

- Clarity of prescription.
- Legibility of the prescription.
- Evidence-based regimens.
- Standardised format.
- A process requiring double-checking of doses and patient eligibility.
- Ongoing review process of the protocols in use.

SPECIFIC REQUIREMENTS OF A CHEMOTHERAPY PROTOCOL

There are many requirements necessary to ensure patient safety and delivery of effective treatment. Some of those listed below are self-explanatory, and others will be discussed in greater detail:

- Accurate identification of the patient and the prescriber.
- Date of administration.
- Patient characteristics such as height and weight.
- A checklist of patient parameters that need to be fulfilled to ensure the safest delivery of the chemotherapy at the time of treatment. Examples include neutrophil count, platelet count, liver function tests, and renal function tests.
- The chemotherapeutic drugs.
- Drug doses and the method for calculating the individual patient's dose.
- Route of administration of each of the drugs.
- The duration of the infusion.
- For intravenous administration, amount and type of administration solution.
- Frequency of administration of each drug per cycle.
- The sequence and scheduling of the drugs.
- Cycle length.
- Number of cycles (if relevant).
- The agents required for the safe delivery of the chemotherapy. Examples include hydration, mesna (ifosfamide), folinic acid (high-dose methotrexate) and premedication prior to paclitaxel.
- Supportive measures to reduce anticipated toxicities associated with these agents such as prophylactic antiemetics, mouth care and G-CSF.

Figure 2.3 is an example of a chemotherapy protocol used at the Royal Marsden Hospital. The protocol system is computerised, and the proforma is printed once the patient's hospital number is entered and the

Pat Num:		Authorising Consultant		The Royal Marsden NHS Trust. **LYMPHOMA UNIT**		Date Calculated →					Published 30.03.2001 by **Version: 1.1**

CHOP

Date of Birth:		Pharmacist				Height (m)					

				Course #	(21 day cycle)	Weight (kg)					

STAPLE SECURELY TO SECTION 3 OF DRUG CHART

						Surface Area (m^2)					Page 1 of 1

Bloods : Hb= g/dL **WBC=** x 10^9/L **Neutrophils=** x 10^9/L **Platelets=** x 10^9/L

Disp/Admin.Record

Admin Date	Admin Time	Drug	Dose	Route	Infusion Duration	Administration Details	Prescriber Signature	Date	Start time	Sign. nurse	Stop time	Sign. nurse
Day 1		Graniseration (2mg if>100kg)	1mg	IV	bolus							
		Cyclophosphamide (750mg/m^2)	mg	IV	bolus	via a fast running drip						
		Doxorubicin (50mg/m^2)	mg	IV	bolus	via a fast running drip						
		Vincrstine (1.4mg/m^2) (maximum dose 2mg)	mg	IV	bolus	via a fast running drip						
		Prednisolone E.C.	100mg	po	od	for 5 days						
TTOs		Allopurinol	300mg	po	od	4/52 (first month only)						
TTOs		Co-trimoxazole	480mg	po	od	Mon, Weds, Fri 3/52						
TTOs		Metoclopramide	20mg	po	tds	for 3 days						
TTOs		Lansoprazole	30mg	po	om	3/52						
TTOs		Corsodyl	5ml	M/W	qds	3/52						
TTOs		Nystatin	1ml	M/W	qds	3/52						

Prescriber's signature:
Date:

Signature of Pharmacist:
Date:

Figure 2.3   Chemotherapy protocol used at the Royal Marsden Hospital.

appropriate protocol chosen. The chemotherapy history of the patient is available to ensure that the correct treatment is being prescribed. The relevant patient parameters such as body surface area are entered, and the prescriber calculates and handwrites the patient's doses of the agents as well as the date of delivery. This is sent to pharmacy who double-checks the prescription, as well as ensuring that the full blood count and other necessary investigations have been performed and are adequate to allow treatment prior to the drugs being dispensed.

The protocol for CHOP has been chosen as an example, as it is a well-recognised and validated regimen in the treatment of non-Hodgkin's lymphoma. All of the drugs have been shown to be active in this tumour type, and improved efficacy in combining these agents is well recognised. The medications needed for supportive care are also included in the protocol (tablets to take out or TTOs), thus ensuring that the patient will receive these at the time of treatment.

The following sections are a discussion of some of the important aspects to consider in the designs of combination chemotherapy and protocols.

The chemotherapy drugs

Chemotherapy protocols are based on the use of a single drug or a defined combination of drugs that have been shown to have activity against particular tumour types. The active drugs and combinations for specific tumour types are discussed in the relevant chapters, and will not be discussed further here.

Dose of the drugs

The dose of a drug or the doses in a combination regimen are determined in dose-escalating studies called phase I studies. The aim of these studies is to find the highest dose that can be delivered safely, called the maximum tolerated dose (MTD). They are generally not designed to determine whether the dose is therapeutic. Efficacy is evaluated in phase II and III studies in specific tumour types. The dose determined is usually based on a formula that then individualises the dose for each patient. (See the Clinical Trials Section for further information.)

Body surface area

For most anticancer drugs the method for calculating the dose for an individual patient is to multiply the predefined dose of the drug by the patient's body surface area (BSA). This formula was derived in 1916 by Du Bois and Du Bois[27] and is calculated using the patient's height and weight. Initially, it was felt to be a good method for standardising drugs, as it was

thought that there was a correlation with BSA and physiological parameters of drug metabolism. The most important parameters in drug metabolism are renal clearance and hepatic function. BSA has been shown to have only a weak correlation with renal clearance, and no correlation with hepatic function.[28] BSA has become the standard method of determining cytotoxic drug dosage. This is principally based on a study showing that the MTD found in the animal studies accurately predicted that for human studies, when normalised to BSA.[29] This study showed only a safe method for calculating the starting dose for a phase I study, but with no validation is used in dose escalating in phase I studies, and has become the principal method of calculating chemotherapy doses in the clinical setting.

For BSA to be a valid method for the safe and effective dosage of chemotherapy, there should be strong correlation between it and the endpoints of toxicity and efficacy. For most chemotherapy agents there is considerable inter- and intrapatient variability in toxicity and tumour response, despite standardisation of the dose by BSA. For many drugs pharmacokinetic parameters have been shown to correlate with toxicity, with area under the time × concentration curve (AUC) the most commonly used measure of drug exposure.[30] Therefore, for BSA to be an appropriate method for safe dosing there must be a strong correlation between BSA and the relevant pharmacokinetic parameters. There are drugs for which BSA is predictive of important pharmacokinetic variables, such as docetaxel,[31] paclitaxel,[32,33] gemcitabine,[34] oral (but not intravenous) busulphan,[32,35] and temozolomide[36] (Table 2.1). There is a weak correlation seen with carboplatin, as carboplatin clearance is dependent on glomerular filtration rate (GFR), which does correlate with BSA, although not as accurately as it does with AUC.[37] However, for most cytotoxic drugs no correlation between BSA and pharmacokinetic parameters has been seen.[32,38–46] (see Table 2.1). There are also some studies suggesting that pharmacokinetic parameters may be important in tumour response for certain tumours, [30,47–50] but other factors such as resistance are much more important.

Other methods of dosing
AUC Carboplatin is an example of a chemotherapy drug for which there is a validated method utilising pharmacokinetic parameters. Calvert et al[37] showed that carboplatin plasma clearance is linearly related to GFR, and that the degree of thrombocytopenia is related to the AUC. They derived a formula for carboplatin dosage that correlates the GFR of the patient with the desired AUC of carboplatin, and this formula has been validated in many studies. (The management

action, the dose that can be delivered and pharmaco-dynamic endpoints such as the toxicity profile or efficacy of a drug. We now consider two examples, 5-FU and paclitaxel, where differing durations of infusions are clinically important.

Preclinical studies with 5-FU suggest that the mechanism of action may differ, depending on the duration of the infusion. Bolus injection of 5-FU leads to inhibition of RNA synthesis, whereas continuous infusion causes inhibition of thymidylate synthase, and thus the mechanisms of resistance may be different, depending on the infusion duration. The effect of the duration of infusion of 5-FU has been investigated in colorectal cancer and has been shown to influence outcomes. Several studies[64,65] have shown that the shorter the bolus injection (1–2 min versus 20 min to 1 hour), the higher the response rate seen. This in part may be due to the higher peak concentration and mean AUC seen with a more rapid delivery of the drug. Continuous infusional 5-FU appears to be more efficacious than bolus injection. The Meta-analysis Group[66] analysed all clinical trials of 5-FU in patients with advanced colorectal cancer over a 10-year period and found a significant improvement in tumour response rates in favour of continuous infusional delivery. There is evidence in advanced colorectal carcinoma suggesting that tumour response is associated with improved survival, and thus the differences in tumour response becomes more important.[66,67] The duration of infusion of 5-FU also modulates the toxicity profile with bolus injection, causing more myelosuppression, and continuous infusion delivery, causing more skin toxicity.

Paclitaxel has been used in many tumour types, utilising many different infusion durations. The duration of infusion has been shown to determine the toxicity profile.[68] Prolonging infusion duration increases the frequency and severity of myelosuppression, suggesting that myelotoxicity may be related to the duration of exposure of the bone marrow to concentrations of paclitaxel above a given threshold. Neurological toxicity is more associated with the shorter duration infusions, suggesting that the peak concentration of paclitaxel is important in the pathogenesis of the neurotoxicity. Paclitaxel is a cell cycle specific agent and there is preclinical evidence to suggest that enhanced cytotoxicity is seen by prolonging exposure of the tumour cells to the drug,[69] but clinical studies to date have not shown significant survival benefit for longer duration infusions.[68,70] Thus, the optimum duration of infusion for paclitaxel is determined more by the toxicity profile than by efficacy.

Drug sequencing and scheduling

With combination chemotherapy, the sequence and schedule in which the various drugs are administered can have significant implications for clinical efficacy and toxicity. Pharmacokinetic, biochemical and cell cycle related interactions between drugs lead to more or less cytotoxicity, depending on the sequence that the drugs are given. When the interaction leads to decreased cytotoxicity (antagonism), it is called 'relative resistance'. Cell cycle mediated resistance is seen where a chemotherapeutic drug is rendered less effective because of accumulation of cells into a phase of the cell cycle in which it is less active, through the action of other drugs given earlier in the combination.

Paclitaxel is predominantly an M phase specific drug, as it stabilises microtubule formation and thus inhibits mitosis. Cisplatin, although not cell cycle specific, appears to be most active when cells are in G_1 phase. In preclinical studies antagonism is seen when cisplatin precedes paclitaxel, as cisplatin causes G_2 arrest and so cells do not enter M phase where paclitaxel is active. When the sequence of drugs is reversed, there is synergistic cytotoxicity. In animal models another important feature of sequence dependence is seen. When cisplatin precedes paclitaxel, severe toxicity is observed, whereas when paclitaxel precedes cisplatin, there is significant prolongation of survival compared to when paclitaxel is given alone.[71] A phase I study of the combination of paclitaxel and cisplatin confirmed the preclinical observation that cisplatin given prior to paclitaxel causes increased toxicity with more severe myelotoxicity.[72] The cause of this increased toxicity may in part be due to pharmacokinetic drug interactions. The administration of cisplatin prior to paclitaxel leads to a marked reduction in the clearance of paclitaxel, and increased myelotoxicity. Animal studies have also shown that the sequence has an effect in terms of neurotoxicity, with cisplatin given before paclitaxel showing additive peripheral neurotoxicity, whereas the reverse sequence afforded relative protection.[73] Another clinically important interaction is that between paclitaxel and doxorubicin, which has shown significant activity in tumour types such as breast cancer. In a study by Holmes et al,[74] paclitaxel was given over 24 hours, either immediately prior or after a 2-day infusion of doxorubicin in patients with metastatic breast cancer. The study design was a crossover such that half of the patients received paclitaxel and then doxorubicin for the first cycle of treatment and the reverse sequence for the second. The other half received the two cycles in the reverse order. This study showed that the peak serum concentration of doxorubicin was significantly higher and the mean doxorubicin clearance significantly lower when paclitaxel preceded doxorubicin. The toxicity (mucosal and myelosuppression) was also significantly higher with this sequence. There are many drugs known to have significant sequence-dependent interactions with the taxanes.[75] Irinotecan and 5-FU have been found in vitro to have a sequence-dependent interaction with synergistic cytotoxicity seen when irinotecan precedes 5-FU.[76] This may in part be due to the position in S phase in which these two drugs are most active.

Interval

The interval between agents may be important for some combinations and, as for sequencing, this may be due either to pharmacokinetic interaction or to cell cycle mediated action, with a delay between drugs allowing synchronisation of cells into the phase for which the subsequent agent is most active. In a phase II study in metastatic breast cancer, patients were treated with paclitaxel and then cisplatin 12 hours later with an overall response rate of 80% (22% CR).[77] This may have been due to synchronisation of the cells into the G_1-S phase in which cisplatin is most active. There are many other drugs such as gemcitabine for which drug interactions are important determinants in deciding on drug scheduling and sequencing.

Duration of chemotherapy cycle

Ideally, chemotherapy would be given on a continuous basis in order to achieve maximal cell kill and lessen the probability of a resistant strain developing. As normal tissue is also affected by cytotoxic drugs, there needs to be an interval to allow recovery of normal tissue. A cycle is defined as a course of chemotherapy and the interval between each cycle is determined by the time taken for the repair of the most sensitive normal tissue (bone marrow and mucosa). The standard timing of cycles every 21–28 days is based on the average time taken for the bone marrow to recover sufficiently to allow further delivery of cytotoxic agents. After damage to stem cells in the bone marrow, the time taken for mature cells to enter the peripheral blood circulation from the bone marrow is about 8–10 days. Leucopenia and thrombocytopenia occur by about days 9–10, with the nadir counts occurring by days 14–18, and recovery by days 21–28. The time interval between cycles can be reduced by accelerating the exit of mature cells from the bone marrow into the peripheral circulation. Growth-stimulating factors, such as G-CSF or granulocyte–macrophage colony-stimulating factor (GM-CSF), can shorten the period of

neutropenia, in some cases allowing cycles with intervals as short as every 2 weeks. These agents, however, do not change the duration of thrombocytopenia, and for drugs such as carboplatin, where thrombocytopenia is the dose-limiting toxicity, the interval required to allow safe retreatment is often 4 weeks.

Total duration of treatment

The number of cycles of treatment that a patient is to receive may depend on the reason for treatment. If the treatment aim is palliative, the number of cycles will depend on the response of the patient to the treatment. If the patient responds, treatment will usually continue until the maximum benefit has been derived, the patient begins to progress through the treatment or toxicity precludes further treatment. Some clinicians advocate the continuation of chemotherapy, in this case to two cycles past the best response, where there is no evidence of the patient beginning to progress. Certain drugs such as the anthracyclines have cumulative toxicity that prevents ongoing treatment with that drug past a certain cumulative dose.

In the adjuvant setting there is an inherent difficulty in determining the optimal number of cycles for a given patient, as response cannot be determined while the patient is receiving treatment. In this case the number of cycles to be delivered must be based on the evidence from clinical studies. There are several tumour groups for which there has been much research into the optimal number of cycles of adjuvant chemotherapy, including breast cancer (CMF), testicular cancer (BEP) and colorectal cancer (5-FU and folinic acid).

Adjuvant treatment in breast cancer using multiple drugs has been shown to improve survival.[78] The most commonly used combination in this setting is CMF (cyclophosphamide, methotrexate and 5-FU). There has been and continues to be considerable debate over the optimal number of cycles. The Early Breast Cancer Trialists' Collaborative Group[78] performed an overview of the published adjuvant studies and found that although there was a non-significant improvement in recurrence rate in patients who had received more than 6 months of adjuvant CMF, there was no survival advantage seen. The IBCSG (International Breast Cancer Study Group) compared three versus six cycles in patients with node-positive breast cancer.[79] At 5 years median follow-up, three cycles was found to be inferior to six cycles, with shorter time to relapse seen. Colleoni et al[80] reported the results of a German Breast Cancer Study Group in a similar cohort, as well as updating the IBCSG study results at a median of 7.9 years. In both studies there was no difference seen in overall disease-free survival or in overall survival.

In patients less than 40 years of age and those with oestrogen-negative tumours, however, there was an increased risk of relapse in those that received treatment of shorter duration.

CONCLUSION

This chapter demonstrates some of the many complicated issues involved in designing chemotherapy regimens. With the introduction of novel agents into the clinical setting there will need to be much research so that their incorporation into combination chemotherapy provides the benefits envisaged.

As discussed in this chapter there are genetic mutations that affect the efficacy and toxicity of many drugs, and in the future determination of these mutations prior to treatment will enter the clinical setting. Although this will provide clinicians with the ability to treat these patients more safely, it will increase the complexity of treatment decisions. Thus, the use of protocols will become more necessary. The protocols will have to be flexible enough to allow modification as new information becomes available, and review of these protocols will need to be regular and frequent. It is entirely possible that in the future chemotherapy regimens will be individualised and dependent on patient and tumour factors. Computerised protocol models that allow the clinician to enter the relevant information and thereby prescribe appropriate treatment may be useful tools.

References

1. Goodman LS, Wintrobe MM, Dameshek W, et al. Use of methyl-bis(beta-chloroethyl)amine hydrochloride for Hodgkin's disease, lymphosarcoma, leukaemia. JAMA 1946; 132:126–132.
2. Farber S, Diamond LK, Mercer RD, et al. Temporary remission in acute leukaemia in children produced by folic acid antagonist 4-amethopteroylglutamic acid (aminopterin). N Engl J Med 1948; 238:787.
3. Luria SE, Delbruck M. Mutation of bacteria from virus sensitivity to virus resistance. Genetics 1948; 28:491–511.
4. Law LW. Origin of resistance of leukaemic cells to folic acid antagonists. Nature 1952; 169:628–629.
5. Goldie JH, Coldman AJ. A mathematical model for relating the drug sensitivity of tumours to their spontaneous mutation rate. Cancer Treat Rep 1979; 63:1727–1733.
6. Skipper HE, Thomson J, Bell M. Attempts at dual blocking of biochemical events in cancer chemotherapy. Cancer Res 1954; 14:503–517.
7. Elion GB, Singer S, Hitchings GH. Antagonists of nucleic acid derivatives. VIII. Synergisms in combinations of biochemically related antimetabolites. J Biol Chem 1954; 208:477–488.
8. Frei E III, Freireich EJ, Gehan E, et al. Studies of sequential and combination antimetabolite therapy in acute leukemia: 6-mercaptopurine and methotrexate. Blood 1961; 18:431–454.
9. DeVita VT Jr, Moxley JH III, Brace KC, et al. Intensive combination chemotherapy and X-irradiation in the treatment of Hodgkin's disease. Proc Am Assoc Cancer Res 1965; 6:15.
10. Skipper HE, Schabel FM Jr, Wilcox WS. Experimental evaluation of potential anticancer agents: XII. On the criteria and kinetics associated with the curability of experimental leukaemia. Cancer Chemother Rep 1964; 35:1–11.
11. Skipper H, Schabel F Jr, Lloyd H. Dose response and tumor cell repopulation rate in chemotherapeutic trials. Adv Cancer Chemother 1979; 1:205–253.
12. Norton L. A Gompertzian model of human breast cancer growth. Cancer Res 1988; 48:7067–7071.
13. Goldie JH, Coldman AJ, Gudauskas GA. Rationale for the use of alternating non-cross-resistant chemotherapy. Cancer Treat Rep 1982; 66:439–449.
14. Bonadonna G, Valagussa P, Santoro A. Alternating non-cross-resistant combination chemotherapy or MOPP in stage IV Hodgkin's disease. A report of 8-year results. Ann Oncol 1986; 104:739–746.
15. Canellos GP, Anderson JR, Propert KJ, et al. Chemotherapy of advanced Hodgkin's disease with MOPP, ABVD, or MOPP alternating with ABVD. N Engl J Med 1992; 327:1478–1484.
16. Day RS. Treatment sequencing, asymmetry, and uncertainty: protocol strategies for combination chemotherapy. Cancer Res 1986; 46:3876–3885.
17. Norton L, Simon R. The Norton–Simon hypothesis revisited. Cancer Treat Rep 1986; 70:163–169.
18. Bonadonna G, Zambetti M, Valagussa P. Sequential or alternating doxorubicin and CMF regimens in breast cancer with more than three nodes: ten year results. JAMA 1995; 273:542–547.
19. Colucci G, Gebbia V, Galetta D, et al. Cisplatin and vinorelbine followed by ifosfamide plus epirubicin vs. the opposite sequence in advanced unresectable stage III and metastatic stage IV non-small-cell lung cancer: a prospective randomized study of the Southern Italy Oncology Group (GOIM). Br J Cancer 1997; 76:1509–1517.
20. Iliadis A, Barbolosi D. Optimizing drug regimens in cancer chemotherapy by an efficacy-toxicity mathematical model. Comput Biomed Res 2000; 33:211–226.

21. Drake R, Anderson B, Persson MA, et al. Impact of an antiemetic protocol on postoperative nausea and vomiting in children. Paediatr Anaesth 2001; 11:85–97.

22. Mitchell KA, Jones EA, Meguid MM, et al. Standardised TPN order form reduces staff time and potential for error. Nutrition 1990; 6:457–460.

23. Peeters M, Koren G, Jakubovicz D, et al. Physician compliance and relapse rates of acute lymphoblastic leukaemia in children. Clin Pharmacol Ther 1988; 43:228–232.

24. Picozzi VJ, Pohlman BL, Morrison VA, et al. Patterns of chemotherapy administration in patients with inter-mediate-grade Non-Hodgkins lymphoma. Oncology (Huntingt) 2001; 15:1296–1306.

25. Pastel DA, Fay P, Lee D. Effect of implementing a cancer chemotherapy order form on prescribing habits for parenteral antineoplastics. Hosp Pharm 1993; 28:1192–1195.

26. Goldspiel BR, De Christoforo R, Daniel CE. A continu-ous improvement approach for reducing the number of chemotherapy related medication errors. Am J Health Syst Pharm 2000; 57(Suppl 4):S4–9.

27. Du Bois D, Du Bois EF. A formula to estimate the approximate surface area if height and weight be known. Arch Intern Med 1916; 17:863–871.

28. Sawyer M, Ratain MJ. Body surface area as a determi-nant of pharmacokinetics and drug dosing. Invest New Drugs 2001; 19:171–177.

29. Freireich EJ, Gehan EA, Rall DP, et al. Quantitative comparison of toxicity of anticancer agents in mouse, rat, hamster, dog, monkey, and man. Cancer Chemother Rep 1966 50:219–244.

30. Gurney H. Dose calculation of anticancer drugs: a review of the current practice and introduction of an alternative. J Clin Oncol 1996; 14:2590–2611.

31. Bruno R, Vivler N, Vergniol JC, et al. A population pharmacokinetic model for docetaxel (Taxotere): model building and validation. J Pharmacokinet Biopharm 1996; 24:153–157.

32. Grochow LB, Varaldi C, Noe D. Is dose normalization to weight or body surface area useful in adults? JNCI 1990; 82:323–325.

33. Verweij J, Bontenbal M, van Zomeren D, et al. Body-surface area is an important determinant in paclitaxel. Proc Am Soc Clin Oncol 2002; 21:124a (abstr 492).

34. Allerheiligen S, Johnson R, Hatcher B, et al. Gemcitabine pharmacokinetics are influenced by gen-der, body surface area (BSA), and duration of infusion. Proc Am Soc Clin Oncol 1994; 13:136 (abstr 339).

35. Gibbs JP, Gooley T, Corneau B, et al. The impact of obesity and disease on busulphan oral clearance in adults. Blood 1999; 93:4436–4440.

36. Hammond LA, Eckardt JR, Baker SD, et al. Phase I and pharmacokinetic study of temozolomide on a daily-for-5-days schedule in patients with advanced solid malignancies. J Clin Oncol 1999; 17:2604–2613.

37. Calvert AH, Newell DR, Gumbrell LA, et al. Carboplatin dosage: prospective evaluation of a simple formula based on renal function. J Clin Oncol 1989; 7:1748–1756.

38. Gurney HP, Ackland S, Gebski V, et al. Factors affect-ing epirubicin pharmacokinetics and toxicity: evidence against using body-surface area for dose calculation. J Clin Oncol 1998; 16:2299–2304.

39. De Jongh FE, Verweij J, Loos WJ, et al. Body-surface area-based dosing does not increase accuracy of predicting cisplatin exposure. J Clin Oncol 2001; 19:3733–3739.

40. Mathijssen RH, Verweij J, de Jonge MJA, et al. Impact of body-size measures on irinotecan clearance: alterna-tive dosing recommendations. J Clin Oncol 2002; 20:81–87.

41. Loos WJ, Gelderblom H, Sparreboom A, et al. Inter-and intrapatient variability in oral topotecan pharma-cokinetics: implications for body-surface dosage regimens. Clin Cancer Res 2000; 6:2685–2689.

42. Cassidy J, Twelves C, Cameron D, et al. Bioequivalence of two tablet formulations of capecitabine and explo-ration of age, gender, body surface area, and creatinine clearance as factors influencing systemic exposure in cancer patients. Cancer Chemother Pharmacol 1999; 44:453–460.

43. Freyer G, Tranchand B, Ligneau B, et al. Population pharmacokinetics of doxorubicin and etoposide and ifosfamide in small cell lung cancer patients: results of a multicentre study. Br J Clin Pharmacol 2000; 50:315–324.

44. Ratain MJ, Mick R, Schilsky RL, et al. Pharmacologically based dosing of etoposide: a means of safely increasing dose intensity. J Clin Oncol 1991; 9:1480–1486.

45. Etienne MC, Chatelut E, Pivot X, et al. Co-variables influencing 5-fluorouracil clearance during continuous venous infusion. A NONMEM analysis. Eur J Cancer 1998; 34:92–97.

46. Teresi ME, Riggs CE, Webster PM, et al. Bioequivalence of two methotrexate formulations in psoriatic and cancer patients. Ann Pharmacoth 1993; 27:1434–1438.

47. Schellens JH, Ma J, Planting AS, et al. Relationship between the exposure to cisplatin, DNA-adduct formation in leucocytes and tumour response in patients with solid tumours. Br J Cancer 1996; 73:1569–1575.

48. Evans WE, Crom WR, Abromowitch M, et al. Clinical pharmacodynamics of high-dose methotrexate in acute lymphocytic leukaemia. Identification of a relationship between concentration and effect. N Engl J Med 1986; 314:471–477.

49. Freyer G, Ligneau B, Tranchand G, et al. The prognos-tic value of etoposide area under the curve (AUC) at first chemotherapy cycle in small cell lung cancer patients: a multicentre study of the Groupe Lyon-Saint-Etienne d'Oncologie Thoracique (GLOT). Lung Cancer 2001; 31:247–256.

50. Milano G, Etienne MC, Renee V, et al. Relationship between fluorouracil systemic exposure and tumor response and patient survival. J Clin Oncol 1994; 12:1291–1295.

51. Stoller RG, Hande KR, Jacobs SA, et al. Use of plasma pharmacokinetics to predict and prevent methotrexate toxicity. N Engl J Med 1977; 297:630–634.

52. Goh BC, Ratain MJ, Berucci C, et al. Phase I study of ZD9331 on short daily intravenous bolus infusion for 5 days every 3 weeks with fixed dosing recommendations. J Clin Oncol 2001; 19:1476–1484.

53. Schellens JHM, Planting AS, Ma J, et al. Adaptive intrapatient dose escalation of cisplatin in patients with advanced head and neck cancer. Anticancer Drugs 2001; 12:667–675.

54. Montazeri A, Culine S, Laguerre B, et al. Individual adaptive dosing of topotecan in ovarian cancer. Clin Cancer Res 2002; 8:394–399.

55. Wilson WH, Grossbard ML, Pittaluga S, et al. Dose-adjusted EPOCH chemotherapy for untreated large B-cell lymphomas: a pharmacodynamic approach with high efficacy. Blood 2002; 99:2685–2693.

56. Lennard L, Lilleyman JS, Van Loon J, et al. Genetic variation in response to 6-mercaptopurine for childhood acute lymphoblastic leukaemia. Lancet 1990; 336:225–229.

57. van Kuilenburg AB, Haasjes J, Richel DJ, et al. Clinical implications of dihydropyrimidine dehydrogenase (DPD) deficiency in patients with severe 5-fluorouracil-associated toxicity: identification of new mutations in the DPD gene. Clin Cancer Res 2000; 6:4705–4712.

58. Iyer I, Das S, Janisch L, et al. UGT1A1*28 polymorphism as a determinant of irinotecan disposition clearance: alternative dosing recommendations. Pharmacogenom J 2002; 2:43–47.

59. Salonga D, Danenberg KD, Johnson M, et al. Colorectal tumors responding to 5-fluorouracil have low gene expression levels of dihydropyrimidine dehydrogenase, thymidylate synthase and thymidine phosphorylase. Clin Cancer Res 2000; 6:1322–1327.

60. Etienne MC, Chazal M, Laurent-Puig P, et al. Prognostic value of tumoral thymidylate synthase and p53 in metastatic colorectal cancer patients receiving fluorouracil-based chemotherapy: phenotypic and genotypic analyses. J Clin Oncol 2002; 20:2832–2843.

61. Shapiro WR, Young DF, Mehta BM. Methotrexate: distribution in cerebrospinal fluid after intravenous, ventricular and lumbar injections. N Engl J Med 1975; 293:161–166.

62. Fernandez CV, Esau R, Hamilton D, et al. Intrathecal vincristine: an analysis of reasons for recurrent fatal chemotherapeutic error with recommendations for prevention. J Pediatr Hematol Oncol 1998; 20:587–590.

63. Markman M. The role of intraperitoneal chemotherapy in the front-line setting. J Clin Oncol 2003; 21 (May 15 suppl):145s–148s.

64. Larrssen PA, Carlsson G, Gustavsson B, et al. Different intravenous administration techniques for 5-fluorouracil. Pharmacokinetic and pharmacodynamic effects. Acta Oncol 1996; 35:207–212.

65. Glimelius B, Jakobsen A, Graf W, et al. Bolus injection (2–4 min) versus short-term (10–20 min) infusion of 5-fluorouracil in patients with advanced colorectal cancer: a prospective randomized trial. Eur J Cancer 1998; 34:674–678.

66. Meta-analysis Group in Cancer. Efficacy of intravenous continuous infusion of fluorouracil compared with bolus administration in advanced colorectal cancer. J Clin Oncol 1998; 16:301–308.

67. Buyse M, Thirion P, Carlson RW, et al. Relationship between tumour response to first-line chemotherapy and survival in advanced colorectal cancer; a meta-analysis. Lancet 2000; 356:373–378.

68. Smith RE, Brown AM, Eleftherios P, et al. Randomized trail of 3-hour versus 24-hour infusion of high dose paclitaxel in patients with metastatic or locally advanced breast cancer: National Surgical Adjuvant Breast and Bowel Protocol B-26. J Clin Oncol 1999; 17:3403–3411.

69. Lopes NM, Adams EG, Pitts TW, et al. Cell kill kinetics and cell cycle effects of Taxol on human and hamster ovarian cell lines. Cancer Chemother Pharmacol 1993; 32:235–242.

70. Holmes FA, Valero V, Buzdar AU, et al. Final results: randomized phase III trial of paclitaxel by 3-hr infusion versus 96-hr infusion in patients (pt) with met breast cancer (MBC). The long and the short of it. Proc Am Soc Clin Oncol 1998; 17:110a (abstr 426).

71. Fujimoto S, Chikazawa G. Schedule-dependent and -independent antitumour activity of paclitaxel-based combination chemotherapy against M-109 murine lung carcinoma in vivo. Jpn J Cancer Res 1998; 89:1343–1351.

72. Rowinsky EK, Gilbert MR, McGuire WP, et al. Sequences of Taxol and cisplatin: a Phase I and pharmacologic study. J Clin Oncol 1991; 9:1692–1703.

73. McKeage MJ, Haddad GG, Ding L, et al. Neuroprotective interactions in rats between paclitaxel and cisplatin. Oncol Res 1999; 11:287–293.

74. Holmes FA, Madden T, Newman RA, et al. Sequence-dependent alteration of doxorubicin pharmacokinetics by paclitaxel in a phase I study of paclitaxel and doxorubicin in patients with metastatic breast cancer. J Clin Oncol 1996; 14:2713–2721.

75. Vigano L, Locatelli A, Grasselli G, et al. Drug interactions of paclitaxel and docetaxel and their relevance for the design of combination chemotherapy. Invest New Drugs 2001; 19:179–196.

76. Mans DR, Grivicich I, Peters GJ, et al. Sequence-dependent growth inhibition and DNA damage formation by the irinotecan–5-fluorouracil combination in human colon carcinoma cell lines. Eur J Cancer 1999; 35:1851–1861.

77. Ezzat M, Raja A, Berry S, et al. A phase II trial of circadian timed paclitaxel and cisplatin therapy in metastatic breast cancer. Ann Oncol 1997; 7:663–667.

78. Early Breast Cancer Trialists' Collaborative Group. Polychemotherapy for early breast cancer: an overview of randomised trials. Lancet 1998, 352:930–942.

79. International Breast Cancer Study Group. Duration and reintroduction of adjuvant chemotherapy for node-positive premenopausal breast cancer patients. J Clin Oncol 1996; 14:1885–1894.

80. Colleoni M, Litman HJ, Castiglione-Gertsch M, et al. Duration of adjuvant chemotherapy for breast cancer: a joint analysis of two randomised trials investigating three versus six courses of CMF. Br J Cancer 2002; 86:1705–1714.

Chapter **3**

Risk management

Joanne Sims

THE FRAMEWORK FOR RISK MANAGEMENT

Clinical governance

In 1997, the UK Government set out a new framework for quality improvement for the National Health Service. The principal aims of the government proposals were to introduce, for the first time, statutory duties in respect of quality and extend the concept of corporate governance (previously only applicable to financial controls) to quality and clinical care.[1]

As part of the new framework, healthcare organisations were charged with ensuring that they had formal arrangements for clinical governance and that standards of clinical practice and treatment are developed, implemented, monitored and maintained. Clinical governance is defined as:

> The framework within which healthcare organisations are accountable for continuously improving the quality of their services and safeguarding high standards of care by creating an environment in which excellence in clinical care will flourish.[2]

Clinical governance is an organisational concept. It requires the development of an organisational paradigm for quality as well as systems and controls that will ensure that the opportunities for quality improvement are identified in all the organisation's services.

Controls assurance

In order to support the clinical governance framework, the UK NHS Executive Health Circular 1998/70 identified the importance of integrating governance with clinical and non-clinical organisational controls.[3] The message was that clinical governance and organisational controls assurance should not be separate stand alone policies. This was further clarified within the Health Circular 1999/123 'Governance in the new NHS Controls Assurance Statements, 1999/2000: Risk Management and Organisational Controls'. The Circular describes how the linkages for clinical governance, controls assurance and risk management should be structured within a healthcare organisation.

The term controls assurance is defined as:

A holistic concept based on best governance practice. It is a process designed to provide evidence that NHS organisations are doing their 'reasonable best' to manage themselves so as to meet their objectives and protect patients, staff, the public and other stakeholders against risks of all kinds.[4]

Measurement of controls assurance standards

In 1999 the UK Government identified the organisational controls assurance standards against which healthcare organisations would be measured. The standards and criteria contained in the control framework 'The NHS Health Circular HSC 1999/123' were drawn from current statutory and mandatory requirements together with relevant best practice guidance.

The aim of the NHS Executive Controls Assurance Standard framework was to draw together all the many facets of clinical and non-clinical risk that underpin clinical governance. As of the 1 April 2000, Trusts were required to submit annual baseline assessment scores, to the NHS Executive, against all of the individual controls assurance standards.[4] These included standards for health and safety; infection control; medical device management; medicines management and risk management.

The Controls Assurance Regimes Assessment Process was abolished in 2004. However, the criteria underpinning the Standards have been incorporated into the new 'Standards for Better Health'.[5]

Risk management

Risk management is seen as the common thread linking clinical governance and wider controls assurance. Risk management has been defined as:

the culture, processes and structures that are directed towards the effective management of potential opportunities and adverse effects[6]

The core risk management standard that has been adopted by the NHS Executive is the Australian Standard for Risk Management AS/NZS 4360:1999. This standard provides a generic guide for the establishment and implementation of the risk management processes within the NHS. The main elements of the process are to systematically identify, analyse, evaluate and treat risks.

Risk management involves reducing the risk of adverse events by systematically assessing and reviewing risks and then implementing practical measures to prevent their occurrence.

In practical terms, controls assurance and clinical governance should go hand in hand, supported by an organisational framework of positive, proactive, risk management. Implementing and maintaining effective systems of financial and organisational control are essential prerequisites for the success of clinical governance and provide a solid foundation upon which to build an environment for quality and excellence.

Studies suggest that healthcare managers understand the definition of risk management but are more vague about strategies for implementation.[7] Managers were found to be passive in their actions towards risk management rather than proactively promoting it. Actions with a statutory requirement, such as health and safety and the control of substances hazardous to health, were more likely to be carried out rather than a review of clinical procedures and clinical risk assessments. The challenges of clinical governance and risk management demand more proactive approaches to effect change and support ongoing clinical quality improvements.[7]

Clinical Negligence Scheme for Trusts

The NHS Litigation Authority (NHSLA) administers a clinical risk-pooling scheme called the Clinical Negligence Scheme for Trusts (CNST). The scheme was created on the 1 April 1995, and was set up to protect trusts against the effects of escalating clinical negligence claims and provide a mechanism for smoothing out the financial risk based on principles of mutuality.[8] CNST is a voluntary scheme open to all trusts and health authorities in England; currently over 400 trusts take part in the scheme.[9] The scheme is funded on a pay as you go basis with member trusts making annual contributions based on their risk and claims profile. Trusts are assessed against compliance with specific clinical risk standards. Specific criteria within the standards include those for risk management, consent, maintaining health records, induction training and competence, clinical care, infection control and clinical incident reporting.[8]

Studies have explored the question of the value of the CNST scheme and whether involvement can make a positive difference to clinical risk management within an organisation.[7,10] The authors propose that trusts should use the CNST standards and related action plans as a benchmark. It is recommended that attention is focused on commitment to strategy, robust systems for managing risk and action to ensure that patient care is improved as a direct consequence.[6,8] The CNST guidelines provide a strategy for undertaking a clinical risk audit of an organisation and the identification and implementation of appropriate action plans.[8]

RISK MANAGEMENT FOR CHEMOTHERAPY SERVICES

Clinical risk management involves identifying what can go wrong in patient care, how and why these events may happen and what can be done to prevent them from recurring. The aim should be to minimise the likelihood ('risk') that an adverse event may occur. This can be achieved by ensuring that healthcare staff are provided with appropriate training, and that effective risk control measures and procedures are in place. Such procedures are likely to include the provision of a safe, clean environment and the selection, use and safety of work equipment and medical devices.

Anticancer chemotherapy agents are by their very nature highly toxic, and are a risk in themselves. Added to the complexity of modern chemotherapy treatments – e.g. the growing use of ambulatory chemotherapy and high-dose regimes – risk management is a significant issue for chemotherapy services.[11]

Risk management therefore needs to consider the control measures required to ensure patient safety as well as the safety of healthcare workers involved in the handling and administration of chemotherapy. The process must involve identifying the points at which risk occurs and the measures in place to reduce them. One half of this process is reactive monitoring of adverse events and near misses. The other half is the proactive analysis of the systems in place and the examination of all of the chemotherapy service pathways. This includes the point at which the prescription in written, through to the preparation, dispensing and administration of the drug.

The aim of the risk management process should be to:

- reduce the risk of adverse exposure to the patient (e.g. via extravasation, sharps injury, spillage or leakage of intravenous infusion)
- reduce the risks of harmful exposure to healthcare staff
- reduce the risk of medication and/or infusion errors
- reduce the risk of equipment malfunction or failure.

Prescription pathways and quality assurance protocols are dealt with in separate chapters. Quality systems such as ISO 9001 support and emphasise the importance of proactive risk management and require the implementation of standardised procedures, clinical protocols, system controls, internal monitoring, training and audit. (See also Chs 2 and 4.)

Clinical incident reporting

A Department of Health review of adverse incidents in healthcare estimated that over 10 000 patients have a serious adverse reaction to their medication each year, £400 million is paid out for clinical negligence claims each year, 5000 patients die from a hospital-acquired infection each year, and between 300 000 and 1.4 million adverse healthcare events occur in hospitals each year.[12]

The primary purpose of adverse incident reporting in clinical risk management is to reduce untoward outcomes and/or injuries to patients and staff. Reporting permits the collection of organisational data and this allows the analysis of trends that may identify organisational, system or environmental problems. Incident reporting policy should be used to pinpoint deficiencies in clinical systems that may need to be improved. If addressed and implemented in a positive way, clinical incident reporting can act as a significant opportunity to eliminate future errors and demonstrate positive risk management.[13]

The CNST Clinical Incident Reporting Standard requires member trusts to have in place 'A clinical incident reporting system that is operated in all medical specialties and department'[8] The core Risk Management Controls Assurance Standard required that:

> Incidents are systematically identified, recorded and reported to management in accordance with an agreed policy of positive, non punitive reporting.[4]

National Patient Safety Agency

In 2000, the Government undertook a large-scale review of incident report systems in healthcare.[12] The report, written by the Chief Medical Officer, outlines the importance of clinical incident reporting within the clinical governance framework. The report concludes that the NHS as a whole currently fails to learn from adverse incident data and that, historically, incident reporting in the NHS had been haphazard and inadequate. In conclusion, the Chief Medical Officer recommends the implementation of standardised incident reporting systems within individual trusts and, the implementation of a national mandatory serious untoward incident reporting database.[12]

In response to the above recommendations, the Government launched the National Patient Safety

Agency (NPSA) in June 2001. The role of the new agency was to implement and operate a national mandatory clinical incident reporting system across the NHS. A further role of the NPSA is to promote organisational learning from adverse incident reporting and provide guidance on incident investigation.

Patient safety incidents

As part of the development of a national mandatory reporting system to improve the quality and safety of patient care, the government have proposed the use of standard definitions for adverse events to enable local and regional comparisons of incidents to be made.[13]

'A Patient Safety Incident' is defined as:

> any unintended or unexpected incident(s) that could have or did lead to harm for one or more persons receiving NHS funded care.[13]

Adverse events are therefore occasions on which patients are potentially harmed in some way by the treatment rather than by the disease. Adverse events may arise from the directly harmful effects of treatment (e.g. extravasation) or the omission of an important aspect of care. They may or may not be preventable.

No harm events

The definition of a Patient Safety Incident includes those that cause 'no harm' (i.e. previously called a 'near miss'). An event can be a prevented incident, or a not prevented incident where no harm occurred.[13]

Implementation of clinical incident reporting systems

To date, clinical incident reporting systems have not been universally applied within healthcare and, as a result, reliable data about risk are very limited. As previously noted, UK government backed research suggests that 300 000 to 1.4 million adverse events might occur each year in the NHS hospital sector, resulting in a £2 billion direct cost in additional hospital days alone.[12] Studies in the USA[13] and Australia[14] have shown that up to 16.6% of patients admitted to hospital suffer an adverse event. A smaller study in two London hospitals revealed 119 adverse events experienced by 110 patients (10.8%).[15]

Studies[12,16–18] examining the strengths and weaknesses of NHS systems for reporting clinical incidents have identified significant barriers for learning from adverse events. The research suggests that the NHS does not learn from adverse healthcare events for a number of reasons, including that:

- adverse events are investigated in terms of identifying individuals at fault rather than looking deeper for process errors
- departments are often isolated and do not get any feedback from incidents reported and therefore receive no incentive to learn from identified errors
- the organisation has too rigid core beliefs and does not recognise the value of reporting, and learning from, adverse events
- the organisation has a poor IT and/or communication strategy
- concerns about confidentiality, reprisal, blame and/or employment prevent reporting.

A successful incident reporting system requires the input to be non-punitive and part of an independent learning culture.[12,16,18]

There should be a standardised reporting policy throughout the organisation based on a common understanding of what factors are important in identifying, assessing and controlling risk. The policy should make reference to standard procedures for reporting and investigating both actual and potential adverse events.[12]

The policy should also use a standard incident report form. The form should gather significant data about the event (e.g. date and time, name and address of patient, patient number, outline of incident, staff involved). The form must clearly state that only fact and not opinion must be recorded and that where serious injury has occurred the reporting must be immediate. The form should also allow for the reporting of equipment failures and near misses.[12,16,18]

In addition, all incidents should be graded for severity and risk and there should be defined categories (e.g. clinical risk definitions) for all the types of incidents to be reported. The involvement of clinical staff in the development of these indicators is vital to their acceptance and use.[18] All healthcare employees should be aware of the organisation's policy and understand the importance of reporting clinical incidents; for example, training should form part of employee induction.[17,18]

A further recommendation is that incident reports should be sent to a central point for collation and placement on a database compatible with the incident report form.[17] The organisation's reporting policy must also allow for rapid, useful and accessible feedback of investigation findings to all stakeholders.[18]

In summary, an effective incident reporting system should include:

- the separation of collection and analysis from disciplinary or regulatory procedures
- collection of information on near misses as well as actual incidents
- rapid, useful, accessible and intelligible feedback to the reporting community
- ease of making a report with user friendly forms
- standard reporting systems within organisations
- a 'no blame' or 'fair blame' culture
- mandatory reporting
- the potential for confidential or anonymised reporting
- the provision of staff training in risk management and incident reporting procedures.

MEDICATION ERRORS

Medication errors can be defined as a failure in the treatment process that harms, or has the potential to harm, a patient.[19] Most cases arise from human error, the frequency of which depends on what procedures staff are following, the complexity of the procedure and the circumstances in which they are trying to complete the task.[19]

Medication errors may include over- or underdosing, incorrect administration (wrong route, drug or patient), incorrect prescription or inadequate pre-treatment assessment. Errors in any of these procedures could lead to an 'adverse drug event'. An adverse drug event is defined as injuries that under optimal care are not a normal consequence of a patient's disease or treatment.[12]

It has been estimated that 6–10% of hospital in-patients experience an adverse drug event, with up to one-third being due to errors.[20] Most of these are low-risk events, with 1–2% causing injury. A further 5% are near misses, i.e. potential adverse drug events that fail to cause injury by chance or because they are detected before the drug is administered.[21] A further study of adverse drug events found that 39% occurred at the prescription stage, 38% at the administration stage and 12% during pharmacy dispensing.[22]

Level of risk in chemotherapy administration

As previously highlighted, the variety of chemotherapy doses used in the treatment of cancer, the necessity of dosage adjustments, the array of administration schedules and the wide variety of infusion devices used to administer chemotherapy are all sources of potential error in chemotherapy administration. The frequency of medication errors and adverse drug events in chemotherapy is unknown. One study of American chemotherapy nurses reported medication errors in 63% of workplaces.[23]

It is important for healthcare organisations to implement a policy on medication error reporting to ensure that adverse events are effectively managed and risk management procedures reviewed.[12]

Intrathecal chemotherapy

Since 1985 at least 13 patients have died or been paralysed as a result of the accidental intrathecal administration of vincristine that was intended for intravenous administration. Two reports on intrathecal injection errors were published in April 2001. One reported on the investigation into the tragic death of a teenager in Nottingham on 2 February 2001. The other on a review of clinical policy and the prevention of intrathecal cancer chemotherapy error. Both reports made important recommendations and are summarized within a government strategy document.[24] A summary of the report's recommendations were:

- A register must be established which lists designated personnel who have been trained and authorised to prescribe, dispense, check or administer intrathecal chemotherapy.
- A formal induction programme must be introduced for all new staff, and training that is appropriate to their role in the prescribing, dispensing, checking or administering of chemotherapy must be provided. Regular training programmes for all professional staff who remain on the register must also be provided.
- All staff involved with chemotherapy must be provided with a written protocol, which reflects both national guidance and additional local information.
- A purpose-designed intrathecal chemotherapy chart must be used.
- Intrathecal chemotherapy drugs must only be issued or received by designated staff.
- Intrathecal drugs must be kept in a lockable designated refrigerator when they cannot be administered immediately.
- Intravenous drugs must be administered before intrathecal drugs are issued, unless intrathecal chemotherapy is being given to a child under general anaesthesia.
- Intrathecal chemotherapy must be administered in a separate, designated area and within normal working hours.
- Checks must be made by medical, nursing and pharmacy staff at relevant stages throughout the administration process.

- All drugs that have life-threatening consequences must be clearly labelled.
- The dilution of intravenous chemotherapy drugs must be standardised.

(See also Ch. 2.)

MEDICAL DEVICE MANAGEMENT

The management of medical devices is an important aspect of risk management. It is a statutory duty to ensure that all work equipment is 'suitable and sufficient' for the work activity and that it is maintained in a safe condition.[25] With respect to 'medical devices', it is important to ensure that they are manufactured to a quality standard: i.e. they are safe to use and they have been designed for the purpose intended.[25,26]

The NHS Executive Controls Assurance Standard for Medical Device Management required healthcare organisations to have in place 'a system which ensures that all risks associated with acquisition and use of medical devices are minimised.'[5] In order to ensure compliance with the standard, healthcare organisations had to implement a medical device policy. The aim of the policy was to ensure that whenever a medical device was used, it must be suitable for its intended purpose, properly understood by the professional using the device and maintained in a safe and reliable condition.[26]

Purchasing new medical devices

The medical device policy includes procedures for the purchase, acceptance, decontamination, maintenance, repair, monitoring and replacement of devices.[23,24]

In order to support policy and procedure implementation, healthcare organisations may find it useful to set up a purchasing advisory or strategy group. The group should include representatives from clinical, engineering and finance departments and should make informed decisions about purchasing policy.[27] The aim of the purchasing policy should be ensure that the organisation maintains continuity in the products used and that they are appropriate for the safety and needs of the users.[27,28]

Training

As well as ensuring that the medical devices used are well designed, safe to use and fit into the organisation's overall strategy for purchasing, it is essential to ensure that users are provided with information, instruction and training in their use.[27,28]

A medical devices policy also identifies arrangements for the training of users, including the provision of information to patients if they are end-users of a device, e.g. wheelchairs or ambulatory chemotherapy devices.

Risk management strategies for chemotherapy should therefore include the implementation of control systems to cover the structured training and retraining of users, equipment maintenance and reporting adverse incidents. User training should be formalised. For example, practical instruction on each type of infusion device used in a clinical unit or home setting should be incorporated into implementation programmes and delivered to all potential users, whatever their grade.[27,28]

New staff, including locums, should not be expected to operate devices until they have received such training. Everyone using infusion systems should keep a training log. Similar logs for the training of patients and/or carers should also be maintained.[27]

Monitoring

The Medical and Healthcare Regulatory Agency (MHRA), formally the Medical Devices Agency, is an executive agency of the Department of Health. Its main function is to ensure that all medical devices and equipment meet the appropriate standards of safety, quality and performance, and comply with the relevant European directives. The MHRA receives reports of adverse incidents related to the use of medical devices from device manufacturers, as part of a mandatory 'vigilance' reporting scheme, and also from healthcare organisations, professional users and/or patients.

Medical devices are involved in a significant number of adverse events, with user error and device failure the principal causes.[29] Table 3.1 outlines the most common causes of user error and device failure in relation to the use of infusion devices.[30]

Clinical governance and risk management arrangements therefore need to incorporate plans for the management of medical devices and, in particular, for chemotherapy, the management of infusion devices. There should be clear lines of accountability enabling any staff member who uses a medical device to know what their responsibilities are within the overall management system.[30,32]

SAFE HANDLING OF CYTOTOXIC DRUGS

The Health and Safety at Work etc. Act 1974 places responsibilities on employers to ensure the safety of their employees and to provide a safe working environment. Individuals have a responsibility under this legislation to ensure that no act or omission on their part leads to an untoward incident or adverse event.

Table 3.1   Types of incidents involving infusion systems

Category of incident	Examples of incident
Storage/packaging	Flat battery due to not charging the pump
	Set packaging damaged – set contaminated
Maintenance	Pump not maintained correctly
Contamination	Fluid ingress into infusion pump. Fluid ingress damaging power cable
Degradation	Set worn out – inaccurate infusion
	Syringe restraining strap perished – siphoning
Damage	Damaged gearbox
	Damage to syringe size sensor
Performance	Infusion pump not performing to specification
Design and labelling	Incorrect instructions
Quality assurance	Incorrect assembly not spotted at manufacturing plant
User errors	Misloading administration set
	Misloading the syringe
	Setting the wrong rate
	Confusing primary and secondary rates
	Not confirming the set rate
	Not confirming the syringe size
	Confusing the pump type
	Not stopping the infusion correctly
	Not confirming the pump mode
	Configuration of the pump

Source: reproduced from Medical Devices Agency,[32] with permission.

Employees are responsible for complying with safety policies and procedures in place for their safety and for the safety of others who may be affected by their work activities.[33]

The Management of Health and Safety at Work Regulations require employers to undertake a formal 'risk assessment' of any activities within the organisation that could lead to a significant risk of injury or ill health.[34] Specific issues that should be considered as part of the risk assessment process include the identification of risks associated with manual handling activities, the use of personal protective clothing, the use of work equipment and the use of substances hazardous to health.

Control of Substances Hazardous to Health

In 1988, the UK Health and Safety Executive introduced the Control of Substances Hazardous to Health (COSHH) regulations. Following a series of amendments, revised regulations were implemented in 1999 and updated in 2002.[35] The COSHH regulations cover a wide range of hazardous substances and include a specific approved code of practice for carcinogens (e.g. cytotoxic drugs). Employers are required to identify hazardous substances in use, the people who may be exposed to them, the control measures in place to ensure safe handling and the contingency measures required to deal with accidental exposure or other adverse events.

The COSHH regulations also require employers to implement adequate control measures to reduce the risk of exposure to the 'lowest level reasonably practicable'. Whilst the regulations recognise the importance of protective clothing, employers should only implement their use when all other safety controls have been considered and, where practicable, implemented. Safety procedures should be documented and this is commonly referred to as a COSHH assessment. The procedures should be made known to all relevant employees and the provision of this information documented.

The COSHH assessments pertinent to cytotoxic drugs include:

1. cytotoxic drug administration
2. cytotoxic drug reconstitution
3. cytotoxic drug spillage
4. disposal of patient by-products following cytotoxic drug therapy
5. cytotoxic waste disposal.

These assessments should be regularly reviewed following the organisation's policy on carrying out assessments. The assessments should identify the safety procedures for the activity, the protective clothing to be worn and details of any appropriate monitoring or health surveillance arrangements. The assessment should also identify appropriate spillage procedures for the activity.

Administration

Cytotoxic drug handling by nursing and pharmacy personnel is an acknowledged occupational hazard.[36] Many antineoplastic drugs inhibit the growth of tumours due to their toxicity towards rapidly proliferating neoplastic tissues. However they have a narrow therapeutic index and are able to damage tissues undergoing cell division. Many cytotoxic drugs have been shown to have mutagenic, teratogenic or carcinogenic properties where no threshold dose can be identified.[37]

A number of experimental studies have suggested that there are serious long-term effects of exposure.

Effects include chromosomal abnormalities[38] and reproductive disorders, including infertility.[36] As a result of these studies, a number of safety measures have been introduced in order to protect all personnel who prepare, administer or handle cytotoxic drugs or waste products.

Primary routes for exposure include absorption through the skin, inhalation or ingestion. Exposure can occur during drug preparation and reconstitution, administration and handling. This can be as a result of aerosolisation of powder or liquid during reconstitution or contact with contaminated equipment used in preparing or administering the drugs.[36,37] Studies have also highlighted the risk of surface contamination of pharmacy-prepared chemotherapy infusion bags and syringes.[39]

Patients may excrete some drugs in their urine or faeces, and therefore staff are exposed when handling and disposing of body waste. Exposure has been reported to result in local effects, caused by direct contact with the skin, eyes and mucous membranes.[36,37,40]

Protective clothing

Protective clothing should be worn during all types of cytotoxic drug handling.[37,40,41] Operator protection should be ensured for all activities involving the handling of cytotoxic drugs, waste materials and contaminated linen and laundry.

There are minimum requirements for the design, type and protection standards afforded by protective equipment. All personal protective equipment should bear a European CE mark (or equivalent).[42] The choice of protective clothing worn will depend on these factors and also the environment in which it is to be worn and the length of time for which it will be worn.[40] All protective clothing should be cleaned, maintained, stored and used according to statutory requirements[42] and local procedures. Appropriate protectiveclothing should be readily available at all times. In accordance with statutory requirements,[35,42] all relevant personnel should receive training in the use of the equipment.

Gloves

Disposable gloves should be worn at all times when reconstituting, administering and handling cytotoxic drugs or when handling the excreta of patients receiving the drugs. They should also be worn when handling any cytotoxic preparations (syringes, infusion bags, tablet packs) and when handling or transporting any samples from patients receiving chemotherapy.[35,43] However, there is still debate as to which

gloves are the most suitable and which offer the best protection; at present there no overall consensus. Studies carried out have attempted to determine glove thickness, particularly the variation in thickness within batches and the permeability of the gloves, and have concluded that no glove material is completely impermeable to every cytotoxic agent.[37,40]

When selecting gloves, consideration should be given to the glove thickness, latex content, the nature of the solvent in which the cytotoxic drug is dissolved and glove flexibility. It is important to weigh the risk of glove permeation and protection against the risk of user discomfort and poor manual dexterity.[44] The use of poor-quality, low-cost gloves should be avoided.[37] The selection of latex gloves should be considered carefully, as use has been linked with sensitisation.[45] Powderfree gloves should be used for handling cytotoxic drugs.[44]

The practice of double-gloving when administering cytotoxic drugs is unnecessary if gloves are of good quality. Double-gloving is usually only required when cleaning up large spills.[44] Regular changing of gloves is common, although the frequency varies from changing them every 30–60 min to changing them at each work session. In all cases, gloves should be changed immediately following known contact with a cytotoxic agent or following puncture.[40,41] Hands should be washed thoroughly before and after use of gloves and a new pair of gloves should be worn for each patient administration.[43]

Goggles/eye protection

Goggles are used to protect the eyes from splashes and any dust particles. Eye protection should be worn whenever reconstituting drugs or dealing with a spillage. Use is also advocated during administration where there is a potential risk of splash. Goggles should fully enclose the eye and conform to EN 166-168 design standards.[44]

Gowns

This category includes gowns, suits, armlets and aprons. Literature supports the use of a disposable gown for cytotoxic administration.[37,40,43]

It has been suggested that gowns should be made of lightweight, low-linting, low-permeability material with a solid front and long sleeves with elasticated or knit closed cuffs. Cuffs should be tucked under gloves.[37,40,46–48] There are many commercially available gowns and suits, although there is no universally accepted material or design. Gowns should be impervious to fluid and bacteria and meet an acceptable quality standard. Some experts recommend the use of Tyvek or Saranex-laminated aprons to provide maximum protection.[44]

When reviewing the types of aprons to be worn, it is important to consider how long they will be worn for and how comfortable they are for the user. The material should not restrict movement in any way and must not adversely affect operator sensation or dexterity.[43,45,48] Studies have suggested that health-care personnel are less likely to wear goggles than gowns or gloves and that this was because goggles were frightening to already stressed and sick patients.[48,49]

The negative effect that protective clothing may have on a patient is an important issue in clinical risk management. Patient and carer's education regarding cytotoxic drug handling is very important in order to ensure that patients and family members understand why precautions are taken.[43]

Masks

Respiratory protection should be worn if there is a possible risk of inhalation or the drug is being pre-pared in an uncontrolled environment. A disposable dust mask or particulate respirator conforming to a BSEN149:1992 standard is recommended. It is impor-tant to ensure that the respiratory protection chosen fits the wearer's face well and a good face seal is main-tained. A range of sizes should be made available.[44] Surgical masks should not be used.[40]

Reconstitution

The essence of the COSHH regulations is to eliminate exposure to any substance hazardous to health.[35] Consideration should therefore be given to the use of a commercial service where the cytotoxic drugs are bought in already prepared. However, this is not always cost-effective or 'reasonably practicable'. In these situations the drug must be reconstituted on the healthcare organisation's premises.

There are a number of possible options when choosing the environment in which to reconstitute cytotoxic drugs. Ideally, in order to ensure compliance with statutory controls and reduce health risks to employees, all reconstitution of cytotoxic drugs should be undertaken within a pharmacy-controlled clean room. The drugs should be prepared by trained pharmacy staff and reconstituted in a vertical class II or III biological safety cabinet with laminar air flow. The cabinets should meet required standards for product and user safety. Standard operating procedures and COSHH assess-ment documentation should be in place for operator protection.[37,43,48,50]

Where it is not 'reasonably practicable' to ensure that cytotoxic drugs are always reconstituted within a pharmacy unit, the use of a mini isolator is advocated.[43,44,47]

The isolator should be situated in a dedicated con-trolled area. Access to the room should be restricted and the reconstitution procedures only undertaken by trained or supervised personnel.[40,41]

Where a mini isolator or satellite pharmacy controlled unit cannot be provided, reconstitution may be undertaken in a ward/clinic room. Although not ideal, occasionally it may be necessary in an emergency situation. In these circumstances, a room that is well ventilated, has a sink with running water and impermeable work surfaces should be utilised. It is important to reduce traffic in the room as far as possible during the procedure in order to minimise interruptions and reduce the risk of contamination.[40,41,43]

The use of a plastic absorbent pad or liner on the work surface or the use of a plastic or stainless steel tray is recommended in order to contain and minimise contamination.[41,47] Protective clothing should be worn and an aseptic technique used throughout the recon-stitution procedure. Ampoules should be handled carefully and the neck of the ampoule covered with a gauze swab and held away from the face when broken.[41] The discarded ampoule should be placed in a sharps bin and disposed of as special waste, in accordance with the UK Special Waste Regulations 1996.[51]

When reconstituting drugs in powder form, care should be taken when adding diluent to vial or ampoules. The drug should be added slowly down the side of the container so that it mixes with the powder and prevents the formation of an aerosol.[40,41,47] The use of filtered venting systems and large-bore needles will help to reduce the risk of aerosol formation by creating a negative pressure in the vial and filtering the air released.[37,40,41,47,48] If air is present in the syringe, it should be held in such a way that the air is near the plunger. The practitioner should simply stop pushing on the plunger when all the drug is expelled and the air is reached. Luer lock syringes should always be used to ensure that there is no risk of disconnection during the procedure.[40,41] Ideally, administration sets should be primed in the reconstitution unit.[47] However, where accidental spillage is possible, infu-sion bags should be connected to intravenous admin-istration sets and primed before adding cytotoxic drug to the infusion solution. If this is not possible, the bag should be laid flat and the administration set spike pushed firmly into it. It may be unsafe to spike a hanging bag because of the risk of splashing or puncturing the side of the bag.[41]

Once reconstituted, the syringe or infusion bag must be labelled according to the organisation's policy.

Details should include the patient's name, hospital number, name and dose of drug, volume of drug, expiration date and time, diluent fluid and storage details.[41]

Spillage and accidental exposure

All personnel involved with handling cytotoxic drugs and cytotoxic waste materials should be aware of the procedures required for dealing with spillages and accidental exposures. Spillage procedures should be identified within COSHH assessment documentation.[35,40,41]

If a cytotoxic drug is spilled onto the clothing of staff or the patient, the piece of clothing should be removed as soon as possible and treated as contaminated linen. If the spill has penetrated clothing and come into contact with the skin of the person, the area must be thoroughly cleansed with soap and large amounts of water.[50] In the case of exposure or splashing into the eye, the eye should be flooded with water or an isotonic eye wash solution for at least 5 minutes.[40,43,48] In the event of any direct exposure of the practitioner, medical attention should be sought and the incident reported to the organisation's occupational health department.[40,41,43] Additional advice should be sought from the pharmacy (drug information) department as appropriate.[43] In all cases, cytotoxic spillage and adverse exposure incidents should be formally documented in accordance with the organisation's local procedures.

Spillage kit

It is recommended that wherever cytotoxic drugs are being reconstituted, administered or handled, a spillage kit is available and that staff are trained in its use.[40,41,47,50] The provision of a spillage kit enables the practitioner to have immediate access to all the necessary equipment, which will help to prevent further contamination of the environment and aid prompt cleaning. The contents of spill kits vary but there are some basic requirements.[40,41,43]

Contents of a spillage kit:

- plastic apron or gown
- plastic overshoes
- disposable armlets
- disposable gloves (two pairs)
- particulate respirator (mask)
- goggles
- disposable clinical waste bags
- paper towels or absorbent pads
- procedure document
- accident form.

Additional equipment that should be readily available and taken to the spillage site, as appropriate, includes a sharps container and a special waste bin.

In the event of a spill, the immediate area should be cleared as far as possible. Protective clothing should be worn, i.e. two pairs of gloves, gown or apron, armlets, overshoes, goggles and, in the event of a powder spill, a good-quality surgical face mask or particulate respirator face mask. Powder spills should be contained with dampened paper towels to prevent dispersal of powder. All spills should be wiped up with absorbent towels, starting from the outside edge and working towards the centre to prevent spread of contamination to a larger area.[50] All contaminated surfaces should be cleaned with cold soapy water at least three times, and dried to remove residual contamination.[47,50]

Waste disposal

In accordance with the COSHH regulations,[35] there should be clear and concise procedures for the safe handling and disposal of cytotoxic drugs and material contaminated by them.

Contaminated needles, syringes, intravenous administration sets and tubing should be disposed of intact and placed in designated 'special waste' sharps containers as complete needle–syringe units to prevent the risk of needlestick or splashing during disconnection. Glass bottles or vials containing residual amounts of cytotoxic agents should also be disposed of in this way. Protective clothing, unless heavily contaminated, e.g. following a spillage, should be placed in a yellow clinical waste bag and should be sealed and labelled according to the institution's policies.[41]

All waste containers should conform to relevant HSE standards and guidance.[51] The most acceptable method of disposal of hazardous waste is by incineration at a licensed site. A registered waste disposal contractor must be used to transport the waste and the appropriate documentation completed.[52]

Contaminated linen should be placed in a red alginate bag followed by a red linen bag to ensure that it is handled correctly by laundry staff. All reusable equipment such as goggles or trays should be washed with soap and water and dried thoroughly.[41]

Cytotoxic drugs can be excreted as unchanged drug or active metabolites in urine, faeces, blood, vomit and even saliva. In order to comply with safe technique and practice, universal precautions should be used and gloves worn whenever handling blood and body fluids of patients receiving cytotoxic therapy.[40,43,50]

Health surveillance

It is essential that a system of health surveillance is provided for staff directly involved in handling cytotoxic drugs. There are no universal standards for health surveillance. It has been suggested that a programme should include a record of the individual's medical history, a physical examination, routine laboratory tests (e.g. full blood count) and annual biological monitoring.[37] However, the value of monitoring levels of drugs and their metabolites is limited due to the wide range of drugs used and the reliability, sensitivity and validation of the test methods available. It has been suggested that there is no data to support a cause and effect relationship between precautionary cytotoxic drug handling and abnormal physical and laboratory findings.[48] It is, therefore, less common for staff to undergo extensive testing.[41] It is important for organisations to develop their own standards for health surveillance in consultation with occupational health advisers.

SUMMARY

- Risk management involves looking systematically at working practices and clinical pathways in order to identify and assess potential risks to patients, staff and others.
- Identified risks can be effectively managed through the implementation of risk control measures such as protective clothing, staff and patient education, training, supervision and documented safety procedures.
- It is essential that any adverse incidents (e.g. medication errors, clinical incidents, cytotoxic spillage) are reported promptly and that the organisation has an open and honest culture for reporting and investigating errors.
- The reporting system should ensure that all staff have access to immediate advice, e.g. from occupational health services, and that there is feedback on the risk management outcomes of an adverse incident investigation.

References

1. Secretary of State for Health. The new NHS modern and dependable. London: HMSO; 1997
2. Department of Health. Clinical governance – quality in the new NHS. HSC 1999/065. London: HMSO; 1999.
3. Department of Health. Corporate governance in the NHS Controls Assurance Statements 1998/1999. HSC 1998/070. London: HMSO; 1998.
4. Department of Health. Governance in the new NHS Controls Assurance Statements, 1999/2000 – risk management and organisational controls. HSC 1999/123. London: HMSO; 1999.
5. Department of Health. Standards for Better Health. London 2004.
6. Standards Australia. Standard 4360:1999 Risk Management. Standards Australia Ltd, 1999.
7. Harris A. Risk management in practice: how are we managing? Br J Clin Govern 2000; 5(3):142–149.
8. NHS Litigation Authority. Clinical negligence scheme for trusts – June 2000 Standards. London: NHSLA; 2000.
9. Lygon M, Secker-Walker J. Clinical governance: making it happen. London: Royal Society of Medicine Press, 1999.
10. Walsh J. The Clinical Negligence Scheme for Trusts. Br J Nursing. 1996; 6(20):1166–1167.
11. Verne J. Anti cancer chemotherapy – time to focus on risk management. Clin Govern Bull 2000; 1(2):5–6.
12. Department of Health. An organisation with a memory. Report of an Expert Group on Learning from Adverse Events in the NHS. London: The Stationary Office; 2000.
13. National Patient Safety Agency. Seven steps to patient safety. London: The Stationary Office; 2004.
14. Brennan T, Leape L, Laird N, et al. Incidence of adverse events and negligence in hospitalized patients. New Engl J Med 1991; 324:370–376.
15. Woloshynowych M, Neale G, Vincent C. Adverse events in hospitalized patients: a pilot study and preliminary findings. Clin Govern Bull 2000; 1(2):2–3.
16. Vincent C, Stanhope N, Crowley-Murphy M. Reasons for not reporting adverse incidents: an empirical study. J Evaluat Clin Pract 1999; 5(1):13–21.
17. Dineen M, Walsh K. Incident reporting in the NHS. Health Care Report 1999; 5(4):20–22.
18. Woods D. Learning from incidents. In: Proceedings of conference on enhancing patient safety and reducing errors in healthcare. California: Amnenberg Center for Health Sciences; 1998.
19. Ferner R, Aronson J. Medication errors, worse than a crime. Lancet 2000; 355:947–948.
20. Bates DW, Cullen DT, Nairn N, et al. Incidence of adverse drug events and potential adverse drug events. Implications for prevention. ADE Prevention Study Group. J Am Med Assoc 1995; 274:20–34.
21. Bates DW, Boyle DL, Vander Vliet MB, et al. Relationship between medication errors and adverse drug events. Implications for prevention. J Gen Intern Med 1995; 10:199–205.
22. Leape LL, Kabcenell AI, Ghandi TK. Systems analysis of adverse drug events. J Am Med Assoc 1995; 274:35–43.
23. Schulmeister L. Chemotherapy medication errors: descriptions, severity and contributing factors. Oncol Nurs Forum 1999; 26:1033–1042.
24. Department of Health. National guidance on the safe administration of intrathecal chemotherapy. London: Department of Health; 2001.

25. Secretary of State. Work Equipment Regulations 1998. London: HMSO; 1998.

26. Secretary of State. Medical Devices Regulations SI No 618. London: HMSO; 2002.

27. Medical Devices Agency (MDA). Medical device and equipment management for hospitals and community based organisations. MDA/DB/901. London: Department of Health; 1998.

28. Medical Devices Agency. Equipped to care. London: Department of Health; 2000.

29. Williams C, Lefever J. Reducing the risk of user error with infusion pumps. Prof Nurse 2000; 6:382–384.

30. Secretary of State. Provision and Use of Work Equipment Regulations SI 2306. London: HMSO; 1998.

31. NMC. Code of Professional Conduct. London: Nursing & Midwifery Council; 2002.

32. Medical Devices Agency. MDA DB20033 Infusion Systems. London: Department of Health; 2003.

33. The Health and Safety at Work etc. Act 1974. HMSO London.

34. Secretary of State. The Management of Health and Safety at Work Regulations 1999. SI No 3242. London: HMSO; 1999.

35. Secretary of State. The Control of Substances Hazardous to Health Regulations 2002. London: HMSO; 2002.

36. Vannis BG, Vollmer W, Labuhn T, et al. Acute symptoms associated with antineoplastic drug handling among nurses. Cancer Nurse 1993; 16(4):288–295.

37. Allwood M. The cytotoxic handbook. 4th edn. Oxford: Radcliffe Medical Press; 2002.

38. Waksvick H, Klepp O, Brogger A, et al. Chromosome analysis of nurses handling cytotoxic agents. Cancer Treat Rep 1987; 65:607–610.

39. Conner T. Surface contamination with antineoplastic agents in six cancer treatment centres in the US and Canada. Pharm J 1999; 263:56.

40. Dougherty L, Lister SE. Manual of clinical nursing procedures. 6th edn. Oxford: Blackwell Science; 2004.

41. Dougherty L. Safe administration of intravenous cytotoxic drugs. In: Dougherty L, Lamb J, eds. Intravenous therapy in nursing practice. Edinburgh: Churchill Livingstone; 1999.

42. Secretary of State. The Personal Protective Equipment (PPE) at Work Regulations 1992. SI 2966. London: HMSO; 1992.

43. Royal College of Nursing. Clinical Practice Guidelines. The administration of cytotoxic chemotherapy. Recommendations. Oxford: RCN; 1998.

44. Ferguson L, Wright P. Administration of chemotherapy. In: Allwood M, ed. The cytotoxic handbook. Oxford: Radcliffe Medical Press; 2001.

45. Medical Devices Agency. Latex sensitisation in the health care setting – (use of latex gloves). DB 9601. London: HMSO; 1996.

46. Occupational Safety and Health Administration: US Department of Labor. Technical manual: controlling exposure to hazardous drugs. TM 1987, Section VI, Ch. 2. Washington: OSHA; 1987.

47. Oncology Nursing Society. Cancer chemotherapy guidelines and recommendations for practice. Pittsburg: Oncology Nursing Press; 1999.

48. Goodman M. Chemotherapy administration: principles and administration. In: Henke Yarbro C, Hansen Frogge M, Goodman SL, et al. Cancer nursing: principles and practice. 5th edn. Boston: Jones and Bartlett; 2000.

49. Health and Safety Executive/Laboratory. Occupational exposure of health workers to cytotoxic drugs: a ward based study. HEF00/05. London: HSE Books; 2000.

50. Vandergift KV. Oncologic therapy. In: Hankin J, Waldman Lonsway RA, Hedrick C, et al. Infusion therapy in clinical practice. 2nd edn. Philadelphia: WB Saunders: 2001.

51. Health and Safety Executive. Safe disposal of clinical waste. London: HSE Books; 1999.

52. The Special Waste Regulations. Statutory Instrument 1996 No 972. London: HMSO; 1996.

Chapter 4

Quality assurance

Andrew Lomath

This chapter deals with the basic concepts of quality assurance and how they are applied to the National Health Service. The basic aim of all quality assurance in the NHS is to improve the patient experience. This is specifically related to experiences in chemotherapy and radiotherapy at the Royal Marsden NHS Foundation Trust. The sections that the chapter is divided into are listed below:

1. Introduction to quality
2. Principles of clinical governance and the Healthcare Commission
3. Cancer quality initiatives
4. Quality management systems
5. Application of ISO 9001:2000 to chemotherapy.

INTRODUCTION TO QUALITY

'What is quality?' is a question that has been tackled by many authors who have come up with varied forms of words to define quality. Basically, quality comes down to 'customer satisfaction': if a customer is satisfied with the product or service then they will come back for a repeat purchase and will recommend the provider to their friends and contacts. This is good quality because the business, whatever its nature, grows and becomes successful.[1,2]

Early concepts of quality evolved from manufacturing industry, where product quality was maintained by inspection, better known as 'quality control'. This relied on the inspection of either all production, as in motor car manufacture, or a sample of production, as in food production, where total sampling would leave no product for sale. During the mid 1900s the concept of 'quality assurance' was developed where 'systems' were put in place to ensure that the specified quality of the final product was delivered. This replaced to some extent the need for the final product inspection. Most manufacturing units now operate a blend of quality assurance and quality control.[3] With the advent of quality assurance non-manufacturing organisations became interested in using the concept to improve their customer relationships; services can have systems and can monitor those systems even when there is no physical end product to test or inspect.

Quality assurance also led to the other key concept of quality, namely continuous improvement.[1,2] This again comes from customer satisfaction. A customer may be satisfied and come back but will often expect the service to be better to keep on coming back (or recommending to friends and contacts). Terms that have been used for ways of working to achieve continuous improvement have included total quality management, quality circles, quality management systems (BS5750 and ISO 9001), six-sigma, the European Foundation for Quality Management business excellence model (often abbreviated to EFQM) and various sets of principles (McKinsey, Ishikawa and others). In the NHS context the Clinical Pathology Accreditation (CPA) for laboratories applies quality assurance principles.

In the NHS the concepts of quality were laid down in 1998 in the document 'A First Class Service – Quality in the new NHS'.[4] This document defined the roles of the National Institute for Clinical Excellence (NICE), National Service Frameworks (NSF) and the CHI, and detailed the concept of clinical governance, effectively quality assurance in the NHS.

National Institute for Clinical Excellence

The main purpose of NICE is to 'give coherence and prominence to information about clinical and cost-effectiveness'. It fulfils this role by producing evidence-based clinical guidelines, assessed on both clinical grounds and cost, and also by disseminating clinical audit methodologies and information on good practice. Membership of this group is drawn from health professionals, the NHS, academics, health economists and patient groups. Recommendations and consultation documents are regularly published and available on the NICE web site. Guidelines for head and neck, breast, haemato-oncology, colorectal and urological cancers have already been published. Guidelines for lung, CNS tumours and sarcoma are still in preparation at the time of going to press.

National Service Frameworks

NSF lay down the standards for care that different groups of patients should expect. These frameworks are drawn up by multi-professional groups; those produced to date are for mental health, coronary heart disease, national cancer plan, treatment of older people, diabetes and children's services. Preparation is in progress on frameworks for renal services and long-term conditions focusing on neurological conditions.

PRINCIPLES OF CLINICAL GOVERNANCE AND THE HEALTHCARE COMMISSION

The Commission for Health Improvement (CHI) was established in 1998 to improve the quality of patient care in the NHS[5]. It carried this out by reviewing the care provided by the NHS Trusts in England and Wales; Scotland has its own regulatory body, the Clinical Standards Board. In April 2004 CHI became the Commission for Healthcare Audit and Inspection (CHAI), also taking on some of the responsibilities of the Audit Commission. Although this body is legally called CHAI it is known as the Healthcare Commission.

The important aspect running through all the original CHI documentation was the emphasis on patient care and continuous improvement.

Clinical governance reviews of NHS Trusts were the major part of CHI's work, with the last reviews being completed in 2005. In order to review clinical governance seven categories were defined, each of which was assessed in every Trust visited. These areas form the basis of clinical governance and are considered in detail below:

- *Patient involvement* – assesses whether patients can have a say in their treatment and how they and patient organisations can have a say in how services are provided.
- *Risk management* – are there systems to understand, monitor and minimise the risks to patients and staff and to learn from mistakes.
- *Clinical audit* – the continual evaluation, measurement and improvement by health professionals of their work and standards they are achieving.
- *Staffing and management* – this covers recruitment, management and development of staff, and includes working environment and effective methods of working.
- *Education and training* – this covers support to enable staff to be competent in doing their jobs, develop their skills and keep up to date with developments in their field.
- *Clinical effectiveness* – the degree to which an organisation is ensuring that 'best practice', based on evidence of effectiveness, is used. Research and development falls under this category.

- *Use of information* – the systems in place to collect and interpret clinical information and to use it to monitor, plan and improve the quality of patient care.

The Healthcare Commission has produced a series of 24 core standards, against which NHS Trusts are expected to carry out self-assessment in autumn 2005. These standards are wider than clinical governance, but embrace all the previous principles with further areas added. There are seven areas into which the core standards are split.

- *Safety* – patient safety is enhanced by the use of healthcare processes, working practices and systemic activities that prevent or reduce the risk of harm to patients.
- *Clinical and cost effectiveness* – treatment is based on evidence base from research.
- *Governance* – this includes both clinical and corporate governance.
- *Patient focus* – healthcare is provided in partnership with patients, their carers and relatives.
- *Accessible and responsive care* – patients receive services as promptly as possible, have choice in access and at no stage experience unnecessary delays.
- *Care environment and amenities* – environments for care are effective and safe for the delivery of treatment and are well maintained and cleaned.
- *Public health* – services are designed and delivered in collaboration with relevant organisations to promote, protect and improve the health of the population.

Fulfilling the requirements of these various standards is key to any quality management system in chemotherapy.

CANCER QUALITY INITIATIVES

The Calman/Hine Report, 'A Policy Framework for Commissioning Cancer Services', published in 1995, set out the forward plan for cancer services with needs for cancer networks to enable high-quality cancer care in specialist centres, local hospitals and through primary and community care.

In September 2000 the NHS Cancer Plan[6] was published. This had four key aims:

- to save more lives
- to ensure people with cancer get the right professional support and care as well as the best treatments
- to tackle the inequalities in health that mean unskilled workers are twice as likely to die from cancer as professionals
- to build for the future through investment in the cancer workforce, through strong research and

through preparation for the genetics revolution, so that the NHS never falls behind in cancer care.

The Manual of Cancer Services Standards,[7] detailing standards for the provision of cancer care, was revised and republished in 2004. These standards have been the subject of peer reviews throughout the cancer service. As well as standards for specific cancer multi-disciplinary teams, this document sets standards for diagnostic services, chemotherapy, radiotherapy, palliative care, education & training, and communication between primary, secondary and tertiary sectors.

Chemotherapy standards concentrate on the safe handling of chemotherapy, training, guidelines/protocols and documentation and checking of prescriptions.

QUALITY MANAGEMENT SYSTEMS

Quality management systems were first formally developed in the defence industry. Application in other types of organisation led, in the UK, to the publication of BS 5750 in 1979. Other countries developed their standards along similar lines. Development of ISO 9000 documentation is shown in Table 4.1.

The ISO formally defines *quality management* as:[8]

the coordinated activities to direct and control an organisation with regard to quality

The ISO 9000 document also details eight quality management principles:[8]

- *Customer focus* – organisations depend on their customers, so should understand their needs and strive to exceed customer expectations.
- *Leadership* – leaders should maintain an environment where everyone can be fully involved in achieving the organisation's objectives.
- *Involvement of people* – people are the essence of any organisation and should be fully utilising their abilities for the organisation's benefit.

Table 4.1 Development of ISO 9000 documentation

Year	Standards published	Standards withdrawn
1979	BS 5750	
1987	ISO 9001, ISO 9002, ISO 9003 (also called BS 5750 parts 1, 2 & 3)	
1994	ISO 9001, 9002 & 9003	BS 5750 all parts
2000	ISO 9001:2000	ISO 9002 & ISO 9003

- *Process approach* – results are achieved more efficiently when activities are managed as a process.
- *Systems approach to management* – understanding interrelated processes as system contributes to effectiveness and efficiency.
- *Continual improvement* of overall performance should be a permanent objective.
- *Factual approach to decision-making* – effective decisions can only be based on accurate data and information.
- *Mutually beneficial supplier relationships* – suppliers are key to the ability to do all of the above.

Although ISO 9001 is widely used, it is by no means the only quality management systems model available. ISO 9001 has the advantage that it can be assessed by independent auditors, who give the award of accreditation to the standard some credibility. Another unrelated system also used in the public sector is the Business Excellence Model, developed by the European Foundation for Quality Management (often abbreviated to EFQM).[9] This model, with its accompanying documentation, assigns scores to a number of business areas and then sets targets for improvement.

All effective quality management systems are ones that consistently meet quality requirements *and* seek to improve continually the effectiveness and efficiency of its activities in meeting those requirements. The mechanism by which this objective may be achieved has been expressed conceptually in various forms of quality cycle (see Refs 10–12 and references therein). The simplest quality cycle, frequently referred to as the Deming cycle, is shown in Figure 4.1.[13]

The Deming cycle is a continuous cycle leading to improvement. Application of this cycle can be demonstrated by the development of the chemotherapy patient pathway. The initial start is at the 'planning' stage to document the pathway; the 'doing' stage is then to produce the document; this is then 'checked' by auditing, resulting in 'action' being taken to correct errors and problems. This can then lead to the cycle starting again with a plan to put the changes into place – hence, a continuous cycle of improvement.

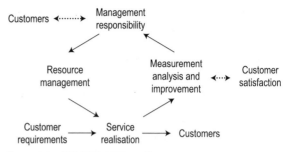

Figure 4.2 ISO 9001:2000 quality management systems model.

ISO 9001:2000 has five major sections (Fig. 4.2):[14]

- quality management systems requirements
- management responsibility
- resource management
- service realisation
- measurement, analysis and improvement.

The quality management systems section details the requirements for the setting up of a quality management system; the remaining four sections can be drawn as a cycle with inputs and outputs to and from customers. This again emphasises the importance placed on meeting customer requirements and hence on increasing customer satisfaction. Customers in the case of the chemotherapy quality management system are the stakeholders, i.e. patients, staff, strategic health authorities, primary care trusts and the general public.

While all of the clauses of the standard have to be satisfied (unless specifically excluded), the key elements of an ISO 9001:2000 system can be summarised as follows:

- All documents in use must be authorised and controlled in some way (date/version number) so that old copies are not used.
- Records must be legible, readily identifiable and retrievable. There must be controls established for identification, storage, protection, retrieval, retention time and disposal.
- Management must review quality and the operation of the system.
- Personnel must be assessed and trained to be fully competent in their roles.
- There must be some control of the 'process' used to deliver the service.
- Customer views, including complaints, must be sought and action taken on those views.
- Relevant equipment must be calibrated.
- Internal audits of the quality management system must be carried out.

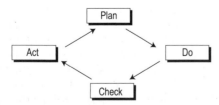

Figure 4.1 Deming quality cycle.

- Nonconformances (adverse incidents and near misses) must be reported and corrective action taken.
- Preventative action (usually as a result of risk assessment) must be part of the system.

Clinical governance/risk management and quality management systems are complimentary to each other: there a few items in each that do not overlap, but on the whole they support each other very well.

APPLICATION OF ISO 9001 TO CHEMOTHERAPY

The application of ISO 9001 to radiotherapy departments in the UK was originally stimulated by a report from the Department of Health working party on quality assurance.[15] In response to serious treatment errors, it was recommended that quality management systems should be implemented in all UK radiotherapy centres. A standard for quality assurance in radiotherapy (QART), modelled closely on the then current ISO 9002, was produced. This was followed by a successful pilot study at two centres[16] and, subsequently, a substantial number of radiotherapy departments or groups serving such departments achieved accreditation to ISO 9002. Some centres obtained accreditation to ISO 9001, which brought in requirements for design control and servicing. The interpretation of these additional requirements could be strongly influenced by the views of the external assessor. For centres that include treatment prescription in the scope of their quality system, design requirements may be implemented in terms of the design of treatments for individual patients. The benefits of the system in radiotherapy have been clearly demonstrated in improving the quality of the service by reduction of errors and the availability of documentation for peer reviews.

In order to implement an ISO 9001 assessable quality management system in chemotherapy, the following steps can be used:

- top management commitment – this is essential because of resources required
- define the scope of the system
- form a multi-disciplinary team covering all areas within the scope
- create the documents required to meet the standard (some of these may already exist)
- apply to an assessment body for external audit
- institute internal audits of the system, including implementation of actions from audits
- external assessment, which will result in an action plan to cover findings

- continuing internal audits and external assessments (usually every 6 months).

Patient pathway

A chemotherapy service registration to ISO 9001:2000 can be achieved by using a patient pathway approach – each step of the pathway has been closely defined with reference to the staff involved, the instruction documents and the methods of recording, storing and transmitting data. The system as developed at the time of writing is restricted to adult patients treated either as day cases or as inpatients and includes all the steps along the pathway from referral to the Royal Marsden Hospital through to final discharge. The pharmacy, laboratory and all areas where chemotherapy is prescribed or administered can be covered within the scope of the system or stand alone. A typical set of steps identified for the chemotherapy pathway is as follows:

1. Patient referred to medical oncologist
2. Initial consultation with doctor
3. Further consultations with doctors, including consent
4. Patient booked/scheduled for chemotherapy administration
5. Preparation for appointment (hospital staff)
6. Patient arrival
7. Blood sample taken and analysed
8. Clinical assessment
9. Chemotherapy prescribed on printed proforma and sent with prescription chart to pharmacy
10. Prescription checked and chemotherapy prepared
11. Chemotherapy dispatched to administration area
12. Chemotherapy received and stored on unit
13. Patient prepared as required, including any further information needed
14. Chemotherapy administered
15. Patient given take home drugs and next appointment booked/confirmed or patient discharged
16. Patient's records stored in relevant place for next visit.

(See also Chapters 8 and 9.)

Areas for improvement are identified from patient's comments, incidents and near misses, audits and staff suggestions. A number of key objectives can be monitored, including the length of time a patient has to wait for chemotherapy administration once the prescription has been approved, time taken for blood results, number of prescribing errors, dispensing errors, equipment failures and completion of correct documentation. Risk assessments are also taking place at all stages along the pathway to identify where preventative action needs to be taken. Implementation of a quality management system will lead to more robust data on which to base improvement decisions and, in the longer term, improved all-round service to patients.

References

1. Oakland JS. Total quality management. Oxford: Butterworth Heineman; 1995.
2. Bank J. The essence of total quality management. Hemel Hempstead: Prentice-Hall; 1992.
3. Oldfield H. UK quality is a vacant lot. Qualityworld 2002; 28:48–50.
4. Department of Health. A first class service. Quality in the new NHS. London: Department of Health; June 1998.
5. Commission for Health Improvement website: www.chi.gov.uk.
6. Department of Health. NHS Cancer Plan. London: Department of Health; September 2000.
7. Department of Health. Manual of Cancer Service Standards. London: Department of Health; 2004.
8. ISO 9000 – 2000 Quality management systems – Fundamentals and Vocabulary, ISO Geneva (also published as BS EN ISO 9000:2000 by BSI, London).
9. EFQM Excellence Model: www.efqm.org.
10. Ellis R, Whittington D. Quality assurance in health care: a handbook. London: Edward Arnold; 1993
11. Øvretveit J. Health service quality: an introduction to quality methods for health services. Oxford: Blackwell; 1992.
12. Gitlow H, Gitlow S. The Deming guide to quality and competitive position. Engelwood Cliffs: Prentice-Hall; 1987.
13. Deming WE. Out of the crisis. Cambridge, Massachusetts: MIT; 1982.
14. ISO 9001 – 2000 Quality management systems – Requirements. Geneva: ISO (also published as BS EN ISO 9000:2000 by BSI, London).
15. Bleehen N. Quality assurance in radiotherapy. Report of Standing Sub-Committee on Cancer. London: Department of Health; 1991.
16. Department of Health. Quality assurance in radiotherapy: a quality management system for radiotherapy. London: Department of Health; 1994.

Chapter **5**

Patient information and education

Beverley van der Molen

INTRODUCTION

Good-quality, appropriate and timely information should be an integral part of cancer care. Through information, individuals can understand the challenges that a cancer diagnosis brings and be able to identify different treatments, alternatives and their consequences. Patient information is an important coping strategy for patients receiving chemotherapy.[1,2] Many patients use information-seeking behaviour as a strategy to cope with a stressful event about which information is limited. [3] Information can promote an individual's psychological well-being and perception of control. Patients are more likely to feel in control when medical information needs have been satisfied and have less psychological control if they feel their needs have not been met.[4-6]

While the majority of patients want to be informed about the medical aspects of their illness and treatment,[4,7-10] they do not necessarily want to actively participate in treatment decision-making. Information can provide individuals with a choice of whether or not they participate in decisions about their care. There is evidence to support the belief that information may help to sustain hopeful attitudes and that individuals who are hopeful are more likely to seek information.[7] Although further research is required to evaluate the effects of information interventions for cancer patients, the literature generally reports positive effects.[11]

PURPOSE OF PATIENT INFORMATION

The functions of patient information[12] are to:

- gain control
- reduce anxiety

- improve compliance
- create realistic expectations
- promote self-care and participation
- generate feelings of safety and security.

With chemotherapy, the right information and support can enable patients to cope more effectively with their treatment, including potential side effects. Some patients may require additional information so that they can understand how chemotherapy works. For instance, an explanation about normal cell division will help with understanding the abnormal or uncontrolled growth that characterises cancer cells. This then leads on to discussing that cancer cells are fast growing and that chemotherapy affects fast-growing cells. If patients understand that other fast-growing cells such as the hair and lining of the GI tract are also affected, they can then start to comprehend why they might experience side effects. This in turn will explain why a break between chemotherapy treatments allows normal cells to recover, since they recover more rapidly than cancer cells. The goal of patient information is to equip patients with enough information to enable them to take as active a role as they wish in the management of their disease and treatment.

POLITICAL BACKGROUND TO PATIENT INFORMATION

The importance of providing information was recognised by the Calman/Hine Report,[13] one of whose general principles was that:

> patients, families and carers should be given clear information and assistance in a form they can understand about treatment options and outcomes available to them at all stages of treatment from diagnosis onwards (Section 3.1.iii).

The NHS Cancer Plan[14] also emphasises the need for patients and their families to receive the information and support required to help them to cope with cancer. Acknowledgement of the need for information and support has been further developed in the Cancer Information Strategy.[15] The strategy picks up on research that shows that many cancer patients feel that the information they are given by health professionals is inadequate. The recommendations for patient-centred information include ensuring the availability of high-quality, publicly accessible information about cancer and cancer services, and improving communication between health professionals and people affected by cancer.

DIFFERENCE BETWEEN PATIENT INFORMATION AND PATIENT EDUCATION

Information in isolation, however, is likely to be of limited value when the meaning and context of the content provided is not clear. Information needs to be understood in order for it to be processed and acted upon. Patient education is more than just the provision of information. Grahn and Johnson[16] state that education 'is a process that takes place over a period of time' and facilitates individuals to actively participate in their health care. Van den Borne[17] describes patient education as 'a systematic learning experience in which a combination of methods is generally used'. Patient education aims to ensure that patients interacting with their carers are able to cooperate effectively in deciding on the care they require and to make their best contribution to that care. Satisfactory patient education has also been shown to benefit providers in terms of reduced number and/or length of hospital stays.[18] A successful education programme is based on formulating mutual learning goals that should be responsive to the participants' individual needs. The goals are to provide knowledge and facts, develop self-care skills, and support desired attitudes and behaviours.[19] Good communication is an essential part of any information exchange.

GIVING INFORMATION

Patients often express dissatisfaction with the information given to them,[20] which may well lead to increased problems with anxiety and coping. It is important not to assume that information provided to a patient will necessarily be understood or retained. Patients are unlikely to process information effectively until they are ready to accept they are living with cancer.[21] There can be considerable variation among individuals as to the stage of their cancer experience that they reach this acceptance. How and when patients come to terms with their diagnosis will have an impact on their information needs. Often, information will need to be repeated several times, checking on each occasion that the information given is at the right level for the patient. Health professionals should encourage patients to ask questions and be responsive to further questions at any time. It can often be helpful to have a family member or friend present when information is given. Just as much thought needs to be given to how information is conveyed as to the information itself. People draw inferences from the meanings communicated as well as the words used and this will determine their level of anxiety. More anxiety will be experienced when meanings are interpreted as threatening.[22]

In addition to the impact of cancer affecting readiness to learn, there are also other potential barriers to understanding and processing information such as communication difficulties, environment and culture (see Barriers to effective patient information section).

Establishing the patient's current level of understanding

The amount of information a patient will require will in part be dependent on where in the cancer continuum chemotherapy treatment is planned. This will indicate the amount of time the patient has had to absorb any information about their cancer diagnosis and treatment plan. Patients often feel overwhelmed with information when they are first diagnosed. If chemotherapy is the first line of treatment, they may still be coming to terms with their diagnosis and need more time as they adapt to the many changes it brings to their lives. When patients have already had other treatments (such as surgery or radiotherapy), they may well have some understanding of their cancer, although not necessarily of chemotherapy.

How much information to provide

Not all patients want the same level of information about their disease and treatment. Many people have limited knowledge about cancer and the health services, and too much information at the beginning can be counterproductive. Incremental information is more likely to be understood and retained. Although a patient may not want information initially, information needs can change over time. As patients become more familiar with their disease and treatment, they may want greater amounts of information. A study by Butow et al[23] showed that single assessments of information needs might be unreliable. Information needs are likely to change when disease status changes and studies show that doctors are not very good at estimating how much information patients want. Therefore it is important to find out what the patient wants to know on a regular basis, rather than making assumptions about what information and support is appropriate to give. It has been well established through studies in a variety of hospital and primary care settings[24] that individuals often do not remember all of the information they are provided with. Information may need to be repeated several times.

When to give information

In a survey of information needs and information-seeking behaviour,[25] patients all wanted basic information about diagnosis, treatment options and side effects.

Differences arose with regard to when patients wanted the information, and in what detail.

Readiness to learn has been identified as an important factor in how patients manage processing information.[26] They need to be both willing to learn and able to use the informational resources available to them. Time needs to be allowed for the impact of diagnosis to be absorbed and patients should be assessed individually, taking into account their current psychological and physical state. Patients are less likely to absorb and retain information when they are overwhelmed by their diagnosis and, equally, physical concerns such as poorly controlled symptoms will also impact on how patients manage information. Key information may need to be given several times before informed consent can be obtained (see Informed consent section).

Provide information in small bites that are relevant to the events taking place, checking frequently that the patient has understood. If too much information is given at one time or it relates to events taking place at a later date, patients will have difficulty in absorbing the most important information. Non-verbal responses can provide clues to an individual's level of understanding. Information may need to be rephrased to ensure clarity.

Barriers to effective patient information

There are several barriers that can influence the effectiveness of patient education.[26] Good communication, which is the key to effective information exchange, can be affected through:

- hearing difficulties
- sight difficulties
- language difficulties
- culture.

Hearing difficulties
Hearing difficulties can add considerable anxiety to an already difficult experience and become a barrier to receiving information. Check whether the patient wears a hearing aid (and is using it). Some people rely on lip-reading and therefore it is essential to ensure that you are facing your patient when you speak and that the light is behind them. It may be necessary to access an interpreter for patients who use sign language such as the British Sign Language or the Deaf Alphabet. Consider the environment when planning a teaching session, as background noise can often be a problem. A quiet room can make a big difference. The concentration needed to take in new facts can be very tiring so give information in 'bite-sized chunks'.

Written information for people with hearing difficulties can be very important to back up verbal information and, where this is not available, ensure that important details are written down. Having a family member or friend present can be reassuring for the patient and ensure that vital information is heard and understood.

Sight difficulties

Written information may have limited value for people with sight difficulties, although it can be possible to enlarge some literature using a photocopier. Some patients may welcome the opportunity to tape record consultations or there may be prerecorded audiocassettes available on different topics.

Language

People who do not have English as their first language will need someone with them who can act as an interpreter. It is important to identify *before* an information exchange that the services of an interpreter will be required, to allow the time for this to be arranged. Ideally, face-to-face interpreting is desirable, although telephone interpreting may be acceptable. It is not good practice to rely on an accompanying family member or friend to take on an interpreting role; however, there may be times when this is unavoidable. Even when family or friends are willing to interpret, this may not always be appropriate as it can be difficult to ensure that the right information is understood as well as being communicated. Understanding spoken English does not necessarily imply understanding of written English. There may be literature available in other languages, although it is likely to be of a generalist nature.

Even when English is the first language, difficulties with reading and writing may not be readily apparent, especially when people are reluctant to admit to them.

Reading requires great concentration for a well person and illness can make the written word seem overwhelming. As listening to information on an audiotape or watching a video can be far less tiring, consider tape recording the information you want to give again, there may be prerecorded audiocassettes available.

Unfamiliar medical terminology can also be a barrier to effective communication. Clarify any terms or technical words that could be unclear, as many people are hesitant to admit they do not understand.

Culture

Culture is an important influence on communication and understanding, and assumptions should not be made as to the impact different cultures will have on an individual. Some of the side effects of cancer treatments such as hair loss from chemotherapy can have more meaning for some cultures than others. If a patient seems reluctant to go ahead with treatment, it is always worth considering if the reluctance is bound in cultural differences.

Information resources

There is a wealth of cancer information material available that people affected by cancer can access. In addition to health professionals, other sources of information include:

- telephone helplines
- written information from cancer charities
- books, magazines and newspapers
- television and radio
- the Internet
- family, friends and other patients.

There does not appear to be consensus amongst people affected by cancer as to what information resources are the most useful. Luker et al[27] found that newly diagnosed women with breast cancer identified the hospital consultant, breast care nurse and written information as the most useful sources of information. In their follow-up study,[28] women's magazines, the hospital consultant and the television and radio were rated the most useful for information. Another study found that information was received from family and friends, the media and other patients with cancer while a smaller number used other sources such as libraries and cancer support groups.[29]

A survey of outpatients[30] found a significant correlation between educational level and active information-seeking from the Internet, medical books and telephone helplines. It has also been suggested that the type of newspaper read by an individual could be an indicator of information needs.[31] In a study looking at personalised computer-based information, 80% of radiotherapy patients said they would prefer 10 min with a nurse specialist or radiographer to computer or booklet information.[32] Manfredi et al's study[33] suggested that people with cancer who contact information services also seek information from several other sources in order to feel they have pursued all their options before making a decision. This behaviour is not a result of availability of information but is an effort to explore all issues or sources prior to decision-making.

The Internet is a rapidly growing source of patient information, but as there is no regulation the quality of information can vary enormously. Information originating from different countries may not be relevant or appropriate in the UK and many people will need guidance in finding accurate and reliable information.

Basic guidelines for searching for information on the Internet include:

- Identifying what information is sought: e.g. cancer treatments or managing the side effects of treatment.
- How to judge a website: the source of information is an indication of its credibility and a site should identify the names of the organisation and contributors. These can range from large organisations such as the Department of Health, hospitals, national charities such as Macmillan Cancer Relief, CancerBACUP, pharmaceutical companies and local cancer support groups to individuals discussing their experience of cancer.
- How to assess the quality of the information: the date of publication or modification will indicate the currency of information and sponsorship of a website by a pharmaceutical company could indicate biased information.

Patients should be encouraged to bring with them any information accessed from the Internet to make further discussion easier.

The format of information

There are three main forms of communicating information.

- verbal
- written
- audio-visual.

Within these formats there can be many variations; however, with all of them, inherent assumptions are often made (see Barriers to effective patient information section).

Verbal

The most frequent method used to convey information is verbally, either on a one-to-one basis or in groups. For information-giving to be effective, it needs to be a two-way process. Interpreting non-verbal body language and using listening skills can help establish that the information communicated has been heard and, more importantly, understood. Many people find that written information, to back up what they have been told, relieves some of the pressure of having to remember everything. Patients often expect health professionals to provide the relevant information necessary for decision-making and, when it is not volunteered, find it difficult to know what questions to ask.

Written

Written information can come in many formats, including leaflets, booklets, magazines and newspapers, books and electronic forms such as CD ROMs and the Internet. The main advantage of most written information is that it is a permanent record for patients and their families which they can refer to at any time.[12] However, information from the Internet is not permanent unless saved and printed. The written form can offer continuity of information and serve as a prompt for further questions and discussion. Written information should not take the place of verbal exchange but enhance it.

Audio-visual

Audio-visual formats include audiotapes and videos, and CD ROMs frequently combine both audio-visual and written formats. Providing patients with audiotapes of consultations with clinicians or other health professionals is one response to the poor retention of verbal information. Findings from studies examining the effect of audiotaping consultations are inconclusive, although they generally suggest that patients find them beneficial.[34] Videotapes are another alternative, with the advantage that they can prepare patients visually for treatment they will be undergoing.[35] Further evaluation of the efficacy of this format is required and one factor likely to determine its place in the future is the cost involved in making a video.

Producing patient information

Producing information materials locally can be a time-consuming process, so it is worth exploring what existing resources could appropriately be used. As much of the widely available information is relatively general, it may need to be supplemented with locally produced specific information. Generally, information from cancer charities is free to patients and carers but there may be a charge for health professionals. Macmillan Cancer Relief has produced a directory of nationally published cancer information materials. An electronic version of the directory is also available on the ChiQ web site:www.hfht.org/macmillan/index.htm.

A useful resource aimed at helping people who want to produce good patient information is the book 'Producing Patient Information: How to Research, Develop and Produce Effective Information Resources'.[36] It offers a step-by-step guide to each stage of the information process, from developing an information policy to writing and disseminating print and electronic materials. Another useful resource available from the Department of Health is the toolkit for producing patient information. It consists of guidance for written patient information and a series of templates to accompany the guidance. The toolkit is available on the NHS identity website at www.nhsidentity.nhs.uk/patientinformationtoolkit/index.htm. Hard copies can be obtained from the NHS Responseline on 0870-155-5455.

The key points to remember when writing patient information leaflets are content, writing style and presentation. Information materials should say why they have been written and the contents should reflect the information needs of the patients and frequently asked questions. Provide contact details for queries. Patient information needs to be:

- clear and understandable
- written in everyday language
- accessible
- evidence based where possible
- sensitive to older people and cultural needs
- cost-effective
- up to date
- appropriate to the patient's stage in the care pathway
- dated when it was written and when it is due for review (if appropriate).

Piloting the leaflets with the intended audience before printing can establish obvious problems at an early stage before too much time or cost has been incurred. In this way, checks can be made to ensure that the language and format used is clear. Equally, piloting the leaflets will establish that the content appropriately reflects the issues health professionals consider important as well as responding to patient-identified issues.

Evaluating patient information

The evaluation of patient information materials should be an ongoing process to assess whether or not they are achieving their intended outcomes and objectives.[37] Written information should be reviewed on a regular basis and take into account:

- new knowledge and changes in practice
- whether the material is accurate and current
- whether the content follows a logical sequence and covers the topics it purports to discuss
- that the style is appropriate for the intended audience, i.e. children, the elderly, ethnic background
- clear illustrations that enhance the text (where appropriate).

When using materials from other sources, it is important to know how they were developed and whether they have been evaluated with patients as well as health professionals. There is no one tool that can be used for assessing patient information materials.

One instrument that concentrates on the content of treatment-related information is DISCERN,[38] developed by the University of Oxford Division of Public Health and Primary Care and funded by the British Library and the NHS Research and Development Programme in 1998. DISCERN consists of 15 questions to help users of consumer health information assess the quality of written information about treatment choices. However, this tool is limited, as it does not assess the evidence base on which a publication is based.[39]

The basic DISCERN criteria states that a good-quality publication about treatment choices will:

1. have explicit aims
2. achieve its aims
3. be relevant to consumers
4. make sources of information explicit
5. make date of information explicit
6. be balanced and unbiased
7. list additional sources of information
8. refer to areas of uncertainty
9. describe how treatment works
10. describe the benefits of treatment
11. describe the risks of treatment
12. describe what would happen without treatment
13. describe the effects of treatment choices on overall quality of life
14. make it clear there may be more than one possible treatment choice
15. provide support for shared decision-making.

Full information about the DISCERN instrument can be found on their website: www.discern.org.uk/

Who is providing the information?

While it is generally the clinician who provides initial information concerning diagnosis and treatment options, other multidisciplinary health professionals also have an important information-giving role. Nurses administering chemotherapy treatment may well encounter questions that concern areas other than treatment-related issues. It is essential to know what other resources are available to provide additional information and support, both hospital- and community-based.

Information for patients receiving chemotherapy

Information provided for patients undergoing chemotherapy treatment should aim to decrease anxiety levels and promote self-care strategies that enable coping. When treatment-related symptoms are managed effectively, patients are more likely to do better both physically and psychologically.[40] However, some patients fear that they may not be given enough information to cope with their disease and treatment.[41]

Increasingly, chemotherapy is given in an ambulatory care setting,[40,42] and this has implications for both patients and health professionals. Patients are more likely to encounter problems resulting from their treatment at home without recourse to the specialist help on hand in an inpatient setting. Health professionals may have more limited time available for patient education, and information exchange has to take place during treatment when there is an expectation that the patient is a willing participant. The limited opportunities for information-giving places greater emphasis on determining an individual's needs on each occasion. Ensure that the patient is given contact details of who they can speak to if they have further questions or concerns, outside of their hospital appointments.

There has been a frequent assumption that health professionals are best placed to know the information needs of people with cancer, both in terms of what to provide and when to provide it.[27,43] However, their perception of information needs have been found to be different to the learning needs expressed by people with cancer.[29,44]

Luker et al[27] found that the information priorities of newly diagnosed women with breast cancer related to their illness and treatment options, which matched similar findings from Davison and Degner[45] regarding men and prostate cancer. The need for full information about side effects has also been emphasised.[46,47]

One area where unmet informational needs have been identified[48] concerns family relationships, particularly when patients rely on family members for support.

Informed consent

The Department of Health[49] introduced new guidance setting out good practice, and the provision of information is central to the consent process. Patients must be given appropriate information about their disease and treatments, stating the risks and benefits of treatments and procedures, to support decision-making in the consent process. Details of the supporting information given to the patient should be documented on the consent forms. To make informed treatment choices, patients need to know the reason for the proposed treatment, how it will affect the cancer, the treatment schedule and potential side effects and lifestyle changes. As to the depth of information required in order for patients to make informed decisions, this will depend on the individual and is likely to be influenced by their educational and cultural background.[5]

While studies have shown that the majority of patients want information, younger people are more likely to want active involvement in the decision-making process.[7,8]

Chemotherapy treatment

The patient should be told why chemotherapy is being given – as primary treatment, adjuvant treatment or palliative treatment. Treatment protocols may be single agents or a combination of drugs. Additional information may be required if the patient is taking part in a clinical trial. Health professionals need to ensure that the information they give out reflects current practice and local policy. Some patients may want to know why they are receiving a particular treatment regime when they know that someone else with the same cancer is receiving something different.

Information should include:

- the names of the drug(s)
- any identifying characteristics, such as 'a red drug given through a vein', or 'a capsule'
- how the drug will be administered.

The chemotherapy schedule

Practical information is important, such as the dates the patient is due to have treatment, what time to arrive and how long they are likely to be at the hospital. Knowing what to expect on the days they receive chemotherapy can help with forward planning. It may be helpful for patients to take a book or some other diversion if there are going to be periods of time waiting, particularly if there is a wait for results of tests to determine that chemotherapy will go ahead. It is equally important to know whether patients can attend on their own or if it is better that they are accompanied. Will hospital transport be needed?

The patient should know:

- who is giving the chemotherapy
- what chemotherapy will be given
- where it will be given
- how it will be given
- what the potential side effects are and what measures to take.

Side effects

Patient information is essential for the prevention and effective management of chemotherapy side effects, and specific information on side effects can enhance self-care and help patients cope.[2,11,42,46,50] A study undertaken by the National Cancer Alliance[46] emphasised the need for full information, especially about side effects. While information about specific side effects is discussed in detail elsewhere in the Management of Toxicity chapters, there are some general guidelines to follow. Patients need to be aware of:

- The immediate and late side effects associated with a drug.
- General reactions to chemotherapy such as fatigue. As patients frequently associate hair loss and nausea and vomiting with chemotherapy, ensure they are also told if they will *not* experience these side effects. Patients can plan around their treatment and make lifestyle changes accordingly, if they know when to expect side effects and how long they might last.
- Recognising the importance of what action to take when side effects do occur. Can self-care strategies be used to help manage symptoms or should the patient seek expert help? Knowing what to do can help reduce anxiety for many patients. The presence or absence of side effects can often be a perceived measure of efficacy by patients.
- Tests that will indicate how well the treatment is working, rather than relying on their assessment of side effects to judge treatment response.

Severe side effects may mean a dose reduction or changing to another regime, which can be extremely distressing for patients, increasing worries that their disease may not be responding to treatment.

For many patients, the use of complementary therapies can be a helpful coping strategy with some symptoms of the disease and treatment.[51] In addition to any complementary therapies available through the hospital/care setting, patients may welcome information about local self-help groups and cancer support centres offering a wider range of complementary therapies.

Self-care skills

Self-care is an important element of health care for patients undergoing treatment and can help with the prevention of side effects as well as their management. Dodd[50] found that patients who had received information on how to manage side effects initiated more effective self-care strategies than those who had not been given information. Informed patients were also more likely to initiate these strategies at an earlier stage of developing symptoms.

Quality of life issues

Patients may want to know whether they can continue to work or carry out their usual activities during their chemotherapy. While it is not always possible to predict how any individual will react to treatment, acknowledging their anxiety will help them to manage it more effectively. If a chemotherapy date clashes with an important diary commitment, can treatment be postponed and if so, by how long? Balancing quality of life issues with probable treatment outcomes is very individual and an important consideration.

CONCLUSION

The value of patient information should not be underestimated. It can help patients to understand the challenges of a cancer diagnosis and give them greater control of their lives. Information can help them cope with both the practical aspects of the illness and chemotherapy, and manage any fears and anxieties they experience.

References

1. Friedman BD. Coping with cancer: a guide for health care professionals. Cancer Nurs 1980; 3:105–110.
2. Manson H, Manderino MA, Johnson MH. Chemotherapy: thoughts and images of patients with cancer. Oncol Nurs Forum 1993; 20(3):527–532.
3. Lazarus RS, Folkman S. Stress, appraisal and coping. New York: Springer; 1984.
4. Sutherland HJ, Llewellyn-Thomas HA, Lockwood GA, et al. Cancer patients: their desire for information and participation in treatment decisions. J Roy Soc Med 1989; 82:260–263.
5. Hack TF, Degner LF, Dyck DG. Relationship between preferences for decisional control and illness information among women with breast cancer: a quantitative and qualitative analysis. Soc Sci Med 1994; 39(2):279–289.
6. Semple CJ, McGowan B. Need for appropriate written information for patients, with particular reference to head and neck cancer. J Clin Nurs 2002; 11:585–593.
7. Cassileth BR, Zupkis RV, Sutton-Smith K, et al. Information and participation preferences among cancer patients. Ann Intern Med 1980; 92:832–836.
8. Blanchard CG, Labrecque MS, Ruckdeschel JC, et al. Information and decision-making preferences of hospitalised adult cancer patients. Soc Sci Med 1988; 27(11):1139–1145.
9. Davison BJ, Degner LF, Morgan TR. Information and decision-making preferences of men with prostate cancer. Oncol Nurs Forum 1995; 22(9):1401–1408.
10. Meredith C, Symonds P, Webster L, et al. 1996 Information needs of cancer patients in west Scotland: cross sectional survey of patients' views. Br Med J 1996; 313:724–727.
11. Ream E, Richardson A. The role of information in patients' adaptation to chemotherapy and radiotherapy: a review of the literature. Eur J Cancer Care 1996; 5:132–138.

12. Mills ME, Sullivan K. The importance of information giving for patients newly diagnosed with cancer: a review of the literature. J Clin Nurs 1999; 8:631–642.

13. Department of Health: Expert Advisory Group on Cancer to the Chief Medical Officers of England and Wales. A Policy Framework for Commissioning Cancer Services. London: HMSO; 1995.

14. Department of Health. The NHS Cancer Plan. Department of Health www.doh.gov.uk/cancer/cancerplan updated 27/09/2000.

15. NHS Information Authority with the National Cancer Director. Towards a cancer information strategy. Cancer Information Strategy Team, NHS Information Authority: www.cancer.nhsia.nhs.uk updated 28/07/2000.

16. Grahn G, Johnson J. Learning to cope and living with cancer. Scand J Caring Sci 1990; 4:173–181.

17. Van den Borne HW. The patient from receiver of information to informed decision-maker. Patient Education and Counselling 1998; 34:89–102.

18. Fernsler J, Cannon CA. The whys of patient education. Semin Oncol Nurs 1991; 7(2):79–86.

19. Adams M. Information and education across the phases of cancer care. Semin Oncol Nurs 1991; 7(2):105–111.

20. Fallowfield L. Quality of life. London: Souvenir Press; 1990.

21. Van der Molen B. Relating information needs to the cancer experience. 2. Themes from six cancer narratives. Eur J Cancer Care 2000; 9:48–54.

22. Teasdale K. Information and anxiety: a critical reappraisal. J Adv Nurs 1993; 18:1125–1132.

23. Butow PN, Maclean M, Dunn SM, et al. The dynamics of change: cancer patients' preferences for information, involvement and support. Ann Oncol 1997; 8:857–863.

24. Ley P. Communicating with patients. Cheltenham: Stanley Thornes; 1988.

25. Leydon GM, Boulton M, Moynihan C, et al. Cancer patients' information needs and information seeking behaviour: in depth interview study. Br Med J 2000; 320:909–1013.

26. Treacy JT, Mayer DK. Perspectives on cancer patient education. Semin Oncol Nurs 2000; 16(1):47–56.

27. Luker KA, Beaver K, Leinster SJ, et al. The information needs of women newly diagnosed with breast cancer. Journal of Advanced Nursing 1995; 22:134–141.

28. Luker KA, Beaver K, Leinster SJ, et al. Information needs and sources of information for women with breast cancer: a follow-up study. J Adv Nurs 1996; 23:487–495.

29. Griffiths M, Leek C. Patient education needs: opinions of oncology nurses and their patients. Oncol Nurs Forum 1995; 22(1):139–144.

30. Carlsson M. Cancer patients seeking information from sources outside the healthcare system. Support Care Cancer 2000; 8:453–457.

31. Jones R, Pearson J, McGregor S et al. Cross sectional survey of patients' satisfaction with information about cancer. Br Med J 1999; 319:1247–1248.

32. Jones R, Pearson J, McGregor S et al. Randomised trial of personalised computer based information for cancer patients. Br Med J 1999; 319:1241–1247.

33. Manfredi C, Czaja R, Buis M, et al. Patient use of treatment-related information received from the Cancer Information Service. Cancer 1993; 71(4): 1326–1337.

34. McClement SE, Hack TF. Audio-taping the oncology treatment consultation: a literature review. Patient Education and Counselling 1999; 36:229–238.

35. Thomas R, Deary A, Kaminski E, et al. Patients' preference for video cassette recorded information: effect of age, sex and ethnic group. Eur J Cancer Care 1999; 8:83–86.

36. Duman M. Producing patient information: how to research, develop and produce effective information resources. London: The King's Fund; 2003.

37. Frank-Stromborg M, Cohen R. Evaluating written patient education materials. Semin Oncol Nurs 1991; 7(2):125–134.

38. Charnock D (Compiler). The DISCERN Handbook. The University of Oxford Division of Public Health and Primary Care and funded by the British Library and the NHS Research and Development Programme, 1998. http://www.discern.org.uk/

39. Jefford M, Tattersall M. Informing and involving cancer patients in their own care. Lancet Oncol 2002; 3:629–637.

40. Dodd MJ, Miaskowski C. The PRO-SELF Program: A self-care intervention program for patients receiving cancer treatment. Semin Oncol Nurs 2000; 16(4):300–308.

41. Rhodes VA, McDaniel RW, Hanson BM, et al. Sensory perception of patients on selected antineoplastic chemotherapy protocols. Cancer Nurs 1994; 17(1):45–51.

42. Sitzia J, Wood N. Patient satisfaction with cancer chemotherapy nursing: a review of the literature. Int J Nurs Stud 1998; 35:1–12.

43. Grahn G. Coping with the cancer experience. I. Developing an education and support programme for cancer patients and their family members. Eur J Cancer Care 1996; 5:176–181.

44. Lauer P, Murphy SP, Powers MJ. Learning needs of cancer patients: a comparison of nurse and patient perceptions. Nurs Res 1982; 31(1):11–16.

45. Davison BJ, Degner LF. Empowerment of men newly diagnosed with prostate cancer. Cancer Nurs 1997; 20(3):187–196.

46. The National Cancer Alliance. "Patient-centred cancer services"? What patients say. Oxford: The National Cancer Alliance; 1996.

47. Lock KK, Willson B. Information needs of cancer patients receiving chemotherapy in an ambulatory setting. Can J Nurs Res 2002; 34(4):83–93.

48. McCaughan EM, Thompson KA. Information needs of cancer patients receiving chemotherapy at a day-case unit in Northern Ireland. J Clin Nurs 2000; 9:851–858.

49. Department of Health. Good practice in consent implementation guide: consent to examination or treatment. London: Department of Health; 2001.

50. Dodd MJ. Self-care for side effects of cancer chemotherapy: an assessment of nursing interventions – Part II. Cancer Nurs 1983; 6:63–67.

51. Bristol Cancer Help Centre. Meeting the needs of people with cancer for support and management. Bristol: Bristol Cancer Help Centre; 1999.

Chapter **6**

Ethical and legal issues

Sarah Jefferies

ETHICAL ISSUES

The fundamental ethical consideration that should underlie both routine medical practice and medical research is respect for the individual patient as a human being. Traditionally, ethical guidelines for treatment and research have been considered separately. This is due to the fact that treatment is generally viewed as not involving interests other than those of the patient, whereas research may involve interests that could distort the doctor–patient relationship.

Informed consent in medical practice

Prior to administering any chemotherapy treatment it is important to obtain valid informed consent (see the dh.gov.uk consent section. www.dh.gov.uk/ PolicyAndGuidance/HealthAndSolicalCareTopics/ Consent/fs/en). The underlying rationale for informed consent is to:

1. safeguard the autonomy and integrity of the individual
2. ensure that the patient plays an active role in the decisions about treatment.

To obtain informed consent:

1. the patient must be capable of giving consent
2. the consent must be given freely.

It is important that all the appropriate information, such as the likelihood of benefits and side effects, has been provided and fully understood. If the consent procedure has not been properly sought – for example, the provision of inaccurate or inadequate information about clinical treatment – this may constitute negligence.

Clinical trials

There are many ethical issues encountered when considering clinical trials. In order to assess the relevant ethical issues for any research proposals it is necessary to decide what makes a clinical trial morally acceptable. This decision raises a whole host of philosophical, legal and ethical questions. Numerous theses have addressed these very issues but three frequently used approaches are given below:[1]

1. *Goal-based approach* – this argues that the researcher believes that the right to do the clinical trial is good, as the outcome is believed to be good. The goal-based question should be considered for each clinical trial and assessed as to whether the design is appropriate to achieve its goal.
2. *Rights-based approach* – this takes into account the views and feelings of the prospective participant. The right to refuse should prevail over any consideration for the public good. This encompasses how the patient is approached and the right not to participate within a clinical trial.
3. *Duty-based approach* – no matter how important the research question, the duty is to the patient. The duty to the patient relates to the risks that the clinical trial may pose and whether these are acceptable for the patient.

Phase I trials

New drugs are researched and developed by the academic and the pharmaceutical industry and then must undergo phase I clinical trials to ascertain maximum dosage and tolerance. For cytotoxic and biological treatments, which clearly cannot be used in healthy individuals, this poses an ethical issue, as the studies have to be performed on cancer patients who are no longer responding to standard treatment. For these patients, it is unlikely that there will be any clinical benefit and there is a significant chance of side effects. From an ethical and legal standpoint it is important that the patient is fully aware of the risks associated with the drug under investigation and that it is unlikely that there will be benefit for themselves but that there may be benefit for others in the future.

Phase II clinical trials

Phase II trials evaluate compounds using data obtained from phase I studies and assess possible therapeutic effect. Although the benefit may be small, from an ethical viewpoint there is some therapeutic justification in having patients participating in such trials.

Phase III/randomised clinical trials

Therapeutic research offers the possibility of benefit to the research subject and to be ethical the patient must expect to receive treatment at least as good as the treatment that would be received as standard medical treatment. This ethical situation is one of equilibrium:

- the new treatment must be believed to be as good as the standard treatment but there is uncertainty as to whether the new treatment is better

Randomised clinical trials are considered to be the 'gold standard' in treatment efficacy research as they carefully define and control as many variables as possible in the treatment process. Random assignment balances groups of patients for factors that could affect the outcome from treatment. If there are factors which are known to impact on outcome, then a stratification process can be put into place to ensure that each arm of the trial is well-balanced for these known factors. (See the Clinical Trials section.)

Much medical research is carried out on standard chemotherapy regimens and compares them to newer combinations in randomised trials. In this setting, patients randomised to the standard regimen may be given extensive information far greater than those in routine medical practice. Each individual patient has different needs and wishes about the information they wish to receive. The vast majority will wish to receive extensive information, whereas a few will not. It is also worth noting that patients participating in randomised trials are likely to be more frequently evaluated and this may result in the outcome being unrealistic in standard practice. (See the Patient Information section.)

Informed consent for clinical trials

Article I.9 of the Declaration of Helsinki[2] outlines that research performed on an individual should only be undertaken after obtaining informed consent. In the UK, key points to consent are outlined by the Department of Health (see dh.gov.uk). For a trial, participant consent should be voluntary, informed, competent and confidential.

Voluntary The consent should not be affected by the desire to please or upset the researcher. Particular care should be taken if the researcher is also the treating physician. Consent to participate in trials should not be induced by financial reward or other perceived benefit.

Informed Sufficient information and time must be provided to enable a potential participant to make a decision based on full understanding of the nature of the research. Information is usually provided both verbally and in written form. If patients are not offered as much information as they reasonably need to make a decision, and in a form they can understand, their consent may not be valid.

Competent   Legally competent subjects understand what is being asked of them and are capable of providing informed consent to participate in research. If a person is unconscious or is unable to give consent or communicate a decision due to his mental or physical condition, then no other person is able to give consent to participate in a clinical trial.[3] Certain situations may arise where it is possible to treat such patients, such as the acutely ill patient (e.g. patients presenting with acute leukaemia), where the treatment is deemed to be in the patient's best interest. 'Best interests' extend beyond medical interests and can incorporate wishes when the patient was competent and current wishes. In certain circumstances a court may authorise medical treatment of an incompetent adult, which in theory could include therapeutic research. In the UK, children of 16 and 17 are legally entitled to give consent to treatment and thus also to therapeutic research. Children under 16 who have the capacity and understanding to take decisions about their own treatment are also able to do so in relationship to therapeutic research. For younger children or those below 16 not competent to decide, persons with parental responsibility can provide consent for therapeutic research. However, the assent of the child is sought. If a competent child consents to a clinical trial, a parent cannot override that consent. Legally, a parent can consent if a competent child refuses, but this would be a rare event in therapeutic research.

Confidentiality   Arrangements must be made to safeguard confidentiality and data should be secured against unauthorised access. No individual should be identifiable from published records without express consent. Research data from which an individual can be identified should not be kept for longer than necessary. All data held electronically is subject to the Data Protection Act.[4]

To improve health care, clinical research must assess new treatments, and an essential component of this research is that the individual participating has been able to give informed consent. The idea of informed consent is widely embraced but in practice the procedure may vary greatly. This topic is excellently discussed in a series of papers published by the British Medical Journal.[5] A recent cross-sectional survey of cancer patients participating in clinical trials found that although there was a high rate of satisfaction with the process of consent there was also lack of knowledge of the degree of risk involved. There was also a lack of understanding that the majority of trials will benefit patients in the future not the participant. Interestingly, this latter point was also not well understood by the providers of the trials.[6]

Conduct of research

It is emphasised by the International Conference on Harmonization[7] good practice guidelines and national guidelines[8] that it is essential that researchers have the appropriate qualifications and clinical competence to carry out the proposed research. The investigator of the trial must ensure that the trial is conducted with the Declaration of Helsinki October 2000 amendment.[9] The European Union has outlined a clinical trial directive that is required to be utilised in all clinical trials by 2004. This outlines that all research involving human volunteers or patients should be conducted to the highest standards. This directive requires detailed documentation and reporting of both academic and pharmaceutical industry trials. Failure to comply with regulations will be a serious offence and provisions will be made for surprise inspections of clinical sites.[10]

Standards of care

When patients are approached for entry into clinical trials, the research may place them at increased risk. Often the degree of risk may not be fully understood until the research has been completed. It is clear that participants must have accurate and detailed information about potential risks and also about possible benefits. Access to such information is essential for good medical care and should dominate medical research.[11] The level of disclosure in clinical trials may be higher than medical practice.

LEGAL ISSUES

There is no law specifically directed at the conduct of clinical research in the United Kingdom. Medicines legislation (Medicines Act 1968) regulates the manufacture and supply of medicinal products in clinical research but does not address the research conduct and also does not apply to phase I trials. For phase I studies, it is necessary to utilise general legislation and legal principles. Research ethics committees have been established to address the ethical and legal issues involved in clinical research.

Local research ethics committees

In the United Kingdom, since 1967, there have been local research ethics committees (LRECs), whose function is to satisfy themselves that research proposals are ethically acceptable in accordance with article I.2 of the Declaration of Helsinki.[2] Each health authority has at least one LREC, on which medical, nursing, other health professionals and lay people sit. LRECs address both the scientific and ethical components of proposed trials. Some health authorities have separate scientific committees that serve as advisory bodies to the LREC committee. For clinical trials that will take place in more than two centres, applications must be submitted to a multi-centre research ethics committee (MREC). Once MREC approval has been granted, the trial also has to obtain LREC approval. Many issues are considered for each research protocol before the committee grants ethical approval.

Information for the research ethics committee

The research protocol should contain an accurate description of the question accompanied by the background literature that has led to the research proposal. Potential risks to which participants may be exposed must be clearly outlined and must be justifiable and kept to an absolute minimum. Details should be outlined on how confidentiality will be maintained both in the method of patient approach and subsequent storage of data. Patients should be 'invited' to participate in research studies. It must be clearly stated that patients are able to decline participation in the research, without giving a reason, and that this will not affect subsequent treatment in any way. The patients participating in the research should understand that they remain free to withdraw at any time, without giving any reason, and that this will not affect subsequent treatment in any way.

Obtaining consent

Procedures for obtaining consent must be assessed by the LREC to ensure they are not coercive or unreasonably induced. Oral explanation of the research procedure is accompanied by written information, and written consent is obtained. Time for reflection should be given to allow consideration of enrolment.

The general principles relating to special groups such as children,[12] adults with special needs and patients with psychiatric illness are that the research should be carried out in competent adults as a preference.

The researcher must be qualified and capable of doing the research. Improved patient care should not be perceived as an inducement to participate in the research study. Payments to patients are generally undesirable and any payments that are made must be fully outlined to the LREC. All payments to doctors should be fully outlined. Payments to doctors on a per capita basis are unethical.

Regulatory bodies

Clinical research using chemotherapy agents sponsored by a company requires either a Clinical Trial Certificate (CTC), a Clinical Trial Exemption (CTX) or a Marketing Authorisation in accordance with the Medicines Act (1968). If the research is doctor-initiated, then referral to the Medicines Control Agency is required to obtain a Doctors and Dentists Exemption (DDX). Research that uses medical devices or radioactivity both have specialist review bodies.

Compensation

The position on compensation for research subjects is outlined by the NHS Executive.[13] Trials sponsored by pharmaceutical companies must comply with the Association of the British Pharmaceutical Industry.[14]

CONCLUSION

Development of treatments for patients relies on the participation of patients in clinical trials.

References

1. Manual for research ethics commitees. London: University of London; 1996.
2. World Medical Association Declaration of Helsinki: recommendations guiding physicians in biomedical research involving human subjects. J Am Med Assoc 1996; 277:925–926.
3. Department of Health. The protection and use of patient information. HSG(96) 18,LASSL(96). London: Department of Health; 1996.
4. The Data Protection Act Guidelines. Wilmslow: Office of the Data Protection Registrar; 1989.
5. Doyal L, Tobias JS. Informed consent in medical research. London:BMJ Books; 2001.
6. Joffe S, Cook EF, Clearly PD, et al. Quality of informed consent in cancer trials: a cross-sectional survey. Lancet 2001; 358;1742–1743.
7. International Conference on Harmonisation of Technical Requirements for Registration of Pharmaceuticals for Human Use. Guideline for Good Clinical Practice. Geneva: IFPMA 1996; 1.
8. The Royal College of Physicians. Guidelines on the Practice of Ethics Commitees in Medical Research involving Human Subjects. London: The Royal College of Physicians. 1996; 3.
9. Declaration of Helsinki October 2000 amendment: http://www.wma.net/e/policy/17-c_e.html).
10. British Association of Research Quality Assurance: http://www.barqa.com
11. Doyal L. Needs, rights and moral duties of clinicians. In: Gillon R, ed. Principles of health care ethics. Chichester: Wiley, 1994:217–230.
12. Local Research Ethics Commitees. HSG (91)5, 1991. London: Department of Health; 1991.
13. NHS indemnity: arrangements for handling clinical negligence claims against NHS staff. HSG(96)48. London: Department of Health; 1996.
14. Clinical trial compensation guidelines. London: ABPI 1991; 1.

Chapter **7**

Measuring the quality of life in palliative chemotherapy

Diane Laverty

INTRODUCTION

The measure of whether curative chemotherapy (i.e. chemotherapy that has the intent to cure a patient of their disease) has been effective is usually related to evidence of tumour response and the overall survival of the patient.[1] In patients receiving palliative chemotherapy, the aim of treatment is different, focusing on the quality of life that the patient is able to achieve. Long-term survival is no longer an issue and the treatment options need to be realistic, taking into account the patient's wishes. It is not unusual for patients to request more chemotherapy as it fosters their concept of hope and gives them the feeling that they are still 'fighting' the disease.[2] The healthcare professional has a responsibility to the patient to be realistic and explain the expected outcomes for treatment in the palliative phase. This is normally that the hope is for stabilisation of the disease and not cure.

QUALITY OF LIFE

The term 'quality of life' has received increasing attention recently, but it has been surrounded by controversy[1,3] due to the issues relating to the fundamental meaning of this concept and the most effective way to measure it.

Quality of life has rarely been defined explicitly but it should ideally include the patient's view – what is possible or ideal[4] – and is always multidimensional (physical, psychological and functional aspects). It should also be remembered that quality of life is a dynamic concept and will change in certain circumstances and situations.[5,6] Quality of life can cover a multitude of issues and, to ensure the validity of any tools used to measure it, most are targeted at a 'population' of patients as opposed to individuals.

Because of the diversity of the assessment, some people believe that quality of life cannot be measured,[1] while others believe that it provides a baseline for decision-making to determine treatment options.[7]

Quality of life measures can be plagued by:

1. high attrition rates
2. poor compliance
3. missing data and lack of conceptual clarity
4. lack of knowledge as to the interpretation and analysis of data
5. the complexity of data collected.

All too often, the results presented give scant information on how symptoms are measured, by whom, when, and for how long. For these reasons it may be easier to measure objective response: e.g. the size of the mass on scanning or duration of survival, as in curative chemotherapy.

For staff to address quality of life issues in palliative chemotherapy there is a need to measure clinical outcome but this does not necessarily have to be done by complete or partial response indicators. The size of the tumour may not show a direct correlation between tumour response and symptom improvement.[8] Nor is it useful to use survival time as an outcome measure, as this may remain undetermined.[7] The measure of quality of life in the patient undergoing palliative chemotherapy is the balance between symptom relief, patient well-being and the side effects of the treatment.

ASSESSMENT TOOLS

Assessment tools should be easy, quick, measurable and clinically relevant (Table 7.1).[9]

There are numerous quality of life tools available. A tool tends to be chosen depending on the purpose of the assessment and the type of patients (e.g. tumour type, symptom problems) that they are being used to measure.[4]

There can be many domains in a tool:

- physical symptoms
- psychological/emotional issues

Table 7.1 Tools used both in curative and palliative chemotherapy

Category	Assessment tool	Characteristics
Symptom control	The Rotterdam Symptom Control Checklist (RSCL)	Originally developed for use in women with breast cancer having first-line chemotherapy.[7] Scoring system is lengthy and difficult for patients who are less well.
Symptom control	The Edmonton Symptom Assessment System (ESAS)	Developed for the assessment of multiple symptoms, completed twice daily by the patient using a VAS[13]
Symptom control	Symptom Distress Scale (SDS)	Completed by patient, usually in the presence of the observer, using a 5 point Likert scale[14]
Symptom control	The Support Team Assessment Schedule (STAS)	Adapted for use in specific settings. Completed once/twice a week and measures the impact of symptoms[15]
Symptom control	Palliative Care Assessment (PACA)	Measures the severity of symptoms from the patient's perspective and the impact on their life and future[16]
Quality of life	The European Organization for Research and Treatment of Cancer QLC-C30 (EORTC QLQ-C30)	Widely used questionnaire that can be adapted for different tumour types.[17] The purpose is to capture the patient's view on their functional ability and overall quality of life. It appears to answer the recommended characteristics of an ideal tool and for this reason it is used in many chemotherapy trials
Quality of life	The Schedule for the Evaluation of Individual Quality of Life (SEIQoL)	Developed to address the relevance of patient's own views and opinions on what quality of life means to them as an individual. Composed of a semi-structured questionnaire that contains 'cues' and then 'weights' these 'cues' in accordance with how much value the individual patient places on each one[18]
Quality of life	The McGill Quality of Life Questionnaire (MQOL)	Measures symptoms and outlook of life and is completed by the patient[19]

VAS, visual analogue scale.

- functional aspects
- spiritual/sexual/social aspects.[10]

It is difficult to focus on all of these domains, so assessment should ideally be patient-focused and judged on what aspects the patients value most of all.[11] This will serve to reflect different patient groups, but in practice may be deemed impossible to do.

Most tools have been widely validated but some authors question how relevant the tools are in addressing important issues such as referring to the 'opportunity cost' where time is spent receiving treatment and the decreased functional ability due to toxicity from the drugs.[12]

CONCLUSION

Evidence shows that it is imperative that assessment in the palliative phase of a cancer journey should be patient-directed and healthcare professionals must ensure that they remain partners in their care.[20] Patient quality of life is paramount when time is limited and a patient's wishes relating to treatment options and care should always be taken into consideration.

Quality of life is an integral means of measuring outcomes of treatment, in terms of addressing cost benefit and, most importantly, in caring for patients when their prognosis may be uncertain but clearly of a short duration.

References

1. Gough IR, Dalgleish LI. What value is given to quality of life assessment by health professionals considering response to palliative chemotherapy for advanced cancer? Cancer 1991; 68(1):220225.
2. Slevin ML, Plant H, Lynch D, et al. Who should measure quality of life, the doctor or the patient? Br J Canc 1988; 57:109–112.
3. Priestman T, Baum M. Evaluation of quality of life in patients receiving treatment for advanced breast cancer. Lancet 1976; 1:899–901.
4. Cella DF, Tulsky DS. Measuring quality of life today: methodological aspects. Oncology (Huntingt) 1990; 4(5): 29–38.
5. DeBoer MF, McCormick LK, Pruyn JFA, et al. Physical and psychological correlates of head and neck cancer; a review of the literature. Otolaryn – Head Neck Surg 1999; 120(3):427–436.
6. Morgan G. Assessment of quality of life in palliative care. Int J Palliat Nurs 2000; 6(8):406–410.
7. Ramirez AJ, Towlson KE, Leaning MS, et al. Do patients with advanced breast cancer benefit from chemotherapy? Br J Canc 1998; 78(11): 1488–1494.
8. Geels P, Eisenhauer E, Bezjak A, et al. Palliative effect of chemotherapy: objective tumour response is associated with symptom improvement in patients with metastatic breast cancer. J Clin Oncol 2000; 18(12):2395–2405.
9. Cohen RS, Mount B. Quality of life in terminal illness: defining and measuring subjective well-being in the dying. J Palliat Care 1992; 8:40–45.
10. Cella DF. Quality of life: concepts and definition. J Pain Sympt Mangt 1994; 9(3):186–193.
11. Osoba D. Lessons learned from measuring health-related quality of life in oncology. J Clin Oncol 1994; 12:608–616.
12. Munro AJ, Sebag-Montefiore D. Opportunity cost: a neglected aspect of cancer treatment. Br J Canc 1992; 65:309–310.
13. Bruera E, Macdonald S. Audit measures: the Edmonton Symptom Assessment System. In: Higginson I, ed. Clinical audit in palliative care. Oxford: Radcliffe Medical Press, 1993:61–78.
14. McCorkle R, Young K. Development of a symptom distress scale. Cancer Nurs 1978; 101:373–378.
15. Higginson I. A community schedule. In: Higginson I, ed. Clinical audit in palliative care Oxford: Radcliffe Medical Press, 1993:34–48.
16. Ellershaw JE, Peat S, Boys LC. Assessing the effectiveness of a hospital palliative care team. Palliat Med 1995; 9(2):145–152.
17. Aaronson NK, Ahmedzai S, Bergman B, et al. The European Organisation for Research and Treatment of Cancer QLQ-C30: a quality of life instrument for use in international clinical trials in oncology. J Natl Canc Inst 1993; 85(5):365–376.
18. Waldron D, O'Boyle CA, Kearney M, et al. Quality of life measurement in advanced cancer: assessing the individual. J Clin Oncol 1999; 17(1):3603–3611.
19. Cohen SR, Mount BM, Strobel MG, et al. The McGill quality of life questionnaire: a measure of quality of life appropriate for people with advanced cancer. A preliminary study of validity and acceptability. Palliat Med 1995; 9(3):207–219.
20. Department of Health. Making a difference. London: HMSO; 1999.

Chapter **8**

Management of the adult patient with cancer receiving chemotherapy

Miriam Wood, Lorraine Hyde and Mave Salter

INTRODUCTION

About 50% of patients with cancer receive chemotherapy, which is determined by the type of cancer and the medical management of the patient.[1] Chemotherapy involves a variety of diagnostic tests, and requires assessments from various members of the multiprofessional team. For the patient receiving chemotherapy, the process of treatment is likely to be for a period of weeks or months and the demands of the timetable of attendance for treatment and possible side effects experienced can make it a very stressful time for patients. A multidisciplinary approach to the delivery of cancer services is required from diagnosis to address the patient's needs and to provide good coordination and communication for those providing treatment and care.[2–6] At the treatment stage of the patient's cancer journey it has been suggested that the following factors are what matters most to patients:[7]

- the speed with which treatment starts
- the nature of the treatment
- the care and support that they are given throughout.

Patients may receive chemotherapy at different stages of the cancer pathway. Chemotherapy may be:

- the main treatment modality to cure the patient, e.g. with leukaemia, lymphoma or testicular cancer, the aim of which is to prolong the patient's survival
- given before or after surgery for cancer (adjuvant/ neoadjuvant)
- given concurrently in combination with other treatment, e.g. radiotherapy (chemoradiation)
- to relieve the patient's symptoms and improve quality of life (palliative).

For some patients, chemotherapy treatment is urgent, due to the type and severity of the patient's symptoms and/or may be a life-saving treatment.[8] For example, spinal cord compression and superior vena cava obstruction are oncological emergencies where chemotherapy may be given to relieve symptoms, whereas acute leukaemia requires urgent chemotherapy to control the disease. In these circumstances patients may have had little time to come to terms with, or think about, their diagnosis or recurrence and the proposed treatment plan. Thus, the provision of information, ongoing support and communication is essential to ensure safe and effective care.[5–9]

As chemotherapy may be administered in the inpatient, day care and outpatient settings or at home, effective coordination of care and good communication is necessary to meet patient's individual needs. The involvement of the appropriate healthcare professionals and services including social services and voluntary agencies to support the patient in the community and/or hospital settings is crucial. Patient-centred care is both challenging and rewarding and its philosophy is based upon the following principles:[3,4]

- taking into account the patients' concerns and choices, their carers and relatives
- the treatment and care plan is tailored to the patient's individual needs
- multiprofessional team working within agreed protocols/guidelines
- coordination of care across primary and secondary settings.

Specialisation in individual types of cancer has been recommended and the effectiveness of specialist care is thought to improve patient outcomes; however, it is not clear if this is true for all types of cancer.[7] A consistent approach to treatment and care for different cancers and ongoing review of care for the individual patient as well as the service itself will facilitate ongoing research and development and improve the patient's experience.[6,10,11]

This chapter focuses upon the management of the adult patient with cancer receiving chemotherapy. Patient assessment for chemotherapy treatment, the process of chemotherapy treatment, continuity of care and the organisation of cancer services in the United Kingdom, in particular England and Wales, are addressed. The challenge for healthcare professionals is to develop chemotherapy services that meet the individual needs of the patient, enabling them to feel supported whilst undergoing treatment. For it is by working in partnership across boundaries to implement the Cancer Plan, that improvements to patient outcomes along the patient pathway, i.e. prevention, screening and investigation, and diagnosis, treatment, palliative care and rehabilitation, will be achieved.[4,6,12] (See Ch. 5.)

> Note: the specific management of the paediatric patients with cancer receiving chemotherapy is covered in Chapter 35, including the organisation of paediatric cancer services in England and Wales.

PATIENT ASSESSMENT FOR CHEMOTHERAPY TREATMENT

For each type of cancer, clinicians use treatment pathways, protocols and guidelines to determine what may be the best possible treatment for the patient's individual circumstances based on the evidence, for example National Institute for Clinical Excellence (NICE) and Improving Outcomes Guidance (IOG).[4,13,14] Patient assessment by different healthcare professionals along the patient's pathway for chemotherapy treatment enables the patient to receive the most appropriate treatment, care and support whilst undergoing treatment.[4] Prior to an individual assessment of the patient's suitability for chemotherapy, the patient's treatment plan should be agreed from a multidisciplinary perspective: i.e. surgeons, radiologists, pathologists, oncologists, nurse specialists and palliative care specialists.[4] The patient's type and stage of cancer will be considered in order to decide the most appropriate treatment for the patient, taking into consideration the aim of treatment: i.e. curative, control of disease or palliative.[15] Members of the multiprofessional team can include psychological support, dietitian, lymphoedema specialist, chaplain, occupational therapist or social worker (to name but a few). The team can make a significant contribution to the patient's experience.[16] The plan of care should be devised with patient-centred goals, and a team approach ensures continuity of care.[5,6]

In oncology care, the multidisciplinary team meeting provides an opportunity to decide the proposed treatment plan within agreed guidelines/protocols (local and national).[4,7,13] It is recognised that not all types of cancers have multidisciplinary team meetings and the need for reorganisation of services and resources to support such an approach is required with the implementation of the Improving Outcomes Guidance.[4–7,10,11] In some cases, the specific needs of the individual patient are discussed at the multidisciplinary meeting, in addition to the cancer treatment plan.[7]

Communication and information-giving

A diagnosis of cancer will invoke fear, uncertainty and disbelief in many patients, rendering them unable to comprehend the implications of their diagnosis and treatment plan.[17] Communicating effectively and building a therapeutic relationship with patients will help the patient to understand the realities of receiving chemotherapy.[17] Effective communication skills are integral to supporting the patient and family and a systematic communication model will assist in this.[8,17]

All healthcare professionals must provide accurate, relevant and sensitive information which allows the patient and family to participate in their care and to take decisions about their treatment options.[18–21] Clarifying whether the patient has a desire for information and also a desire to participate in decision-making is necessary to determine how the patient wishes to be involved in the decision-making process.[18,22] By involving the patient and their family in all aspects of the treatment plan it has been suggested that the patient's sense of empowerment is enhanced.[10,11]

It is important that the doctor and nurse provide the patient and carer with a full explanation and relevant written information of:

- the rationale for blood tests and other investigations
- the aim of chemotherapy
- the type of chemotherapy
- the length of hospital stay
- the expected side effects of treatment (immediate, short-term and long-term side effects)
- self-care measures to manage side effects, toxicities and complications
- the possible impact on family relationships and lifestyle
- emergency contact numbers of the medical team and when they should be contacted.

It is recognised that the patient's readiness to learn and ability to retain information will vary and that the information required over time will differ, as will the impact on family relationships and the support required by both the patient and their family.[4,9,17,23,24] (See Ch. 5.)

Consent

Informed consent is integral to the decision-making by the patient as to whether or not to undergo treatment.[20,21] The nursing and medical team should liaise closely in order to ensure that the patient has received a full explanation of all aspects of the treatment plan. It is important to remember that the patient and family may need time to comprehend all of the information that has been given. The impact of treatment on the patient and family must be considered in relation to the benefits and risks involved.[25–27]

When a full explanation of the treatment has been given, in conjunction with any relevant written information, the patient is in a position to give consent to the treatment. Consent should be given in writing and is valid only if it has been given fully, voluntarily and freely. Patients should receive a copy of the consent form, which should have an explanation of the treatment, its benefits and risks, and contact information, and the consent should be documented in the medical notes. Consent is an ongoing process and the patient's understanding and agreement should be sought on an ongoing basis.[25,27–29] (See Chs 5 and 6.)

Diagnostic tests

Before chemotherapy treatment can begin, the patient needs to understand that a range of tests may need to be performed to ensure that they are fit enough for treatment, taking into account any co-morbid illnesses, as well as the stage of their disease. For the patient, the number of diagnostic tests prior to chemotherapy treatment can be daunting. Most patients will undergo many diagnostic tests, including blood tests, biopsy, X-ray and scans, and may have undergone previous treatments such as surgery.[30]

In general, diagnostic tests are related to:

- assessment of the disease, or the patient's response to treatment
- the safe decision-making for treatment.

Diagnostic tests will depend on the type of chemotherapy treatment and may include:

- blood samples, to assess the haematological function of the patient
- renal function – e.g. cisplatin can cause nephrotoxicity (see Ch. 40, Medical section)
- cardiac function, i.e. electrocardiogram – e.g. anthracyclines can cause cardiotoxicity
- lung function – e.g. bleomycin can cause pleural damage
- radiological investigations, e.g. X-ray and scans, to determine stage of disease
- histology, to confirm diagnosis and in some cases response to treatment.

(For side effects see Chs 24 (renal sections), 28 and 29: see also Ch. 40, Medical section.)

Clinical trials

Clinical trials are an integral part of the clinical management of the patient with cancer.[4] When the medical team are deciding the most appropriate treatment plan for the patient, it is important to consider if the patient is eligible to participate in a clinical trial.[4,31] The type of trial will depend on the patient's stage of disease and whether they have received any previous cancer therapies. While it may not be appropriate to enrol a newly diagnosed patient into a phase I trial of a new drug, a phase III trial comparing two established treatments may be appropriate and help to expand the evidence base of chemotherapy treatment.

Many teams include a research nurse, who will play a pivotal role to support the patient undergoing chemotherapy.[32] The patient and their family will require explanations regarding the nature of the trial and the concept of randomisation, which are given in language that is unambiguous and easy to understand.[25]

There are a number of regulations and organisations that oversee and support research trials in the UK. They provide advice and guidelines on good clinical practice that must be adhered to at all times.[33] The key organisations that provide coordination and support of cancer research in the UK are:[4]

- National Cancer Research Institute (NCRI)
- National Cancer Research Network (NRCN)
- National Translational Cancer Research Network (NTRAC).

(See Chs 6 and 8.)

Assessment and supportive care

The medical assessment of the patient will determine the patient's general health status, assessing the patient's fitness for chemotherapy, including the patient's performance status, e.g. Karnofsky or ECOG (Eastern Cooperative Oncology Group) assessment criteria.[34] A change in the patient's performance status helps the doctor to decide the intensity of the planned treatment. If the patient has a poor physical status, irrespective of age, it may be a reason to modify the dose to chemotherapy drug(s), or not to treat. The decision will be dependent on the type and stage of the cancer at diagnosis and the aim of treatment (Box 8.1).[15] Cancer in the elderly (over 65 years old) accounts for approximately 60% of all newly diagnosed cancers, and co-morbidity and functional status impact upon patient outcomes.[35–37]

Cancer is still feared by the public and oncology health professionals alike.[38] People's fears may be

---

Box 8.1 Performance status and treatment decision-making[15]

Example 1
For patients diagnosed with leukaemia their performance status may be poor; however, in order to cure the patient, it is imperative the chemotherapy treatment is initiated.

Example 2
For patients with metastatic breast cancer, if their performance status is poor – e.g. ECOG performance status of 3 – a discussion with the patient as to the potential benefits and risks of treatment is essential to decide whether chemotherapy treatment is appropriate.
See also Chs 14 and 47.

---

related to the fact that people of different ages are affected by cancer and the unpredictable course of the disease.[39] Misconceptions about cancer should be identified and addressed, as this may have considerable impact on the patient's quality of life.[39] In a study of patients' fears of the possible side effects of chemotherapy, it was found that their fears changed over time during the chemotherapy treatment, with some of their fears lessening and the level of importance of their fears had altered. The changes in the patients' fears were thought to be in response to the provision of adequate management of side effects.[40]

Each patient's experience of cancer will be different and how the disease, treatment and prognosis affect quality of life will be unique to the individual.[41] The psychosocial impact of a cancer diagnosis should be addressed, and a holistic approach to care that addresses the physical, psychological, social and spiritual aspects of the patient's life should be made. [6,8,42,43] Systematic assessment of chemotherapy-related problems (Box 8.2), as well as addressing the patients' needs from their perspective, is integral to meeting the patient's needs.[6,44–46] It is acknowledged that physical assessment skills are not straightforward and that, with new ways of working, nurses will need to develop their skills accordingly.[47]

Various assessment tools to assist healthcare professionals to gain the relevant assessment data/information to plan the patient's care have been developed.[44,48–51] The timing of assessment and the method, e.g. face to face or by telephone for specific patient groups and different regimens, should also be addressed.[52] Some symptoms are visible and the

Box 8.2   Assessment for chemotherapy[46]

1. Pre-chemotherapy assessment
   A Physical evaluation
      (i) Pertinent past history
         (a) Diagnosis and disease presentation
         (b) Concomitant health conditions and allergies
      (ii) System review
         (a) Pertinent laboratory data (haematopoietic function)
         (b) Neurological function
         (c) Oral cavity and integumentary status
         (d) Cardiovascular function
         (e) Respiratory function
         (f) Urological function
         (g) Gastrointestinal function
         (h) Sexual function
         (i) Dermatological status
      (iii) Presence of prior cancer therapy toxicities
         (a) Surgery
         (b) Radiation therapy
         (c) Chemotherapy
   B Psychosocial evaluation
         (a) Knowledge of cancer and chemotherapy
            • Dispel myths
            • Address feelings of anxiety and fear
         (b) Prior (personal) experience with chemotherapy
         (c) Support system and significant others
         (d) Informed consent
   C Patient/family education
2. Post-chemotherapy assessment
   A Review assessment as above for changes
      (i) Tumour response
      (ii) Status improvements
      (iii) Abnormal findings
   B Management of side effects
   C Patient/family education

patient, and encouraging the patient to articulate their concerns, professionals will be facilitated to support the patient in an appropriate way.[45,51] It has been suggested that nurses focus on the physical and technical aspects of chemotherapy and do not adequately address the patient's psychological problems and emotional needs.[56,57] The use of a short patient questionnaire (Fig. 8.1) in the outpatient setting to clarify the patient's concerns prior to the patient's consultation was shown to be helpful in addressing the patient needs by encouraging communication and facilitating staff–patient relationships.[58]

Telephone assessment and triage is a way to provide patient assessment and support and has been found to be effective.[59–62] An audit of telephone calls for advice to a cancer nurse specialist highlighted their role in the provision of psychological support, symptom management and treatment advice.[63] The introduction of patient-held records or care diaries has been advocated as beneficial to patients, facilitating communication between patients and the various healthcare professionals involved in their care.[64–66]

Assessment should provide information from which the healthcare professional is able to take decisions about the appropriate interventions and outcomes to be achieved. Prioritising care needs should be based upon their severity or whether they are of major concern to the patient. Appropriate referrals to other member of the multiprofessional team and community teams or other agencies should be made to meet the patient's needs. The patient's needs and level of support required will change over time and the need for ongoing assessment and support throughout chemotherapy treatment should not be underestimated.[17,44,46,51,59]

Supportive care has been described as care that:

> … helps the patient and their family to cope with cancer and treatment of it – from pre-diagnosis, through the process of diagnosis and treatment, to cure, continuing illness or death and into bereavement. It helps the patient to maximise the benefits of treatment and to live as well as possible with the effects of the disease. It should be given equal priority alongside diagnosis and treatment.[43]

Supportive care encompasses the following: self-help and support, user involvement, information-giving, psychological support, symptom control, social support, rehabilitation, complementary therapies, spiritual support, palliative care and end-of-life and bereavement care.[43] The challenge for local services is to review whether they are able to support patients

healthcare practitioner can observe these easily, whilst others rely on a detailed assessment in order to elicit the true experiences of the patient.[46] The patient's perception of their symptoms may vary from that of the doctor or nurse,[53] and the professional may not acknowledge the intensity of the symptoms in the same way as the patient.[44,51,53] Nurses' awareness of what the patient views as stressors whilst undergoing chemotherapy treatment differs also.[54]

Patient self-assessment tools specific to the clinical setting and patient needs have been advocated.[44,51,55] By clarifying 'how much the symptom bothers' the

In order that we can provide you with a better service, we would like to know of any concerns that you may have about your illness and treatment since we last saw you. Please remember to answer all of the questions.

Name   Date of birth   Date

Please tick

	Concerns	No concerns
The illness itself (what it is, is it better, etc.)	☐	☐
Treatment for the illness	☐	☐
How I have been physically	☐	☐
Not being able to do things	☐	☐
My job	☐	☐
Finances	☐	☐
Feeling upset or distressed	☐	☐
Feeling different from other people	☐	☐
How I feel about myself as a man or woman	☐	☐
My relationship with my partner	☐	☐
Support I have	☐	☐
Transport to and from hospital	☐	☐

Office use only   Assessed prior to appointment

Figure 8.1   Concerns checklist.[58]

in relation to the NICE guidelines and to clarify whether staff training needs have been addressed as well as organisation of services.[67] However, the value of complementary therapies, which may enhance the sense of well-being for some patients, has been described positively by one patient: 'Chemotherapy removed from my life all the things that made it pleasurable . . . but the massage was something nice that happened in the daily round of unpleasantness'.[68]

Toxicity assessment and symptom management

The doctor, nurse and members of the multidisciplinary team have an important role in toxicity assessment and managing symptom control. It is essential to undertake toxicity assessment prior to each course of treatment to measure the toxic effects of treatment. Dose modifications or treatment delays may be required in order to ensure patient safety and health. Common toxicity assessment criteria have been developed to ensure standardised assessment of toxicities and to determine the appropriate interventions.[34,46]

The clinician will assess the toxicity of the chemotherapy treatment and the patient's symptomatic and clinical response to treatment as evidenced by the patient's history, physical examination, diagnostic tests and radiological investigations.[69] The monitoring and support of the patient should also be based upon possible causes of death, be that from the disease or complications of disease. For example, in leukaemia the major cause of death is bleeding and infection and, by detecting complications early, patient outcomes will be improved.[70,71] (See Sec. 2 for side effects and Chs 12 and 14 for protracted venous infusion of chemotherapy and palliative care, respectively.)

Response to treatment

The focus of the assessment of the patient's response to chemotherapy differs for individual patients, and will depend on:[34,72]

- the expected aim of treatment, e.g. cure, control of the disease or symptom control
- the type of malignancies, i.e. solid tumours or haematological malignancies
- the individual patient's circumstances and health over time.

The clinician will determine whether the patient should receive further cycles of chemotherapy based on indices of response, which may be objective, such as size of tumour, or subjective, such as patient's symptoms and general health status (Table 8.1). The relative importance of these indices depends on the role of the chemotherapy. If the aim of treatment is

Table 8.1   Indices of response[34,72]

Type	Assessment process
Clinical	Signs – direct measurement of tumour, photographs, e.g. fungating tumours
	Symptoms – the patient's experience, e.g. breathlessness, cough, pain, appetite, weight, bowel actions
	Quality of life – designed to try to provide more objective data. Aspects that may be monitored include the social impact of the disease and treatment, e.g. work, relationships, infertility
Serological	Blood tests help to stage the disease, measure disease response or indicate complications of the disease or treatment and are checked with each chemotherapy cycle.
	For example:
	• full blood count, e.g. haematological malignancy, or if there is marrow involvement and complications of the treatment, e.g. neutropenia
	• liver function tests (LFTs), e.g. metastatic breast cancer
	• immunoglobulins, e.g. myeloma
	• tumour markers in different cancers, e.g. CA125 for ovary, PSA for prostate, CEA for colorectal, AFP, beta-hCG for teratoma, CA 19.9 for pancreas, CA 15.3 for breast and 5-HIAA for carcinoid
	A lowering in the level of the tumour marker suggests a response to treatment, whereas increasing levels suggests a relapse.
	In chronic B-cell leukaemia, the absence of systemic symptoms, lymphadenopathy, hepatosplenomegaly and a normal blood count indicates a complete response in relation to the standard response criteria[73]
Radiological	Radiological investigations help to stage the disease by:
	• identifying the site of disease
	• the size and extent of disease.
	Response may be measured by the tumour dimensions and complications identified during treatment:
	• plain X-rays, e.g. chest X-ray for lung cancer or lung metastases, mammograms for breast cancer, bone X-ray for bone tumours
	• ultrasound, e.g. primary breast tumours
	• CT scan, e.g. solid tumours
	• MRI scan, e.g. rectal cancer
	• bone scans – response may take months, so not very helpful
	• PET scan – may be helpful to demonstrate a response at an earlier stage than other methods and if any areas of abnormality remains on the CT scan or MRI scan and it is not clear whether the abnormality is active tumour or fibrous/scar tissue
	Radiological response is defined using the RECIST criteria (Table 8.5) for solid tumours[74]
Histological	A diagnosis of cancer is needed in all patients prior to treatment to determine the site of disease, the nature and subtype of malignancy and prognostic features, e.g. vascular invasion. Histological investigations helps in deciding the treatment options and is the most accurate indicator of response. The degree of response often correlates with prognosis; however, it is rarely practical. Examples of assessing histological response are bone marrow in haematological malignancy, after neoadjuvant chemotherapy in breast or rectal cancer or osteosarcoma
Survival data	Helpful in deciding the most appropriate treatment for an individual patient based upon population survival data

See also Medical sections of Section 3 and Chapter 14.

CA, cancer antigen; CEA, carcinoembryonic antigen; AFP, alpha fetoprotein; hCG, human chorionic gonadotrophin; 5-HIAA, 5-hydroxyindoleacetic acid; CT, computed tomography; MRI, magnetic resonance imaging; PET, positron emission tomography.

curative, then the blood tests and scans are a more important indicator of response than the patient's clinical symptoms. If the aim of treatment is palliative in nature, then improvement or deterioration in the patient's symptoms related to their cancer is a more important indicator of response than blood tests or scans.[34]

PRESCRIPTION, PREPARATION AND ADMINISTRATION OF CHEMOTHERAPY

There is an extensive range of chemotherapy protocols/regimens, the choice of which is dependent upon tumour type and patient fitness.[75,76] Local guidelines and protocols for chemotherapy will determine the accountability and responsibilities of different health-care professionals and all staff must:

- be familiar with the guidelines and protocol
- ensure that they are familiar with normal blood count values within the context of the protocol and that the blood count is checked prior to chemotherapy
- ensure any other relevant test results need to be checked – e.g. urea and electrolytes and renal function
- record the height and weight of the patient in order to determine the body surface area so that the dose of chemotherapy may be calculated.

The different roles and responsibilities of the medical staff who prescribe and the pharmacist and the nursing staff highlight the complexity of chemotherapy, and information as to the many different types of regimens helps to support the clinicians both as a reference and as an aid to learning.[76] Algorithms for the checking of prescriptions have been developed (Fig. 8.2) that clearly identify responsibilities of the doctor, nurse and pharmacist to ensure that the correct chemotherapy regimen is prescribed and administered safely.[77] (See also Chs 2 and 3.)

The role of the oncology pharmacy service

The role of the pharmacist and pharmacy technicians is essential in the delivery of chemotherapy services.[78] Their contribution to patient care is both clinical and technical in nature:[79,80]

- participation in the development of local guidelines and protocols, e.g. Hospital Drug & Therapeutics Committee and the local cancer network
- implementation of national guidelines and protocols
- preparation of protocols (proforma checklist) and development of electronic prescriptions
- preparation of chemotherapy drugs and work-sheets on how to prepare the drugs, including compatibility, labelling, expiry dates and storage conditions
- checking of the drugs to ensure the prescription complies with the protocol
- patient advice and support, e.g. nausea and vomiting, counselling, medicines information
- staff training and support
- provision of information to staff, e.g. Cytotoxic Drug Information Guide
- risk assessments.

Chemotherapy is prepared in cytotoxic reconstitution units designed for the safe preparation of sterile injectable cytotoxic drugs. Out of hours chemotherapy should only be reconstituted in certain circumstances, e.g. life-threatening oncological emergency. Chemotherapy should be transported in appropriately labelled containers and stored appropriately. Cytotoxic drugs are dispensed for individual patients and must be locked in medicine cupboards or designated refrigerators.[6,79,80]

The introduction of new therapies or newly approved drugs by NICE requires a systematic approach to address funding of these drugs and the reorganising of services, e.g. workload and communication between the primary and secondary setting.[81,82] For example, with the increase in oral chemotherapy, less time is spent on reconstituting intravenous chemotherapy and more time on the dispensing of the oral chemotherapy and the production of patient information leaflets and treatment diaries. Pharmacy services have had to reorganise their work practices in relation to education of primary care professionals and patients to minimise the risks of oral chemotherapy.[83] Nurse- or pharmacist-led clinics to monitor patients on oral chemotherapy have been developed.[82] Medicines information help lines are thought to be beneficial as, after discharge, patients may seek advice about their medicines; however, more research is required in this area.[84] (See Ch. 3.)

Chemotherapy administration

For safe administration, it is essential that the following steps occur:

- provision of information to the patient and checking of the patient's understanding about the treatment and its potential side effects or complications
- patient height and weight and calculation of the body surface area
- clarification of the patient's fitness for chemotherapy on the day of administration
- patient consent
- the chemotherapy prescription must be dated, legible and signed by a medical practitioner
- the prescription must be checked by the pharmacist to ensure that it is appropriate, including the supportive care measures such as hydration and antiemetics
- the chemotherapy drug(s) must be prepared and dispensed according to the chemotherapy preparation procedures
- the safe handling of the chemotherapy drug(s) during the preparation, their transportation and storage.

As with the administration of any medication, the nurse must be aware of normal dose ranges, routes of

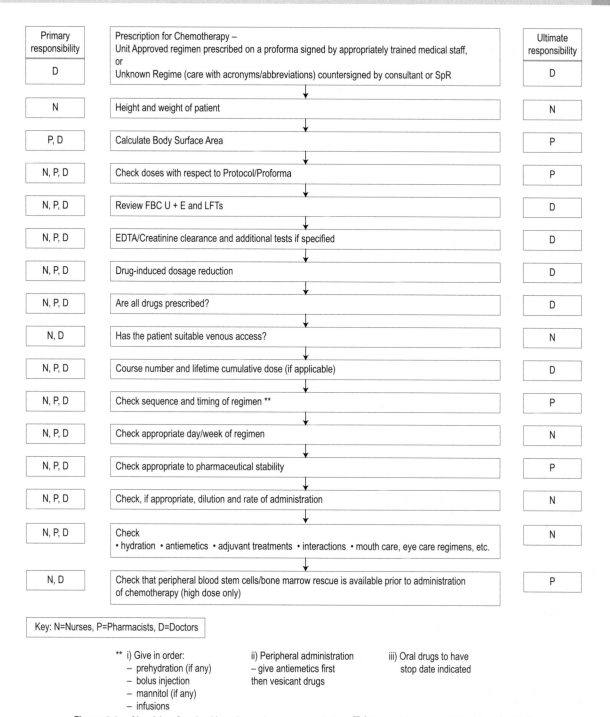

Primary responsibility	Prescription for Chemotherapy – Unit Approved regimen prescribed on a proforma signed by appropriately trained medical staff, or Unknown Regime (care with acronyms/abbreviations) countersigned by consultant or SpR	Ultimate responsibility
D		D
N	Height and weight of patient	N
P, D	Calculate Body Surface Area	P
N, P, D	Check doses with respect to Protocol/Proforma	P
N, P, D	Review FBC U + E and LFTs	D
N, P, D	EDTA/Creatinine clearance and additional tests if specified	D
N, P, D	Drug-induced dosage reduction	D
N, P, D	Are all drugs prescribed?	D
N, D	Has the patient suitable venous access?	N
N, P, D	Course number and lifetime cumulative dose (if applicable)	D
N, P, D	Check sequence and timing of regimen **	P
N, P, D	Check appropriate day/week of regimen	N
N, P, D	Check appropriate to pharmaceutical stability	P
N, P, D	Check, if appropriate, dilution and rate of administration	N
N, P, D	Check • hydration • antiemetics • adjuvant treatments • interactions • mouth care, eye care regimens, etc.	N
N, D	Check that peripheral blood stem cells/bone marrow rescue is available prior to administration of chemotherapy (high dose only)	P

Key: N=Nurses, P=Pharmacists, D=Doctors

** i) Give in order:
  – prehydration (if any)
  – bolus injection
  – mannitol (if any)
  – infusions

ii) Peripheral administration
  – give antiemetics first
  then vesicant drugs

iii) Oral drugs to have
  stop date indicated

Figure 8.2   Algorithm for checking chemotherapy prescriptions.[77] (Adapted from Royal Marsden Hospital).

administration, side effects of chemotherapy and an understanding of contraindications prior to its administration.[85] Knowledge and understanding of how to manage complications or adverse events following administration of chemotherapy, e.g. extravasation of vesicant chemotherapy drugs and anaphylaxis, is essential.[86,87]

Designated wards with the necessary equipment in which chemotherapy may be administered by appropriately trained nurses are crucial for patient safety. Equipment should include resuscitation equipment, drugs for the management of emergencies, extravasation kit, spillage kit, eyewash/access to running water, emergency bell and waste disposal equipment. Any medical device, e.g. infusion pumps, should be checked and maintained according to the agreed specifications and used by staff that have been trained to use the equipment.[6,87]

There are two routes of administration (Table 8.2):

- systemic – aims to destroy the primary malignancy site and distant metastases
- regional – delivers the cytotoxic drug in high concentrations to the disease area whilst minimising systemic concentrations and thus side effects.

The route of chemotherapy administration will depend on:

- the tumour type
- the cytotoxic drug
- bioavailability
- the condition of the patient's venous access
- the patient's age, health status and wishes.

There is specific literature available and online resources to support learning more about both individual chemotherapy drugs and factors to take into consideration when prescribing, preparing, checking or administering a chemotherapy drug or protocol/regimen.[75,76,79,80,88–92] For this reason, this section will provide an introduction only to routes of administration and summarise factors for special consideration. For specific information as to the procedures to follow

for administration of cytotoxic drugs see References 87 (pp 228–256) and 93. (See also Chs 10, 12 and 14.)

Oral route

Oral chemotherapy is increasing and may be taken by the patient at home, e.g. capecitabine.[14] There are several oral anticancer therapies commercially available. Capecitabine was one of the first to impact on changing the patient pathway and experience.[81,82,94]

Subcutaneous or intramuscular

Very few cytotoxic drugs are administered via this route. It may be used in the community for maintenance therapy. Platelet count should be above $50 \times 10^9/L$ prior to administration.

Intravenous

The majority of chemotherapy drugs are given via the intravenous route. (See also Ch. 10.)

Intra-arterial

Very few cytotoxic drugs are administered via this route.

Intrapleural

Any pleural effusion should be drained to dryness before administering chemotherapy. The chemotherapy drug is usually instilled via a chest drain by the doctor. The patient is asked to rotate on each side, back and front, to distribute the drug throughout the chest. The patient may require analgesia for the procedure.

Intrathecal/intraventricular

Administration is by medical staff with specific training, and drugs are prescribed, prepared and administered according to national and local guidelines. Specific national guidance has been issued in relation to intrathecal chemotherapy in order to avoid life-threatening consequences if the wrong drug is administered via the intrathecal route. An intrathecal register is held of the staff (doctors, pharmacist and nurses) who are competent to be involved with intrathecal chemotherapy.[95]

Intravesical

The patient is catheterised and their bladder emptied prior to the instillation of the drug. After instillation, the catheter is withdrawn unless there is a reason for the catheter to remain in situ. Dependent on the drug, the patient is asked to hold the drug in their bladder for 1 hour prior to passing urine. The patient should be advised about increasing their fluid for a 24-hour period and that their urine may be cloudy. They

Table 8.2 Routes of chemotherapy administration[87]	
Systemic route	Regional route
Oral	Intra-arterial
Subcutaneous	Intrapleural
Intramuscular	Intrathecal/Intraventricular
Intravenous	Intravesical
	Intraperitoneal
	Topical

should be advised to report immediately to the hospital or community staff, e.g. district nurse or general practitioner, if they suffer from any discomfort or inability to pass urine.

Intraperitoneal

Ascites should be drained to dryness before administering chemotherapy. The chemotherapy injection or infusion should be warmed to body temperature prior to instillation via an ascitic drain. After slowly injecting the drug or instilling the drug as prescribed, the ascitic drain is clamped and left in situ for 1–3 hours. The ascitic drain is then unclamped and removed after drainage is complete. Accurate recording of fluid balance should be made during the procedure. The patient may require analgesia for the procedure.

Hyperthermic intraoperative intraperitoneal chemotherapy may be given for the rare condition pseudomyxoma peritonei if the tumour has features of mucinous adenocarcinoma.[96]

Topical

Topical cytotoxic therapy is only suitable for superficial skin lesions and is usually applied daily or twice daily.

Documentation

Effective documentation of care is essential for patient safety, continuity of care, good communication and quality care (Fig. 8.3).[6,44,50,51,79,80,97–99]

Key aspects of documentation in the patient pathway include:

- the decisions taken at the multidisciplinary team meeting
- treatment plan and aim, i.e. curative, adjuvant, neoadjuvant, palliative
- patient consent, including information given
- patient assessment and any risk factors identified
- investigations to be performed prior to starting course of chemotherapy and those to be performed prior to each cycle of chemotherapy

- prescription, supply and administration of chemotherapy, including supportive drugs and route of administration
- location and condition of administration access site, including the type and size
- adverse events, e.g. extravasation, errors and spillage
- response to treatment and toxicity assessment, including any dose modifications and whether these are permanent in nature
- whether the course of treatment was completed, and if not, the reasons and the doses administered
- symptom management
- patient education and support, including emergency numbers and contact details as to who to contact for complications of chemotherapy, e.g. infection
- supportive care, including community care
- discharge plan and follow-up.

Document control of any preprepared documents used to support treatment decision-making and care are essential to ensure that the most up-to-date document is referred to in practice by clinical staff, e.g. National Guidance and local policies and procedures.[79]

The analysis of mistakes in a fair blame culture encourages positive system change, recognising the complexity of the decision-making by different professionals in the administration of chemotherapy.[100] (See also Consent section above; Chs 12 and 14 for protracted venous infusion of chemotherapy palliative care, respectively; Sec. 3, Medical sections; and Chs 6 and 9 for ethical issues and clinical trials, respectively.)

PRIMARY AND SECONDARY CARE – TRANSFER OF CARE

Collaboration between hospital and community services (health and social care) must be an integral part of cancer services,[2] especially as the patient spends the majority of their time at home when undergoing cancer treatments.[4] Specific patient groups have been recognised as requiring specific support, e.g. the elderly patient who lives alone with a poor prognosis[101] (Box 8.3).

Healthcare, social care services, the independent sector and voluntary agencies should work together. Inadequate communication networks and a lack of interpersonal cooperation between hospital and community have been identified as contributing to problems with discharge.[101] Careful liaison (Table 8.3) between the primary and secondary care setting to

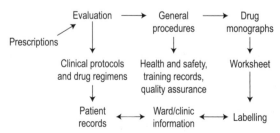

Figure 8.3   Documentation required for cytotoxic services.[100]

Box 8.3   Patients with particular care needs in the community

- Live alone
- Are frail and/or elderly
- Have care needs which place a high demand on carers and carers find difficulty coping
- Have a limited prognosis
- Have a serious illness, and who may be returning to hospital for further treatments
- Have a continuing disability
- Have learning difficulties
- Have mental illness or dementia
- Have dependants
- Have limited financial resources
- Are homeless or living in poor housing
- Do not have English as their first language
- Require aids/equipment at home
- Have been in hospital for an 'extended stay'

Source: Adapted from Department of Health.[114]

ensure patient support along the patient pathway is crucial,[113,114] especially as more patients are undergoing chemotherapy at home by NHS or private healthcare services.[16,81,82,102–106] It has been suggested that the role of the district nurse in relation to a patient who has had a cancer-related hospital admission is often unclear and that further service development and evaluation should be undertaken.[107] In a small study,

Table 8.3   Roles and responsibilities in discharge planning

Hospital staff	Community staff
Needs assessment of patient and carer	Community assessment
Appropriate referrals	A clear picture of the home situation
Interdisciplinary collaboration	How a patient looks/feels/manages
Flow of information	Provide holistic care – physical, social and psychological:
Patient and carer education	1. care of vascular access device
Documentation – patient and carer and community teams	2. recognising and managing side effects and complications of treatment
	Interdisciplinary collaboration

district nurses felt that they did have a role in the care of people receiving palliative chemotherapy and felt that they should be involved at an early stage in the patient's care; however, the need for more education about chemotherapy and the patient's care plan was highlighted.[108]

Discharge planning

Effective, safe discharge planning should be patient/carer-focused.[101] Discharge from hospital can be a major life event for both patient and carer and good-quality discharge should not be a matter of chance.[109] The patient should receive support during treatment and active involvement of patients and carers is central to successful discharge planning. Discharge planning is the process of identifying the patient's needs and developing a plan of care for a patient who is transferred from one environment to another. Discharge planning should commence on the initial contact with patients.[101] Consideration of the patient's prognosis and circumstances will also be a part of the decision-making process. If the patient has an estimated prognosis of less than 3 months or he has a complex, unpredictable, rapidly deteriorating or unstable medical condition, then the patient is eligible for continuing NHS healthcare.[101,110]

Common questions from the patient's perspective[101] that should be addressed include (see p. 39):

- What do they think is wrong with me?
- If I need help how much will it cost and how will I get it?
- How would it help me?
- I haven't got room for that equipment – do I need to have it and how will I use it?
- How can I use my bathroom if it's upstairs?
- How can I do my shopping?
- Can I get transport to go there?
- What are the risks and benefits of the alternatives?
- How long will I have to stay in hospital?
- Can I drive/work/look after my family afterwards?
- Maybe I would like to talk it over with my family before I decide?

It should be recognised that the patient needs and coping styles may differ from their family[111,112] and, if appropriate, a carer's assessment (Box 8.4) should be made.[101]

Information about discharge arrangements should be disseminated between professionals and patients/carers, with the latter being provided with written information of ongoing care.[101,114]

Box 8.4 Carer's need assessment (see p. 44)[101]

- Care-giving tasks
- How to get help and advice
- Information about care workers
- Information about mental illness
- Involvement in planning of treatment and care
- Support for carers
- Relationships with the person you care for
- Family and friends
- Money
- Your well-being
- Stigma and discrimination
- Risk and safety
- Choice of care
- Other issues

Home chemotherapy

It may be necessary to set up chemotherapy services at home and mechanisms to ensure safe practice should be developed. Due to the complexity and small number of studies into the costs, patient preferences and outcomes, the role of home chemotherapy is unclear.[94,113,115,116] For certain groups of patients, e.g. the elderly or the patient who is psychologically distressed, home chemotherapy may be an appropriate option and would enable patients to receive their care at home.[113] It has been suggested that patients are more satisfied with their care and have an increased compliance with treatment at home.[113,116] In a small study of community nurses' attitudes and concerns about home chemotherapy, the need for appropriate policies and procedures to be in place was highlighted. The district nurses held differing views as to their role: some felt the role was more technical in nature, e.g. changing and flushing of infusion lines, whereas others felt the role involved ongoing patient assessment, managing and reporting adverse events, contributing to the management of side effects and providing patient support. The provision of education to support the changing role of the district nurses and the availability of resources to support this change in practice were also highlighted.[117]

Careful assessment of the patient's condition and home circumstances is necessary to ensure:[116,117]

- patient and nurse safety
- safe transportation of cytotoxic drugs
- procedures to manage emergency situations are in place, e.g. extravasation, anaphylaxis, cardiac/respiratory arrest and spillage of cytotoxic drugs

- arrangements with pharmacy services and the accessing/checking of drugs are agreed
- safe administration of cytotoxics at home by staff trained in chemotherapy administration
- relevant contact numbers for patient and family
- follow-up care arrangements are made.

Follow-up care

Follow-up care will be dependent on the type of cancer and the patient's specific treatment plan. Research into the most effective type of follow-up care for cancer patients and whether it makes a difference to the patient's quality of life or survival is of a greater priority in recent years.[118-123] Follow-up care that incorporates alleviating symptoms and psychosocial support may be more appropriate for some cancers, e.g. lung cancer, than a follow-up model which is focused upon the detection of recurrence and disease progression.[124,125] The reorganisation of services and research into the effectiveness of nurse-led clinics, including follow-up and the type of follow-up that is most appropriate for the patient, are areas for ongoing research.[125-128] In addition, research into the issues of cancer survivorship and the long-term effects of chemotherapy are being addressed more proactively in cancer care.[129,130]

ORGANISATION OF CHEMOTHERAPY SERVICES

Chemotherapy services involve access to specialised multidisciplinary teams with an oncologist or a haematologist with specialised training in haematological oncology. In England and Wales, chemotherapy services are organised in the cancer unit or cancer centre within a cancer network. The cancer unit will treat patients with the commoner cancers – breast, lung and colorectal – and the cancer centre will treat patients with less common cancers, and high-dose, experimental and complex chemotherapy. In a cancer unit, patients receive chemotherapy in one of three types of chemotherapy services, which are organised according to the type of cancer and the level of service available (Table 8.4).[131] By determining the patient pathway for patients receiving chemotherapy, standardisation, consistency of care and service improvements will be facilitated.[6,11,13,137,138]

Staff training and competence

Patients should receive their chemotherapy treatment and care by specialist staff (doctors, pharmacists and nurses) who have received specific competency-based

Table 8.4 Types of chemotherapy services in district general hospitals[131]

Cancer unit	Type I	Type II	Type III
Non-surgical specialist cancer services	Consultation service with outpatient chemotherapy and inpatient services. First-line treatment for common cancers, particularly adjuvant chemotherapy for breast and colorectal cancers	Consultation service with outpatient chemotherapy	Consultation service only
Population	Large catchment population	Large catchment population	Small catchment population
Travel time to cancer centre	Long travel time	Short travel time	Short travel time
Site-specific and general oncology clinics	+	+	+
Multidisciplinary team	+	+	+
Outpatient chemotherapy	+	+	–
Specialised chemotherapy nurses (trained in the rationale and use of chemotherapy and in the administration of intravenous chemotherapy)	+	+	–
Pharmacy for cytotoxic drug preparation	+	–	–
Chemotherapy ward	+	–	–
24-hour on-site oncology cover	+	–	–
Patient self-referral for complications of treatment and for prompt treatment of oncological emergencies	+	+	–
Psychosocial support and palliative care	+	+	+

training about chemotherapy practice.[2–6,95] Many cancer centres/units have recognised the role of specialised nurses or intravenous therapy teams in chemotherapy delivery. An improvement in patient outcome has been noted when specialised nursing services perform a venous access assessment at the beginning of chemotherapy treatment.[86,93] Guidelines for safe practice include venepuncture, peripheral venous cannulation, insertion of central venous catheters and chemotherapy.[86] Nurses should be satisfied that they have the necessary knowledge to administer the chemotherapy safely. Nurses should also be able to know what actions to take in the event of an extravasation and anaphylaxis. The safe administration of cytotoxic chemotherapy depends upon strict adherence to guidelines and ongoing education and development in cancer care.[86,132–134] (See Chs 10 and 13 for intravenous management and infection control, respectively; Ch. 15 for anaphylaxis; and Ch. 4 for quality assurance.)

Standards of care

The performance of chemotherapy services (Box 8.5) are assessed as part of the cancer services standards[5,6] and waiting times for start of treatment are being monitored.[4,135] The patient's experience of care and the systems of care to achieve clinical effectiveness and risk management is integral to the clinical governance.[136]

In the UK there are several national guidelines which are related to chemotherapy practice:

- Clinical Practice Guidelines: The Administration of Cytotoxic Chemotherapy[132]
- Chemotherapy Guidelines Clinical Oncology[35]
- Standards for infusion therapy[86]

- NeLH Cancer Guidelines[13]
- NICE Technology Appraisals Approved Cancer Drugs[14]
- Manual of Cancer Services Standards[5,6]
- National Guidance on the Safe Administration of Intrathecal Chemotherapy[95]

By auditing and monitoring practice against the standards which are evidence based, clinicians are able to develop ways of improving practice.[136–142] It is recognised when implementing guidelines and standards that clinicians must use their clinical judgement when applying to the individual patient and that there should be ongoing review of practice. The importance of individualised care is integral to holistic care; however, standards enable practice to be reviewed.[136] Changing roles and reorganisation of services in order to meet the patient's needs has been demonstrated in practice, although this may be challenging and require considerable consultation.[143,144] Changes in the delivery of chemotherapy, e.g. oral chemotherapy, has necessitated the development of nurse-led services,[82] or changes in the delivery of the service.[145–148] Different indicators and processes of care have been reviewed, e.g. waiting times, patient satisfaction and support, and the role of self-care activities and managing side effects following education.[71,140,145,148–151]

Prompt reporting of problems will facilitate patient safety, comfort and support.[136] The provision of the 'Chemotherapy Toolkit' to facilitate service improvements across cancer networks by the Cancer Services Collaborative has enabled improvements to the delivery of chemotherapy services and improvements to multidisciplinary working.[4,10,11,152] (See also Chs 3 and 4.)

The treatment protocols should be evidence-based. For certain cancers, specific guidance on clinical outcomes based on the evidence has been developed, clarifying the role of chemotherapy as part of the treatment plan.[4] There are several chemotherapy drugs which have now been approved for their clinical effectiveness and cost-effectiveness.[13,14] The different tumour groups have ongoing evidence-based guidance (Improving Outcomes Guidance – IOG)[4] with the expectation that:

- patient experience and outcomes will be improved
- services with specialist multidisciplinary teams will be established
- peer review assessment of services against measurable national standards will occur to enable quality improvement and team working.

(See also Ch. 2.)

The reorganisation of chemotherapy services is ongoing for a number of reasons:[5–7,13,14]

- advances to chemotherapy treatment occur, e.g. new drugs, oral chemotherapy
- new guidelines and protocols are implemented, e.g. NICE Guidelines, intrathecal chemotherapy, staff education and training
- changes to service delivery, e.g. day care or outpatient chemotherapy, home chemotherapy
- changes to staff roles, e.g. nurse-led care, medicines information help lines
- national cancer datasets to ensure consistency of information collection.

The audit of services, local organisational guidelines and national standards are recommended in addition to national monitoring of standards and waiting times for treatment.[5–7,13,14] Benchmarking of cancer services in the 1990s highlighted that chemotherapy day case episodes increased considerably and it was recommended that activity and outcomes of treatment should be undertaken in a systematic fashion.[153] There has been a rapid expansion of chemotherapy services and a review of services nationally is underway to:[4]

- benchmark chemotherapy services
- explore the future capacity and demand, including the anticipated ratio of intravenous and oral chemotherapy administration

- provide a competency framework for staff involved in chemotherapy delivery
- revise national standards on chemotherapy.

(See also Chs 3 and 4.)

Health outcomes and financial management

Improved information about chemotherapy treatment and its outcomes is seen as essential to the decision-making process for allocation of resources and planning of services.[4] Healthcare Resource Groups (HRGs) is the way in which activity data is collected in the same way and then analysed to establish how resources are used and the planning of services and to evaluate performance. Chemotherapy HRGs capture the cost of the prescribed chemotherapy drugs and associated drugs, e.g. anti-emetic drugs. The cost of hotel, nursing and general ward costs are allocated in the inpatient and day case HRGs. Outpatient chemotherapy will be allocated as a separate entry in outpatient nursing.[154]

The initial costing of chemotherapy treatment, i.e. (HRGs), has been undertaken in relation to solid tumours and this is to facilitate the financial management of care in England.[154] Further costing of HRGs for haematological cancer is planned for 2003/2004.[15] The linking of HRGs to a specific patient group who have similar interventions and expected outcomes has started in breast cancer in the context of Health Benefit Groups (HBGs).[155] A 'Healthcare Framework' (Fig. 8.4) has been developed to look at the overall outcomes of treatment and care for the population, to facilitate the decision-making for future service developments and patient management.[156]

The need for more information to determine future financial management is highlighted by a population-based assessment of hospitalisations for toxicity from chemotherapy in the United States. In this population-based assessment the rates of hospitalisation were greater from standard treatments than that found in clinical trials.[157] Population data of this kind are not available in the United Kingdom at this time; however, with the data collated from the cancer networks and the cancer information services, data should be more readily available to make these comparisons, i.e. cost of chemotherapy treatment and the management of chemotherapy toxicity.[158]

CONCLUSION

The management of the patient receiving chemotherapy requires coordination of services and multiprofessional teams working together to meet the needs of the patient. The increasing demand for chemotherapy and changing approaches to treatment require that organisations across the cancer network must continue to evolve, taking into account any national guidelines/protocols.

Chemotherapy may be just one aspect of the patient's care pathway, and the importance of supportive care with effective transfer of care between primary and secondary care should be considered with specific reference to the key aims of the NHS Cancer Plan:[4]

- assessment and early diagnosis
- improving communication between primary and secondary care
- improving patient experience at all stages in the care pathway
- palliative care.

The challenge to continue to improve the patient's experience is essential and ongoing, and future

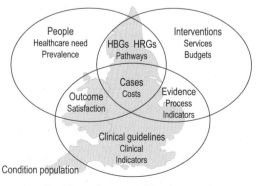

Figure 8.4 Healthcare Framework.[156]

Table 8.5 Criteria of radiological response

Criteria	Description
CR (complete response)	Disappearance of all target lesions
PR (partial response)	At least 30% decrease in the sum of the longest diameter of target lesions
PD (progressive disease)	At least 20% increase in the sum of the longest diameter of target lesions, or the appearance of new lesions
SD (stable disease)	Neither sufficient shrinkage for partial response nor sufficient increase for progressive disease

developments depend on:[4,43,159]

- identifying patient outcomes and the efficacy of chemotherapy treatment for different types of cancer
- the patient's quality of life
- enabling the patient and family to access appropriate supportive care
- the organisation of cancer services and the ongoing monitoring of performance standards
- staff training and education to provide specialist services
- research and development.

RECIST CRITERIA

RECIST stands for **R**esponse **E**valuation **C**riteria in **S**olid **T**umours[74] and are criteria of radiological response. For the target lesion, i.e. all measurable lesions up to a maximum of 5% of the organ, and 10 in total, representative of all involved organs, the longest diameter is measured. The sum of the longest diameter of target lesions is calculated. The presence or absence of non-target lesions (non-measurable disease) is noted throughout treatment (Table 8.5).

References

1. Royal College of Physicians. The Cancer Patient's Physician: recommendations for the development of medical oncology in England and Wales. London: RCP; 2000 http://www.rcplondon.ac.uk/pubs/brochures/pub_print_cpp.htm Accessed online 3 Feb 2004

2. Calman KD, Hine D. A Policy Framework for Commissioning Cancer Services: A Report by the Expert Advisory Group on Cancer to the Chief Medical Officers of England and Wales. London: DoH; 1995. http://www.dh.gov.uk/PublicationsAndStatistics/Publications/PublicationsPolicyAndGuidance/PublicationsPolicyAndGuidanceArticle/fs/en?CONTENT_ID=4071083&chk=%2Bo6fka Accessed online 3 Feb 2004

3. Department of Health. The NHS Cancer Plan: a plan for investment, a plan for reform. London: DoH; 2000 http://www.dh.gov.uk/PublicationsAndStatistics/Publications/PublicationsPolicyAndGuidance/PublicationsPolicyAndGuidanceArticle/fs/en?CONTENT_ID=4009609&chk=n4LXTU Accessed online 3 Feb 2004

4. The NHS Cancer Plan Progress Report. The NHS Cancer Plan three year progress report maintaining the momentum. London: DoH; 2003. http://www.dh.gov.uk/PublicationsAndStatistics/Publications/AnnualReports/DHAnnualReportsArticle/fs/en?CONTENT_ID=4064827&chk=3ReuSO Accessed online Dec 2003

5. NHS Executive. Manual of Cancer Services Assessment Standards. London: DoH; 2000. http://www.dh.gov.uk/PublicationsAndStatistics/Publications/PublicationsPolicyAndGuidance/PublicationsPolicyAndGuidanceArticle/fs/en?CONTENT_ID=4002999&chk=/BiOBs Accessed online 3 Feb 2004

6. Department of Heath. Manual for Cancer Services 2004. London: DOH; 2004. http://www.dh.gov.uk/PolicyAndGuidance/HealthAndSocialCareTopics/Cancer/fs/en Accessed online July 2004

7. Commission for Health Improvements. National Service Framework Assessments No. 1 NHS Cancer Care in England and Wales. London: CHI; 2001 http://www.chi.nhs.uk/cancer/index.htm Accessed online 3.Feb 2004

8. Cassidy J, Bissett D, Spence RAJ. Oxford handbook of oncology. Oxford: Oxford University Press; 2002:240–258.

9. NHS Modernisation Agency. Cancer Services Collaborative Improvement Partnership Improving Communication in Cancer Care, 2003. http://www.modern.nhs.uk/cancer/5629/Improving%20Communications%20booklet.pdf Accessed online July 2004

10. NHS Modernisation Agency. Cancer Services Collaborative Toolkit – Service Improvement Guide. London: Hayward Medical Communications; 2001. http://www.ebc-indevelopment.co.uk/nhs/chemotherapy/index.html

11. NHS Modernisation Agency. Chemotherapy Toolkit. London: Hayward Medical Communications; 2002. http://www.modern.nhs.uk/cancer/5628/5732/Chemotherapy%20-%202003.doc

12. Lane C, Kelly V, Clarke D. Cancer networks: translating policy into practice. In: Clarke D, Flanagan J, Kendrick K, eds. Advancing nursing practice in cancer and palliative care. Basingstoke: Palgrave Macmillan; 2002:238–254.

13. National electronic Library for Health National Service Frameworks (NSF) Zones – Cancer – a directory of resources Guidelines and Care Pathways Online. Available: http://www.nelh.nhs.uk/nsf/cancer/guidelines.htm 3 Nov 2003.

14. NICE Technology Appraisals Approved Cancer Drugs Online. Available: http://www.nice.org.uk/catta1.asp?c=153O 3 Nov 2003.

15. Skeel RT (ed.). Selection of treatment for the patient with cancer. In: Handbook of cancer chemotherapy. 6th edn. Philadelphia: Lippincott, Williams & Wilkins; 2003:46–50.

16. Steele S. A team approach to palliative chemotherapy Cancer Nurs Pract 2002; 1(2):22–26.

17. Webb C, Wood M. Communication and assessment. In: Lister S, Dougherty L, eds. The Royal Marsden Hospital of clinical nursing procedures. 6th edn. Oxford: Blackwell; 2004:16–42.

18. Fallowfield L. Participation of patients in decisions about treatment for cancer. Br Med J 2001; 32:1144.

19. Sainio C, Lauri S. Cancer patients' decision-making regarding treatment and nursing care. J Adv Nurs 2003; 41(3):250–260.

20. Say R, Thomson R. The importance of patient preferences in treatment decisions – challenges for doctors. Br Med J 2003; 327:542–545.

21. O'Connor AM, Mulley AG Jr, Wennberg JE. Standard consultations are not enough to ensure decision quality regarding preference-sensitive options. J Natl Cancer Inst 2003; 95(8):570–571.

22. Thome B, Dykes AK, Gunnars B, et al. The experiences of older people living with cancer. Cancer Nurs 2003; 26(2):85–96.

23. McCaughan E, Thompson KA. Information needs of cancer patients receiving chemotherapy at a day case unit in Northern Ireland J Clin Nurs 2000; 9(6):851–858.

24. The 'Patient Experience Quick Guide'. NHS Modernisation Agency available: http://www.modern.nhs.uk/cancer 3 Feb 2004.

25. Department of Health. Reference guide to consent for examination or treatment. London: DoH; 2001. http://www.dh.gov.uk/PublicationsAndStatistics/Publications/PublicationsPolicyAndGuidance/PublicationsPolicyAndGuidanceArticle/fs/en?CONTENT_ID=4006757&chk=snmdw8 Accessed online 3 Feb 2004

26. Ferns H. Campto effective and flexible chemotherapy for advanced colorectal cancer. Int J Palliat Nurs 2003; 9(7):290–297.

27. Lister S, Rees E. Context of care. In: Lister S, Dougherty L, eds. The Royal Marsden Hospital of clinical nursing procedures. 6th edn. Oxford: Blackwell; 2004:1–15.

28. General Medical Council. Seeking patients' consent. The ethical considerations. London: GMC; 1998.

29. Nursing and Midwifery Council. Code of Professional Conduct. London: NMC;2002.http://www.nmc-uk.org/nmc/main/publications/codeOfProfessionalConduct.pdf Accessed online 3 Feb 2004

30. Griffin-Brown J. Diagnostic evaluation, classifications & staging. In: Yarbro CH, Goodman M, Frogge MH, et al, eds. Cancer nursing principles and practice. 5th edn. Boston: Jones & Bartlett; 2000:214–239.

31. Daugherty CK. Impact of therapeutic research in informed consent and the ethics of clinical trials: a medical oncology perspective. J Clin Oncol 1999; 17(5):1601–1617.

32. Ocker BM, Pawlik Plank DM. The research nurse role in a clinic-based oncology research setting. Cancer Nurs 2000; 23(4):286–294.

33. World Medical Association. Declaration of Helsinki: ethical principles for medical research involving human subjects. WMA General Assembly Washington: WMA; 2002. http://www.wma.net/e/ethicsunit/helsinki.htm. Accessed online 3 Feb 2004

34. Skeel RT (ed.). Systematic assessment of the patient with cancer and long-term complications of treatment. In: Handbook of cancer chemotherapy. 6th edn. Philadelphia: Lippincott, Williams & Wilkins; 2003:26–45.

35. Royal College of Radiologists. Chemotherapy (Guidelines). Clin Oncol 2001; 13:S215. Available online from: http://www.rcr.ac.uk/upload/ChemotherapyGuideline2001.pdf

36. Otto SE (ed.). Chemotherapy. In: Oncology nursing. 4th edn. St Louis: Mosby; 2001:638–683.

37. Boyle DA. Cancer in the elderly: key facts. Oncol Support Care Quart 2003; 2(1):6–21.

38. Miller M, Kearney N, Smith K. Measurement of cancer attitudes: a review. Eur J Oncol Nurs 2000; 4(4):233–245.

39. Purandare L. Attitudes to cancer may create a barrier to communication between the patient and caregiver. Eur J Cancer Care 1997; 6(2):92–99.

40. Passik SD, Kirsh KL, Rosenfield B, et al. The changeable nature of patients' fears regarding chemotherapy: implications for palliative care. J Pain Sympt Manage 2001; 21 (2):113–120.

41. MacDonald BH. Quality of life in cancer care: patient's experiences and nurses' contribution. Eur J Oncol Nurs 2001; 5(1):32–41.

42. Barsevick AM, Much J, Sweeney C. Psychosocial responses to cancer management. In: Yarbro CH, Goodman M, Frogge MH, et al, eds Cancer nursing principles and practice. 5th edn. Boston: Jones & Bartlett; 2000:1529–1549.

43. NICE. Guidance on cancer services: improving supportive and palliative care for adults with cancer. 2004. http://www.nice.org.uk

44. Brown V, Sitzia J, Richardson A, et al. The development of the Chemotherapy Symptom Assessment Scale (C-SAS): a scale for the routine clinical assessment of the symptom experiences of patients receiving cytotoxic chemotherapy. Int J Nurs Stud 2001; 38(5):497–510.

45. Anderson H, Espinosa E, Lofts F, et al. Evaluation of the chemotherapy patient monitor: an interactive tool for facilitating communication between patients and oncologists during the cancer consultation. Eur J Cancer Care 2001; 10(2):115–123.

46. Langhorne M, Barton-Burke M. Chemotherapy administration: general principles for nursing practice. In: Barton-Burke M, Wilkes GM, Ingwersen KC, eds. Cancer chemotherapy a nursing process approach. 3rd edn. Boston: Jones & Bartlett; 2001:608–644.

47. Price CIM, Han SW, Rutherford IA. Advanced nursing practice: an introduction to physical assessment. Br J Nurs 2000; 9(22):2292–2296.

48. Pickett RR. Outpatient Oncology Chemotherapy Documentation Tool. Oncol Nurs Forum 1992; 19(3):515–517.

49. Weiss Behrend S. Documentation in the ambulatory setting. Semin Oncol Nurs 1994; 10(4):264–280.

50. Senior Smith G, Richardson A. Development of nursing documentation for use in the outpatient setting. Eur J Cancer Care 1996; 5:225–232.

51. Dikken C. Benefits of using a chemotherapy symptom assessment scale. Nurs Times 2003; 99(39):50–51.

52. Kelly DF, Faught WJ, Holmes LA. Ovarian cancer treatment: the benefit of patient telephone follow-up post-chemotherapy. Can Oncol Nurs J 1999; 9(4)175–178.

53. Tanghe A, Evers G, Paridaens R. Nurses' assessments of symptom occurrence and symptom distress in chemotherapy. Eur J Oncol Nurs 1998; 2(1):14–26.

54. Parsaie FA, Golchin M, Asvadi I. A comparison of nurse and patient perceptions of chemotherapy treatment stressors. Cancer Nurs 2000; 23(5):371–374.

55. Hirshfield-Bartek J, Hassey Dow K, Creaton E. Decreasing documentation time using a patient self-assessment tool. Oncol Nurs Forum 1990; 17(2):251–255.

56. Dennison S. An exploration of the communication that takes place between nurses and patients whilst cancer chemotherapy is administered. J Clin Nurs 1995; 4(4):227–233.

57. Uitterhoeve R, Duijnhouwer E, Ambaum B, et al. Turing toward the psychosocial domain of oncology nursing: a main problem analysis in the Netherlands. Cancer Nurs 2003; 26(1):18–27.

58. Dennison S, Shute T. Identifying patient concerns: improving the quality of patient visits to the oncology out-patient department – a pilot audit. Eur J Oncol Nurs 2000; 4(2):91–98.

59. Anastasia PJ, Blevins MC. Outpatient chemotherapy: telephone triage for symptom management. Oncol Nurs Forum 1997; 24(1):13–22.

60. Korcz IR, Moreland S. Telephone prescreening. Cancer Pract 1998; 6(5):270–275.

61. Chobanuk J, Pituskin E, Kashuba L, et al. Telephone triage in acute oncology. Can Nurse 1999; 95(1):30–32.

62. Wilson R, Hubert J. Resurfacing the care in nursing by telephone: lesson from ambulatory oncology. Nurs Outlook 2002; 50(4):160–164.

63. Twomey C. Telephone contacts with a cancer nurse specialist. Nurs Stand 2000; 15(3):35–38.

64. Lecouterier J, Crack L, Mannix K, et al. Evaluation of patient-held record for patients with cancer. Eur J Cancer Care 2002; 11:114–121.

65. The 'Patient-held Records Toolkit'. NHS Modernisation Agency. Available: http://www.modern.nhs.uk/cancer 3 Feb 2004.

66. Sharp L, Laurell G, Tiblom Y, et al. Care diaries. Cancer Nurs 2004; 27(2):119–126.

67. Richardson A. Cancer care. Improving supportive and palliative care for adults with cancer. Nurs Times 2003; 99(39):49.

68. Izod D. Personal experience. A patients' perspective. Complement Ther Nurs Midwifery 1996; 2(3):66–67.

69. Camp-Sorrell D. Chemotherapy: toxicity management. In: Yarbro CH, Frogge MH, Goodman M, et al. Cancer nursing principles and practice. 5th edn. Boston: Jones & Bartlett; 2000:444–486.

70. Murphy-Ende K, Chernecky C. Assessing adults with leukemia. Nurse Pract 2002; 27(11):49–60.

71. Coleman EA, Coon SK, Mattox SG, et al. Symptom management and successful outpatient transplantation for patients with multiple myeloma. Cancer Nurs 2002; 25(6):452–460.

72. Holmes S (ed.). Chemotherapy as a treatment for cancer. In: Cancer chemotherapy: a guide for practice. 2nd edn. Dorking: Asset Books; 1997:62–76.

73. Roberts BE. Peripheral N-cell lymphoproliferative disorders in lymph nodes, spleen, blood and bone marrow. In: Child JA, Jack AS, Morgan GJ, eds. The lymphoproliferative disorders. London: Chapman & Hall Medical; 1998:183–283.

74. Therasse P, Arbuck SG, Eisenhauer EA, et al. New guidelines to evaluate the response to treatment in solid tumours. J Natl Cancer Inst 2000; 92(3):205–216.

75. Dearnley D, Judson I, Root T. Handbook of adult cancer chemotherapy schedules. Oxon: TMG Healthcare Communications; 2002.

76. Summerhayes M, Daniels S. Practical chemotherapy. Abingdon: Radcliffe Medical Press; 2003.

77. DTAC Guidelines. Drug & Therapeutics Advisory Committee Prescribing Guidelines, August 2004. London: Royal Marsden Hospital; 2004:143–144.

78. The British Oncology Pharmacy Association. The NHS Cancer Plan and the pharmacy contribution to cancer care. http://www.bopa-web.org/Publications/OncologyPharmacy.pdf Accessed online July 2004

79. Allwood M, Stanley A Wright P (eds). The cytotoxic handbook. 4th edn. Abingdon: Radcliffe Medical Press; 2002.

80. Marc Guidelines. Available: http://www.marcguidelines.com/uk

81. Deery P, Faithfull S. Developing a patient pathway to deliver a new oral chemotherapy. Prof Nurse 2003; 19(2):102–106.

82. Harrold K. Development of a nurse-led service for patients receiving oral capecitabine. Cancer Nurs Pract 2002; 1(8):19–24.

83. The British Oncology Pharmacy Association. Position statement on safe practice and the pharmaceutical care of patients receiving oral anticancer chemotherapy. British Oncology Pharmacy Association; January 2004. http://www.bopa-web.org/Publications/oralchemofinal.htm

84. Hands D, Stephens M, Brown D. A systematic review of the clinical and economic impact of drug information services on patient outcome. Pharm World Sci 2002; 24(4):132–138.

85. Nursing and Midwifery Council. Guidelines for administration of medicines. London: NMC; 2002. http://www.nmc-uk.org/nmc/main/publications/adminOfrMedicines.pdf Accessed online 2 Feb 2004.

86. Royal College of Nursing. Standards of infusion therapy. London: Royal College of Nursing; 2003.

87. Dougherty L, Hyde L, Haq S. Drug administration cytotoxic drugs. In: Lister S, Dougherty L, eds. The Royal Marsden Hospital of clinical nursing

procedures. 6th edn. Oxford: Blackwell Publishing; 2004:228–256.

88. Lilly Oncology. Cytotoxic drugs. 5th edn. Lilly; 1997.

89. Chu E, DeVita VT. Physicians' cancer chemotherapy drug manual. Boston: Jones & Bartlett; 2001.

90. Wilkes GM, Ingwersen K, Barton-Burke M. Oncology nursing drug handbook. Boston: Jones & Bartlett; 2003

91. British National Formulary. BNF 47, March 2004. London: British Medical Association and Royal Pharmaceutical Society of Great Britain http://bnf.org/ Accessed online July 2004

92. Electronic Medicines Compendium. 2004. Available online http://www.medicines.org.uk/ Accessed online July 2004

93. Goodman M. Chemotherapy: principles of administration. In: Yarbro CH, Frogge MH, Goodman M, et al. Cancer nursing principles and practice. 5th edn. Boston: Jones & Bartlett; 2000:385–443.

94. Hayward T. Setting up chemotherapy service at home. Cancer Nurs Pract 2002; 1(3):22–25.

95. Health Service. Circular HSC 2003/010. Updated national guidance on the safe administration of intrathecal chemotherapy. London: DoH; 2003. http://www.dh.gov.uk/PublicationsAndStatistics/ LettersAndCirculars/HealthServiceCirculars/ HealthServiceCircularsArticle/fs/en?CONTENT_ID= 4064931&chk=JA/pnL

96. Witham G. Pseudomyxoma peritonei. Nurs Times 2003; 99(39):30–32.

97. Steele S, Carruth AK. A comprehensive interdisciplinary chemotherapy teaching documentation flowsheet. Oncol Nurs Forum 1997; 24(5):907–911.

98. Nursing and Midwifery Council. Guidelines for records and record keeping. London: NMC; 2002. http://www.nmc-uk.org/nmc/main/publications/ guidelinesForRecordskeep.pdf Accessed online 3 Feb 2004

99. Heidt C, Matthias D. A closer look at chemotherapy errors. Nurs Manage 2001; 32(11):36–38.

100. Shaw R, Stanley A. Aspects of service operation. In: Allwood M, Stanley A, Wright P, eds. The cytotoxic handbook. 4th edn. Abingdon: Radcliffe Medical Press; 2002:64.

101. Department of Health. Discharge from hospital: pathway, process & practice. London: Stationery Office; 2003. http://www.dh.gov.uk/ PublicationsAndStatistics/Publications/Publications PolicyAndGuidance/PublicationsPolicyAndGuidanc eArticle/fs/en?CONTENT_ID=4003252&chk=CKj7ss Accessed online 3 Feb 2004

102. Vooght S, Richardson A. A study to explore the role of community oncology nurse specialist. Eur J Cancer Care 1996; 5:217–224.

103. McIllmurray MB, Cummings M, Hopkins E, et al. Cancer support nurses: a co-ordinating role in cancer care. Eur J Cancer Care 1998; 7:125–128.

104. Macduff C, Leslie A, West B. Ambulatory chemotherapy: towards best community practice. J Comm Nurs 2001; 15(7)24–26.

105. Pattison J, MacRae K. Cancer care, part 4: home chemotherapy: NHS and independent sector collaboration. Nurs Times 2002; 98(35):34–35.

106. Wright K, Myint A. The colorectal clinical nurse specialist role in chemotherapy. Hosp Med 2003; 64(6):333–336.

107. Wilson K, Pateman B, Beaver K, et al. Patient and carer needs following a cancer-related hospital admission: the importance of referral to the district nursing service. J Adv Nurs 2002; 38(3):245–253.

108. Andrew J, Whyte F. The experiences of district nurses caring for people receiving palliative chemotherapy. Int J Palliat Nurs 2004; 10(3):110–118.

109. Department of Health. The hospital discharge workbook: a manual on discharge practice. London: Stationery Office; 1994. (In: Salter M. Discharge planning. In: Lister S, Dougherty L, eds. The Royal Marsden Hospital Manual of clinical nursing procedures. 6th edn. Oxford: Blackwell Publishing; 2004:170–183.)

110. Department of Health. Continuing care: NHS and local councils' responsibilities. London: Department of Health; 2001. http://www.dh.gov.uk/ assetRoot/04/01/26/87/04012687.pdf Accessed June 04

111. Jens GP, Chaney HS, Brodie KE. Family coping, styles and challenges. Nurs Clin N Am 2001; 36(4):795–808.

112. Flanagan J. Clinically effective cancer care: working with families. Eur J Oncol Nurs 2001; (5)3:174–179.

113. Taylor H. Chemotherapy at home – a case study. Pharm J 2003; 270(7240):372–373.

114. Salter M. Discharge planning. In: Lister S, Dougherty L, eds. The Royal Marsden Hospital of clinical nursing procedures. 6th edn. Oxford: Blackwell Publishing; 2004:170–183.

115. King MT, Hall J, Caleo S, et al. Home or hospital? An evaluation of costs, preferences and outcomes of domiciliary chemotherapy. Int J Health Serv 2000; 30(3):557–579.

116. Borras JM, Sanchez-Hernandez A, Navarro M, et al. Compliance, satisfaction, and quality of life of patients with colorectal cancer receiving home chemotherapy or outpatient treatment: a randomised controlled trial. Br Med J 2001; 322:826–828.

117. Gavin N, How C, Condliffe B, et al. Cytotoxic chemotherapy in the home: a study of community nurses' attitudes and concerns. Br J Comm Nurs 2004; 9(1):18–24.

118. Schneider M. Follow-up of cancer. Cancer Futures 2003; 2:11.

119. Chaigneau XP. Follow-up following treatment for primary breast cancer. Cancer Futures 2003; 2:12–14.

120. Schneider M. Follow-up of resection of colorectal cancer. Cancer Futures 2003; 2:14–17.

121. Westeel V. Follow-up after complete resection of non-small-cell lung cancer. Cancer Futures 2003; 2:17–21.

122. Dufresne A, Guardiola E. Follow-up of ovarian carcinoma after primary therapy. Cancer Futures 2003; 2:21–24.

123. Dolivet G. Follow-up of head and neck cancer. Cancer Futures 2003; 2:24–27.

124. Moore S, Corner J, Fuller F. Development of nurse-led follow-up in the management of patients with lung cancer. NT Res 1999; 40(6):432–447.

125. Cox K, Wilson E. Follow-up for people with cancer: nurse-led services and telephone interventions. J Adv Nurs 2003; 43(1):51–61.

126. Earnshaw JJ, Stephenson Y. First two years of a follow-up breast clinic led by a nurse practitioner. J R Soc Med 1997; 90(5):258–259.

127. Loftus LS, Weston V. The development of nurse-led clinics in cancer care. J Clin Nurs 2001; 10(2):215–220.

128. Taylor K, Cardy C. Colorectal cancer – development of a nurse led follow-up clinic. Cancer Nurs Pract 2003; 2(7)25–29.

129. Aziz NM, Rowland JH. Trends and advances in cancer survivorship research: challenge and opportunity. Semin Radiat Oncol 2003; 13(3):248–266.

130. Gaze MN, Wilson IM. Late effects of cancer treatment – the cost of cure. In: Gaze MN, Wilson IM, eds. Handbook of community cancer care. London: Greenwich Medical Media; 2003:97–102.

131. Royal College of Physicians. Cancer Units improving quality in cancer care. A report of the Joint Collegiate Council for Oncology, London; 2000. http://www.rcplondon.ac.uk/pubs/wp_cu_hom.htm

132. Royal College of Nursing. Clinical practice guidelines: the administration of cytotoxic chemotherapy, Volume 1 – Recommendations; Volume 2 – Technical report. London: Royal College of Nursing; 1998.

133. Oncology Nursing Society. Cancer chemotherapy guidelines and recommendations for practice. Pittsburgh: Oncology Nursing Press 1999; III.

134. Royal College of Nursing. A framework for adult cancer nursing. London: Royal College of Nursing; 2003.

135. Health Service. Circular HSC 2001/012. Cancer waiting times achieving the NHS Cancer Plan waiting times targets. London: DoH. http://www.dh.gov.uk/PublicationsAndStatistics/LettersAndCirculars/HealthServiceCirculars/HealthServiceCircularsArticle/fs/en?CONTENT_ID=4004478&chk=7YDhN9 Accessed online Nov 2003

136. Wright J, Hill P. Clinical governance. Edinburgh: Churchill Livingstone; 2003.

137. Cancer Services Collaborative 'Improvement Partnership'. NHS Modernisation Agency. Available: http://www.modern.nhs.uk/cancer 3 Feb 2004

138. Cancer Services Collaborative 'Improvement Partnership'. Chemotherapy TOP TIPS NHS Modernisation Agency. Available: http://www.modern.nhs.uk/cancer/5628/5732/16564/Chemo%20Top%20Tips_v2.pdf Accessed online 3 Feb 2004

139. Sitzia J, Wood N. Patient satisfaction with cancer chemotherapy nursing: a review of the literature. Int J Nurs Stud 1998; 35(1-2):1–12.

140. Sitzia J, Wood N. Development and evaluation of a questionnaire to assess patient satisfaction with chemotherapy nursing care. Eur J Oncol Nurs 1999; 3(3):126–140.

141. Grocott P, Richardson A, Ambaum B, et al. Nursing in colorectal cancer initiative – the audit phase part 1. Development of the audit tool. Eur J Oncol Nurs 2001; 5(2):100–111.

142. Grocott P, Richardson A, Ambaum B, et al. Nursing in colorectal cancer initiative – the audit phase part 2. Content validity of the audit tool and implications of the standards set for clinical practice. Eur J Oncol Nurs 2001; 5(3):165–173.

143. Mun LY, Ping CM, Fai WK, et al. An evaluation of the quality of a chemotherapy administration service established by nurses in an oncology day care centre. Eur J Oncol Nurs 2001; 5(4):244–253.

144. Perrett S. Improving haematology care in Wales. Nurs Stand 2002; 16(31):39–42.

145. Burns JM, Tierney KD, Long GD, et al. Critical pathway for administering high dose chemotherapy followed by peripheral blood stem cell rescue in the outpatient setting. Oncol Nurs Forum 1995; 22(8):1219–1224.

146. Alllsop A, Sheppard S. Providing patient choice: a nurse-led haematology outpatient service 2002; 18(2):112–125.

147. Baly N, Cairns J, Chisholm J, et al. Research into the workload and roles of oncology nurses within an outpatient oncology unit. Eur J Oncol Nurs 2002; 6(1):6–14.

148. Wallis M, Tyson S. Improving the nursing management of patients in a hematology/oncology day unit: an action research project. Cancer Nurs 2003; 26(1):75–83.

149. White NJ, Given BA, Devoss DN. The advanced practice nurse: meeting the information needs of the rural cancer patient. J Cancer Educ 1996; 11(4):203–209.

150. Gruber M, Kane K, Flack L. A 'perfect day' work redesign in a chemotherapy and infusion center. Oncol Nurs Forum 2003; 30(4):567–568.

151. Kearney N. Classifying nursing care to improve patient outcomes: the example of WISECARE. NT Res 2001; 6(4):747–756.

152. Kerr D, Bevan H, Gowland B, et al. Redesigning cancer care. Br Med J 2002; 324:164–166.

153. Richards MA, Parrott JC. Tertiary cancer services in Britain: benchmarking study of activity and facilities at 12 specialist centres. Br Med J 1996; 313:347–349.

154. NHS Information Authority (NHSIA). Chemotherapy HRGs definitions manual Version 3.1. NHS Information Authority; 2001.

155. NHS Information Authority (NHSIA). 2003. Accessed online http://www.nhsia.nhs.uk/casemix/pages/hbg.asp

156. NHS Information Authority (NHSIA). 2003. Accessed online http://www.nhsia.nhs.uk/casemix/pages/projects/hcf_info.asp

157. Du XL, Osbourne C, Goodwin JS. Population-based assessment of hospitalizations for toxicity from chemotherapy in older women with breast cancer. J Clin Oncol 2002; 20(24) 4636–4642.

158. NHSIA. Cancer Information Services. London: NHS Information Authority; 2003. Available online from: http://www.nhsia.nhs.uk/cancer/pages/relevant/ncdoutline.asp

159. Richardson A, Miller M, Potter H. Developing, delivering and evaluating cancer nursing services: building the evidence base. NT Res 2001; 6(4):726–735.

Chapter **9**

Clinical trials

Hilary Hollis

INTRODUCTION

For a new compound to become a recognised and established cancer treatment, a series of trials need to be carried out. Initially, in the laboratory, preclinical studies are carried out on human cancer cell lines and in animal studies to assess a compound's biological activity and predicted side effects.[1] Many compounds are screened for their potential anticancer activity, but few make it through to further clinical trials. It is estimated that for every 10 000 compounds screened only 5–8 investigational drugs proceed to trials in humans.[1] The alternative to large-scale screening is to utilise our understanding of cellular biology and biochemistry in order to design drugs that attack specific targets, e.g. enzymes that regulate cellular proliferation.[2] Drug development in humans occurs though a series of trials that can be spilt into four phases. Each phase requires a different trial design in order to demonstrate the safety and effectiveness of the chemotherapy drug under investigation.

PHASE I CLINICAL TRIALS

Phase I clinical trials are the first use of an investigational drug in humans. Most anticancer drugs are too dangerous to give to healthy volunteers, so phase I trials with these drugs are offered to patients who have advanced cancer for whom no other effective treatment exists.[3] A phase I trial aims to:

- establish the maximum tolerated dose (MTD) using a specific schedule of administration
- identify the dose-limiting toxicity (DLT) of the drug
- define the pharmacology of the drug by establishing the drug's absorption, distribution, metabolism and excretion.

Historically, the starting dose in phase I trials has been one-tenth of the MTD in the most sensitive animal species in which toxicological studies have been performed.[4] Three patients are treated at this dose level and observed for acute toxicity for one course of treatment before any more patients are entered. If no irreversible, life-threatening or fatal toxicities occur, 3 more patients are treated at the next dose level, and this continues according to the modified Fibonacci sequence in which ever-higher escalation steps have ever-decreasing relative increments (e.g. dose increases of 100%, 65%, 50%, 40% and 30–35% thereafter). Dose escalation is continued in cohorts of 3 until the MTD is reached; however it is the next lower dose from the MTD that becomes the recommended dose for further evaluation.[5]

This standard approach to phase I trials has been criticised. First, with 3 patients entered at each dose level, substantial numbers of patients are treated at doses that are subsequently found to be subtherapeutic. Secondly, these trials take a long time to complete, especially when the starting dose is far below the MTD.[4,5] New approaches to phase I trial design are being examined, although it must be remembered that ultimately they must result in precise determination of the phase II dose, as to complete a trial quickly but inaccurately is of no benefit.

On completion, a phase I trial will provide a description of toxicities experienced, the severity of these toxicities and a starting dose for future studies, but not the response of the tumour to the drug. As the overall response rate in phase I trials is lower than 5%, it has been suggested that the patient entering a phase I trial is motivated by the hope of a response, the desire to help others and the fact that they are cared for by experts.[6,7] However, Cox[8] found that, while initially this was the case, as patients progressed through the trial it became apparent to them that their hope was unrealistic, the trial demands were unanticipated, care by experts meant they were passive recipients and they experienced lack of continuity of care.

The lack of antitumour activity in a phase I trial does not provide sufficient evidence for a new compound to be considered inactive. However, a phase I drug should not continue in clinical trial if there are serious or unmanageable toxicities or if difficulties arise in administering the drugs to humans. On completing a phase I trial to determine the starting dose, phase II trials begin to define the cancers in which the drug is active in humans.[9]

PHASE II CLINICAL TRIALS

A phase II clinical trial is designed to determine the anticancer activity of an investigational drug against specific types of tumours. Phase II trials therefore act as a screen so that only those drugs showing the most promise for a particular tumour type are taken forward to be tried in large numbers of patients in a phase III trial.[10] The tumour types for a phase II trial are identified through screening of investigational drugs against panels of cultured human cell lines, based on the biochemical/pharmacological data or the suggestion of antitumour activity in a particular tumour type in a phase I trial. In addition, a phase II trial provides the chance to modify the recommended dose and identify any further toxicities of the drug based upon the experience of treating a patient population more similar to a phase III trial population than a phase I.

The trial design that is typically used for a phase II trial of an investigational cytotoxic drug is a single-arm study: i.e. no randomisation and all eligible patients receiving the investigational drug at the dose established in the phase I trial. Historical experience is used to define the response rates required to generate interest in pursuing development of the investigation drug into phase III trials. Thus, one might look for a 20% versus 5% response rate for a drug in a cancer where therapeutic options have limited effectiveness; however, in a cancer where the current response rate is 30%, the investigational drug may be expected to achieve a 50% response rate.[10] Using this design, other end points can be used to establish the effectiveness of treatments and these could be progression-free survival, quality of life or specified improvement in pain or performance status. There is a need for good statistical design to identify the required numbers of patients to allow statistically meaningful conclusions to be drawn about the investigational agent under study.

Patients treated in a phase II trial have received prior treatment for their disease and have progressed or been refractory to existing standard treatment. As in a phase I study, the toxicity of the trial treatment may outweigh the benefits of a possible treatment response;[9] therefore, patients' experiences are similar to those being treated on a phase I trial. Cytotoxic drugs shown to be effective in a phase II trial will then be taken forward into larger phase III trials.

PHASE III CLINICAL TRIALS

A phase III trial aims to establish the usefulness of the investigational drug in the treatment of the specified cancer through large randomised controlled trials (RCTs), comparing the new treatment with the current standard treatment. Phase III trials are usually major undertakings that involve many institutions and hundreds or thousands of patients. Patients able to participate in these trials have usually received no previous therapy or a limited number of previous therapies.

Allocation of patients to receive different treatment by random selection is used in an attempt to ensure that any differences that occur between those receiving the new rather than the standard treatment have happened by chance. Optimal sample size in a phase III trial is determined by the ability to detect a previously defined level of difference between the two groups being studied. Overall, the smaller the predefined difference, the larger the sample size will have to be to be sure that it will detect small but medically significant differences if they exist.[11,12]

Many patients find the concept of randomisation difficult to understand and accept with its associated uncertainty.[13] For those patients who want to select the treatment they will receive rather than be assigned their treatment as part of the randomisation process, participation in an RCT is not possible. There are some suggestions of poor recruitment to RCTs occurring as a result of this. RCTs are accepted as the most reliable way to compare therapies; however, if patients are to be recruited to such trials, cancer clinicians need to assist them with the decision-making process when they are faced with the uncertainty of an RCT. The provision of detailed information about the trial, including risk benefits and time to consider options and consult more widely, should be given.[13]

The inclusion of quality of life measurement and health economic analysis as part of phase III trial design has become an increasingly commonplace requirement. The selection of the most appropriate end point in such trials is important and although cure is desirable in advanced cancer this is not achievable, so quality of life may be a more rational criteria for comparison of treatment modalities.[2] Health economic analysis has become more important, with the National Institute for Clinical Excellence (NICE) requiring new treatments to be evaluated for not only clinical effectiveness but also cost-effectiveness.

PHASE IV CLINICAL TRIALS

The phase IV trial seeks to monitor adverse effects of a new drug after it has been approved for marketing. These studies tend to be carried out on large numbers of patients, but minimal data is collected. The most widely used type of phase IV study is post-marketing surveillance.[3]

NEW APPROACHES TO CANCER TREATMENT TRIALS

Increased understanding of the biology and biochemistry of cancer cells is leading to the development of new drugs, both cytotoxic and cytostatic, and the design of clinical trials for such therapies presents a challenge. In the future, trial design may move away from the more traditional approach outlined here; however, new trial designs themselves will need to be tested to ensure the utility of these new approaches.[5,10] Our overall aim must be to ensure that clinically useful new agents are not rejected and, likewise, ineffective agents are discarded. In this way those people with cancer will receive the best treatment currently available.

References

1. Jenkins J, Hubbard S. History of clinical trials. Semin Oncol Nurs 1991; 7(4):228–234.
2. Carmichael J. Current issues in cancer: cancer chemotherapy: identifying novel anticancer drugs. BMJ 1994; 308(6939):1288–1290.
3. Di Giovanna I, Hayes G. Principles of clinical research. Petersfield: Wrightson Biomedical; 2001.
4. Simon R, Freidlin B, Rubinstein L, et al. Accelerated titration designs for Phase I clinical trials in oncology. J Natl Cancer Inst 1997; 89(15):1138–1147.
5. Eisenhauer EA, O'Dwyer PJ, Christian M, et al. Phase I clinical trial design in cancer drug development. J Clin Oncol 2000; 18(3):684–692.
6. Decoster G, Stein G, Holdener E. Responses and toxic deaths in Phase I clinical trials. Ann Oncol 1990; 1:175–182.
7. Braverman AS. Medical oncology in the 1990s. Lancet 1991; 337:901–902.
8. Cox K. Researching research: patients' experiences of participation in phase I and II anti-cancer drug trials. Eur J Oncol Nurs 1999; 3(3):143–152.
9. Gross J. Clinical research in cancer chemotherapy. Oncol Nurs Forum 1986; 13(1):59–65.
10. Korn EL, Arbuck SG, Pluda JM, et al. Clinical trial designs for cytostatic agents: are new approaches needed? J Clin Oncol 2001; 19(1):265–272.
11. Sylvester R. An introduction to the statistical design of phase III cancer clinical trials. Eur Urol 1997; 31(suppl 1):65–71.
12. Sylvester R, Van Glabbeke M, Collette L, et al. Statistical methodology of Phase III cancer trials: advances and future perspectives. Eur J Cancer 2002; 38 (suppl 4):162–168.
13. Daugherty CK. Impact of therapeutic research in informed consent and the ethics of clinical trials: a medical oncology perspective. J Clin Oncol 1999; 17(5):1601–1617.

Chapter 10

Intravenous management

Lisa Dougherty

VASCULAR ACCESS DEVICES

A vascular access device (VAD) is a device that is inserted either into a vein or an artery, via the peripheral or central vessels, to provide for either diagnostic or therapeutic purposes. There are many VADs available (Table 10.1) that allow for cancer patients' vascular access device, therapy and quality of life needs and their care and management will differ (Table 10.2).[1]

Types of device

Winged infusion device
A winged infusion device or 'butterfly' is a steel needle with a short section of tubing attached that can be used to give bolus injections intravenously. Steel needles are associated with a greater risk of extravasation[2,3] and so are never used for the administration of vesicant drugs.

Peripheral cannula
A cannula is a flexible tube containing a needle (stylet), that may be inserted into a blood vessel.[4] It is usually inserted in the peripheral veins of the lower arm (Fig. 10.1). It is indicated for short-term therapies of 3–5 days or for bolus injections or short infusions in the outpatient/day unit setting.[5]

Peripheral cannulae are usually easy to insert and have few associated complications – the most common being phlebitis (either mechanical or chemical), which often results in the need for cannulae to be removed and resited every 72–96 hours.[6–13]

Midline catheter
A midline catheter is a peripheral device inserted into an antecubital vein, where the tip is advanced along the vein of the upper arm up to 20 cm, but is not

Table 10.1 Vascular access devices

Device	Insertion site	Duration	Method of delivery	Complications	Comments
Winged infusion device	Peripheral veins of lower arm	For bolus injections only	For bolus injections only	Infiltration	Not to be used for vesicant drug administration
Peripheral cannula	Peripheral veins of lower arm	72–96 hours	For bolus and infusion	Phlebitis, infiltration, extravasation	
Midline catheter	Antecubital veins	2–4 weeks	For bolus or infusions	Phlebitis, leakage	Not to be used for vesicant drug administration
Peripherally inserted central catheter	Antecubital veins	Weeks to months	For all types of delivery	Phlebitis, dislodgement, occlusion	Requires weekly dressing and flushing
Non-tunnelled central venous catheter	Jugular, subclavian	7–10 days	For all types of delivery	Infection	
Skin-tunnelled catheter	Jugular, subclavian, femoral	Months to years	For all types of delivery	Infection, thrombosis	
Implantable port	Subclavian, femoral	Months to years	For all types of delivery	Occlusion, extravasation	Requires access by a non-coring needle Only requires flushing monthly

Table 10.2   Care and management of VADs[1,16,33]

Device	Dressing	Patency
Peripheral cannulae	Gauze and tape after each manipulation or transparent dressing usually changed when cannula resited unless soiled	5 ml 0.9% sodium chloride daily
Midline	Transparent dressing changed every 5–7 days or as necessary	Heparinised saline (50 IU heparin in 5 ml 0.9% sodium chloride weekly)
PICC	Transparent dressing changed every 5–7 days or as necessary	Heparinised saline (50 IU heparin in 5 ml 0.9% sodium chloride weekly)
Non-tunnelled CVC	Transparent dressing changed every 5–7 days or as necessary	5–10 ml 0.9% sodium chloride after each use
Skin-tunnelled CVC	Sutures removed: I week (top suture); 3 weeks exit site suture. Cover with transparent dressing. Thereafter no dressing required unless patient requests – then change daily if gauze	Open-ended catheters – heparinised saline (50 IU heparin in 5 ml 0.9% sodium chloride) weekly. Valved catheters – 10 ml 0.9% sodium chloride weekly
Implanted port	Support needle with gauze and cover with transparent dressing when accessed. No dressing when not accessed	Heparinised saline (500 IU heparin in 5 ml 0.9% sodium chloride) once a month

extended past the axilla (Fig. 10.2).[5,9,10,14] It does not enter the central venous circulation and can be left in situ for 2–4 weeks.[14] It is ideal for patients without accessible peripheral veins in the lower arm or with a minimal number of adequate vessels available for administration of therapy. Midline catheters are used for moderate duration (less than 6 months)[7] or for therapy of more than 5 days to preserve peripheral veins for future use and increase patient comfort, e.g. for antibiotics.

The midline catheter also provides venous accessibility, along with an easy insertion at the antecubital fossa,[15,16] when the use of a central venous catheter (CVC) is contraindicated, e.g. head and neck surgery. As the catheter tip does not terminate beyond the proximal aspect of the limb being used, X-ray verification is not usually required. The main problem associated with midline catheters is mechanical phlebitis and there is a restriction on the type of solutions/drugs that may be administered: i.e. vesicant or hyperosmolar

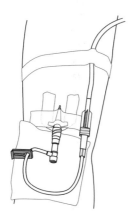

Figure 10.1   Peripheral cannula.

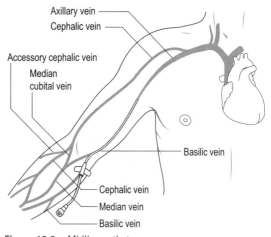

Figure 10.2   Midline catheters.

solutions should not be administered via midline because of the risk of damage should the drugs extravasate.[7,9,10,17,18]

Central venous access devices

Peripherally inserted central catheter   A peripherally inserted central catheter (PICC) is a catheter that is inserted via the antecubital veins in the arm and is advanced into the central veins, with the tip located in the lower third of the superior vena cava (SVC)[10,19,20,21] (Fig. 10.3). It is available as a single- or dual-lumen catheter. PICCs are indicated when:

- there is a lack of peripheral access in the lower arm
- for infusions of vesicant, irritant, parenteral nutrition or hyperosmolar solutions
- for long-term venous access (months)
- for patients with needle phobia to prevent repeated cannulation
- some patients may prefer a PICC to a tunnelled catheter
- the clinician may prefer a patient to have a PICC instead of a skin-tunnelled catheter due to risks of haemorrhage or pneumothorax.[16,22]

The PICC has many advantages over other central venous access devices – mainly because the risks associated with CVAD placement, such as pneumothorax, haemothorax, cardiac arrhythmia and air embolism, are eliminated.[5,14,16] In addition, PICCs have also been shown to reduce catheter sepsis and to reduce patient discomfort and also provide a reliable form of access.[16,20] However, there are contraindications for inserting a PICC, such as the inability to locate suitable antecubital veins and anatomical distortions from surgery, injury or trauma, e.g. scarring from mastectomy, lymphoedema, burns, etc., which may prevent advancement of the catheter to the desired tip location.[22]

Non-tunnelled central venous catheter   A non-tunnelled central venous access device enters through the skin directly into a central vein and is not tunnelled.[5] This type of CVAD allows for administration of multiple therapies, as the catheters can have up to five lumens. These catheters are indicated for short-term therapy of a few days up to several weeks (if left in situ longer than 10–14 days they must be either replaced over a guide wire or removed and reinserted). They can be used for central venous pressure readings and inserted when there is an absence of peripheral veins.[5,23] The catheter is usually inserted via the jugular or subclavian vein, and complications include pneumothorax, infection, haemorrhage or dislodgement.[23,24]

Skin-tunnelled catheter   A skin-tunnelled catheter ('Hickman' catheter), is a catheter that lies in a subcutaneous tunnel exiting midway from the anterior chest wall, while the tip of the catheter lies at the junction of the SVC and right atrium or within the SVC or upper right atrium.[5,25] (Fig. 10.4). It is the most frequently used catheter for long-term venous access.

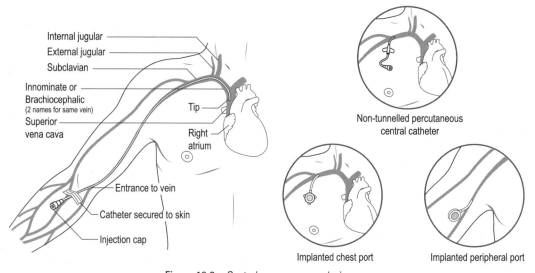

Figure 10.3   Central venous access devices.

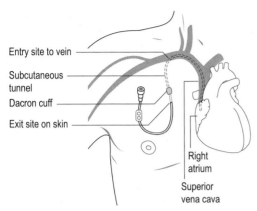

Entry site to vein

Subcutaneous
tunnel

Dacron cuff

Exit site on skin

Right
atrium

Superior
vena cava

Figure 10.4   Skin-tunnelled catheter.

The purpose of the tunnel is to distance the entry site of the catheter into the vein from the exit site on the skin, so providing a barrier to infection.[5,16,24] A cuff made of Dacron is positioned in the subcutaneous tunnel, allowing granulation of surrounding tissue, which forms a barrier to invading organisms and also reduces the risk of dislodgement.[7] The cuff should be sited at least 5 cm from the entry site.[16,26] The catheter currently used at the Royal Marsden NHS Trust has a cuff that is situated 22 cm from the top of the bifurcation. This measurement may assist the practitioner in locating the cuff during removal of the catheter. However, the distance of the cuff from the bifurcation may vary according to the type of catheter.

Implantable ports   An implantable port is a totally implanted vascular access device consisting of a portal body attached to a silicone catheter. These are implanted subcutanously, usually on the chest wall or in the antecubital area, and require access by a needle. It is a long-term venous access device which can remain in place for a number of years.[5,16,27]

Ports require minimal care of the site, except when accessed. This is done using a special non-coring needle that can remain in place for up to 7 days.[5,16,24] The needle should be supported by gauze and covered by a transparent dressing to avoid needle dislodgement, as this has been shown to be the most frequently documented cause of extravasation.[28–30]

The main advantages over external CVADs appear to be less risk of infection and less interference with daily activities (which may be related to reduction in manipulations, as it only requires monthly flushing). There is also less threat to body image.[27,28,31]

One disadvantage of a port is the discomfort associated with accessing the port (especially if placed deeply or in a difficult area to access), although this can be overcome with the use of topical local anaesthetic cream.

Prior to accessing a port, the practitioner must have knowledge and the skill to insert the most appropriate type of needle into the port,[27] as a wrongly placed needle could lead to extravasation of drugs.[27,28,30,32] As small syringes can create high pressure within the catheter, most manufacturers recommend the use of 10 ml syringes or larger to prevent excessive pressure being exerted, which could result in separation of the catheter from the portal body. (See also Ch. 13)

ADMINISTRATION OF CYTOTOXIC DRUGS

Methods of administration

The choice of method for administration of a cytotoxic drug is based upon:

- the type of drug
- the pharmacological considerations (such as stability or the need for dilution in a certain volume of fluid)
- the degree of potential venous irritation
- whether the drug is a vesicant or not and
- the type of device in situ.

There are three methods by which cytotoxic drugs may be administered:

- direct bolus injection
- bolus injection via the side arm of a fast-running infusion of 0.9% sodium chloride
- infusion.

Direct bolus injection

The rationale for administering a drug as a direct bolus injection is that it allows the integrity of the vein to be assessed and the signs and symptoms of extravasation or infiltration may be detected earlier. Direct bolus injection allows the immediate discontinuation of the injection and investigation and appropriate management of the problem. The main difficulty with this method is that it can increase the risk of venous irritation due to the constant contact of the drug with the vein. This, in turn, can result in pain, making it difficult to distinguish between venous spasm and extravasation.[33] (See Extravasation section.)

Bolus injections via side arm

Bolus injections can also be administered via the side arm of a free flowing infusion of 0.9% sodium chloride. This ensures greater dilution of irritant drugs and aids rapid circulation away from the insertion site. Bolus injections can also allow the practitioner to observe for early signs and symptoms of infiltration or extravasation. However if the veins are small or if a small-gauge cannula is in situ, there will not be a brisk flow of the infusate and the drug may back up the administration set tubing. Bolus injections also require the practitioner to clamp off the administration set tubing and pull back on the syringe to check for blood return, as well as continually checking the flow of infusate.

Infusion

Administering drugs as an infusion allows increased dilution of the drug, thereby reducing the chemical irritation. Dilution may also be necessary due to the side effects that could occur if the drug was given too rapidly as a bolus, e.g. hypotension or hypoglycaemia.[16] Infiltration and extravasation may be subtle and difficult to detect until a large volume has infiltrated, particularly if the patient is sedated and unable to report sensations associated with extravasation. It should be noted that due to the risk of extravasation, giving vesicants as an infusion into a peripheral vein should be avoided.[16] Blood return cannot be assessed on a regular basis as for injections, and the longer the infusion the greater the possibility of the device becoming dislodged and an infiltration or extravasation occurring.

When vesicants are given as infusions via a central venous access device, it is recommended that an external catheter, e.g. a tunnelled catheter, is used rather than an implantable port. This is because ports are associated with a greater incidence of extravasation, especially with long infusion times. Where appropriate, the patient can be taught to check the needle in the port at least three times a day.[13]

Steps of administration

Preparation of the patient

Cytotoxic drugs must be administered by specially trained practitioners.[1,7,16] The practitioner must be satisfied that the patient has been given a full explanation regarding side effects that may occur during or following administration and that the patient has given consent to receive the treatment. Appropriate laboratory results, e.g. full blood count and renal function tests, should be within acceptable levels and the prescription should be dated, legible and signed. Protocols and dosage should also be checked and the appropriate supportive therapies such as prehydration and antiemetics should be administered.[1,7,16]

Equipment

Protective clothing should be worn and its necessity explained to the patient. Aseptic technique should be followed throughout the administration procedure. All syringes and infusion bags should be checked for any leakage or contamination and the details on the labels should correspond with the prescription chart and the patient. Only intravenous administration sets and syringes with Luer lock fittings should be used to minimise the risk of accidental disconnection during administration. (See Chs 3 and 13.)

Checking patency

Drugs may be administered via a winged infusion device, a peripheral cannula or a central venous access device. If the patient has an established peripheral cannula in situ, the dressing should be removed and the site should be assessed for redness, pain or tenderness. Patency of the cannula must be checked by withdrawing blood and then flushing, using 5–10 ml of 0.9% sodium chloride to ensure no resistance to the flow of fluid. This also allows the practitioner to observe for any swelling or for the patient to report any feelings of pain or discomfort.

The practitioner administering intravenous cytotoxic drugs will need to be aware of the immediate effects such as local allergic reaction, cold sensation along the vein or drugs that may affect the future condition of the peripheral veins. The practitioner must be able to recognise and differentiate the local side effects, e.g. venous spasm, from more serious complications, e.g. extravasation, and respond appropriately.

Commencing administration

The drugs should be administered in the correct order: i.e. vesicant cytotoxic drugs first.[1,16,33] This is because vascular integrity decreases over time of administration and the vein is most stable and least irritated at the start of administration. The initial assessment of vein patency is also more accurate and the patient's awareness of changes is more acute. At least 5–10 ml of 0.9% sodium chloride should be used to flush in between each drug to avoid mixing and chemical interactions, unless the drug is only compatible with 5% glucose, e.g. liposomal doxorubicin. Gently aspirating blood ('blood return') to check for patency should be performed every 2–4 ml, especially when administering a vesicant and assessing for any swelling.[16,27,33–36] If attaching an administration set for an infusion, ensure all the connections are secure and the administration set is taped to the patient. This is to prevent the tubing being pulled, causing discomfort for the patient, and to minimise the risk of the cannula moving out of the vein.

Observation and completion

The site should be monitored throughout the bolus injection to check for signs of infiltration, extravasation or leakage at the site. This will ensure the prompt recognition and management of any complication, thus minimising local damage and preserving venous access for future treatment.[1,33] A gauze swab should be kept at connecting points in case of any spillage of cytotoxic drug, which may result in contamination of patient and/or practitioner.[37] Once the drugs have been administered, a final flush of 5–10 ml of 0.9% sodium chloride should be given to ensure the drug is flushed out of the device, tubing and the vein. On completion, waste should be disposed of according to the institution's policy. Documentation must be carried out immediately after completion of bolus administration to prevent duplication of treatment and include the following:

- a start and stop time for infusions
- any adverse reactions.

LOCAL EFFECTS

Pain at the insertion site

A number of cytotoxic drugs are irritants or vesicants. During administration, chemical irritation by a drug can result in venous spasm, causing a dull ache or pain at the insertion site and along the vein. This can often be confused with symptoms of extravasation. Therefore it is important that the practitioner has knowledge of the drugs that are likely to cause pain as well as methods to prevent and relieve the pain. Drugs that are known to cause pain include doxorubicin, epirubicin, dacarbazine, cytosine, vinorelbine, thiotepa, streptocozin and BCNU.[7,16,37–39] Where possible, the drug should be diluted and given either as an infusion, preferably via a CVC, or administered slowly via the side arm of a fast-running infusion of 0.9% sodium chloride. Local heat, in the form of a heat pack, can be applied above the peripheral cannula to relieve the spasm. The application of a glycerol trinitrate (GTN) patch distal to the cannula (Fig. 10.5) encourages vasodilation and results in better dilution and more rapid circulation away from the insertion site, thus reducing venous spasm.[40]

Local allergic reaction or 'flare reaction'

Some drugs cause a red streak or flush from the insertion site along the vein. This is called a flare reaction and is caused by a venous inflammatory response to histamine release (Table 10.3).[34,41] Flare is usually associated with red-coloured drugs such as doxorubicin and epirubicin, and occurs in about 3–6% of cases.[3,42] This reaction is characterised by a red streak or blotchiness and may result in the formation of small wheals, having a similar appearance to a nettle rash. A flare

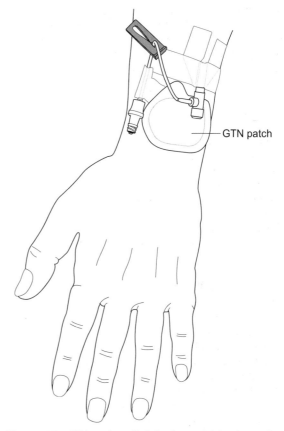

GTN patch

Figure 10.5 GTN patch applied distal to a peripheral cannula.

reaction does not cause pain, although the area may feel itchy and the reaction usually subsides within 30–45 min without treatment .[1,3,7,27] However, the reaction responds well within a few minutes to the application of a topical steroid or an intravenous injection of hydrocortisone.[16] The chance of a local allergic reaction occurring can be reduced by diluting the drug or by administering via the side arm of an infusion.

Discoloration of the veins/hyperpigmentation

This is not an immediate side effect but one that can progressively become evident and may influence the availability of peripheral veins for vascular access. There is an increased incidence in patients with greater pigmentation and it may be associated with exogenous trauma/post-inflammatory changes or areas of increased vasodilation.[7] It is more common when alkylating and antitumour antibiotics, e.g. 5-fluorouracil (5FU), vinblastine, chlormethine (mustine) and dactinomycin, are administered. The exact mechanism is unknown but it may result from direct stimulation of the melanocytes. It has been suggested that the use of

Table 10.3   Management of signs and symptoms of local peripheral effects[16]

Complication	Signs and symptoms	Management
Flare reaction	Blotchiness Itching Hive-like urticaria Stinging sensation of heat Rapid appearance of wheals	Usually subsides without treatment Topical application of steroids IV hydrocortisone
Infiltration	Swelling Tightness/discomfort Coolness of skin Leakage at VAD site	Warm compress to alleviate discomfort and help absorb infiltration Elevation of limb
Extravasation	Burning stinging pain No blood return Absence of free flow Swelling	Follow extravasation procedure according to type of drug

heating pads or warm compresses to aid vasodilation should be avoided during the administration of the causative drugs[7] as this may increase the incidence. It usually disappears 2–3 months after completion of treatment and appears to cause no other adverse effects.[33]

Cold sensation

The patient may complain of a cold sensation along the vein that is often related to the difference between the temperature of the drug (often stored in a fridge) and the patient's circulation. However, some drugs specifically cause a cold sensation, e.g. vinca alkaloids, and the patient should be informed and reassured that this is normal.

Chemical phlebitis

This can result from repeated administration of irritant drugs through peripheral cannulae and can make it more difficult for the practitioner to locate a suitable vein for cannulation and therefore the safe administration of cytotoxic drugs. The incidence is increased when combinations of irritant or vesicant drugs are administered. Early signs include pain, local erythema, oedema, a sensation of warmth and discoloration of the venous pathway. The patient may suffer discomfort and in some extreme cases the skin may become taut and stretched as the vein becomes cord-like, and this can lead to restricted use of the limb.[16,33] Knowledge of the drugs with the potential for phlebitis will enable all preventative measures to be applied at the time of administration. These include:

- diluting the drugs (if pharmaceutically acceptable)

- administering the drug slowly with frequent flushing with 0.9% sodium chloride
- application of warmth to the area to aid vasodilation.

The use of a small-gauge cannula in a large vein with good blood flow will increase the dilution drug and encourage rapid circulation away from the insertion site. However, if this is a recurring problem, it may be necessary to reassess the patient's venous access and consider the use of a CVAD.

EXTRAVASATION

Infiltration is the inadvertent administration of a non-vesicant drug out of the venous system into the surrounding tissues.[7] Extravasation is defined as the inadvertent administration of a vesicant drug out of the venous system into the tissues. A vesicant is an irritant drug that has the potential to cause blistering, severe tissue damage, and even necrosis if extravasated, and usually requires some form of management.[6,27] An irritant drug can cause local sensitivity and, if it infiltrates, it can cause local inflammation and discomfort but no long-term damage (see Table 10.3).[7,36]

Incidence

Extravasation is one of the most serious complications associated with administration of intravenous cytotoxic drugs,[43] with an incidence estimated of between 0.1 and 6% in patients receiving peripheral chemotherapy.[44,45] This may not reflect the true incidence, as extravasation may not be recognised or reported.[7,36,46] The incidence appears to be higher in children[47] and with implantable ports, often as a result of needle dislodgement.[7,30]

Risk factors

There are certain factors that increase the risk of extravasation occurring:

1. The inability to communicate appropriately, e.g.
   - neonates
   - infants
   - young children
   - comatose or sedated patients
   - confused patients
   - very restless patients.
2. Vascular impairment and reduced vascular integrity, e.g.
   - in the elderly
   - patients with Raynaud's disease
   - radiation areas
   - multiple attempts at venepuncture
   - cardiac disease
   - obstructed venous drainage
   - lymphoedema
   - superior vena cava syndrome[48]
   - fragile, sclerosed, thrombosed and small veins.
3. Lack of knowledge and skill level of the person performing cannulation and administering the drugs.[27,43,45,49]

Pathogenesis

When an extravasation occurs:

- fluid leaks into the tissue
- the tissue is compressed due to the restricted blood flow
- this in turn reduces the amount of oxygen to the site and lowers the cellular pH
- there is loss of capillary wall integrity, an increase in oedema and eventual cellular death.

This is further compounded by the chemistry of an extravasation and whether the drug binds to DNA or not.

Drugs that do not bind to DNA

Drugs that do not bind to DNA tend to inhibit mitosis and often cause immediate damage. However, they are quickly metabolised and inactivated. The type of injury that results is similar to a burn and can result in ulceration. These drugs tend not to erode down to deeper structures and normal tissue healing occurs within 3–5 weeks. These injuries rarely require any surgical intervention. Examples of drugs in this group are the vinca alkaloids.[50]

Drugs that bind to DNA

Drugs that do bind to DNA can cause immediate damage that is followed by an indolent and progressive tissue necrosis. This ongoing damage is due to a process of endocytosis, whereby the DNA-binding drug is taken up by the cell, which results in the cell's death. When the cell dies, its membrane ruptures and the drug is released to be taken up by a neighbouring cell, thereby perpetuating the process of tissue death.[50–52] This results in the cell losing its ability to heal spontaneously and explains the prolonged effect.[47] Drugs in this group include chlormethine (mustine) (nitrogen mustard), which tends to bind rapidly to the tissues and cause immediate injury, and the drugs in the antibiotic family, e.g. doxorubicin, daunorubicin, and mitomycin C.

Clinically, most experience has been gained and many studies have been performed on the most common and widely used cytotoxic vesicant drug – doxorubicin. It has been found that there is a positive correlation between the concentration of doxorubicin and the extent of ulceration. The active drug has been isolated from wounds from 3–5 months after a doxorubicin extravasation.[47,48,50] Under ultraviolet light, tissue containing doxorubicin glows a dull red and this helps to identify the area of injury.[50]

Stages of damage

The first suggestion of an extravasation of doxorubicin may be a burning sensation, although local discomfort does not always occur in the initial stages. The pain can be quite severe and last minutes, hours or even days, but will eventually subside.[16,50]

In the following weeks, the tissue will become reddened and firm and the skin may blanch when pressure is applied, suggesting infection or local irritation.[50] Necrosis may become obvious as early as a few days, depending on the size of the area of extravasated drug.[50] If the area is small, the redness gradually reduces over a few weeks. If the extravasation is large, a small necrotic area will appear in the centre of the red skin. Once necrosis occurs, surgical debridement is indicated. If this is not performed, a thick black eschar will result, surrounded by a rim of red painful skin. When the eschar is removed, deep subcutaneous necrosis is often found. The key feature of doxorubicin ulceration is that it is often progressive and may lead to extensive joint stiffness and neuropathy.[50]

Extravasation syndrome

It has been suggested that there are three types of extravasation syndrome, [36] although the management of types I and II is the same:

- Pre-extravasation syndrome often involves little or no leakage of vesicants but particularly severe phlebitis and/or local hypersensitivity, together with a number of other local risk factors such as difficult cannulation resulting in multiple punctures. This is an indication that patients may be more susceptible to extravasation and may be candidates for a central venous access device instead of continuing on peripheral devices.
- Type I extravasation injuries cause a blister and have a defined area of firmness around the site of injury. They are usually associated with bolus injections where pressure of the injection is applied when administering the drugs.
- Type II extravasations are differentiated by a diffuse, 'soggy' type of tissue injury, where dispersal into intracellular space has occurred. These are usually associated with gravity infusions or bolus injections through the side arm of an infusion.

Selection of vein and device

A vesicant drug should never be administered via a winged infusion device as it has been shown that the incidence of extravasation is greater when steel needles are used than with plastic cannulae.[2,3] Choice of site for cannulae is firstly the forearm,[16,36,44] then the dorsum of the hand. Veins on the dorsum of the hand are not ideal due to the lack of subcutaneous tissue and the proximity of tendons and joints to the skin. The latter could be damaged if extravasation occurs and severe problems associated with movement have been reported following ulceration in this area.[48,50,53] Siting over joints should be avoided as tissue damage in this area may limit joint movement in the future. Veins in the antecubital fossa are in close proximity to nerves and arteries and if drugs extravasate in this area it is often difficult to detect and there is a greater risk of damage to local structures such as nerves and tendons. Therefore, these veins should be avoided and are best left for venepuncture and collection of blood samples.

Location

The best location is the proximal forearm over the flexor and extensor muscle bulk; however, these veins are often not easily accessible or have been used extensively.[50,53] It is recommended that a large straight vein in the dorsum of the hand is preferable to a smaller vein in the forearm. Veins that have been previously used for blood sampling or have multiple punctures are not suitable due to increased risk of leakage of the drug from the old venepuncture sites. If a cannulation has been unsuccessful, then a different vein, and if

possible in the opposite limb, should be used. If this is not possible, then a site in the same vein may be selected but it should be proximal to the previous puncture.[6,44,53]

The cannula must be securely fixed and it is essential that the insertion site is visible throughout the administration. Venous patency must always be checked with at least 5–10 ml of 0.9% sodium chloride prior to administration of a vesicant and the area assessed for pain and swelling. If patency is questioned, the device should be removed and resited.

Use of an existing device

A pre-existing peripheral device should not be used for vesicant drug administration if:

- the IV cannula was placed more than 24 hours earlier
- the area or insertion site is red, swollen or painful or there is any evidence of infiltration
- the cannula is sited over or around the wrist (or over a joint)
- if blood return is sluggish or absent or
- infusion fluid is flowing erratically and seems positional.

However, if the fluid runs freely, there is a good and consistent blood return and the site is free of swelling, pain and redness, the device may be used to avoid the need for the patient to undergo another cannulation.[33]

Skill of the practitioner

The key to preventing extravasation is good venous assessment and using methods to improve venous access. The practitioner should be proficient at performing cannulation[35,36,43,44] before attempting to cannulate for vesicant drug administration, as well as being knowledgeable about the signs and symptoms of extravasation. Multiple attempts after failure to cannulate a vein should be discouraged and inexperienced practitioners should not attempt to cannulate difficult veins.[44,46] If a practitioner does not feel confident in his ability or is unsuccessful after one or two attempts at cannulation, he should seek assistance of an experienced colleague. Any patient who consistently requires frequent attempts to successfully obtain peripheral vascular access should be considered for a CVAD. Early recognition and prompt action comes from ensuring only skilled and knowledgeable practitioners administer vesicant drugs.[35,36,44,59]

Preparation of the patient

All patients should be informed about the drugs being given, any anticipated side effects and the risks of extravasation. They should be advised not to move the limb that has the cannula in situ during administration of a bolus injection, and should be instructed to report immediately any pain, burning or unusual sensations. Adequate information given to patients will ensure early recognition and cooperation as the patient is the first to notice pain.[3,16,27,35,36] If the patient cannot verbalise the discomfort, they should be observed closely for other signs of pain, e.g. facial expressions. If the dressing is not transparent, then the site should be exposed to enable adequate visualisation of the site and the device must be checked for patency.

Signs and symptoms

Pain
A burning or stinging pain is usually the first signs of an extravasation. However, this sensation must be distinguished from venous spasm or a feeling of cold that can occur with some cytotoxic drugs. It must also be remembered that, although rare, extravasation can occur in the absence of pain. Pain can occur as a result of vesicant drugs extravasating from both peripheral and central venous access devices. Patients may complain of pain around the cannula site, along the catheter tunnel or around the port site. This may be a result of cannula dislodgement, split catheter, needle dislodgement or poor needle placement in a port.[27,30,53] Any change in sensation warrants further investigation.

Swelling
The vascular access device site should be constantly assessed for signs of swelling. Swelling may not be immediately obvious if the patient has a cannula sited in an area of deep subcutaneous fat, in a very deep vein or if the leak is via the posterior vein wall.

Erythema
Erythema is not usually present at the time of extravasation but often occurs within a few hours. Erythema during a bolus injection usually indicates flare.

Absence of blood return
Peripheral blood return should be checked at regular intervals during drug administration, although blood return does not guarantee vein patency and any change should be investigated. If no blood return is the only sign, it should not be regarded as an indication of a non-patent vein. A vein may not bleed back for a number of reasons, such as the cannulae being situated in a small vein that collapses when the syringe plunger is pulled back, or excess fluid from an infusion preventing blood from pooling at the tip of the cannula. In a CVAD, fibrin sheath formation may also prevent blood return.[16,24,27,36,54] Any change in blood flow should be investigated.

Other signs
During an infiltration or extravasation, there may be a reduction or absence of flow rate of an infusion or resistance felt on the plunger of the syringe when administering a bolus injection.[34,36] If any signs or symptoms are present or there is any doubt that the drug is not being administered as it should, then the drug should be discontinued immediately.[7,16] The patency of the device should be checked with a syringe of 0.9% sodium chloride, although if an extravasation has occurred this may result in further spread of the drug into the tissues.

Management of extravasation

One of the main aims when administering vesicant cytotoxic drugs is to prevent extravasation. However, despite the skill of the practitioner, extravasations do occur and the emphasis should be on immediate recognition and prompt management. It is these two factors which will ameliorate the serious consequences of an extravasation injury. Sometimes it is difficult to detect if an extravasation has occurred, but the literature stresses that in the event of a suspected extravasation it is better to assume the drug has extravasated and act accordingly.[16]

The management and treatment of extravasation is a complex and controversial one but comprehensive treatment and expert advice must be available as early as possible following an extravasation. Ideally this should occur within 10 min of the event, certainly within 1 hour and definitely within 24 hours.[36] After 24 hours, management will no longer be aimed at preventing injury but rather damage limitation. Whatever form of treatment is chosen it should not cause further damage, or in the case of misdiagnosis of an extravasation, cause any damage.[36] (See also Ch. 11.)

Withdrawing the drug
Once an extravasation is suspected, clinicians agree that the infusion or administration should be stopped immediately, followed by aspiration of any remaining drug in order to reduce the size of the lesion.[7,16,34,36,46,50] However, aspiration is only possible during bolus injections and in practice may achieve little and is often distressing for the patient.[36,44]

Removing the device
Some authors suggest that the device be left in situ in order to instill the antidote through the device

and into the surrounding tissues, thus infiltrating the area where the extravasation has occurred.[7,16,36,46] However, it has also been recommended that the device be removed as it is felt that the antidote may push the vesicant drug further into the tissues.[1,34,45,50]

Warm/cold packs and antidotes

There appears to be two main courses of treatment:

- localise and neutralise
- spread and dilute.[36]

Localise and neutralise In order to localise the extravasated drug, the recommended course would be to apply a cold pack to the area to cause vasoconstriction. Vasoconstriction reduces the locally destructive effects by reducing the local uptake of the drug by the tissues, decreasing local oedema and slowing the metabolic rate of the cells as well as reducing local pain.[16,45,55] There is no consensus on how long the pack should be left in situ; however, some suggest 15 min four times a day[7,16,44,45,50] for up to 24–48 hours.[7,44,45]

Spread and dilute It appears that warmth is beneficial in managing the extravasation of non-DNA-binding vesicant drugs. It is used after the antidote has been administered in order to increase blood supply and thereby increasing the dispersion and absorption of the antidote into the subcutaneous tissues. The increased blood supply may also help to promote healing by increasing metabolic demands and reducing cellular destruction.[7,16] The use of warmth is recommended for vinca alkaloid extravasation and should be applied 15–20 min four times a day for 24–48 hours.[1,7,37]

There are two main types of antidotes: those with the aim to neutralise the drug, e.g. 0.9% sodium chloride and hyaluronidase;[45] or to dilute the drug and reduce subsequent local inflammation, such as the use of steroid injections and/or cream, e.g. dexamethasone or hydrocortisone.[36] Data now discourages use of locally injected steroids, as there is little evidence to support their use.[44,55] Topical antidotes aim to minimise skin inflammation and erythematous reactions. Application of 99% dimethyl sulfoxide (DMSO) has been found to be beneficial in treating doxorubicin and mitomycin C extravasations. The recommended topical application is 1–2 ml applied to the site every 6 hours.[36,55] Hyaluronidase is an enzyme that destroys tissue cement, aiding in reduction or prevention of tissue damage by allowing rapid diffusion of the extravasated fluid and promoting drug absorption. The usual dose is 1500 IU administered following vinca alkaloid extravasations.[34,45,55] However, 0.9% sodium chloride has also been used successfully to limit the effects of vinca alkaloid extravasation by diluting the concentration of the drug.[42,46]

Some centres have a list of antidotes for each vesicant drug and some suggest the use of no antidotes.[50] There are also various degrees of conservative treatments, i.e. the use of observation and/or antidotes, but not requiring surgical intervention.

Elevation of the extremity

The elevation of the extremity is recommended for up to 48 hours to minimise oedema. Some advocate the importance of elevation,[7,50] following the application of an ice pack. Movement should also be encouraged to prevent adhesion of damaged areas to underlying tissue, which could result in restriction of movement.[1]

Surgical intervention

Some centres suggest that a plastic surgery consultation should be performed as part of the immediate management procedure.[16] The need for early surgical intervention with excision of the area (particularly with doxorubicin) helps to stop progression of cellular destruction, thereby minimising damage.[42] However, the requirement for surgery is probably based on the size and location of the extravasation as well as the type of drug that has been extravasated.[7,34,42] Excision should include removal of all indurated, reddened, oedematous and pale tissue with a margin of normal-appearing tissue.[48]

'Saline flush-out' technique and the use of liposuction

It has been suggested that the use of 0.9% sodium chloride flushing performed within the first 24 hours is a less traumatic and more cost-effective procedure than surgery.[44,56] The 'saline flush-out' technique involves a number of small stab incisions, through which 0.9% sodium chloride is flushed in order to facilitate the cleansing of any drug from the subcutaneous tissues. It is advocated for use with DNA-binding vesicants such as doxorubicin.[3] Liposuction involves making a small incision alongside the extravasation under local or general anaesthetic and using a blunt-ended liposuction cannula, aspirating extravasated material and subcutaneous fat. Both methods have shown that, used early, the majority healed without any soft tissue loss at all.[44,56]

Identification and demarcation of the area can be achieved by the use of fluorescence microscopic analysis.[57] Photographs are useful as well as marking the area of extravasation with an indelible marker to observe for an increase or decrease in swelling and redness.

Further points

Most extravasations occur via peripheral cannula and most management procedures reflect this; however, the consequences of an extravasation from a CVAD are more serious and require immediate consultation with the medical team.

Consideration must also be given to the management of mixed vesicant extravasation, which are usually given via the central venous route, in terms of which drug to treat with which antidote. It is recommended to act in accordance with the drug that possesses the most deleterious properties.[3]

Patients should always be informed when an extravasation has occurred and an explanation of what has happened as well as what is required in order to manage the situation. Following the management of the extravasation, an information sheet should be given to the patient, instructing the patient what signs and symptoms to observe for and when to contact the hospital during the follow-up period.[1,33]

Consequences of untreated or poorly managed extravasation

The consequences of an untreated or poorly managed extravasation can be extensive and result in a necrotic ulcerated injury but such injuries can be minimised through careful preparation, administration and monitoring. An injury can have an impact on the patient's ability to work and function normally, both socially and emotionally. This is particularly so if the extravasation injury occurred over a joint, limiting mobility and even resulting in permanent disability. As a result of the injury, the patient may suffer from pain, which in turn may lead to problems with working, sleeping and the general ability to cope with the treatment.

An extravasation injury may affect the patient's long-term prognosis, as they may not be able to continue therapy in order to allow the wound time to heal. If patients suffer myelosuppression during treatment, the wound becomes a potential area for infection. If the patient is debilitated through the injury, this could also result in secondary medical problems.

There are also costs to the patient and family in time, money and their overall health and quality of life. This is especially true if a patient cannot resume work due to disability or the requirement for time off for plastic surgery. There may be costs involved in surgery, both to treat the injury and to repair the damage

cosmetically, and repeated hospitalisations may be necessary.[16] One consequence of extravasation could be litigation. Practitioners are now being named in malpractice allegations in the UK and extravasation injuries are an area of increasing concern.[3,5,29,30,32] Therefore, it is imperative that an evidence-based management procedure is in place wherever vesicant drugs are to be administered. (See also Extravasation Wounds Aetiology & Management section.)

The use of extravasation kits

The use of an extravasation kit and policy is recommended.[1,33,36] An extravasation kit is particularly useful in areas where vesicant cytotoxic drugs are administered, as it enables staff to have immediate access to a step-by-step guide to management, as well as having all the required equipment to hand.

The kit should remain uncomplicated in order to avoid confusion (especially as the practitioner will be anxious), but comprehensive enough to meet all reasonable needs.[36] The instructions should be clear and easy to follow and the use of a flow chart is an easy way of enabling staff to follow the management procedure. Kits will be assembled according to the particular needs of the individual institution.

Documentation and reporting

Documentation of an extravasation is vital for a number of reasons. An extravasation is an accident and must be reported and fully documented. The patient will require follow-up care and the documentation must be available to all practitioners involved in the follow-up. Information about extravasation will be used for statistical purposes and may also be required in the case of litigation.[16,29,36,45,58]

The documentation should contain the following aspects:

- patient details
- the drug given
- the method used, e.g. bolus or infusion
- type of device, e.g. cannula, CVC
- diagram to indicate the location and size of the area
- the appearance of the area
- any signs and symptoms felt by the patient/ observed by the practitioner
- interventions performed (step by step)
- photographs if ordered
- any referrals to plastic surgeons
- follow-up/further action taken
- date, time and signature of practitioner.

References

1. Dougherty L, Lister S. The Royal Marsden manual of clinical nursing procedures. 6th edn. Oxford: Blackwell Science; 2004.
2. Tully JL, Friedland GH, Baldrini LM, et al. Complications of intravenous therapy with steel needles and teflon catheters: a comparative study. Am J Med 1981; 70:702–706.
3. How C, Brown J. Extavasation of cytotoxic chemotherapy from peripheral veins. Eur J Oncol Nurs 1998; 2(1):51–58.
4. Anderson KN, Anderson LE (eds). Mosby's pocket dictionary of nursing, medicine and professions allied to medicine. 1995 UK edition. London: Mosby.
5. Perucca R. Obtaining vascular access. In: Hankin J, Lonsway RAW, Hedrick C, et al., eds. Infusion therapy in clinical practice. 2nd edn. Philadelphia: WB Saunders; 2001:338–397.
6. Perdue L. Intravenous complications. In: Hankin J, Lonsway RAW, Hedrick C, et al., eds. Infusion therapy in clinical practice. 2nd edn. Philadelphia: WB Saunders; 2001:418–445.
7. Oncology Nursing Society. Cancer chemotherapy guidelines and recommendations for practice. Pittsburgh: Oncology Nursing Press; 1999.
8. Homer LD, Holmes KR. Risks associated with 72 and 96 hour peripheral IV catheter dwell times. J Intraven Nurs 1998; 21(5):301–305.
9. Hadaway L. Peripheral IV therapy in adults. Self study workbook. Georgia: Hadaway Associates, 2000.
10. Intravenous Nursing Society (INS). Standards for infusion therapy. INS and BD USA, 2000.
11. Taylor MJ. A fascination with phlebitis. JVAD 2000; 5(3):24–28.
12. Royal College of Nursing Guidance for Nurses giving intravenous therapy. London: RCN; 1999.
13. Springhouse Corporation. Handbook of infusion therapy. Pennsylvania: Springhouse; 1999.
14. Carlson KR. Correct utilisation and management of peripherally inserted central catheters and midline catheters in the alternate care setting. J Intraven Nurs 1999; 22(6S):S46–S50.
15. Goetz AM, Miller J, Wagener MM, et al. Complications related to intravenous midline catheter usage. J Intravenous Nurs 1998; 21(2):76–80.
16. Weinstein SM. Antineoplastic therapy in Plumers principles and practice of IV therapy. 7th edn. Philadelphia: JB Lippincott; 2000.
17. Banton J, Leahy Gross K. Assessing catheter performance – 4 years of tracking patient outcomes of midline, midclavicular and PICC line program. J Vasc Access Devices 1998; 3(3)19–25.
18. Frey AM. IV therapy in children. In: Hankin J, Lonsway RAW, Hedrick C, et al., eds. Infusion therapy in clinical practice. 2nd edn. Pennsylvania: WB Saunders; 2001:561–591.
19. Goodwin M, Carlson I. The peripherally inserted catheter: a retrospective look at 3 years of insertions. J Intraven Nurs 1993; 16(2)92–103.
20. Gabriel J. 1999 Long term venous access. In: Dougherty L, Lamb J, eds. Intravenous therapy in nursing practice. Edinburgh: Churchill Livingstone; 1999.
21. Todd J. Peripherally inserted central catheters. Prof Nurse 1998; 13(5):297–302.
22. Macrae K. Hand held Doppler's in central catheter insertion. Prof Nurse 1998; 14(2):99–102.
23. Simcock L. The use of central venous catheters for IV therapy. Nurs Times 2001; 97(18):34–35.
24. Springhouse Corporation. Intravenous therapy made incredibly easy. Philadelphia: Lippincott, Williams & Wilkins; 2002.
25. Davidson T, Al Mufti R. Hickman central venous catheters in cancer patients. Cancer Topics 1997; 10(8):10–14.
26. Stacey RGW, Filshie J, Skewes D. Percutaneous insertion of Hickman type catheters. Br J Hospital Med 1991; 46:396–398.
27. Goodman M. In: Henke Yarbro C, Hanssen Frogge M, Goodman M, et al., eds. Chemotherapy: principles of administration cancer nursing. Boston: Jones and Bartlett; 2000:385–443.
28. Camp-Sorrell D. Implantable ports: everything you always wanted to know. J Intraven Nurs 1992; 15(5):262–273.
29. Camp-Sorrell D. Developing extravasation protocols and monitoring outcomes. J Intraven Nurs 1998; 21(4):232– 239.
30. Schulmeister L. A complication of vascular access device insertion. J Intraven Nurs 1998; 21(4):197–202.
31. Bow EJ, Kirkpatrick MG, Clinch JJ. Totally implantable venous access ports systems for patients receiving chemotherapy for solid tissue malignancies. J Clin Oncol 1999; 17(4)1267.
32. Schulmeister L, Camp-Sorrell D. Chemotherapy extravasation from implanted ports. Oncol Nurs Forum 2000; 27(3):531–560.
33. Dougherty L. Obtaining peripheral access. In: Dougherty L, Lamb J, eds. Intravenous therapy in nursing practice. Edinburgh: Churchill Livingstone; 1999.
34. Vandergrift KV. Oncologic therapy. In: Hankin J et al, eds. Infusion therapy in clinical practice. 2nd edn. Philadelphia: WB Saunders; 2001.
35. McCaffrey Boyle D, Engleking C. Vesicant extravasation: myths and realities. Oncol Nurs Forum 1995; 22(1):57–65.
36. Stanley A. Managing complication of chemotherapy. In: Allwood M, Stanley A, Wright P, eds. The cytotoxic handbook. 4th edn. Oxford: Radcliffe Medical Press, 2002.
37. Reymann PE. Chemotherapy: principles of administration in cancer nursing. In: Groenwald SL, Goodman M,

Frogge MH, et al, eds. Cancer nursing. Boston: Jones and Bartlett; 1993:293–330.

38. Eli Lilley. Cytotoxic chemotherapy. 5th edn. 1997.

39. Rittenberg CN, Gralla RJ, Rehmeyer TA. Assessing and managing venous irritation with vinorelbine tartrate. Oncol Nurs Forum 1995; 22(4):707–710.

40. Hecker J. Improved techniques in IV therapy. Nurs Times 1988; 84(34):28–33.

41. Curran CF, Luce JK. Extravasation doxorubicin from vascular access devices. Sel Cancer Ther 1991; 6:103–107.

42. Heckler FR. Current thoughts on extravasation injuries. Clin Plastic Surg 1989; 16(3):557–563.

43. Beason R. Antineoplastic vesicant extravasation. J Intraven Nurs 1990; 13(92):111–114.

44. Gault D, Challands J. Extravasation of drugs. Anaesth Rev 1997; 13:223–241.

45. CP Pharmaceuticals. How quickly could you act? Wrexham: CP Pharmaceuticals; 1999.

46. Cox K, Stuart-Harris RA, Addini G, et al. The management of cytotoxic drug extravasation: guidelines drawn up by a working party for the clinical oncological society of Australia. Med J Australia 1988; 148:185–189.

47. Doyle A. Oncologic therapy. In: Terry J, Baranowski L, Lonsway RA, et al, eds. Intravenous therapy: clinical principles and practices. Philadelphia: WB Saunders; 1995:249–274.

48. Banerjee A, Brotherson TM, Lamberty BGH, et al. Cancer chemotherapy agent induced perivenous extravasation injuries. Postgrad Med J 1987; 63:5–9.

49. Schulman R, Drayman S, Harries M, et al. Management of extravasation of IV drugs in CL injectable drug administration. Oxford: Blackwell Science; 1998.

50. Rudolph R, Larson DL. Etiology and treatment of chemotherapeutic agent extravasation injuries: a review. J Clin Oncol 1987; 5(7):1116–1126.

51. Montrose PA. Extravasation management. Semin Oncol Nurs 1987; 3(2):128–132.

52. Kara M, Ross DC. Severe soft tissue necrosis after extravasation of mitoxantrone case report. Can J Plastic Surg 1998; 6(4):204–206.

53. Gullo LS, Wood SM. IV vesicants: How to avoid extravasation. Am J Nurs 1993; April:42–45.

54. Mayo DJ. Fibrin sheath formation and chemotherapy extravasation: a case report. Support Care Cancer 1998; 6:51–56.

55. Bertolli G. Prevention and management of extravasation of cytotoxic drugs. Drug Safety 1995; 12(4):245–255.

56. Gault DT. Extravasation injuries. Br J Plastic Surg 1993; 46:91–96.

57. Dahlstrom KK, Chenoufi HL, Daugaard S. Fluorescence microscopic demonstration and demarcation of doxorubicin extravasation. Cancer 1990; 65:1722–1726.

58. Irving V. Managing extravasation injuries in preterm infants. Nurs Times Plus 2001; 97(35)40–46.

59. Nursing and Midwifery Council. Code of Professional Conduct. London: NMC; 2002.

Chapter **11**

Extravasation wounds: aetiology and management

Wayne Naylor

AETIOLOGY

The extravasation of a vesicant drug may cause severe tissue damage that results in the formation of a non-healing necrotic ulcer. This area of tissue damage may result in significant pain, cosmetic disfigurement, nerve damage, loss of function of a limb or even necessitate amputation.[1-3] Drugs commonly associated with severe tissue necrosis are dactinomycin, daunorubicin, doxorubicin, mitomycin C, vinblastine and vincristine.[4] Both paclitaxel (Taxol) and mitoxantrone (mitozantrone) have also been reported to cause considerable tissue damage should extravasation occur.[5,6] The most common sites of serious extravasation wounds are the dorsum of the hand, the forearm and the foot, as these areas have little soft tissue to protect underlying nerves and tendons.[7,8]

ULCER FORMATION

Generally, ulceration forms over a period of a few days to weeks, with maximal tissue damage evident after 2–3 weeks post extravasation.[9] Extravasation wounds may be complicated by tissue ischaemia related to endothelial damage and thrombosed vessels.[9] Ulcer formation is normally preceded by redness, swelling and superficial skin loss at the site of extravasation. This is followed by progressive induration and the development of a necrotic ulcer that may contain slough and/or dry black eschar (Fig. 11.1).[7] Ulcers may become wider and deeper over a period of weeks or months and involve underlying structures such as tendons and nerves.[3] Extravasation wounds resulting from DNA-binding drugs often show a lack of spontaneous healing that may be influenced by a reduced inflammatory response and deficiency in wound contraction.[6,8]

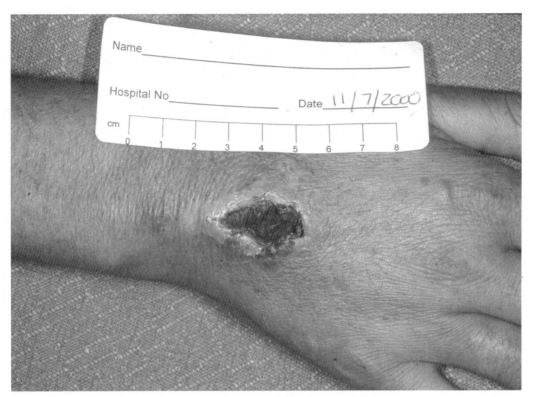

Figure 11.1 Extravasation wound showing black eschar.

TREATMENT

Following initial local treatment to remove or neutralise the extravasated drug, wound management should be guided by the characteristics of the wound. For partial- or full-thickness skin loss, a dressing that protects the wound and maintains a moist wound environment should be chosen. Examples include semi-permeable films (e.g. Tegaderm, Opsite Flexi-Grid), hydrocolloid sheets (e.g. Granuflex, Comfeel, Tegasorb) or hydrogel sheets (e.g. Geliperm, Hydrosorb, Novogel).[1,10] If slough or eschar is present in the wound, then this should be removed to encourage wound healing. This will also allow for better inspection of the wound and assessment of the extent of tissue damage.[11] Suggested methods of debridement are given in Table 11.1.

A more recent non-invasive method of managing extravasation wounds involves using a hydrogel (e.g. Granugel, Intrasite Gel, Nu-Gel) enclosed in a polythene bag with the affected limb being secured within the bag. This method has been particularly successful for injuries to the feet or hands of babies

and small children and should be instituted as soon as the injury occurs.[2,12]

Severe necrosis that is accompanied by continued pain indicates the need for surgical intervention and a referral to a plastic surgeon should be made.[3,7,8] The usual treatment is wide excision of all affected tissue, with the defect being repaired using a delayed split skin graft or flap.[9,12]

An integral part of managing any wound is documentation. Apart from documenting the circumstances surrounding the extravasation incident, a formal wound assessment should be undertaken if an ulcer develops. The assessment should document:

- the position and size of the wound
- the amount and type of tissue present
- the amount and type of exudate, odour, bleeding and pain
- the extent and spread of erythema.[1,12]

It may be useful to photograph the wound to track the course of the injury and evaluate the effectiveness of treatment.[1]

Table 11.1   Methods of wound debridement

Method	Description
Surgical debridement	This method of debridement is useful for deep necrosis and is performed under general anaesthetic by a skilled surgeon.
	Surgical debridement is considered the best method for the removal of necrotic tissue but may be unsuitable for patients who are unfit for anaesthesia.
Sharp debridement	Sharp debridement may be undertaken by a healthcare professional competent in this form of treatment.
	It is usually performed at the patient's bedside using scissors and scalpel. Useful for loose, superficial necrotic tissue only
Autolytic debridement	This is the body's natural debridement method for removing dead tissue and is suitable for wounds where surgical or sharp debridement is inappropriate.
	The autolytic process is enhanced by maintaining the wound in a moist environment. This may be achieved by the use of hydrogels (in both gel and sheet form) or occlusive dressings, such as hydrocolloids or semi-permeable films
Enzymatic debridement	This method is useful for wounds where autolytic debridement is proving ineffective.
	The most commonly used enzyme preparation in the UK is Varidase, which contains two enzymes, streptokinase and streptodornase, that break down necrotic tissue
Larval therapy	Also known as biosurgery, this method of debridement involves the application of fly larvae (maggots) to moist necrotic wounds.
	The larvae produce powerful enzymes that break down necrotic tissue and they also cleanse the wound of bacteria
Other treatment options	Sterile honey or sugar paste may be used to treat necrotic wounds as they will debride necrotic tissue and also destroy bacteria.
	Topical negative pressure assisted closure or vacuum therapy can be used on moist necrotic wounds where it will remove necrotic tissue and excess wound fluid. It may also reduce the bacterial load on the wound and encourage the formation of granulation tissue.

References

1. Stoios N. Prevention of extravasation in intravenous therapy: a review of the research evidence. Nuritinga 1999; 2. Online. Available: http://www.healthsci.utas.edu.au/nursing/nuritinga/vol2/stoios.html 21 November 2000.

2. Thomas S, Rowe HN, Keats J, et al. The management of extravasation injury in neonates World Wide Wounds 1997. Online. Available: http://www.worldwidewounds.com/1997/october/Neonates/NeonatePaper.html 21 August 2000.

3. Montrose PA. Extravasation management. Semin Oncol Nurs 1987; 3(2):128–132.

4. Ramu A. Compounds and methods that reduce the risk of extravasation injury associated with the use of vesicant antineoplastic agents. Baylor College of Medicine 1996. Online. Available: http://research.bcm.tmc.edu/OTA/techs/tech-96-30.html 21 November 2000.

5. Herrington JD, Figueroa JA. Severe necrosis due to paclitaxel extravasation: case report. Pharmacotherapy 1997; 17(1):163–165.

6. Kara M, Ross DC. Severe soft tissue necrosis after extravasation of mitoxantrone: case report. Can J Plastic Surg 1998; 6(4):204–206.

7. Murhammer JM. Management of intravenous extravasations. Virtual Hospital: P & T News, University of Iowa Health Care 1996. Online. Available: http://www.vh.org/Providers/Publications/PTNews/1996/12.96.PTN.html 24 November 2000.

8. Rudolph R, Larson DL. Etiology and treatment of chemotherapeutic agent extravasation injuries: a review. J Clin Oncol 1987; 5(7):1116–1126.

9. McCaffrey Boyle D, Engelking C. Vesicant extravasation: myths and realities. Oncol Nurs Forum 1995; 22(1):57–67.

10. Mulder GD, Haberer PA, Jeter KF. Clinicians pocket guide to chronic wound repair. Pennsylvania: Springhouse Corporation; 1999.

11. Naylor W, Laverty D, Mallett J. The Royal Marsden Hospital handbook of wound management in cancer care. Oxford: Blackwell Science; 2001.

12. Bale S, Jones V. Wound care nursing: a patient centred approach. London: Baillière Tindall; 1997.

Chapter **12**

Protracted venous infusion of chemotherapy (ambulatory chemotherapy)

Sally Legge

RATIONALE FOR PROTRACTED VENOUS INFUSION

Chemotherapy brings about tumour kill by interrupting the cell cycle and hence replication and tumour growth.[1] Chemotherapy agents are only active for a certain period of time following their administration as they are broken down and excreted. Many chemotherapy agents are cell cycle phase-specific, attacking the cell during a short period of the replication process. 5-Fluorouracil (5-FU), the most commonly used chemotherapy agent for protracted venous infusion, has a short half-life of only 10–20 min and is S-phase specific.[2] Therefore, either frequent or continuous administration increases the cells exposed to the chemotherapy during the active phase. Clinical trials have demonstrated that there is an increased tumour response in patients with colorectal cancer receiving protracted venous infusion (PVI) 5-FU (22%) in comparison to bolus administration (14%).[3] PVI 5-FU has been adopted, in combination with other chemotherapy, for the treatment of cancers such as ovarian and breast cancer. The aim of combining PVI 5-FU with other cytotoxic agents is to bring about a multi-phase attack on the cell cycle to increase tumour kill.

It has also been discovered that 5-FU acts as a radiosensitiser[4] and concomitant chemoradiation is now part of clinical trials for certain gastrointestinal cancers, e.g. rectal cancer.

Rationale for protracted venous infusion chemotherapy in the community

The duration of protracted venous infusion varies from 2 days to 4 days, given cyclically, or may be an infusion given continuously over a period of

3–6 months. It is therefore not desirable, practical or economical for patients to remain in hospital for such long periods. PVI chemotherapy also offers patients the opportunity to become fully involved in their own care and to return home or to work within a short period of time. Community support is available through district nurses, Macmillan nurses and general practitioners. Care of PVI chemotherapy on an outpatient basis has now become an accepted and established practice[5] and is employed by many centers.

PATIENT SELECTION CRITERIA

Patient selection for treatment should be a team decision between the doctor, nurse and patient. The medical evaluation of eligibility for treatment focuses on the histological type, stage and site of the disease and the patient's general health.[6] Two commonly used physical assessment tools are the World Health Organisation and the Karnofsky scales which measure the performance status (PS) of the patient (Table 12.1). The patient's performance status should preferably be 0, 1 or 2 to be able to receive this chemotherapy.

Also taken into account is the overall aim of the treatment, whether it is possible to cure the patient or at best provide palliation, and the patient's ability to withstand side-effects of the regimen. If the patient is offered the opportunity to take part in a clinical trial, further specific trial inclusion criteria has to be adhered to.

Patients receiving PVI chemotherapy need to be involved in their own care. Some self-care is an absolute necessity. Therefore, patient and family agreement to participate in care together with careful patient selection and assessment are essential.

Assessing the ability and suitability of the patient for PVI chemotherapy

It is generally the role of the nurse to evaluate the patient's cognitive skills, physical abilities and emotional state. When assessing a patient, consideration should be given to the various factors that influence learning ability and styles. Literacy, coping mechanisms, emotional state, anxiety, motivation, fatigue and culture all have an impact on learning.[7] Specifically, when assessing a patient for PVI chemotherapy, the ability to care for and manage a central venous access device (CVAD), ambulatory pump and potential side effects of the chemotherapy while at home must be included. Therefore, assessment of the patient should include:

- *Ability to manage the equipment:* dexterity is essential to ensure that the patient can use the equipment effectively and safely.
- *Ability to follow instructions:* reading abilities, sight and hearing and the ability to understand and follow written instructions.
- *The home environment:* the availability of a shower, bath or adequate washing facilities is necessary for good general hygiene. A telephone is necessary as this allows the patient to access immediate advice to cope with problems such as in the case of infection.
- *Home support:* support of family, friends and community services are an essential part of successful care.
- *The psychological status of the patient:* patients need to be motivated and willing to participate in their own care or have a partner, friend or relative who will assist with the necessary care.

Table 12.1 Karnofsky and WHO performance measures

Karnovsky condition	Scale	WHO Scale	Condition
Normal, no complaints	100	0	Normal activity
Able to carry on normal activity	90	1	Symptoms – normal activity
Cares for self. Unable to carry on normal active work	70	2	Symptomatic – spends some time in bed – less than 50% of the day
Requires considerable assistance and frequent medical care	50	3	Needs to be in bed more than 50% of the day
Severely disabled. Hospitalisation indicated	30	4	Unable to get out of bed
Dead	0	5	Dead

Sources: Karnofsky DA, Abelmann WH, Craver LF, et al. The use of the nitrogen mustards in palliative treatment of carcinoma. Cancer (Philad.) 1948; 1:634; WHO Handbook for Cancer Treatment. (1979) WHO offset Publication No. 48. Geneva: World Health Organisation; 1979.

Insertion of a vascular access device and receiving chemotherapy can be frightening; therefore, care and assessment should encompass both physical and psychological aspects. Including the patient and nominated family members or friends in the discussion when assessing the patient is important. The support of others may influence the level of self-care the patient can participate in. Often a particular friend or member of the family will be a key person who relates to the nurse.[8] Through this person, information and advice flow between family, patient and healthcare professional. Inclusion of family members or friends in teaching sessions can facilitate communication and learning. Families often learn together by interpreting and collating information and sharing experiences.[8]

Patient education programme

The patient and his family will need to learn and develop new skills to acquire a new language and new knowledge to cope with a PVI infusion of chemotherapy.[9] Education given on an individual basis will allow the patient's own special needs to be considered. The nurse educating the patient needs to be aware of and adapt to the patient's needs and preferred learning style.[10] Generally, patients have been shown to prefer interactive and one-to-one communication with printed material to support the information given.[10] A well-structured teaching programme will provide the patient with concise and relevant information. This will ensure that all the necessary areas of care are discussed with the patient. Visual aids, audio-taping and computer-assisted learning all contribute and have been found to be helpful in the patient's learning process.[11] Headings for a suggested teaching programme are given below.

Care of the central venous access device

- Explanation of CVAD placement
- Signs and symptoms of potential complications
- Management of the potential complications
- How to avoid complications
- Care of insertion sites
- Maintaining patency of the CVAD lumen(s).

Care of the ambulatory pump

- How the pump works
- Alarm facilities
- Battery reliability and change
- Troubleshooting
- Where to obtain further supplies of equipment.

Care of the chemotherapy

- Information about the chemotherapy regimen
- Renewing the chemotherapy reservoir bag
- Signs and symptoms of potential side effects
- Management of the potential side effects of chemotherapy.

Contact names and numbers

- Names and telephone numbers of the patient's nurse and medical team during working hours
- Names and telephone numbers of who to call for out-of-hours advice: i.e. a specific ward nurse in charge or the on-call doctor
- Where possible, name and telephone number of the patient's district nurse.

Anxiety can inhibit the ability to hear, understand and remember information. It is important to carefully select the time and environment of teaching sessions to try and reduce unnecessary stress from interruptions, noise and lack of privacy. Information needs to be repeated and re-enforced over a period of time during the patient's admission. (See also Ch. 5.)

Levels of self-care

The amount of self-care taken on by the patient should be discussed and agreed with the patient and his family. Below are three suggested levels of self-care for patients using a battery-operated pump such as a WalkMed 350.

Minimum level of self-care

- Able to clamp closed catheter lumens
- Able to turn off pump
- Understands and able to call hospital for advice immediately if side effects or complications occur.

Moderate level of self-care

- Above plus:
- Able to manage pump alarms (if appropriate)
- Able to check and carry out daily dressing to the insertion site following catheter placement.

Maximum level of self-care

- Above plus:
- Able to safely change chemotherapy reservoir bags
- Able to safely flush catheter lumens to maintain catheter lumens.

Whatever the level of care chosen and achieved, community support is crucial. A totally self-caring patient will still require initial supervision, whereas others will need regular advice and help. Therefore, it is essential to set up ongoing support from the community nurse and general practitioner (GP) prior to the patient's discharge. Telephone intervention from the nurse can help to improve adherence with treatment and limit the effect of any occurring problems.[11]

THE AMBULATORY PUMP

The choice of the ambulatory pump delivering small volumes of solution may differ from hospital to hospital. There are different types of pumps to choose from: mechanical battery-operated devices, totally implantable systems or disposable elastomeric pumps are available. The criteria for pump selection should include reliability, accuracy of delivery, simplicity of use, size and weight and also cost-effectiveness.[12] As these pumps are used in the community, it is important that they are reliable and require the minimum maintenance.[13] Whatever the device chosen, written information should be provided with respect to problem-solving for any alarm functions or faults in the pump. A 24-hour telephone advice line should be available for help in solving problems and reassuring the patient.[14]

VASCULAR ACCESS

Two types of vascular access devices are commonly used to administer a protracted infusion of chemotherapy: a skin-tunnelled catheter (STC) or a peripherally inserted central catheter (PICC) may be placed. Chapter 10 sets out the various intravenous routes, catheters available and the care needed. Ideally, the patient may be offered a choice of catheter placement; however, this is not always possible due to either resources or anatomical limitations. When selecting a vascular access route and device for PVI chemotherapy, certain criteria must be considered: i.e. infection risk, the security of placement, irritation to a vein from a continuous infusion and simplicity of care of the device.

Peripherally inserted central catheter

PICCs require a weekly change of dressing[15] and will require a bandage to reduce the risk of catching the extension tube on clothing. When bathing, the PICC exit site needs to be kept dry by covering the area with a waterproof wrap. For the patient, dressing the PICC can be difficult with only one hand. The help of a district nurse, relative or friend may be needed. The exit site should be examined regularly when the dressing is changed to check for any signs of complications.[15] The patient, family and district nurse will need specific advice regarding the flushing solution and frequency necessary to maintain catheter patency.

Skin-tunnelled catheter

A common site for an STC to exit the skin is either mid chest or mid abdomen – the latter for a CVAD placed in the femoral vein, which allows the patient to have both hands free and to be able to see the exit site. This allows the patient to change his own dressing, which is usually weekly if a transparent dressing is used. Sutures placed at the entry site and exit site are removed at 7 and 21 days, respectively, after which dressings are no longer required. The two recommended dressings are either a transparent dressing, e.g. Opsite IV 3000, to be changed every 5–7 days, or sterile gauze changed daily.[15,16] Patients may allow the exit site to get wet in a shower, being diligent to ensure that the wound sites are dried well with a clean towel. A chlorhexidine solution in 70% alcohol has been shown to be the preferred cleaning solution for the STC exit site. There is some discussion as to the flushing solution to be used and frequency of flushing.[17] Lumens not in constant use need to be flushed. The lumen receiving the PVI chemotherapy does not require weekly flushing. (See also Ch. 10.)

Management of and signs and symptoms of potential catheter complications

To ensure that best care is given, patients who are participating in self-care will need to know and be able to recognise the signs and symptoms of catheter complications. Knowledge has been shown to affect the experience of the patients with cancer by creating a sense of control.[18] It is important that patients understand the reason for reporting these symptoms immediately to their medical team. In particular, patients receiving immunosuppressive chemotherapy will be at great risk of septicaemia, which can, if not treated promptly, be fatal. Although knowledge is not a guarantee to best self-care behaviour, it is not at all possible without the correct knowledge.[19] Table 12.2 lists the possible problems and action needed for care of CVADs. (See also Ch. 10.)

CHEMOTHERAPY AGENTS

Spillage

As mentioned previously, the most commonly used chemotherapy agent is 5-FU. However, other agents

Table 12.2   Problems and action needed for the care of CVADs

Problems	Signs and symptoms	Action plan
Skin infection at the insertion sites	Redness, swelling, pain or discharge from the site	Swab discharge. Check patient's temperature Report to doctor. Oral or intravenous antibiotics may be necessary
PICCs only – phlebitis or mechanical irritation commonly happens with 24–48 hours or within 1 week of insertion	Redness, swelling and pain occurring at the insertion site or along the route of a PICC	Apply warmth to the area. Assess over next 72 hours: if not resolved, remove catheter
Systemic infection	Rigor with or without fever (38°C). May occur shortly after flushing of the catheter	Take cultures – centrally from catheter and peripherally from insertion site. Refer to doctor. Intravenous antibiotics and likely removal of catheter
Superior vena cava, subclavian or axillary vein thrombosis	Pain, generalised swelling, redness and warmth is located in the shoulder, neck or arm on the side of the catheter insertion	Refer to doctor for Doppler ultrasound to confirm diagnosis. Anticoagulation therapy needed and possible removal of catheter
Displacement of or damage to catheter	Localised swelling, pain and possible difficulties with infusion or flushing of the catheter. Increased length of catheter at insertion site, no blood return.	Refer to doctor for possible X-ray to check catheter integrity using radio-opaque dye
Occlusion of catheter lumen	Difficulty flushing catheter, no blood return	Ascertain cause of occlusion. If occluded by a drug seek further advice. If thrombotic, normal saline using a 10 ml syringe may clear the blockage either by using a gentle push-pull technique or a negative pressure method with a 3-way tap. Otherwise, instillation of a fibrinolytic agent may help.

such as vincristine and doxorubicin (both vesicants) may also be used. Whatever the agent used, it is important that all care is taken to reduce the risk of spillage, particularly if the agent is a vesicant. Information and advice should be given to the patient with respect to what to do in these circumstances, according to local policy. The Royal College of Nursing Clinical Practice Guidelines (1998) provide general procedures for dealing with spillage.[20]

Management of and signs and symptoms of chemotherapy side effects

5-Fluorouracil may cause stomatitis, diarrhoea and planta-palmer erythema (PPE), the most common side effects,[21] or nausea, hair thinning and coronary artery spasm, which are less likely. Side effects and chemotherapy toxicities are covered in Section 2. These side effects may occur at any time during the infusion. If action is taken promptly, the side effects can be controlled and limited. If it is not possible to resolve or maintain the degree of the side effects the patient will be advised to discontinue with the 5-FU infusion, for approximately 7 days, until the adverse effects have resolved. The infusion may then be recommenced at a newly prescribed adjusted dose. Vincristine and doxorubicin will cause bone marrow suppression, hair loss, nausea and vomiting, discoloured red urine and less commonly peripheral neuropathy. Nurses are in an ideal position to ensure that the patient's experience of chemotherapy is not fraught with discomfort and difficulty.[22] Good patient assessment, education, home support and access to medical advice ensure that the best care is available to the patient. Prompt reporting of problems will limit the overall effect, discomfort and anxiety to the patient and family.

DISCHARGE PLANNING

Before leaving hospital, plans and decisions should be made about how patient needs can be met.[23] Discharge planning and follow-up care are crucial to the success of ambulatory chemotherapy for the patient and family. As suggested earlier, full patient and family involvement should be encouraged at the introduction of the chemotherapy regimen in outpatients.

A multidisciplinary approach should be taken, including an assessment of the patient's and carer's needs and the resources required, and clearly defined areas of responsibilities should be agreed.[24] Once the patient's chemotherapy regimen has been chosen, contact should be made with the district nurse to ascertain she is able to support the patient in the community. Full and detailed patient information should be provided as soon as possible to the district nurse, together with any additional specific information required: e.g. chemotherapy agents, their side effects and management. Further support may be offered to the district nurse in the form of a visit to the hospital or for the specialist hospital nurse to visit the community to provide further education. Contact names and telephone numbers should also be provided. Below is a suggested list of information and equipment to be sent out to the community with the patient:

- A detailed discharge letter to the district nurse, stating the dose, rate and name of drug infusion; potential side effects of chemotherapy agents; care of the venous access device and potential complications; contact names and telephone numbers of in and out-of-hours advice; and advice in case of spillage
- A letter or discharge summary to the GP from the hospital nurse, advising the GP immediately that the patient is at home and has commenced PVI chemotherapy via a central venous access, and contact telephone names and numbers. A more detailed discharge summary should be sent out from the medical team.
- Dressings for central venous access insertion, as needed.
- Equipment to flush the central venous device, as needed.
- Sharps box.
- Medications.

Discharge planning should be an integral part of care, as it can have a profound impact on the patient's treatment outcome and experience.[25]

References

1. Wilkies G. Potential toxicities and nursing management. In: Burke MB, Wilkes GM, Ingwersen K, et al., eds. Cancer chemotherapy a nursing process approach. 2nd edn. Boston, Massachusetts: Jones & Bartlett; 1996:97–185.

2. Algren J. Principles of chemotherapy in gastrointestinal cancer In: Ahlgren JD, Macdonald JS, eds. Gastrointestinal oncology. Philadelphia: Lippincott; 1992:39–49.

3. Hansen RM, Ryan L, Anderson T, et al. Phase III study of bolus versus infusional fluorouracil with or without cisplatin in advanced colorectal cancer. J Natl Cancer Inst 1996; 88:668–674.

4. Algren C, Grem J. Antimetabolities. In: DeVita VT Jr, Hellman S, Rosenberg SA, eds. Cancer: principles and practice of oncology. 5th edn. Philadelphia: Lippencott-Raven; 1997:437–452.

5. Nightingale C, Norman A, Cunningham D, et al. A prospective analysis of 949 long-term central venous access catheters for ambulatory chemotherapy in patients with gastrointestinal malignancy. Eur J Cancer 1996; 33(3):398–403.

6. Garvey E, Kramer R. Improving cancer patients adjustments to infusion chemotherapy: evaluation of a patient education program. Cancer Nurs 1983; Oct:373–378.

7. Treacy JT, Mayer DK. Perspectives on cancer patient education. Semin Oncol Nurs 2002; 16:47–56.

8. Friesen P, Pepler C, Hunter P. Interactive family learning following a cancer diagnosis. Oncol Nurs Forum 2002; 29(6):981–987.

9. Chrystal C. Administering continuous vesicant chemotherapy in the ambulatory setting. J Intraven Nurs 1997; 20(2):78–88.

10. Chelf JH, Deshler AMB, Kay MSW, et al. Learning and support preferences of adult patients with cancer at a comprehensive cancer centre. Oncol Nurs Forum 2002; 29(5):863–867.

11. Chelf JH, Agre P, Axelrod A, et al. Cancer-related patient evaluation: an overview of the last decade of evaluation and research. Oncol Nurs Forum 2002; 28(7):113–1147.

12. Woolens. Infusion devices for ambulatory use. Prof Nurse 1996; 11(10):689–695.

13. Dolan S. Intravenous flow control and infusion devices. In: Dougherty L, Lamb J, eds. Intravenous therapy in nursing practice. Edinburgh: Churchill Livingstone; 1999:195–222.

14. Daehler MA, DeCicco C, Frey AM, et al. Antineoplastic therapy. In: Weinstein S, ed. Plumer's principles and practice of intravenous therapy, 7th edn. Philadelphia: Lippencott; 2000:474–560.

15. Young GP, Alexeyeff M, Russell DR. Catheter sepsis during parenteral nutrition: the safety of long-term opsite dressings. J Parenteral Enteral Nutr 1998; 12(4):365–370.

16. Cook J. Central venous catheters: preventing infection and occlusion. Br J Nurs 1999; 3(15):981–988.

17. Masoorli S. Cost containment program for IV Nursing. Paper presented at 7th NAVAN Conference, Washington, DC, 1993.

18. Fieler VK, Wlasowicz GS, Mitchell ML, et al. Information preferences of patients undergoing radiation therapy. Oncol Nurs Forum 1996; 23:1603–1608.

19. Dodd MJ. Self-care: ready or not. Oncol Nurs Forum 1997; 24(6):983–990.

20. Royal College of Nursing (RNC). Clinical Practice Guidelines: the administration of cytotoxic chemotherapy (recommendations and technical report). Harrow: Nursing Standard Publications; 1998.

21. Miller S. Stomatitis and oesophagitis. In: Yasko J, ed. Nursing management of symptoms associated with chemotherapy. 4th edn. Bala Cynwyd: Meniscus Health Care Communications; 1998:63-76.

22. Tange A, Evers G, Paridaens R. Nurses's assessments of symptom occurrence and symptom distress in chemotherapy patients. Eur J Oncol Nurs 1998:14–16.

23. Department of Health. The patient's charter. London: Stationary Office; 1995.

24. Bristow O, Stickney C, Thompson S. Discharge planning for continuity of care. No. 21-1604. New York: National League of Nursing; 1986.

25. Mallet J, Dougherty L. Discharge planning. In: The Royal Marsden Hospital manual of clinical nursing procedures. 5th Ed. Oxford: Blackwell Science; 2000:200–206.

Chapter **13**

Infection control

Sarah Hart

CHAPTER CONTENTS

INTRODUCTION

Patients with cancer have an increased risk of infection;[1] the degree of risk depends on the clinical manifestations of the cancer,[2] as well as the chemotherapy or radiotherapy that is given to treat the cancer. Infection remains of major concern in the management of patients with haematological malignancies such as lymphoma, leukaemia and myeloma. These patients will develop direct damage to the bone marrow by the abnormal cancer cells, which will result in cellular and humoral immune deficiency.[3] This risk will be increased as the treatment of haematological malignancies inevitably affects replicating bone marrow progenitor cells,[4] as well as the malignant cells. This damage will increase the patient's risk of infection.[5]

For patients with solid tumours such as lung, pancreas and bowel, risk of infection is directly attributed to the presenting signs and symptoms of the solid tumour. For example, obstruction of bronchial tree, urinary, alimentary or biliary tract, or damage to anatomical barriers such as skin and mucosal membranes, which damage the body's natural defence against infection.[6] The treatment for solid tumours is generally not as severe or as prolonged as in patients with haematological malignancies. Therefore, the risk is directly related to the underlying malignancy, the severity of the impairment to the patient's immune defence mechanisms and the combination of surgical techniques, radiotherapy and chemotherapy that is used to treat the solid tumour.[6]

The spectrum of infection occurring in cancer patients will differ from general hospitalised patients, with infections such as cytomegalovirus, *Pneumocystis carinii* and aspergillosis being of increased risk. These infections, coupled with the classic pathogens known to cause infections in hospitalised patients, means that constant observations for the first signs of infection, prompt medical evaluation and early commencement of antimicrobial therapy are essential if signs and symptoms are present that suggest infection has occurred.

Healthcare associated infection

Approximately 9% of inpatients acquire an infection during their hospital stay that was neither present nor incubating when the patient entered hospital. Such infections are termed healthcare associated infection (HAI).[7] This is the equivalent to at least 100 000 infections in 1 year. Studies identifying rates of infection in neutropenic patients found that the overall rate was 48.3 per 100 neutropenic patients, or 46.3 per 1000 days at risk. Bloodstream infections were found to be the most common infection, at 13.5 per 100 neutropenic patients.[8] Healthcare associated bacteraemia rates varied between specialties, the highest rates occurring in general intensive care and the haematology wards. A surveillance of healthcare associated bacteraemia found that central lines caused 31% and peripheral lines 7% of all bacteraemias.[9]

Inpatients with HAI incur costs 2.9 times greater than those without infection. Similarly, following discharge from hospital, patients with HAI make more visits to their general practitioner than uninfected patients do.[10] Treating catheter-related infections has been particularly associated with a profound increase in resource use.[11]

It has been suggested that as many as 30% of all HAI can be prevented through effective infection control measures,[12] although a 10% reduction is a more achievable figure.[10] This 10% reduction in the national observed incidence rate would still release resources valued at £93.06 million. The Department of Health[7] acknowledges that some patients die each year as a result of HAI. Although many of these deaths occur in patients already dying from other causes and/or in patients whose infections were not preventable, a proportion of these deaths are avoidable. It has been estimated that as many as 5000 inpatients die as a direct result of HAI, with HAI a substantial contributing factor in a further 15 000 deaths.[13]

IMMUNOCOMPROMISED PATIENTS

The risk of patients acquiring an infection is influenced by their susceptibility to infection. Although neutropenia is significantly associated with chemotherapy, other factors that need to be taken into considerations include:

- age, with the very young and old having an increased risk of infection due to their maturing or waning immunity
- other diseases affecting the immune system
- invasive procedures
- presence of a medical device
- length of stay in hospital.[13]

Besides surgery, cancer treatments often involve invasive procedures and the use of medical devices – these may be urinary catheters, feeding or tracheotomy tubes. However, the most common invasive procedure and device will be related to phlebotomy and intravenous (IV) therapy. Wilkinson[14] suggested that between 18% and 80% of general hospital admissions would require IV intervention. Elliott[15] estimated that as many as 200 000 central venous catheters were used annually in the United Kingdom.

Immunocompromised patients can become infected with pathogens that can infect people with a normal immune response, as well as from opportunist microorganisms that usually do not cause disease in a healthy person. It is important to undertake a risk assessment to evaluate the immune status of a patient prior to and during cancer therapy and therefore the risk of the patient acquiring an infection. The risk assessment would, for example, evaluate the extent of mucositis or diarrhoea, or the presence of pressure sores or skin lesions, which increase the risk of acquiring an infection. Risk assessments ensure that practical measures can be adopted to reduce the likelihood of infection. An example of a risk of infection assessment is shown in Table 13.1.[16]

SOURCES OF INFECTION

Endogenous and exogenous infection

The source of infection may be from endogenous infection (originating from or within the body) or

Table 13.1   Risk assessment for chemotherapy

Activity/hazard	Examples of associated hazards	Associated assessments & procedures to reduce risk	Likelyhood of injury rating 1 = Improbable 2 = Remote 3 = Possible 4 = Probable 5 = Certain	Severity rating 1 = Negligible 2 = Minor 3 = Major 4 = Permanent 5 = Fatal	Risk rating number (F × S)
Neutropenia. Risk of infection	• Invasive procedures, i.e. IV devices • Mucositis • Diarrhoea • Existing medical conditions, i.e. diabetes, dental, caries, pressure sores • Infected or colonized with resistant microorganisms, i.e. MRSA., VRE	• Compliance with: Infection control policies Nursing procedure manual Antibiotic policy • Handwashing before and after patient care • Maintain high standard of patients' personal hygiene • Close observation • Specialist medical and nursing support • Protective isolation facilities • Barrier nursing of infected patients • Use of aseptic technique • Maintain clean environment • Provision of a clean diet • Safe use of medical devices • Educated, informed patients and visitors	3	5	15

exogenous infection (originating from outside the body). Exogenous infections can be caused by intrinsic (bacteria present in a medical device, for example) or extrinsic contamination (originating from outside – e.g. hands of the healthcare worker).

Endogenous infection can be due to transfer of microorganisms:

• From one area of the patient's body where they are causing infection, e.g. a wound infection.
• From the person's normal flora. For example, *Staphylococcus aureus* can colonise a person's nose without causing any symptoms of infection, but can cause infection in other areas, e.g. an IV catheter entry site.

It has been estimated that 40–60% of microorganisms responsible for infection originate from the patient's endogenous flora.[17]

Exogenous infection implies cross-infection, and involves microorganisms that originate outside the patient's body. Exogenous infection may be caused by:

• unclean equipment
• the environment or
• microorganisms transferred from other patients, visitors or staff.

Microorganisms can be passed by direct or indirect contact or the airborne route. It has been estimated that 20–40% of infections are due to cross-infection.[17]

Intrinsic and extrinsic contamination

Intrinsic contamination occurs prior to the use of equipment and can be present in items such as medical devices, infusion fluids, IV administration equipment, dressings, lotions or creams. Contamination may be due to faulty manufacture, despite the extremely high standard of production. It is essential that all equipment used during invasive procedures, such as IV fluids and drugs, are sterile, non-pyrogenic and particle-free.[18] Contamination can also occur following damage to the packaging, due to poor packaging, poor transport and poor storage, as the packaging maintains the cleanliness or sterility of the equipment. All equipment must be stored safely to comply with recommendations in the Health Technical Memorandum 71.[19] All adverse incidents involving medical devices that cause unexpected or unwanted effects involving the safety of patients, users or other persons have to be reported to the Medical Devices Agency.[20]

Extrinsic contamination can occur at any time during an invasive procedure. Within IV therapy, this may be during insertion, use or removal of the IV device and the infusion equipment. It is generally as a result of poor practice, e.g. during catheter manipulation or preparation and administration of infusates.[21] Frequent manipulation of the catheter increases the risk of catheter infections.[22] Prevention includes thorough handwashing before and after each patient contact, appropriate preparation of the insertion site, careful preparation and administration of infusates and the use of an aseptic technique.[23] The expertise and practices of the person involved in providing care[22] can also be a risk factor for contamination, and adequate training must be provided.[24]

ROUTES OF INTRAVENOUS CATHETER INFECTION

Extraluminal, intraluminal and haematogenous seeding routes of infection

Most cytotoxic drugs are given via the IV route, and IV devices are the most commonly used invasive medical device and are essential in the management of patients with cancer.[25] Due to the invasive nature and frequency of use, IV catheters are associated with significant patient mortality and morbidity.[26]

There are three main routes by which microorganisms gain entry and cause infection. These are:

- extraluminal
- intraluminal
- haematogenous seeding.

Extraluminal catheter-related infection is caused either by microorganisms that contaminate the outside of the catheter during insertion or migrate along the catheter tract. These microorganisms may originate from:

- patient skin that contaminates the catheter during insertion
- contaminated dressing covering the insertion site
- contamination of the intravenous devices and equipment hub (entry ports) during use from the

hands of the healthcare worker, patient or the environment.

Studies suggest that skin and hub colonisation are the major determinants for catheter-related infections.[27] A positive skin microbiology culture is useful for assessing catheter colonisation.[28]

Intraluminal catheter-related infection is caused by microorganisms migrating down the inside of the catheter. This may be from contaminated infusate, injections or the intravenous device entry points, e.g. the catheter hub.[29]

Haematogenous seeding is contamination of the catheter from microorganisms from another site carried to the catheter by blood. An example is bacterial translocation from the gastrointestinal tract via the blood, causing systemic dissemination of microorganisms.[30]

Indirect, direct and airborne transmission of infection

Immunocompromised patients are at increased risk of acquiring infection. Although some endogenous infections cannot be avoided, exogenous infections can be avoided.

Microorganisms can be transmitted in hospital by several routes, and consideration has to be made on how to prevent their spread. The routes are as follows:

- Indirect contact involves the patient coming into contact with contaminated equipment or the environment.
- Direct contact involves direct body surface to body surface contact, which allows the physical transfer of microorganisms between patients or between patients and healthcare workers.
- Airborne transmission of microorganisms can occur between one patient and another, or from one site to another site of the same patient. An example includes methicillin-resistant *Staphylococcus aureus* (MRSA),[31] which can colonise the environment[32] and be transferred during procedures such as bedmaking[33] and drawing the bedside curtains.[34]

Indirect contact can be significantly reduced by:

- Handwashing before and after patient contact.
- Use of an aseptic technique.
- Correct use of single-use disposable equipment such as syringes, needles and dressings. Single-use equipment should never be reused.[35]
- Careful cleaning of equipment before being used on another patient. General equipment such as tourniquets or monitoring devices while not needing to be sterile, must be clean. Scissors or instruments for sterile procedures must be clean and sterile.[36]

- Maintaining a clean environment to prevent contamination, e.g. dirty handwash basins and baths contaminating staff, the patient or any invasive device.

Direct contact can be significantly reduced by:

- Careful handwashing before and after patient contact.[23,37]
- Use of an aseptic technique.[24]
- High standard of patient's personal hygiene. In particular, handwashing after going to the toilet and before meals.

Airborne transmission of microorganisms can be reduced by:

- clean well-maintained environment[38]
- the use of filtered air conditioning[39]
- adequate supplies of clean equipment such as linen
- careful bagging and removal of used linen and waste.

MRSA, for example, is a major cause of bacteraemia[9] and wound infections[40] and has the ability to survive for long periods in the environment[41] and on sterile goods packaging.[42] MRSA can be transferred by the direct route, the indirect route and the airborne route.

PROTECTIVE ISOLATION

Historical perspectives

High-dose chemotherapy regimens, in particular pre-transplant conditioning therapy, causes severe immunosuppression. Prevention of infection during this time is essential. Traditionally, protective isolation has been used to eliminate sources of infection to protect the patient during this time, so increasing the chances of recovery.[43]

Controversy continues, related to the degree of protection necessary for immunocompromised patients. The Centers for Disease Control and Protection (USA)[44] suggested that patients highly susceptible to infection require special attention, to reduce the risk of infection. However, they stated that protective isolation would not prevent endogenous infections, which were the most common infection amongst immunocompromised patients, stressing that such patients should be cared for using:

- routine good patient care techniques
- single room accommodation
- segregation from infected patients
- compliance to handwashing policies.

In the 1970s and 1980s many researchers undertook trials attempting to evaluate protective isolation. It was suggested that although protective isolation

seemed to reduce the incidence of bacterial infection,[45] long-term survival was not improved. The exception to this was in the cases of patients with aplastic anaemia, who received their bone marrow transplantation in protective isolation and were seen to develop less graft versus host disease (GvHD).[46] (See Ch. 62.)

Poe and colleagues[47] surveyed 91 bone marrow transplant units and found that all units used some type of protective environment, although wide variations were found. They concluded that national standards were required.

Currently, the increase in transplantation with peripheral blood cells, which has significantly reduced the neutropenic period following transplantation, is an effective measure for prevention of severe infections associated with prolonged neutropenia.[48] A study involving bone marrow transplant patients who were allowed out of their single rooms to go home found that patients continued on dietary restrictions and antibiotic prophylaxis, and that infection rates compared favorably with strict isolation care. These researchers concluded that in some institutions bone marrow transplantation may be safely completed without the patient being continuously confined in hospital.[49]

Levels of protective isolation

Infection remains the most significant complication for patients with haemato-oncology malignancies during high-dose chemotherapy regimens. The risks persist once the patient has been discharged from hospital and can continue for most patients for as long as 1 year, but for those with GvHD it can continue for longer.[50,51]

It is known that the period of neutropenia following peripheral blood stem cell transplantation is shorter than that following bone marrow transplantation; however, this has little effect on the incidence and mortality of infections.[51] It is therefore important that the healthcare workers, the patients and their carers adopt practices that reduce the risk of infection. Protective isolation is designed to prevent transmission of microorganisms. Emphasis is on cleanliness and handwashing.

The British Clinical Haematology Task Force[52] defined four levels of care required for the management of adult patients with haematological malignancies. These are given in Table 13.2.

Such care requires increased specialist expertise, staffing levels and resources. Resources include equipment, laboratory and radiotherapy facilities, pharmacy, support services, research and suitable ward provision and bed numbers. Emphasis is placed on suitably trained, experienced staff who have access to a clinical nurse specialist and single room accommodation for neutropenic patients.

Table 13.2   Haematology patient levels

Level of care	Type of patient and therapy	Type of accommodation
Level 1	General haematology patients, i.e. chronic leukaemia, multiple myeloma	Flexible number of specific haematology beds available on a general medical ward, with one room for neutropenic patients
Level 2	Remission induction in acute myeloid and lymphoblastic leukaemia	Specific haematology beds with a number of singles with ensuite facilities
Level 3	Peripheral stem cell and bone marrow autologous transplants	Specific haematology beds with a number of singles with ensuite facilities in a unit that performs at least 10 transplants a year to maintain expertise
Level 4	Related allogeneic bone marrow transplants and autologous transplants using total body irradiation	Single rooms with ensuite facilities, preferably with positive pressure filtered air, and a designated kitchen area

The Croner's Health Service Risks Management and Practice special report[53] supports the view that special arrangements are required for patients susceptible to infection, suggesting that single room, ensuite toilet facilities with air flow under positive pressure are required.

As gaps exist in the knowledge related to the value of protective isolation, differences in opinion do occur. However, certain issues related to neutropenic patients' care have been reviewed: for example, Pattison[54] reviewed the provision of clean food for neutropenic patients in the UK and found wide variation in practice, with little documented evidence on the use and effectiveness of clean diets, with a move away from stringent sterile diet towards a more relaxed well-cooked diet. Smith and Besser[55] reviewed dietary restrictions in 156 American centres and found similar differences in practices and suggested that nursing protocols for neutropenic dietary restrictions should be based on research findings.

Research has explored patients' feelings following protective isolation. The four main concerns were 'being shut in', 'coping with the experience', 'being alone', and 'maintaining contact with the outside world'. All patients did not enjoy the experience but accepted the importance of the restrictions.[56] A small sample of patients undergoing autologous bone marrow transplant found that levels of anxiety were higher before admission to hospital than during or after discharge from hospital.[57] Studies that interviewed patients 12 months after bone marrow transplantation found that they perceived their physical and psychosocial functioning as rather good.[58] Provision of written and individualised information, improved communication and better facilities to relieve boredom may help in reducing or preventing negative feelings to isolation[59] as well as family and friends receiving more guidance on ways to provide support to patients in

isolation.[60] It has been suggested that nurses need to take more initiative to gain insight and a greater understanding of the patient's illness and treatment.[61]

INFECTION ASSOCIATED WITH INTRAVENOUS DEVICES

Infection has been identified as a potentially life-threatening complication of IV therapy[62] and is especially a risk for those patients treated with aggressive chemotherapy.[48] Surveillance of hospital-acquired bacteraemias found that central IV catheters were the commonest source of infection.[9]

Catheter-related infections

Complications from catheter-related infections include:

- phlebitis
- entry-site infection
- tunnel infection
- bloodstream infection
- endocarditis.[63]

Organisms associated with IV devices include:

- *Staphylococcus* spp.
- enterococci
- *Candida* spp.[63]

Infection from Gram-negative bacteria

Gram-negative microorganisms such as *Klebsiella* spp., *Enterobacter* spp., *Serratia* and *Pseudomonas aeruginosa* can survive and multiply in water and dirt, contaminating hands as well as moist areas of the hospital environment such as drains and cracked surfaces of baths and sinks. These organisms can cause both intrinsic and extrinsic contamination. Cleaning and drying of the environment and equipment, plus correct disinfection and sterilisation of IV equipment, can reduce bacterial contamination.

Infection from Gram-positive bacteria

Staphylococcus epidermidis followed by *S. aureus* are the most frequently isolated microorganisms involved in catheter-related infection.[63] Similarly, *S. aureus* followed by *S. epidermidis* are the major causes of hospital-acquired bacteraemia.[9]

Gram-positive organisms such as *S. aureus* and *S. epidermidis* can survive drying and can be spread by unwashed hands and airborne transmission in dust. These organisms are the major causes of extrinsic contamination. Careful cleaning of the environment with the use of damp dusting and vacuum cleaning methods can reduce the risk of contamination. However, the most important aspect of the prevention of contamination of IV devices is thorough handwashing before and after patient contact.

DIAGNOSIS OF INFECTION

Early recognition of infection, rapid detection of the causative microorganisms and prompt initiation of appropriate therapy are essential.[64] Rigors following the use of a catheter are highly suggestive of a catheter-related infection. Early recognition and treatment of infection improves outcomes.

Catheter insertion sites should be observed at least daily for signs of infection.[63] Clinical signs and symptoms of infections should be carefully evaluated.

Catheter-related infection can be divided into:

- localised infection evidenced by fever, pain, tenderness, oedema and cellulitis at the site or along the subclavian tunnel
- systemic infection that is not limited to a particular site and includes bacteraemia and septicaemia, chills, fever, headaches, tremors, nausea, vomiting, abdominal pain, hyperventilation and shock.

Clinical detection of catheter-related infections may be difficult but should always be suspected when there are signs and symptoms of infection that cannot be contributed to another cause.

Attempts should be made to make a microbiological diagnosis when infection is suspected.[63] For catheter site infections, microbiology swabs should be obtained for culture and sensitivity testing. For catheter infections, blood cultures should be taken from a separate peripheral vein and from the catheter, and the results compared. If blood cultures from the catheter are positive and the peripheral vein cultures are negative, or if the catheter blood cultures have a significant increase in bacterial colonies compared

with the peripheral vein blood cultures, this suggests a catheter-associated infection.[64]

Catheter-related infections often require the removal of the catheter. The tip of the catheter should be aseptically cut off and sent to microbiology for culture and sensitivities.[65] Tip line cultures provide valuable information, especially when taken in conjunction with blood cultures.[66] Research continues to evaluate the use of an endoluminal brush to sample the distal catheter tip without removing the catheter.[67,68]

TREATMENT OF INFECTION

Antibiotic therapy should be commenced promptly when a neutropenic patient develops signs of infection,[69] as granulocytopenia is the single most important risk factor for infection in the cancer patient.[70] When deciding on the most appropriate antibiotic therapy, considerations have to include both the possibility of Gram-negative, Gram-positive and fungal microorganisms. Other factors that need to be considered include dosage, cost, the drug's serum levels and the antimicrobial sensitivity of the microorganism.[71] When the antibiotic sensitivity pattern are known, and if signs of infection persists after 48 hours, the antibiotics need to be reviewed.[72] Advice can be obtained from the hospital's antibiotic guidelines (Box 13.1) or from the consultant microbiologist.

Treatment regimes have to be extended in neutropenic patients with a residual focus of infection.

The increasing prevalence of antimicrobial-resistant organisms is causing concern,[73] because it makes infections more difficult to treat and increases the length and severity of illness and periods of infectiousness.[74] The five key, inter-related elements to the control antimicrobial resistance are:

- Surveillance to monitor what we are doing.
- Appropriate use of antimicrobial drugs, to discourage overuse and misuse. This reduces the exposure of microorganisms to inappropriate antimicrobial agents.
- Effective infection control to reduce the spread of infection (whether drug resistant or not), therefore reducing the use of antimicrobial agents.
- Improved diagnostic practices to guide drug prescribing.
- Promoting education and behaviour changes amongst clinicians, and informing consumers about the uses and limitations of antimicrobial drugs.[74]

PRINCIPLES OF INFECTION CONTROL

Clinical governance, quality assurance measures, the Medical Devices Agency, Medical Device Strategy

Box 13.1 The Royal Marsden Hospital Antibiotic Guidelines

Correct and in use in The Royal Marsden NHS Trust November 2004.

Up-to-date local guidelines or policy should be considered before commencing antibiotics. Alternatively, advice can be sought from the consultant microbiologist.

Empirical antibiotic therapy will be initiated for patients satisfying the criteria for neutropenic sepsis.

Neutropenic sepsis is defined as patients with, or expected to have due to recent chemotherapy or presenting with an acute haematological malignancy such as ALL or AML, an absolute granulocyte count of less than or equal to $< 0.5 \times 10^9/l$ who have one of the following:

- fever of greater or equal to 38.5°C on one occasion or greater or equal to 38°C on two or more occasions separated at least by an hour during a 12-hour period
- patients with the above neutropenic criteria with documented clinical deterioration thought to be due to sepsis, regardless of patient's temperature such as:
  - development of shock, with a systolic blood pressure of less than 90 mmHg or a decrease of more than 50 mmHg in a hypertensive patient
  - an acute respiratory distress syndrome in a patients with arterial hypoxia and bilateral diffuse infiltrates on chest X-ray
  - disseminated intravascular coagulation
  - multiple organ failure.

If still febrile after 48 hours:
Consider adding further antibiotics.

If still febrile after 96–120 hours:
Consider change in antibiotics.

Duration of therapy

1. In patients with mild neutropenia or expected to be neutropenic for <7 days:
   - significant causative bacterial isolate identified – treat for a minimum of 7 days
   - no significant causative bacterial isolate identified – treat until patient has been apyrexial for 3 days, then stop.

Antibiotic therapy can be changed to appropriate oral therapy when becomes apyrexial or shows marked improvement in clinical condition or fever.

2. Patients with severe neutropenia or expected to be neutropenic for >7 days:
   - significant causative bacterial isolate identified - treat for a minimum of 14 days or until patient neutrophil count is $>0.5 \times 10^9/l$
   - no significant causative bacterial isolate identified – until patient neutrophil count is $>0.5 \times 10^9/l$.

The patient can be changed to appropriate oral therapy or IV monotherapy when he has been apyrexial for 4 days.

3. Patients responding to empirical antifungal therapy should continue therapy until the patient's neutrophil count is $>0.5 \times 10^9/l$, if there is no good evidence of fungal infection.

4. *Staphylococcus aureus* septicaemia. IV antibiotics should be given for at least 14 days and then reassess. This applies regardless of the patient's neutrophil count.

Specific cases
Intravascular catheter-related infections
In neutropenic sepsis, if catheter infection is suspected, a swab of the site.

Blood cultures from peripheral site and all lumens should be taken and empirical therapy started with the addition of a glycopeptide.

In the neutropenic patient, the catheter should be removed if the line infection is caused by:

- *Bacillus* spp.
- Gram positive bacilli
- Vancomycin resistant enterococci
- or relapse or worsening infection.

committees and the Infection Control Committee all play an important part in obtaining compliance to infection control principles.

Health authorities are required to protect the public's health by controlling communicable disease and infection. The Department of Health requires the chief executive of every NHS trust to ensure that effective infection control arrangements are in place, with managerial interest at a strategic level and commitment and support of senior management essential.[75]

The principal objective of infection control is to prevent avoidable infection. However, if an infection does occur, it should be recognised early and appropriate treatment commenced, to improve patient outcome and reduce the risk of cross-infection.

The following infection control principles are relevant in reducing the incidence of infection in patients receiving chemotherapy:

- handwashing
- maintaining a clean hospital environment
- aseptic technique
- care of IV and other invasive devices
- monitoring of the patient for signs of infection or decreased immunity.

Handwashing

Handwashing is one of the most important procedures for preventing the spread of infection. Evidence shows that contaminated hands can be responsible for transmitting infection [76] Hands have also been seen to contaminate IV equipment.[77] Hand decontamination prior to insertion of a peripheral venous catheter has been seen to significantly reduce infection (Table 13.3).[78] Handwashing before and after patient contact is essential.[3]

Soaps and antibacterial solutions can cause irritation and allergic dermatitis. Prevention is essential, as breaks in the skin of the hands can increase the risk of infection to both the worker and the patient.[81] An outbreak of surgical wound infection has been attributed to a nurse with dermatitis.[82] The use of fragrance-free soap products[83] and the use of an alcoholic handrub are simple interventions to reduce the prevalence of sore hands.

Caution should be adopted when using handcream, as it has been suggested that communal handcream may become contaminated in use,[84] and that some handcreams which contain anionic emulsifying agents reduce the effects of chlorhexidine.[85]

Before handwashing, all jewellery must be removed.[23] A wedding ring is the exception. Although studies have concluded that keeping rings on may put the patient at risk from the unwashed skin under the ring,[86] staff are naturally reluctant to remove wedding rings.[87] Sleeves must be rolled back to expose wrists and forearms, nails must be short and clean, and nail varnish and false nails that inhibit effective handwashing are not to be used.[88] As wet surfaces transfer microorganisms more effectively than those that are dry, hands must be dried carefully after handwashing.[89] Hands must be washed when gloves have been removed.[90]

Compliance with handwashing policies

Most studies demonstrate that rates of handwashing compliance are less than 50%,[91] with nurses and nursing assistants more compliant than doctors.[92] One of the factors that contributes towards poor compliance to handwashing policy is the lack of adequate and appropriate handwashing facilities.[57] Non-touch water taps are being installed to reduce cross-contamination. Concerns have been raised related to the low amount of water that flows through non-touch taps,

Table 13.3	Hand decontamination
Type of solution	Rationale for use
Soap and water	Effective in removing transient microorganisms and makes hands socially clean. To be used when coming on and going off duty, following a visit to the toilet and before eating and drinking
Alcoholic-based handrub	More effective in decontaminating hands than soap and water, but does not remove physical dirt or soiling. Very effective quick methods of hand decontamination when hands are visually clean. Especially useful when staff to patient ratio is low[79]
Aqueous antiseptic solutions (most commonly chlorhexidine or povidone-iodine).	Suitable for surgical handwashing when there is a need to remove or destroy transient microorganisms and reduce detachable resident microorganisms. Surgical handwashing is essential before all surgical and invasive procedures, e.g. operating theatre procedures such as insertion of a central line. Hands must be rinsed and dried carefully after use[80]

which could provide an ideal growth condition for microorganisms.[93]

It is thought that education can improve compliance with handwashing policy,[94] but it has been found that often there is no retention of good effect.[90,95] The Infection Control Nurses Association (2000) suggests that hand hygiene can be improved by:

- effective communication related to the importance of infection control
- constant creative and innovative education to all staff
- adequate and conveniently placed facilities
- visual reminders
- commitment by managers to improve resources.

Maintenance of a clean hospital environment

- The hospital environment must be visibly clean, free from dust and dirt
- Equipment used for more than one patient, i.e. drip stand, must be cleaned following each use
- Statutory requirements related to safe disposal of clinical waste, laundry and pest control should be met
- All staff involved in hospital hygiene must be suitably trained and supervised.[76]

Aseptic techniques

A strict aseptic technique is required to be used for all placements of intravenous devices.[74] The correct implementation of an aseptic technique has been seen to reduce the incidence of catheter-related infection.[24,96] For the insertion of a central venous access device (CVAD), this includes sterile gown, sterile drapes and gloves.[23,97] The regular review of procedures and initiatives to improve and maintain aseptic techniques procedures and policies have been seen to reduce catheter-related infections.[98]

CHOICE OF EQUIPMENT

Intravenous catheters

It is essential that medical devices and equipment used to support the care and treatment of patients are suitable for the task they are being used for. Therefore, all medical devices and equipment should be:

- Evaluated fully before purchase.
- All users of the equipment must be trained in its use and its maintenance.[20]
- Appropriate decontamination facilities and compatible decontamination agents should be available before new devices are purchased.[99]

- Single-use medical devices must never be reused.
- Any adverse incidents associated with a medical device must be reported to the Medical Devices Agency: e.g. a faulty catheter that has to be replaced increases the number of invasive procedures, which sequentially increases the risk of infection.[100]

Peripheral intravenous catheters

Surveillance suggests the risk of phlebitis and/or infection with peripheral lines is associated with:

- what the catheter was used for
- the duration in situ
- part of a surveillance study and
- whether an infusion pump was used.[101]

The risk of complications occurring with peripheral IV devices increases with time. It is recommended that peripheral IV devices are removed and resited at 72 hours.[102] This is supported by Pearson,[63] who also suggests that peripheral catheters inserted under emergency conditions, where lapses in aseptic technique may have occurred, should be replaced every 48–72 hours.

Later studies do not support removing and resiting peripheral catheters at 72 hours, suggesting that low-risk patients will generally have completed their IV therapy by 72 hours. This means that only high-risk patients continue to require cannulation, and resiting the catheter at 72 hours does not significantly reduce the risk of phlebitis. This is because a restarted catheter has been seen to have significantly higher risk of complications in its first 24 hours than does an initial catheter.[103,104]

Central venous access devices

Approximately 20 000 CVADs are used in the UK each year and it has been estimated that 5800 cases of catheter bloodstream infections occur annually.[23] Neutropenia is associated with a significant risk of infection related to long-term tunnelled central venous catheters.[16] Complications such as clot formation[105] necessitate extra manipulation of the catheter, increasing the risk of infection.[106]

Non-tunnelled central venous catheter

Non-tunnelled CVADs are placed percutaneously by puncturing the patient's skin, or by a surgical cut-down through the patient's skin to obtain access to a blood vessel. These catheters have a high risk of infection.[107] Infection is probably due to the easy access of skin organisms to the transcutaneous tract, plus these catheters are difficult to secure and dress.

Tunnelled central lines

Tunnelled central catheters have a tunnelled section of the catheter under the skin of the chest wall before it enters the central vein. The catheter is held in place in the tunnel by a Dacron cuff, which anchors the catheter securely in position and allows the stitches to be removed 14–21 days following insertion. The Dacron cuff and the tunnel prevent the passage of microorganisms along the tunnel, so reducing the risk of infection.[23,63]

Peripherally inserted central venous catheters

Using a peripherally inserted central catheter (PICC) device, long-term and short-term venous access can be obtained for adults and children.[108] This provides a cost-effective and convenient venous access by cannulating a peripheral vein in the arm.[109] Using a scrupulous aseptic technique and a knowledgeable selection of the insertion site,[110] this can be easily undertaken at the bedside.[111] A study has shown that PICCs have a significantly higher length of stay and lower incidence of phlebitis.[112] A further study concluded that PICCs have an acceptable complication rate in patients with leukaemia,[113] but further trials are required before PICCs can be considered an alternative to tunnelled central venous catheters.[114]

Midline catheters

Midline catheters are a type of peripheral device introduced into an antecubital vein. By using a larger vein, this device can remain in situ for extended periods of time depending on the type of catheter material, which reduces the number of invasive procedures the patient undergoes. Once in situ, a midline catheter is managed as a central line.[115] The risk of infection has been found to be low,[116] providing a safe method of IV access for a patient with limited peripheral vein access who needs extended IV therapy.[117]

Implantable ports

Implantable ports are implanted subcutaneously with the catheter tunnelled under the skin until it reaches the desired venous access point. The skin is sutured closed, providing a barrier to infection.[118]

Catheter lumens

It has been suggested that infection can be reduced by the use of a single-lumen CVAD (unless multiple ports are essential for the management of the patients).[23, 63] This opinion is not fully supported. Farkas and colleagues[119] found no difference in the incidence of infection between the single- and triple-lumen catheters, while the need for repeated invasive procedures to insert peripheral access was dramatically reduced when multiple lumens were available.

Type of catheter material

The relationship between infection risk and catheters made from materials such as polyurethane and silicone is not conclusive.[23,63] The use of antimicrobial-impregnated CVAD for adult patients requiring short-term CVAD and who are at risk of developing an infection is recommended.[63] This type of catheter is less likely to be colonised by microorganisms, and is therefore less likely to be a source of infection.[120]

Choice of site

It is important that the best insertion site for the patient is sought, as the site is a factor in the risk of infection. The subclavian is the site of choice rather than the jugular or femoral sites, unless medically contraindicated.[63] An association has been found between contamination and infection of an IV catheter in a femoral site.[121,122] The internal jugular poses a similar risk because of contamination from oropharyngeal secretions and the difficulty of anchoring the catheter.[23]

Table 13.4   Infection control for inserting intravenous devices

Device	Environment	Cleaning solution	Personal protective equipment
Peripheral line	Bedside	Alcoholic chlorhexidine gluconate solution	Gloves
Non-tunnelled CVAD	Bedside	Alcoholic chlorhexidine gluconate solution	Sterile gloves, gown
Tunnelled CVAD	Operating theatre	Alcoholic chlorhexidine gluconate solution	Full sterile theatre clothing and drapes
PICC	Bedside	Alcoholic chlorhexidine gluconate solution	Sterile gloves, gown
Midline	Operating theatre	Alcoholic chlorhexidine gluconate solution	Sterile gloves, gown
Implantable port	Operating theatre	Alcoholic chlorhexidine gluconate solution	Full sterile theatre clothing and drapes

CVAD, central venous access device; PICC, peripherally inserted central catheter.

Insertion

Optimum aseptic techniques must be adopted during the insertion of an IV device. For the insertion of a CVAD this includes a sterile gown, gloves and a large sterile drape.[23]

The insertion site should be cleaned with an alcoholic chlorhexidine gluconate solution and the solution must be allowed to dry before inserting the catheter (Table 13.4). The routine application of antimicrobial ointment to the catheter site prior to insertion is not recommended.[23]

Intravenous teams

An IV team comprises nurses and phlebotomists who are specially trained in all aspects of IV therapy, and are responsible for safe and successful IV practice. This involves clinical practice as well as education and service development tasks.[123] Studies have shown that the use of IV teams decreases the incidence of IV-related morbidity and mortality,[124] and improves the quality of patients' care.[125]

SURVEILLANCE OF INFECTION

Surveillance is an essential component in the prevention and control of infection in hospitals. The main objectives of surveillance is to prevent outbreaks of infection, or if infection does occur, that it is detected early in order to allow timely investigation and treatment.[7]

Surveillance includes the assessment of:

- type of infection, i.e. wound, IV line
- type of microorganism
- consultant or medical or surgical unit involved
- number of infections
- significance and outcome
- measures that were most effective in controlling the infection
- policies or procedures that need to be reviewed to ensure this or similar infections do not occur in the future.

Surveillance involves:

- collecting
- collation
- analysis
- interpretation of the data
- dissemination of information for action to those people who need to know.
- formal reports compiled for the Hospital Infection Control Committees' meetings and reports
- for some infections, such as MRSA bacteraemias, this may also include reporting to national surveillance schemes.

Regular feedback of surveillance data is associated with a decrease in infection rates, suggesting that this knowledge improves staff compliance with precautions.[98]

UNIVERSAL BLOOD AND BODY FLUIDS PRECAUTIONS

Universal precautions

Universal precautions emphasises the need to apply blood and body fluid precautions universally to all persons, regardless of their known or presumed infection status; they must be implemented at all times,[126] although it is unlikely that all accidents can be prevented.[127,128] Universal precaution measures involve those procedures that are necessary to prevent the spread of infection. This may be related to barrier precautions, such as wearing gloves when handling blood and body fluids, or adopting safe techniques when handling waste, used equipment and especially in the safe disposal of used needles. Most incidents results from a failure to follow recommended procedures,[76] particularly during disposal of a used sharp.[129]

Needlestick injuries

All healthcare workers must be informed and educated about the possible risks from occupational exposure to blood and body fluids, and they must be aware of the importance of seeking urgent advice following an accident or incident. Training is essential to ensure everyone is aware of how to report incidents, as many incidents go unreported[130] and staff exposed to blood and body fluids are not always aware of the risks from needlestick injuries.[131]

Poor organisation and high work load are associated with increased numbers of needlestick accidents. Needlestick injuries can be reduced following action by:

- the employer
- the healthcare worker.

The employer:

- eliminate the use of needles where safe and effective alternative needleless systems are available
- analyse accidents to identify hazards and injury trends
- ensure users are properly trained
- modify work practices that pose hazards
- promote safety awareness
- establish procedures for reporting and follow-up of all injuries
- ensure staffing levels are sufficient to allow staff to work safely.[132]

The healthcare worker:

- participate in training and educational events
- sharps must never be passed directly from hand to hand
- handling of sharps must be kept to a minimum
- needles must not be recapped
- needles must not be bent or broken prior to disposal
- needles and syringes must not be disassembled by hand prior to disposal
- used sharps must be immediately disposed of into a sharps disposal container that conforms to national standards (UN3291 and BS7320 Standards)
- sharps bins must be located in a safe position to facilitate immediate disposal of used sharps
- sharps bins must not be overfilled or placed on the floor.
- consider the use of needle-prevention devices, which need to be evaluated for their effectiveness, acceptability, impact on patient care and cost benefit.[76]
- thoroughly wash hands and other surfaces that are contaminated with blood and body fluids.

Needleless intravenous systems have been developed to prevent needlestick injury, and while there was initial concern over possible increased infection rates,[133] later studies indicated that there was no evidence of increased incidence of infection.[134]

Needlestick injury can be the cause of transmission of infections such as human immunodeficiency virus (HIV), hepatitis B and hepatitis C.[135]

Human immunodeficiency virus exposure

The risk of HIV transmission is 3 per 1000 percutaneous exposures and 1 per 1000 mucocutaneous exposures.[76] There is no reported risk following contamination of intact skin.

A risk assessment has to be undertaken following an exposure with HIV-contaminated blood and body fluids, to evaluate the significance of the accident. Four factors have to be considered:

- extent of injury – deep injury presents increased risk
- whether device was bloodstained
- injury with a needle that had been placed in the patient's artery or vein
- status of the source patient – in a terminally ill HIV-positive patient the HIV viral load is likely to be higher than a more fit person.

If the risk is considered to be significant, postexposure prophylaxis of a combination of antiretroviral drugs should be offered to the injured person immediately. Local policies and protocols must be devised, with the antiretroviral drugs, help and support available 24 hours of the day.[136]

Hepatitis B exposure

All healthcare workers should be vaccinated with hepatitis B vaccine and obtain antibody levels of >10 mIU/ml 3 months after the third dose of vaccine. Following an accident with hepatitis B blood or body fluids, individuals who have already been successfully vaccinated should be given a booster dose of vaccine unless a booster has been given within the last year.

Persons who have never been vaccinated or were unsuccessfully vaccinated should be given human hepatitis B immunoglobulin (HBIG); a second dose of immunoglobulin should be administered 1 month after the first dose.

The effectiveness of hepatitis B vaccination programmes could be further improved by ensuring vaccination schedules are completed.[137]

Hepatitis C exposure

Infection with hepatitis C virus (HCV) is estimated to affect 3% of the world's population. An average transmission rate of 1.8% following percutaneous injury has been reported.[138] The risk is related to the type and size of the inoculum, route of transmission and the titre of virus.[139] Those healthcare workers conducting exposure-prone procedures on HCV-positive patients do not seem to be at higher risk than other healthcare workers.[140]

No vaccine or prophylaxis is available to prevent HCV.[141] Following a needlestick injury, the source patient should be tested for hepatitis C. Healthcare workers exposed to known HCV-infected sources should be followed up at 6, 12 and 24 weeks after exposure.

Personal protective equipment

Personal protective equipment (PPE) is used to protect staff and to reduce the opportunities for transmission of microorganisms in hospital. Personal protective equipment is only used where risks cannot be adequately controlled by other means. Guidance is included in the Personal Protective Equipment at Work Regulations.[142] The decision to use or wear protective equipment must be based upon a risk assessment of the level of risk related to the specific patient care task or intervention (Table 13.5).

When choosing PPE, it is essential that the manufacturer's specifications are checked to ensure the PPE is suitable for the task.

Table 13.5 Use of personal protective equipment

Type of protective clothing	Use
Gloves	Worn when handling blood, body fluids, chemicals and drugs
Plastic disposable apron	Worn to protect the wearer from organisms from the patient and to prevent transmission to other patients by clothing. Plastic aprons should be worn as a single-use item for one patient contact and then discarded. Hands must be washed following removal of the apron
Non-sterile gowns	Worn when the area of contamination is expected to be larger than that covered by the plastic apron
Sterile gown	Worn during the insertion and removal of a central IV device
Overshoes	Worn when spillage of blood, body fluid or cytotoxic drugs has occurred to protect the environment from further contamination and to protect the wearer's footwear
Eye and face protection	Worn when there is a risk of airborne spread of blood, body fluids, drugs or chemicals

Gloves

The use of gloves has increased. There are four main indications for the use of gloves:

1. To protect hands from contamination with blood, body fluids and microorganisms. Boxed clean gloves are generally the most suitable and cost-effective choice.
2. To reduce transmission of microorganisms from staff hands to the patient: e.g. during insertion of central lines. Sterile gloves and the use of a surgical aseptic technique are essential.
3. To reduce transmission of microorganisms from staff hands to the patients: e.g. during flushing of an IV device. Although the use of an aseptic technique is the most important issue in the prevention of cross-infection, gloves are generally worn when spillage of blood is anticipated or cytotoxic drugs are being administered.
4. To protect staff and the patients when handwashing facilities are not available. Generally in such cases boxed clean gloves are appropriate.

Gloves must conform to European Community (CE) Standards (1995). The use of a powder to assist in the donning of gloves is harmful, and is associated with risks to the patients as well as the risk of the development of allergies for the wearer.[143,144] Gloves of an acceptable quality must be available in all clinical areas.[145]

Safe handling of hazardous drugs

Safe limits of time and amount of exposure to many potential hazardous drugs is unknown, which means that full precautions on safe handling of hazardous drugs at all times is essential. Precautions and safe practice should be adopted during:

- transport
- storage
- reconstitution
- administration
- disposal of waste
- handling blood or body fluid of patients who are receiving cytotoxic drugs.

Occupational Health must be informed and will provide support following exposure to cytotoxic drugs.[146]

HEALTHCARE WORKERS EDUCATION AND TRAINING

It is essential that all staff receive infection control education and training:[76] in particular, related to IV practice.[147] All staff must receive orientation, training and supervision with IV policies and procedures to ensure competency.[148] It is suggested that the gap between actual and expected IV therapy knowledge and skills can be extremely wide.[149] Training programmes should be multidisciplinary and be part of continuous education programmes.[150] British guidelines for the preparation of nurses for intravenous administration have been produced which provide guidance of training and assessment of individuals involved in IV therapy.[151] Interactive infection control computer-assisted learning software programs are available and have proved to be a convenient and effective way for users to gain evidence-based infection control practice understanding.[152]

AUDIT

The effective monitoring of infection control practices is important and has been seen to have an impact on practice and infection rates.[153] Examples of audit tools are available[62,154,155] which allow practices to be reviewed, thereby facilitating improvements that may in turn reduce infection rates.

The use of a benchmarking process also provides a structured approach to sharing and comparing practice, and enables healthcare workers to identify best practice and to develop action plans to remedy poor practice.[156]

References

1. Tsiodras S, Samonis G, Keating MJ, et al. Infection and immunity in chronic lymphocytic leukaemia. Mayo Clin Proc 2000; 75(10):1039–1054.

2. Yuen KY, Woo PC, Hui CH, et al. Unique risk factors for bacteraemia in allogeneic bone marrow transplant recipients before and after engraftment. Bone Marrow Transplant 1998; 21(11):1137–1143.

3. Burgoyne T, Knight A. Myelodysplastic syndromes. In: Grundy M, ed. Nursing in haematological oncology. Edinburgh: Baillière Tindall; 2000:21–30.

4. Van Der Meer JWM. Defects in host defence mechanisms. In: Rubin RH, Young LS, eds. Clinical approach to infection in the compromised host. 3rd edn. New York: Plenum; 1994:33–66.

5. Glauser MP, Calandra T. Infection in patients with haematologic malignancies. In: Glauser MP, Pizzo PA, eds. Management of infection in immunocompromised patients. London: WB Saunders; 2000:141–188.

6. Rolston KVI. Infections in patient's with solid tumours. In: Glauser MP, Pizzo PA, eds. Management of infection in immunocompromised patients. London: WB Saunders; 2000:117–140.

7. Department of Health. Hospital infection control: guidance on the control of infection in hospitals. London: Department of Health; 1995.

8. Carlisle PS, Gucalp R, Wiernik PH. Nosocomial infections in neutropenic cancer patients. Infect Control Hosp Epidemiol 1993; 14(6):320–324.

9. Public Health Laboratory Service. Surveillance of hospital acquired bacteraemia in English hospitals 1997–2002. London: Public Health Laboratory Service; 2003.

10. Plowman R, Graves N, Griffin M, et al. The socio-economic burden of hospital acquired infection. London: Public Health Laboratory Service; 2000

11. Dimick JB, Pelz RK, Consunji R, et al. Increase resource use associated with catheter-related bloodstream infection in the surgical intensive care unit. Arch Surg 2001; 136(2):229–234.

12. Haley RW, White JW, Culver DH. The efficacy of infection surveillance and central programs in preventing nosocomial infection in US hospitals. Am J Epidemiol 1985; 121(2): 182–205.

13. Taylor K, Plowman R, Roberts JA. The challenge of hospital acquired infection. National Audit Office. London: The Stationery Office; 2001.

14. Wilkinson R. Nurse's concerns about I.V. therapy and devices. Nurs Stand 1996; 10(35):35–37.

15. Elliott TS. Line-associated bacteraemias. Commun Dis Rep Rev 1993; 3(7):R91–R95.

16. Howell PB, Walters PE, Donowitz GR, et al. Risk factors for infection of adult patient with cancer who have tunnelled central venous catheters. Cancer 1995; 75(6):1367–1375.

17. Weinstein RA. Epidemiology and control of nosocomial infections in adult intensive care patients. Am J Med 1991; 91(3B):179S–184S.

18. Sani M. Pharmacological aspects of intravenous therapy. In: Dougherty L, Lamb J, eds. Intravenous therapy in nursing practice. Edinburgh: Churchill Livingstone; 1999:117–138.

19. National Health Service Estates. Infection control in the built environment. London: Department of Health; 2002.

20. Medical Devices Agency. Equipped to care. London: MDA; 2000.

21. Al-Rabea AA, Burwen DR, Eldeen MA, et al. *Klebsiella pneumoniae* bloodstream infection in neonates in a hospital in the Kingdom of Saudi Arabia. Infect Control Hosp Epidemiol 2000; 19(9):674–679.

22. Polderman KH, Girbes AJ. Central venous catheter use. Part 1: mechanical complications. Intens Care Med 2002; 28(1):1–17.

23. Department of Health. Guidelines for preventing infections associated with the insertion and maintenance of central venous catheters. J Hosp Infect 2001; 47(supplement):S47–S67.

24. Medical Devices Agency. Selection and use of infusion devices for ambulatory application. DB 9703. London: MDA; 1997.

25. Waghorn DJ. Intravascular device-associated systemic infection: a 2 year analysis of cases in a district general hospital. J Hosp Infect 1994; 28(2):91–101.

26. Eggimann P, Pittet D. Overview of catheter-related infections with special emphasis on prevention based on educational programs. Clin Microbiol Infect 2002; 8(5):295–309.

27. Moro ML, Vigano EF, Cozzi Lepri A. Risk factors for central venous catheter-related infections in surgical and intensive care units. The Central Venous Catheter-Related Infection Study Group. Infect Control Hosp Epidemiol 1994; 15(4):253–264.

28. Guidet B, Nicola I, Barakett V, et al. Skin versus hub cultures to predict colonisation and infection of central venous catheter in intensive care patients. Infection 1994; 22(1):43–48.

29. Sitges-Serra A, Pi-suner T, Garces JM, et al. Pathogenesis and prevention of catheter-related septicaemia. Am J Infect Control 1995; 23(5):310–316.

30. Carter LW. Bacterial translocation: nursing implications in the care of patients with neutropenia. Oncol Nurs Forum 1994; 21(5):857–865.

31. Rao GG. Risk factors for the spread of antibiotic-resistant bacteria. Drugs 1998; 55(3):323–330.

32. Wagenvoort JH, Sluijsmans W, Penders R.J. Better environmental survival of outbreak vs. sporadic MRSA isolates. J Hosp Infect 2000; 45(3):231–234.

33. Shiomori T, Miyamoto H, Makishima K, et al. Evaluation of bedmaking-related airborne and surface methicillin-resistant *Staphylococcus aureus* contamination. J Hosp Infect 2002; 50(1):30–35.

34. Ayliffe GAJ, Fraise AP, Geddes AM, et al. Control of hospital infection. A practical handbook. 4th edn. London: Arnold; 2000.

35. Medical Device Agency. The reuse of medical devices supplied for single use only. DB 9501. London: MDA; 1995.

36. Medical Device Agency. Medical devices and equipment management: repair and maintenance provision. DB 2000 (02). London: MDA; 2000.

37. Infection Control Nurses Association (ICNA). Guidelines for hand hygiene. ICNA in collaboration with Deb. Edinburgh: Fitwise; 1997.

38. Association of Domestic Managers & Infection Control Nurses Association. Standards for environmental cleanliness in hospitals. Edinburgh: Fitwise; 1999.

39. Johnson E, Gilmore M, Newman J, et al. Preventing fungal infections in immunocompromised patients. Br J Nurs 2000; 9(17):1154–1164.

40. Banbury MK. Experience in prevention of sternal wound infections in nasal carriers of *Staphylococcus aureus*. Surgery 2003; 134(5 Suppl):S18–22.

41. Oie S, Kamiya A. Survivial of methicillin-resistant *Staphylococcus aureus* (MRSA) on naturally contaminated dry mops. J Hosp Infect 1996; 34(2):145–149.

42. Dietze B, Rath A, Wendt C, et al. Survival of MRSA on sterile packaging. J Hosp Infect 2001; 49(4):255–261.

43. Jameson B, Gamble DR, Lynch J, et al. Five year analysis of protective isolation. Lancet 1971; 1(7708):1034–1040.

44. Centers for Disease Control and Protection. Guidelines for isolation in hospital. Infect Control (special supplement) 1983; (4):325.

45. Klein BS, Perloff WH, Dennis GM. Reduction of nosocomial infections during pediatric intensive care by protective isolation. N Engl J Med 1989; 320(26):1714–1720.

46. Buckner CD, Clift RA, Sanders JE. Protective environment for marrow transplant recipients. Ann Intern Med 1978; 89:893–901.

47. Poe SS, Larson E, McGuire D. A national survey of infection prevention practices on bone marrow transplant units. Oncol Nurs Forum 1994; 21(10):1687–1694.

48. Kolbe K, Domkin D, Derigs HG, et al. Infectious complications during neutropenia subsequent to peripheral blood stem cell transplantation. Bone Marrow Transplant 1997; 19(2):143–147.

49. Russell JA, Poon M, Jones AR, et al. Allogeneic bone-marrow transplantation without protective isolation in adults with malignant disease. Lancet 1992; 339(8784):38–40

50. Hiemenz JW, Green JN. Special consideration for the patient undergoing allogenic or autologous BMT. In: Pizza PA, ed. Hematology/oncology clinics of North America. Infectious complications in the immunocompromised host. Philadelphia: WB Saunders; 1993: 961–1002.

51. Kibbler CC, Prentice G. What is the risk of infection in patients undergoing peripheral blood stem cell transplantation? Curr Opin Infect Dis 1996; 9:215–217.

52. British Clinical Haematology Task Force. Guidelines on the provision of facilities for the care of adult patients with haematological malignancies (including leukaemia and lymphoma and severe bone marrow failure) Clin Lab Haematol 1995; 17:3–10.

53. Croner's Health Service Risks Special Report. Infection control isolation precautions. Surrey: Croner Publications, 1998; Issue No 25.

54. Pattison AJ. Review of current practices in clean diets in the UK. J Hum Nutr Diet 1993; 6:3–11.

55. Smith LH, Besser SG. Dietary restrictions for patients with neutropenia: a survey of institutional practices. Oncol Nurs Forum 2000; 27(3):515–520.

56. Campbell T. Feelings of oncology patients about being nursed in protective isolation as a consequence of cancer chemotherapy treatment. J Adv Nurs 1999; 30(2):439–447.

57. Gaston-Johansson F, Foxall M. Psychological correlates of quality of life across the autologous bone marrow transplant experience. Cancer Nurs 1996; 19(3):170–176.

58. Wettergren L, Langius A, Bjorkholm M, et al. Physical and psychosocial functioning in patients undergoing autologous bone marrow transplantation – a prospective study. Bone Marrow Transplant 1997; 20(6):497–502.

59. Ward D. Infection control: reducing the psychological effects of isolation. Br J Nurs 2000; 9(3):162–170.

60. Cohen MZ, Ley C, Tarzian AJ. Isolation in blood and marrow transplantation. West J Nurs Res 2001; 23(6):592–609.

61. Gaskill D, Henderson A, Fraser M. Exploring the everyday world of the patient in isolation. Oncol Nurs Forum 1997; 24(4):695–700.

62. Elliott TS, Faroqui MH, Tebbs SE, et al. An audit programme for central venous catheter-associated infections. J Hosp Infect 1995; 30(1):181–191.

63. Pearson ML. Hospital Infectious Program Centers of Disease Control and Prevention (HICPAC). Guidelines for prevention of intravascular device related infections. Am J Infect Control 1996; 24(4):262–293.

64. Correa L, Pittet D. Problems and solutions in hospital-acquired bacteraemia. J Hosp Infect 2000; 46(2):89–95

65. Elliott TS, Moss HA, Tebbs SE, et al. Novel approach to investigate a source of microbial contamination of central venous catheters. Eur J Clin Microbial Infect Dis 1997; 16(3):210–213.

66. Peacock SJ, Eddleston M, Emptage A, et al. Positive intravenous line tip cultures as predictors of bacteremia. J Hosp Infect 1998; 40(1):35–38.

67. Van Heerden PV, Webb SA, Fong S, et al. Central venous catheters revisited – infection rates and an assessment of the new fibrin analysing system brush. Anaesth Intens Care 1996; 24(3):330–333.

68. McLure HA, Juste RN, Thomas ML, et al. Endoluminal brushing for detection of central venous catheter colonisation – a comparison of daily vs single brushing on removal. J Hosp Infect 1997: 36(4):313–316.

69. Meunier F. Infections in patients with acute leukaemia and lymphoma. In: Mandell GL, Bennett JE, Dolan R, eds. Principles and practice of infectious diseases. New York: Churchill Livingstone; 1995:2675–2685.

70. Pizzo PA. Empirical therapy and prevention of infection in the immunocompromised host. In: Mandell GL, Bennett JE, Dolan R, eds. Principles and practice of

infectious diseases. New York: Churchill Livingstone; 1995:2686–2695.

71. Correa L, Pittet D. Problems and solutions in hospital acquired bacteraemia. J Hosp Infect 2000; 46(2)89–95.

72. Yinnon AM, Schlesinger Y, Gabbay D, et al. Analysis of 5 years of bacteraemia: importance of stratification of microbial susceptibility of source of patients. J Infect 1997; 35(1):17–23.

73. Department of Health. Standing Medical Advisory Committee Subgroup on Antimicrobial Resistance. The path of least resistance. London: Department of Health; 1998.

74. Department of Health. UK antimicrobial resistant strategy and action plan. London: Department of Health; 2000.

75. National Audit Office. The management and control of hospital acquired infection in acute NHS Trusts in England. London: The Stationery Office; 2000.

76. Department of Health. Standard principles for preventing hospital-acquired infections. J Hosp Infect 2001; 47 (supplement):S21–S37.

77. Calop J, Bosson JL, Croize J, et al. Maintenance of peripheral and central intravenous infusion devices by 0.9% sodium chloride with or without heparin as a potential source of catheter microbial contamination. J Hosp Infect 2000; 46(2):161–162.

78. Hirschmann H, Fux L, Podusel J, et al. The influence of hand hygiene prior to insertion of peripheral venous catheters on the frequency of complications. J Hosp Infect 2001; 49(3):199–203.

79. Karabey S, Derbentli S, Nakipoglu Y, et al. Handwashing frequencies in an intensive care unit. J Hosp Infect 2002; 50(1):36–41.

80. Gould D. The significance of hand-drying in the prevention of infection. Nurs Times 1994; 90(47):33–35.

81. Borgatta L, Fisher M, Robbins N. Hand protection and protection from hands: hand-washing, germicides and gloves. Women Health 1989; 15(4):77–92.

82. Beck-Sague CM, Chong WH, Roy C, et al. Outbreak of surgical wound infections associated with total hip arthroplasty. Infect Control Hosp Epidemiol 1992; 13(9):526–534.

83. Wilkinson SM. Effects of infection control measures on skin of health care workers. Commun Dis Public Health 2000; 3(4):305–306.

84. Gould D. Infection control. Making sense of hand washing. Nurs Times 1994; 90(30):63–64.

85. Walsh B, Blackmore PH, Drabu YJ. The effect of hand-cream on the antibacterial activity of chlorhexidine gluconate. J Hosp Infect 1987; 9(1):30–33.

86. Hoffman PN, Cooke EM, McCarville MR, et al. Microorganisms isolated from skin under wedding rings worn by hospital workers. Br Med J 1985; 290(6463):206–207.

87. Bernthal E. Wedding rings and hospital-acquired infection. Nurs Stand 1997; 11(43):44–46.

88. Hoffman PN, Wilson J. Hand hygiene and hospitals. PHLS Microbiol Dig 1994; 11(4):211–261.

89. Gould D, Chamberlain A. Gram-negative bacteria. The challenge of preventing cross infection in hospital wards: a review of the literature. J Clin Nurs 1994; 3(6):339–345.

90. ICNA. Guidelines for preventing intravascular catheter-related infection. Edinburgh: Fitwise; 2000.

91. Harris AD, Samore MH, Nafziger R, et al. A survey on handwashing practices and opinions of healthcare workers. J Hosp Infect 2000; 45(4):318–321.

92. Pittet D, Hugonnets S, Harbarth S, et al. Effectiveness of a hospital-wide programme to improve compliance with hand hygiene. Lancet 2000; 356(9238):1307–1312.

93. Halabi M, Wiesholzer-Pitt M, Schober J, et al. Non touch fittings in hospitals: a possible source of Pseudomonas aerginosa and Legionella spp. J Hosp Infect 2001; 49(2):117–121.

94. Gould D. Nurses' hand decontamination practice: results of a local study. J Hosp Infect 1994; 28(1):15–30.

95. Moongtui W, Gauthier DK, Turner JG. Using peer feedback to improve handwashing and glove usage among Thai health care workers. Am J Infect Control 2000; 28(5):365–369.

96. Bull DA, Neumayer LA, Hunter GC, et al. Improved sterile technique diminished the incidence of positive line cultures in cardiovascular patients. J Surg Respir 1992; 52(2):106–110.

97. Maki DG. Yes, Virginia, aseptic technique is very important: maximum barrier precautions during insertion reduce the risk of central venous catheter-related bacteremia. Infect Control Hosp Epidemiol 1994; 15(4 pt 1):227–230.

98. Maas A, Flament P, Pardou A, et al. Central venous catheter-related bacteraemia in critically ill neonates: risk factors and impact of a prevention program. J Hosp Infect 1998; 40(3):211–224.

99. Medical Devices Agency. Compatibility of medical devices and reprocessing equipment with decontamination agents. MDA SN2001(28). London: MDA, 2001.

100. Medical Devices Agency. Medical devices – reporting adverse incidents and disseminating safety warnings. SN2002(01). London: MDA, 2002.

101. Curran ET, Coia JE, Gilmour H, et al. Multi-centre research surveillance project to reduce infection/phlebitis associated with peripheral vascular catheters. J Hosp Infect 2000; 46(3):194–202.

102. Maki DG, Ringer M. Risk factors for infusion-related phebitis with small peripheral venous catheters. A randomized controlled study. Ann Intern Med 1991; 114(10):845–854.

103. Homer LD, Holmes KR. Risks associated with 72 and 96 hours peripheral intravenous catheter dwell times. J Intraven Nurs 1998; 21(5):301–305.

104. Lai KK. Safety of prolonging peripheral cannula and IV tubing from 72 hours to 96 hours. Am J Infect Control 1998; 26(1):66–70.

105. Barzaghi A, Dell'Orto M, Rovelli A, et al. Central venous catheter clots: incidence, clinical significance

and catheter care in patients with hematologic malignancies. Pediatr Hematol Oncol 1995; 12(3):243–250.

106. Mahieu LM, De Dooy JJ, Lenaerts AE, et al. Catheter manipulations and the risk of catheter-associated bloodstream infection in neonatal intensive care unit. J Hosp Infect 2001; 48(1):20–26.

107. Seifert H, Cornely O, Seggewiss K, et al. Bloodstream infection in neutropenic cancer patients related to short-term nontunnelled catheters determined by quantitative blood cultures, differential time to positivity, and molecular epidemiological typing with pulse-field gel electrophoresis. J Clin Micro 2003; 41(1):118–123.

108. Crowley JJ, Pereira JK, Harris LS, et al. Peripherally inserted central catheters: experience in 523 children. Radiology 1997; 204(3):617–621.

109. Camara D. Minimizing risks associated with peripherally inserted central catheters in the NICU. Am J Matern Child Nurs 2001; 26(1):17–21.

110. Neuman L, Murphy BD, Rosen MP. Bedside placement of peripherally inserted central catheters: a cost-effectiveness analysis. Radiology 1998; 206(2):423–428.

111. Griffiths VR, Philpot P. Peripherally inserted central catheters (PICCs): do they have a role in the care of critically ill patients. Intensive Crit Care Nurs 2002; 18(1):37–47.

112. Snelling R, Jones G, Figueredo A, et al. Central venous catheter for infusion therapy in gastro-intestinal cancer. A comparative study of tunnelled centrally placed catheters and peripherally inserted central catheters. J Intraven Nurs 2001; 24(1)38–47.

113. Strahilevitz J, Lossos IS, Verstanding A, et al. Vascular access via peripherally inserted venous catheter (PICCs): experience in 40 patients with acute myeloid leukaemia at a single institution. Leuk Lymphoma 2001; 40(3–4):365–371.

114. Duerksen DR, Papineau N, Siemens J, et al. Peripherally inserted central catheters for parenteral nutrition: a comparison with centrally inserted catheters. J Parenter Enteral Nutr 1999; 23(2):85–89.

115. Mermel LA, Parenteau S, Tow SM. The risk of midline catheterization in hospitalized patients. A prospective study. Ann Intern Med 1995; 123(11):841–844.

116. Goetz AM, Miller J, Wagener MM, et al. Complications related to intravenous midline catheter usage. A 2-year study. J Intraven Nurs 1998; 21(2):76–80.

117. Carlson KR. Correct utilization and management of peripherally inserted central catheters and midline catheters in the alternate care setting. J Intraven Nurs 1999; 22(6 suppl):S46–50.

118. Camp-Sorrell D. Implantable ports. J Intraven Nurs 1992; 15(5):262–273.

119. Farkas JC, Liu N, Bleriot JP, et al. Single-versus triple-lumen central catheter-related sepsis: a prospective randomized study in a critically ill population. Am J Med 1992; 93(3):277–282.

120. Maki DG, Stolz SM, Wheler S, et al. Prevention of central venous catheter-related bloodstream infection by use of an antiseptic-impregnated catheter. A randomized, controlled trial. Ann Intern Med 1997; 127(4):257–266.

121. Goetz AM, Wagener MM, Miller JM, et al. Risk of infection due to central venous catheters: effect of site placement and catheter type. Infect Contr Hosp Epidemiol 1998; 19(11):842–845.

122. Harden JL, Kemp L, Mirtallo J. Femoral catheters increase risk of infection in total parenteral nutrition patients. Nutr Clin Path 1995; 10(2):60–66.

123. Dougherty L. The benefits of an IV team in hospital practice. Prof Nurse 1996; 11(11):761–763.

124. Miller JM, Goetz AM, Squier C, et al Reduction in nosocomial intravenous device-related bacteraemia after institution of an intravenous therapy team. J Intraven Nurs 1996;19(2)103–106.

125. Scalley RD, Van CS, Cochran RS. The impact of an IV team on the occurrence of intravenous-related phlebitis. A 30 month study. J Intraven Nurs 1992; 15(2)100–109.

126. Center of Disease Control and Prevention. Perspectives in disease prevention and health promotion update: universal precautions for prevention of transmission of human immunodeficiency virus, hepatitis B virus, and other bloodborne pathogens in health-care settings. MMWR 1988; 37(24):377–388.

127. Cheng FK, Ford WL, Cheng SY, et al. Occupational risk of acquiring HIV infection through needlestick injuries. Clin Perform Qual Health Care 1995; 3(3)147–150.

128. Gershon RM, Vlahov D. HIV infection risk to health care workers. Am Ind Hyg Assoc J 1990; 51(12):A802–806.

129. Jagger J, Bently MB. Injuries from vascular access devices: high risk and preventable. J Intraven Nurs 1997; 30(6S):S33–S39.

130. Ramsay ME. Guidance on the investigation and management of occupational exposure to hepatitis C. PHLS Advisory Committee on blood born viruses. Community Disease Public Health 1999; 2(4):258–262.

131. Diprose P, Deakin CD, Smedley J. Ignorance of post-exposure prophylaxis guidelines following HIV needlestick injury may increase the risk of sero conversion. Br J Anaesth 2000; 84(6):767–770.

132. Clarke SP, Sloane DM, Aiken LH. Effects of hospital staffing and organizational climate on needlestick injuries to nurses. Am J Public Health 2002; 92(7):1115–1119.

133. Danzig LE, Short IJ, Collins K, et al. Blood stream infections associated with a needleless intravenous infusion system in patients receiving home infusion therapy. JAMA 1995; 273(23):1962–1964.

134. Hanchett M, Kung LY. Do needleless intravenous systems increase the risk of infection? J Intraven Nurs 1999; 22(3):117–121.

135. Garces JM, Yazbeck H, Pi-Sunyer T, et al. Simultaneous HIV and hepatitis C infection following a needlestick injury. Eur J Clin Microbiol Infect Dis 1996; 15(1):92–94.

136. Department of Health. HIV post-exposure prophylaxis: guidance from the UK Chief Medical Officers' Expert Advisory Group on AIDS. London: Department of Health; 2000.

137. Brotherton JM, Bartlett MJ, Muscatello DJ, et al. Do we practice what we preach? Health care worker screening and vaccination. Am J Infect Control 2003; 312(3):144–150

138. Stevens AB, Coyle PV. Hepatitis C virus: an important occupational hazard? Occup Hazard (Lond.) 2000; 50(6):377–382.

139. Beltrami EM, Williams IT, Shapiro CN, et al. Risk and management of blood-borne infection in health care workers. Clin Microbiol Rev 2000; 13(3)385–407.

140. Thorburn D, Dundas D, McCruden EA, et al. A study of hepatitis C prevalence in health care workers in the West of Scotland. Gut 2001; 48(1):116–120.

141. Lanphear BP. Transmission and control of bloodborne viral hepatitis in health care workers. Occup Med 1997; 12(4):717–730.

142. Health and Safety Executive. Personal protective equipment at work regulations (EEC Directive). London: HMSO; 1992.

143. Medical Devices Agency. Latex sensitivities in the health care setting – the use of latex gloves. DB (96) 01. London: HMSO; 1996.

144. Medical Devices Agency. Latex medical gloves (surgeons and examinations) powdered latex gloves medical gloves (surgeons and examination). London: MDA: 1998.

145. Infection Control Nurses Association (ICNA). Glove usage guidelines. Edinburgh: Fitwise; 1997.

146. Power LA, Anderson RW, Cortopassi R, et al. Update on safe handling of hazardous drugs: the advice of experts. Am J Hosp Pharm 1990; 47(5):1050–1060.

147. O'Grady NP, Alexander M, Dellinger EP, et al. Guidelines for the prevention of intravasular catheter-related infections. Centers for Disease Control and Prevention. MMWR Recomm Rep 2002; 51(RR-10):1–29.

148. Rudzik J. Establishing and maintaining competency. J Intraven Nurs 1999; 22(2):69–73.

149. Hadaway LC. Developing an intraactive intravenous education and training program. J Intraven Nurs 1999; 22(2):87–93.

150. Dolan S. Intravenous flow control and infusion devices. In: Dougherty L, Lamb J, eds. Intravenous therapy in nursing practice. Edinburgh: Churchill Livingstone; 2000:195–222.

151. Dougherty L, Lamb J (eds). Intravenous therapy in nursing practice. Edinburgh: Churchill Livingstone; 2000: 481–486.

152. Desai N, Philpott-Howard J, Wade J, et al. Infection control training: evaluation of a computer-assisted learning package. J Hosp Infect 2000; 44(3):193–199.

153. Askew C. Auditing problems. Nurs Times 1993; 89(10):68–72.

154. Glenister HM, Taylor LJ, Bartlett CLR, et al. An evaluation of surveillance methods for detecting infections in hospital inpatients. J Hosp Infect 1993; 23(3):229–242.

155. Millward S, Barnett J, Thomlinson D. A clinical infection control audit programme: evaluation of an audit tool used by infection control nurses to monitor standards and assess effective staff training. J Hosp Infect 1993; 24(3):219–232.

156. Department of Health. Essence of care. Patient-focused benchmarking for health care practitioners. London: HMSO; 2001.

SECTION 2

Management of toxicity

Toxicities are a major factor in the patient's experience of chemotherapy treatment. This section covers a variety of the common and unusual side effects of treatment. We begin with an overview of toxicity from the perspective of symptom control in palliative care and cover acute and common toxicities, working through to less common and long-term toxicities.

Chapter **14**

Palliative care and the patient undergoing chemotherapy

Anna-Marie Stevens

INTRODUCTION

The role of chemotherapy in palliative care is a contentious issue.[1] There has always been a small percentage of people receiving chemotherapy in palliative care and over the last decade the likelihood of the palliative care team being involved in patients receiving chemotherapy has increased.[2] Symptom control is only one part of palliative care and can and should be accessed for patients who have uncontrolled symptoms. The role of palliative care for the patient having chemotherapy is explored and some guidance is offered on the control of the most common symptoms that patients may experience, which provides a good introduction to some of the toxicities that are discussed later.

PALLIATIVE CARE

Palliative care is referred to as:

> the active total care of patients whose disease is not responsive to curative treatment. Control of pain and other symptoms, and of psychological, social and spiritual problems is paramount. The goal of palliative care is achievement of the best quality of life for patients and their families. Many aspects of palliative treatment can also be applied earlier in the course of the illness in collaboration with anticancer therapy.

This definition goes on to explain that:

> palliative care affirms life and regards dying as a normal process, neither hastens nor postpones death, provides relief from pain and other distressing symptoms and integrates the psychological and the spiritual aspects of care.[3]

Palliative care has traditionally been associated with the last few weeks of life, a time when symptoms and psychological distress are often present and can be more difficult to control.[4] Patients should be able to access palliative care services at any time of their disease trajectory. It is evident that with new anticancer treatments available for patients, there is a probability that patients will live longer. Additionally, they need to access the services of a palliative care team for support or for issues relating to symptom control; hence the need for collaboration in patient care between the specialities of oncology and palliative care.

CHEMOTHERAPY AND PALLIATIVE CARE

Palliative chemotherapy is occasionally perceived as being futile and causing more unnecessary distress to the patient. There is clinical evidence available of the benefits in palliating symptoms in certain malignancies. Over a decade ago literature referred to the fact that in patients with non small cell lung cancer that has already spread there is a possibility that they will respond to chemotherapy. A response rate of 80% was found in some cases, with a small number of patients surviving for 2 years.[5] Further literature suggests that 78% of patients received symptomatic benefit from pleural effusions following chemotherapy.[6] Chemotherapy has been found to benefit many other patients symptomatically in other studies.[7–10] The provision of palliative care services up until the last decade has focused on the end stages of life, whereas now the focus of attention is on the presence of need rather than life expectancy.[11]

Palliative medicine stresses the importance of the patient maintaining control of his destiny and the importance of symptom control in achieving that objective.[12] It is fair to say that there is nothing wrong in considering any form of treatment that will help this process. Palliative radiotherapy has a role and so does palliative systemic therapy in many circumstances.

In considering the patient for palliative chemotherapy it is worthwhile revisiting the cardinal points of medical ethics:[12]

1. to do good
2. to minimise harm
3. to foster patient autonomy
4. to ensure a fair distribution of resources.

To do good while minimising harm

While it is clearly in the patient's interest to access treatments that will relieve symptoms and have a positive effect on quality of life, most therapies are not without some degree of side effect. When offering pharmacological interventions to improve symptoms or to offer psychological support, this appears to be a straightforward measure to palliate symptoms and produce better outcomes for the patient. However, the advocacy of surgery, radiotherapy and chemotherapy can raise more problematic ethical issues. Ethical issues are often easier to address when treatment protocols are formally planned and contain clear patient/family information and consent mechanisms.

Patient autonomy

Patients may often choose to go down the line of palliative chemotherapy to ensure that they have explored every option open to them that may give them a better quality of life, or for some lengthen their prognosis. On occasion, family members can also become involved in pushing the medical staff to 'try one last time'. Some of the unrealistic goals can be overcome with clear guidelines from the outset as well as the availability of staff to answer questions of the patient and family.

Palliative care research

Patients have two main interests in research. The first issue relates to the fact that patients often feel that in participating in research will ensure that they have access to the most up-to-date treatment. Secondly, patients often wish to make a contribution through their illness experience to the well-being of others.[13] Involvement of palliative care patients in cancer research is now a frequent event and the recruitment of palliative care patients into research studies is likely to continue to rise.

Fair distribution of resources

There has been much discussion in the media acknowledging patient reports of not always having access to the same cancer services depending on their geographical location. In some areas, patients have felt they have been denied access to some chemotherapy regimes and have found difficulty in being referred to other cancer centres where other forms of treatment may be used. The implementation of the NHS Cancer Plan[14] and the introduction of guidelines relating to the National Institute for Clinical Excellence (NICE) will hopefully ensure in the future that equity of treatments, irrespective of where the patient lives, will become an issue of the past.

TRANSITION TO PALLIATIVE CARE

As already mentioned, palliative care can be accessed at any stage of the patient's cancer journey. However, when active anticancer therapy is no longer an option for the patient it is often suggested that the day-to-day care of the patient is taken over by a palliative care team. It is imperative that this transition is undertaken sensitively.[15] The reasons for any cessation of treatment should be fully explained to the patient with the patient's family if this is what the patient wants. It will need to be made clear that stopping of anticancer treatment does not mean that the patient will be left to face the future alone. Although a cure of the disease is no longer possible, it should be highlighted that the quality of the patient's life will be the focus of care.

CHEMOTHERAPY AND ITS EFFECT ON SYMPTOMS

The most commonly reported symptoms by patients undergoing chemotherapy involve nausea, vomiting, peripheral neuropathy, symptoms associated with bone marrow depression such as mucositis and, depending on the drugs used, constipation may be prevalent.

Correct effective management of any symptom induced by any cause begins with assessment, as shown in Table 14.1.

General principles of symptom management

Evaluation

Ascertain what has been tried so far   This is helpful in considering which treatment strategy to employ first. It is necessary to explore any current treatment option used to ensure that any pharmacological intervention used has been optimised before any new therapy is commenced.

Ascertain how the symptom is affecting the patient's quality of life   Some questions that may help in identifying the impact of any symptom include:

1. When did you first experience the symptom?
2. Have you ever experienced anything like it before?

3. Is there anything we have tried so far that makes it feel better/worse?
4. Is there any pattern that you have noticed to the symptom?

Explanation

Explaining the potential reasons for the disease can be beneficial for the patient, as it reduces the fear of the unknown as well as reducing some of the psychological impact of the symptom on the patient. Demystifying symptoms for the patient is often the first step towards eradicating them.[16]

Discuss treatment options with the patient

Where possible, an open discussion should take place between the staff and the patient to ensure that the patient feels as included as he wants to be.

Management of symptoms

It is suggested that the management of symptoms often involves a combination of pharmacological and non-pharmacological therapies. Depending on the clinical area that the patient is having treated, it is important to remember non-pharmacological interventions such as relaxation, visualisation, acupuncture and other complementary therapies which may help in the management of the symptoms that the patient is experiencing.

When considering the treatment of a recurring or persistent symptom with pharmacological interventions, the drug should be administered on a regular basis and not as needed. Where possible, the drug treatment should be kept straightforward and reviewed to evaluate the intervention used.[16] In considering the use of drug treatment for the management of nausea for the patient undergoing chemotherapy, it is likely that treatment successfully used in the hospital will need to be carried on at least for the first few days. Staff often have access to self-medicating charts for use by

Table 14.1   Assessment of symptoms

Evaluation	Explanation	Management	Monitoring	Attention to detail
Diagnosis of each symptom before treatment	Explanation to the patient before, during and after treatment	Individualised treatment at all times	Continual review of the efficacy of treatment	Listen carefully to the patient's description of the symptom as well as not making assumptions

Source: adapted from Twycross and Wilcock.[12]

patients that clearly set out the time of day medications need to be taken, the name of the medication, the dose and an area for additional comments, i.e. side effects of the medication to look out for. Relevant contact numbers can also be added to self-medication charts should the patient have any queries when at home.

SYMPTOM CONTROL IN THE PATIENT UNDERGOING CHEMOTHERAPY: NAUSEA/VOMITING, ORAL PROBLEMS AND CONSTIPATION

There is overwhelming evidence to suggest that emesis secondary to chemotherapy is caused by a range of stimuli.[17] Nausea and vomiting are well-observed potential side effects of many anticancer drugs. Uncontrolled emesis affects quality of life, including physical, spiritual, psychological and social well-being.[18]

There are three well-defined stages of anticancer induced emesis:[19]

1. Acute: occurring usually during or within hours of chemotherapy (0–24 hours).
2. Delayed: occurring usually between 24 and 72 hours post chemotherapy.[20]
3. Anticipatory: occurring usually before treatment.

In clinical practice 5-HT$_3$ (5-hydroxytryptamine or serotonin) antagonists (ondansetron, granisetron, tropisetron) provide the benchmark therapy for stopping chemotherapy-induced emesis. The use of these antiemetics is largely based on increasing understanding of emetic pathways. The rule of pharmacological interventions in palliative care is that drugs should be given orally if possible and on a regular basis for a persisting problem. There are contraindications, however, when a patient is so nauseated that to take medications by mouth is not possible or in some cases the patient has intractable vomiting and is unable to absorb medications via the oral route. Many regimes of antiemetics given for chemotherapy are given intravenously. If this is not possible, a subcutaneous syringe driver can be considered. In some instances if a patient does not wish to have a subcutaneous syringe driver commenced, then antiemetic suppositories can be considered.

Syringe driver

Battery-controlled syringe drivers are convenient and portable: not only can they be used in the hospital setting but they can also be used in the home. The advantages of this method include:

1. Better control of nausea and vomiting, as this method will ensure drug absorption.
2. Generally reloaded once in a 24-hour period.
3. Reduces the number of repeated single injections.
4. Does not interfere with patient's activity, as this is a portable system that the patient can mobilise with. This system can, if necessary, be maintained at home and does not necessitate hospital admission.

Table 14.2 is a suggestion of pharmacological interventions that may help chemotherapy-induced nausea and vomiting.

Table 14.2   Pharmacological interventions that may help chemotherapy-induced nausea and vomiting

Cause	Features	Antiemetic	Dose	Consider
Chemotherapy-induced	Acute or delayed	Granisetron Dexamathasone	1 mg bd po/iv 4 mg tds po/iv	May cause constipation Consider usual side effects with steroids, particularly insomnia if given late in the day
		Metoclopramide	10–20 mg po/sc or 30–120 mg over 24 h via a subcutaneous syringe driver	
		Domperidone	10–20 mg qds po or 30–60 mg qds pr	
		Levomepromazine	6.25–25 mg po or can be given in a 24 h continuous syringe driver	Can cause drowsiness

Source: adapted from Department of Palliative Medicine, Guidelines for symptom control (unpublished data). Royal Marsden Hospital, 2002.

It has been suggested that the role of lorazepam in the treatment of chemotherapy-induced nausea and vomiting should be considered in the management of this symptom. It is recommended that where standard therapy has failed and anticipatory emesis persists, the addition of lorazepam can significantly improve emesis control. The need to assess patients prior to each cycle of chemotherapy or before each new challenge of treatment will alert the professional as to whether using lorazepam as an adjuvant will be helpful in the management of this symptom.

Oral symptoms

The following sections consider the various causes and treatments for oral discomfort and are based on local guidelines: Guidelines for symptom control (unpublished data, 2002), Department of Palliative Medicine, Royal Marsden Hospital.

Fungal infections
Candida is typically seen as white oral plaques, but may be present in other forms. It can be represented as a red tongue or generalised stomatitis. Use:

- nystatin 2 ml qds for prophylaxis
- fluconazole 50 mg od or 100 mg iv for 1 week or single-dose 150 mg (moderate to severe infections)
- ketoconazole 200 mg od for 1 week (need to be careful regarding drug interactions).

Viral
Viral ulcers are often herpetic and require systemic antiviral therapy:

- aciclovir 200 mg 4 hourly for 1 week.

Bacterial
This is often associated with malignant disease in the oral cavity:

- requires treatment with systemic antibiotics
- a pungent smell suggests anaerobic infections necessitating treatment with metronidazole.

Oral pain
1. Treat the underlying cause, e.g. infection.
2. Systemic analgesics.
3. Aspirin mouthwash (1 or 2 × 300 mg soluble tablets dissolved in water qds). This can be mixed with mucilage to aid adherence to the hypopharnyx.
4. Topical coating agents (sucralflate) for an ulcerated mucosa.
5. Orabase to cover and protect large ulcers, combination with triamcinolone (Adcortyl in Orabase) may be helpful in painful ulcers.

6. Local anaesthetic agents lidocaine (lignocaine) 2% gel (Instillagel) applied qds or lidocaine (lignocaine) spray.
7. Topical morphine (Oramorph mouthwash)

These interventions are guidelines only. Each clinical area may have its own local treatments, depending on chemotherapy agents being used and cost. What is important is to, where possible, ascertain from the patient a description of the problem in the oral cavity, use evidence-based interventions where possible and review the interventions on a regular basis.

Constipation

Constipation can occur for several reasons. Drug-induced constipation can be a result of chemotherapy agents. Some patients may have the problem of additional strong painkillers that may add to this problem.

Guidelines for the prescription of laxatives are based on local guidelines
An accurate history is essential for the diagnosis and effective management of constipation.
Inquiry should be made about:

- frequency and consistency of stools
- abdominal discomfort/bloating
- mobility and diet
- emotional factors such as being able to maintain dignity and privacy in getting to the toilet.

In patients with a history of diarrhoea, care needs to be taken to distinguish between true diarrhoea and overflow caused by faecal impaction.
In some cases, if diagnosis remains uncertain, an abdominal X-ray to ascertain the cause may be indicated.
Consider causes of constipation and where possible treat or prevent:

- drugs that may cause constipation
- immobility of patients
- dehydration
- low-fibre diet
- hypercalcaemia
- spinal cord compression.

Classification of laxatives
Table 14.3 gives a classification of laxatives.

Treatment guidelines
Treat underlying causes by non-pharmacological methods. Where possible, encourage:

- oral fluids

Table 14.3 Classification of laxatives

Type of laxative	Notes	Preparation	Special instruction
Bulk-forming	These agents act by retaining water so the stool remains large and soft, thus stimulating peristalsis	Isphaghula husk (Fybogel)	Patients with strictures or partial obstruction must be cautious as intestinal obstruction could occur, if insufficient quantities of fluid are taken
Stimulant	Cause water and electrolytes to accumulate in the intestines and stimulate motility through direct contact of the agent and the mucosa	Dantron (component of co-danthramer and co-danthrusate) Senna – tablets/liquid Bisacodyl – tablets/liquid Glycerine suppository – rectal Phosphate enema – chronic constipation	This group should be avoided in bowel obstruction as they can exacerbate colic
Mixed stimulants and softeners	2 in 1 preparations	Co-dantramar – liquid/capsules Dantron and poloxamer available in normal and strong strengths Dioctyl	Alert patients to orange/brown change in urine. Can cause perianal irritation avoid when patient has a catheter or is incontinent Mild stimulant
Softeners	Attract/retain water in intestinal lumen increasing intraluminal pressure	Milpar (liquid parafin and magnesium hydroxide) Docusate Arachis oil enema	Long-term use of softeners can cause gut granulomata and lipoid pneumonitis **Avoid if patient has nut allergy, plus it is expensive**
Osmotic	Agents act in the intestinal tract by increasing stimulation of fluid secretion and motility	Lactulose Phosphate enema Microlax enema Magnesium sulphate mixture	Can cause bloating, flatulence and abdominal discomfort. Patients often find sweet taste difficult to tolerate. Is used in the case of hepatic encephalopathy as it induces a low pH which discourages the proliferation of ammonia-producing organisms For rapid bowel evacuation, use with caution

- diet modifications
- increased mobility.

General points
All patients on opioids should have an appropriate laxative commenced.
Titrate doses of laxatives as necessary after assessment of the patient response to a particular laxative.

There is evidence to suggest that there is no proven correlation between increasing doses of opioids requiring escalating doses of laxatives. Necessary increases in the laxative will depend on the patient's response.

Avoid mixing two laxatives of the same type, i.e. stimulants.

Chronic constipation
- First line: non-pharmacological interventions – encourage fluid intake, review diet and increase mobility where possible.
- Second line: Milpar 10–20 ml bd. Senna 2–4 tablets bd on a regular basis.
 Senna tablets or liquid should only be used in association with a softening agent such as Milpar to prevent colic.
 Co-danthramer capsules 1–4 tablets bd
 or
 Co-danthramer liquid 10–20 ml bd
 Co-danthramer forte 1–4 capsules bd for those patients who have persistent constipation.

Co-danthramer use is inappropriate in patients who are incontinent, as the dantron can cause superficial skin irritation and excoriation

- Third line: docusate 2–4 tablets bd

Rectal measures   Rectal impaction – first line:

- Glycerine suppositories × 2
- Microlette enema
- Phosphate enema

Colonic impaction – high arachis oil enema overnight followed by a phosphate enema the following morning. Repeat process until a result.

If there is still no result, consider prokinetics – erythromycin, cisapride.

Use under the guidance of the palliative care team.

Other options include cathartic agents:

- Picolax
- Citramag
- Klean-Prep.

Magnesium salts should only be used in conjunction with enemas after an abdominal X-ray has excluded intestinal bowel obstruction.

Bowel obstruction   If bowel obstruction, stop all stimulant laxatives as these will exacerbate colic.

Continue with softening agents, i.e. Milpar/docusate. Use glycerine suppositories to relieve faecal impaction. Lidocaine (lignocaine) gel can be administered topically prior to the insertion of the enema to ease the procedure for the patient.

For patients with colonic inertia:

- keep stool soft, i.e. Milpar 10–20 ml bd
- bisacodyl suppositories every 3rd day.

CONCLUSION

This chapter, although not exhaustive, has tried to give an overview of the most common symptoms in the patient undergoing chemotherapy. It has also tried to offer insight into how the principles of palliative care can be applied to patients undergoing chemotherapy who are at any stage of their disease trajectory. The important aspects must always be to listen to the patient, select an appropriate management plan, explain the suggested plan to the patient and review on a regular basis. There are many aspects of the palliative care approach to the management of this group of patients that can be employed to ensure a better quality of life for the patient, irrespective of whether the patient is at the beginning or coming towards the end of the cancer journey.

References

1. McGrath P, Kearsley JH. Is there a better way? Bioethical reflections on palliative cytotoxic drug use. Palliat Med 1995; 9:269–271.
2. Macdonald N. Principles governing the use of cancer chemotherapy in palliative medicine. In: Doyle D, Hanks G, Macdonald N, eds. Oxford textbook of palliative medicine. Oxford: Oxford University Press; 1997:105–107.
3. World Health Organisation. Cancer pain relief and palliative care. Technical Report Series 804. Geneva, 1990.
4. Penson J, Fisher R. Palliative care for people with cancer. London: Edward Arnold; 1991.
5. Spiro SG. Management of lung cancer. BMJ 1990; 301:1287–1288.
6. Bonnefoi H, Smith IE. How should cancer presenting as a malignant effusion be managed? Br J Cancer 1996; 74(5):832–835.
7. Pagnoncelli D, Vianna LB. The use of chemotherapy in palliative care. Palliat Med 1992; 6:341–342.
8. Tannock IF, Boyd NF, De Boer G, et al. A randomised trial of two dose levels of cyclophosphamide, methotrexate, and fluorouracil chemotherapy for patients with metastatic breast cancer. J Clin Oncol 1988; 6:1377–1387.
9. Henderson IC. Breast cancer. In: Murphy GP, Lawrence W, Lenhard RE, eds. American Cancer Society textbook of clinical oncology. Atlanta: American Cancer Society; 1995:214.
10. Russell JA. Cytotoxic therapy – pain relief and recalcification. In: Stoll BA, Parbhoo S, eds. Bone metastasis: monitoring and treatment. New York: Raven Press; 1983:354–368.
11. Gaebler S. Chemotherapy: the palliative role. Eur J Palliat Care 1998; 5:144–147.
12. Twycross R, Wilcock A. Symptom management in advanced cancer. 3rd edn. Oxford: Radcliffe Medical Press; 2002.
13. Macdonald N. The interface between oncology and palliative medicine. In: Doyle D, Hanks G, Macdonald N, eds. Oxford textbook of palliative medicine. Oxford: Oxford University Press; 1997:11–17.
14. Department of Health. The NHS Cancer Plan. London: Department of Health; 2001.
15. Doyle D, Hanks G, Macdonald N. Oxford textbook of palliative medicine. Oxford: Oxford University Press; 1997.
16. Twycross R. Symptom management in advanced cancer. 2nd edn. Oxford: Radcliffe Medical Press; 1997.
17. Cooper R, Gent P. An overview of chemotherapy-induced emesis highlighting the role of lorazepam as adjuvant therapy. Int J Palliat Nurs 2002; 8:331–335.
18. Grant M. Nausea and vomiting, quality of life and the oncology nurse. Oncol Nurs Forum 1997; 24:20–32.
19. Hogan C, Grant M. Physiologic mechanisms of nausea and vomiting in patients with cancer. Oncol Nurs Forum 1997; 24:8–12.
20. Gandara DR. Progress in the control of acute and delayed emesis induced by cisplatin. Eur J Cancer 1991; 27:9–11.

Chapter **15**

Chemotherapy-associated anaphylaxis

Corinne Rowbotham

INTRODUCTION

Anaphylaxis is a rapid and often life-threatening reaction that may be precipitated by many chemotherapy drugs (Table 15.1). The term, derived from 'ana' meaning without and 'phylaxis' meaning protection, was first used in the early 20th century by Portier and Richet to describe the fatal effect of re-injecting venom into dogs that had previously tolerated the poison.[1]

PATHOPHYSIOLOGY[2]

The inappropriate activation of mast cells (and their circulating counterparts, basophils) is the key event in anaphylaxis (Fig. 15.1).[2] This activation occurs when either the drug binds to IgE antibodies located on the mast cell surface (anaphylactic reaction) or triggers the enzymatic cascade of plasma proteins known as the complement system, releasing the biologically active anaphylatoxins C3a and C5a (anaphylactoid reaction). In the more common anaphylactic reaction a drug may cross-react with pre-existing IgE antibodies or bind avidly to specific IgE antibodies produced from previous exposure to the drug.

Once activated, mast cells release pre-formed and newly synthesised pharmacologically active compounds, including histamine, heparin, platelet activating factor (PAF), leukotrienes, prostaglandins and kinins. These compounds produce the bronchoconstriction, vasodilatation and increased capillary permeability that are responsible for the clinical features of anaphylaxis.

It must be appreciated that all of these events are normal immunological and inflammatory responses. Anaphylaxis is the result of the inappropriate and

Table 15.1   Cytotoxic drugs that may precipitate anaphylactic reactions

Drug	Frequency
Asparaginase	25–44%
Amsacrine	Case reports
Bleomycin	Case reports
Carboplatin	5–15%
Cisplatin	Up to 20%, increases with total exposure
Cyclophosphamide	Case reports
Cytarabine	Case reports
Dacarbazine	Case reports
Daunorubicin	1–5%
Docetaxel	Up to 30% unpremed. 5% premed
Doxorubicin	<1–5%
Epirubicin	<1–5%
Etoposide	3%
Fluorouracil	Case reports
Idarubicin	1–5%
Ifosfamide	Case reports
Melphalan	2–5%
Methotrexate	Case reports
Mitomycin	Case reports up to 10%
Mitoxantrone (mitozantrone)	Case reports
Chlormethine (mustine)	Case reports
Oxaliplatin	Case reports
Paclitaxel	Up to 40% unpremed. 2–5% premed
Pentostatin	Case reports
Teniposide	Case reports up to 13%
Vinblastine	Case reports

Source: reproduced with permission of Allwood et al.[5]

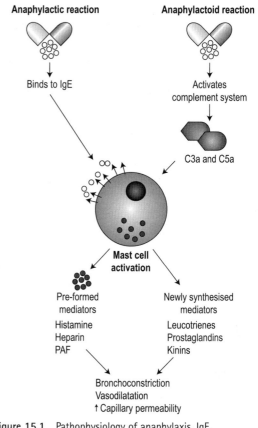

Figure 15.1   Pathophysiology of anaphylaxis. IgE, immunoglobulin E; PAF, platelet activating factor.

often widespread overstimulation of these responses by the offending drug.

CLINICAL FEATURES[3,4]

The clinical presentation of anaphylaxis depends on the severity of the reaction and the route of administration of the offending drug: onset is usually rapid but can be delayed for up to 30 min. Unexplained anxiety and unease may be the earliest indications that a patient is developing an adverse reaction. If the offending drug is given orally, the predominant features are mucosal with oral, facial and laryngeal oedema. If given intravenously, reactions range from localised urticaria and pruritis to severe bronchospasm with hypotension and circulatory collapse (anaphylactic shock). Other features include sneezing, flu-like symptoms, metallic taste, light-headedness and dizziness, tightening in the chest and palpitations.

MANAGEMENT

An acute anaphylactic reaction is a medical emergency and the outcome will depend on the rapidity of treatment. Adrenaline (epinephrine), an alpha and beta-adrenergic agonist, is the key drug and can prevent serious life-threatening reactions from developing. It reverses vasodilation and decreases capillary permeability and musosal oedema (alpha-adreno-receptor mediated effects) as well as dilating bronchial smooth muscle, relieving bronchospasm (beta-adrenoreceptor mediated effect). Chlorphenamine (chlorpheniramine) (Piriton), an H_1 receptor antagonist or antihistamine, blocks the effects of histamine the major mediator released in anaphylaxis. Finally, corticosteroids (hydrocortisone) continue to modulate the immune response after the short-lived effects of adrenaline (epinephrine) have subsided.

The recommended emergency management of a patient experiencing an anaphylactic reaction is as follows:[6]

- Stop the offending drug but maintain peripheral intravenous access.
- Maintain airway and administer oxygen via re-breathing facemask.
- Summon help.
- Begin regular, frequent measurements of pulse and blood pressure and respiratory rate.
- If the patient is hypotensive, lay them in a supine position. If they are experiencing respiratory difficulties and are not hypotensive, nurse them in an upright position.
- Administer emergency drugs:
  - Adrenaline (epinephrine) 500 µg (0.5 ml of a 1:1000 solution) aliquots intramuscularly, repeated every 5 min, according to patient response. If there is real doubt about the adequacy of the circulation and intramuscular absorption, adrenaline (epinephrine) 500 µg (5 ml of a 1:10 000 solution) can be given by slow intravenous injection with extreme caution.
  - Chlophenamine (chlopheniramine) 10–20 mg by intramuscular or slow intravenous injection.
  - Hydrocortisone 100–300 mg by intramuscular or intravenous injection.
- Provide reassurance and information throughout to both patient and his family.
- Carefully document assessment, intervention and patient response and ensure the patient's reaction to the offending drug is officially documented to prevent future administration.

CONCLUSION

Anaphylaxis is an uncommon reaction that may be precipitated by many chemotherapy drugs. Its severity ranges from irritating reactions at intravenous injection sites to life-threatening laryngeal oedema, bronchospasm and anaphylactic shock. All professionals should be aware of the clinical features of anaphylaxis and be familiar with local protocols for its immediate management. They should take time to prepare their patients at the start of their chemotherapy, discussing the symptoms of anaphylaxis as well as possible side effects of the drugs they are to receive.

References

1. Green T, Gardiner P. The immune system part I: anaphylaxis. Nurs Times 1997; 93:60–63.
2. Roitt IM, Delves PJ. Hypersensitivity. In: Roitt IM, ed. Roitt's essential immunology. 10th edn. Oxford: Blackwell Scientific Publications; 2001:322–348.
3. Nendick M. Anaphylactic reactions during chemotherapy. Prof Nurse 1999; 14(8):553–556.
4. Ewan P. ABC of allergies: anaphylaxis. BMJ 1998; 316:1442–1445.
5. Allwood M, Stanley A, Wright P (eds). Managing complications of chemotherapy. In: The cytotoxics handbook. 4th edn. Oxford: Radcliffe Medical Press; 2002:119–194.
6. British National Formulary. Allergic emergencies. In: BNF No 47, March 2004. London: British Medical Association and Royal Pharmaceutical Society of Great Britain; 2004:156–158.

Chapter **16**

Nausea and vomiting

Moira Stephens

INTRODUCTION

Nausea and vomiting remains as one of the most frequent side effects of cancer chemotherapy, despite advances in antiemetic treatment.[1,2] Nausea and vomiting may be related to one or more of the following causes:

- the cancer treatment (chemotherapy or radiotherapy)
- the cancer itself
- other factors (chemical, drug, central nervous system, vestibular, visceral).

Patients typically view control of nausea as more important than control of vomiting, while physicians and nurses judge vomiting control to be more important to antiemetic efficacy than nausea control.[2]

PATHOPHYSIOLOGY

Our knowledge of the physiology of nausea and vomiting is incomplete. Research regarding chemotherapy-related emesis in adults has grown over the last 20 years, but much less has been learned about nausea.[3]

There are a number of mechanisms responsible for nausea and vomiting (Fig. 16.1).

The chemoreceptor trigger zone (CTZ) in the fourth ventricle of the brain is activated by substances within the blood and cerebrospinal fluid.

Once these receptors are stimulated, signals are relayed to the vomiting centre in the brainstem, a network of neuroanatomic connections. This interprets the input from other structures and sends impulses to motor nuclei, which leads to vomiting and nausea.

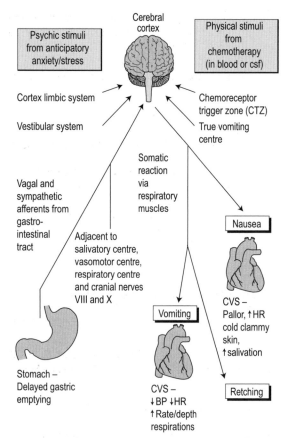

Figure 16.1 Mechanisms of cancer-related nausea and vomiting.

Emetic stimuli act on dopamine receptors within the CTZ and include:

- drugs such as hormones, opioids and chemotherapy agents
- hypercalcaemia
- toxins from pathogens
- tumour breakdown products.

Visceral disturbances cause nausea and vomiting and may be due to:

- distension
- constipation
- obstruction from the tumour compressing or obstructing the gastrointestinal tract or other abdominal organs.

(See also Ch. 17.)
Vestibular causes include:

- motion-induced nausea and vomiting
- some drugs, such as opioids, aspirin and alcohol

- tumours affecting the vestibular system (such as intracranial lesions, metastases to the base of skull and acoustic neuroma).

(See also Ch. 53.)
Other factors:

- pain
- infection
- emotional responses, either alone, or in conjunction with another cause.

(See also Chs 13 and 14.)

EPIDEMIOLOGY AND RISK FACTORS

Acute nausea and vomiting occurs immediately after chemotherapy administration. Optimal emetic control in the acute phase is essential to prevent nausea and vomiting in the delayed phase.

Delayed emesis typically occurs after 24 hours and following highly emetogenic chemotherapy, either given as a single agent or in combination. Delayed emesis seems to be partially mediated by 5-HT$_3$ (5-hydroxytryptamine or serotonin) antagonists, and granisitron has shown efficacy in delayed emesis.

Anticipatory nausea and vomiting generally occurs after several cycles of chemotherapy but may occur after one course. Certain sights, sounds or smells become cues and the patient will vomit prior to receiving the chemotherapy. Patients at risk of anticipatory vomiting (Table 16.1):

- female patients
- patients under 40 years
- patients receiving high doses of cisplatin
- patients with a prior susceptibility to vomiting, such as with motion sickness.[4]

Table 16.1 Emesis risk factors – favourable and non-favourable (not including emetic potential of drug given, Table 16.2) [5-12]

Favourable risk factors	Non–favourable risk factors
Male	Female
State of relaxation	Anxious
Initial course of chemotherapy	Subsequent courses of chemotherapy
Chemotherapy administered as inpatient	Chemotherapy administered as outpatient
History of high alcohol intake	Younger patient
Timely administration of appropriate antiemetics	Insufficient or ill-timed antiemetic administration

Table 16.2   Assessing the emetogenicity of a regime – risk of emesis with single or combination cytotoxic regimes[13]

Low risk: regimens containing one or more of the following	Moderate risk: regimens containing one of the following ± any low risk agents NB. Regimens containing 2 or more of these agents should be treated as high risk	High risk: regimens containing one or more of the following
5-Fluorouracil	Amsacrine	Busulfan >40 mg
Asparaginase	Cyclophosphamide (po)	Carboplatin
Bleomycin	Cyclophosphamide <750 mg/m^2	Carmustine
Busulfan	Cytarabine <1 g/m^2	Cisplatin
Chlorambucil	Docetaxel	Cyclophosphamide ≥750 mg/m^2
Cladribine	Etopside	Cytarabine ≥1 g/m^2
Fludarabine	Fotemustine	Dacarbazine
Fluoropyrimidines (po)	Gemcitabine	Dactinomycin
Hydroxyurea	Ifosfamide <1.5 g/m^2	Daunorubicin
Melphalan (po)	Melphalan <100 mg/m^2	Doxorubicin
Mercaptopurine (po)	Methotrexate >50 mg/m^2	Epirubicin
Methotrexate ≤50 mg/m^2	Mitomycin	Idarubicin
Thioguanine (po)	Paclitaxel	Ifosfamide ≥1.5 g/m^2
Thiotepa	Procarbazine (po)	Irinotecan
Vinblastine	Raltitrexed	Lomustine
Vincristine	Topotecan	Melphalan 100 mg/m^2
Vindesine		Mitoxantrone (mitozantrone)
Vinorelbine		Chlormethine (mustine)
		Oxaliplatin
		Pentostatin
		Streptozocin
		Temozolamide

Chemotherapeutic agents have variable emetic potential (Table 16.2) and not all patients will experience nausea and vomiting, and if they do so, will experience it in varying degrees of severity. Studies have demonstrated a number of potentially predictive factors:

- women vomit more readily than men
- younger patients are more susceptible
- anxiety exacerbates nausea and vomiting following treatment
- emesis may be more easily controlled following the first dose of chemotherapy; however, this may be due to the effect of anticipatory vomiting.
- a history of high alcohol intake has been shown to reduce the likelihood of sickness following chemotherapy.[5]

MANAGEMENT OF NAUSEA AND VOMITING

Pharmacological

Three major categories of drugs are used to treat nausea and vomiting associated with cancer chemotherapy. These are:

- serotonin or 5-HT$_3$ antagonists such as ondansetron or granisetron
- dopamine antagonists such as metoclopramide
- corticosteroids, which are often effective in combination with another antiemetic such as dexamethasone.

Patients treated with combination therapy of ondansetron and dexamethasone received better relief from cisplatin-induced nausea and vomiting than those receiving ondansetron alone.[14] For this reason, standard regimes of corticosteroids have been devised, matched to the emetic potential of drugs (Table 16.3 and Box 16.1). There are also miscellaneous antiemetics such as antihistamines (H$_1$, e.g. cyclizine, and H$_2$, e.g. ranitidine, cannabinoids, benzodiazepines and anticholinergics.[15,16] See also Ch. 14.)

Although nausea and vomiting is treatable, it is better to take a prophylactic approach, both for the benefit of the patient's experience and in order to reduce the potential for anticipatory vomiting in the future.

Non–pharmacological

A number of non-pharmacological interventions have been used effectively but evidence of efficacy remains largely anecdotal:

Table 16.3 Common antiemetic protocols according to the emetic potential of drugs[11]

Low emetic risk	Moderate emetic risk	High emetic risk
Regular antiemetics not routinely required If necessary, metoclopramide 10 mg iv prior to chemotherapy If symptoms develop, then metoclopramide 10–20 mg po tds or domperidone 10–20 mg tds/qds	**First-line schedule** Prior to chemotherapy dexamethasone 8 mg iv ± metoclopramide 10–20 mg iv Then: dexamethasone 4 mg po tds for 2–3 days, with metoclopramide 10–20 mg po tds/qds or domperidone 10–20 mg tds/qds **Antiemetics should be prescribed regularly to prevent delayed emesis**	**First-line schedule** Prior to chemotherapy: granisetron 1 mg iv (2 mg if >100 kg) Then: dexamethasone 4 mg po tds for 2–3 days, with metoclopramide 20 mg po tds/qds or domperidone 20 mg tds/qds Antiemetics should be prescribed regularly to prevent delayed emesis Granisetron 1 mg po od for 2–4 days may be considered if vomiting occurs in the acute phase
	Second-line schedule If antiemetics fail in the acute period (i.e. 1st 24 hours or before chemotherapy complete Next cycle, prior to chemotherapy give: dexamethasone 8 mg iv granisetron 1 mg iv (2 mg if >100 kg) Then: as above	**Second-line schedule** Inadequate control in the acute period (i.e. 1st 24 hours or before chemotherapy complete) Add high-dose dopamine antagonist (metoclopramide 20 mg iv/po qds or levomepromazine 6.25–12.5 mg sc/iv or 6–12 mg po od–bd) Add lorazepam 1 mg iv/po/sl stat if nausea is anticipatory Threshold effect for granisetron is likely. Exceptionally, a second dose may be given, however, this may not increase efficacy once all 5-HT3 receptors are saturated.

Box 16.1   Failure of emetic control[13]

If delayed nausea and vomiting after moderately or highly emetic regimens are not adequately controlled by the above recommendations, the following options should be considered. Evaluate how poor emetic control is first, as a change of antiemetic regimen may not be superior.

Evaluate the antiemetic regimen for appropriateness:

- dexamethasone is the most useful agent in preventing delayed emesis
- ensure antiemetics cover the full period of delayed nausea; dexamethasone duration may be increased to 5 days
- to ensure absorption, consider the use of suppositories, e.g. cyclizine, domperidone or prochlorperazine (if rectal route is not contraindicated) or s/c or iv routes
- consider concurrent disease and medication factors
- in anticipatory vomiting, give lorazepam 1 mg po/sl the evening before and the morning of the chemotherapy.

For breakthrough treatments consider:

- levomepromazine 6.25–25 mg/day iv/sc or 6–24 mg po in 2 divided doses
- or cyclizine 50 mg po/iv/sc
- or haloperidol 1.5–3mg od-bd po/iv/sc.

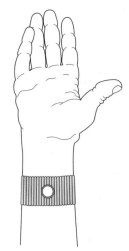

Figure 16.2   Seaband in situ.

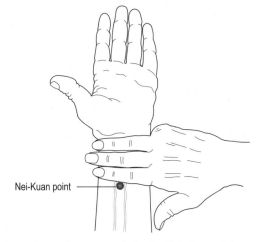

Nei-Kuan point

Figure 16.3   Acupressure, indicating Nei-Kuan point.

1. Exercise has been shown to be useful, and in one controlled study of exercise conducted in 42 patients with breast cancer, those patients in the experimental group undertaking aerobic exercise three times a week for 10 weeks reported significant decreases in nausea.[17]
2. Evidence supporting cognitive-behavioural interventions is uncertain. However, since anxiety potentially may exacerbate nausea and vomiting, interventions to reduce anxiety may be beneficial and although they cannot control nausea and vomiting alone, they make a contribution to patient well-being and comfort. Patients receiving supportive interventions have reported feeling more in control, hopeful, powerful, relaxed and less afraid.[18]
3. Dietary changes may be recommended, and although evidence is again largely anecdotal, recommendations include:

   - offering clear liquids
   - ginger, ginger beer
   - soda water
   - dry toast
   - avoidance of hot foods, as they may have a more pronounced odour.

Acupressure and the use of 'seabands' (Fig. 16.2) have been shown in a number of clinical trials to be beneficial.[19–21]

The acupressure point for emesis is located on the inside of the wrist, three digit widths above the crease of the wrist joint between the two tendons, and is referred to as the Nei-Kuan point (Fig. 16.3).

CONCLUSION

The key elements in attempting to control nausea and vomiting in the patient undergoing chemotherapy include:

- knowledge of the drugs to be administered
- the timely administration of prophylactic antiemetics if indicated
- a prepared prescription of 'as required' antiemetics
- knowledge of the patient and his experience
- establishing a therapeutic relationship with the patient
- a calm and supportive atmosphere
- the availability of resources and advice for the patient.

References

1. Osoba D, Zee B, Pater J, et al. Determinants of postchemotherapy nausea and vomiting in patients with cancer. J Clin Oncol 1997; 15(1):116–123.
2. Morrow GR, Roscoe JA, Hickok JT, et al. Nausea and emesis: evidence for a biobehavioral perspective Support Care Cancer 2002; 10(2):96–105.

3. Groenwald SL, Goodman M, Frogge MH, et al (eds). Cancer symptom management. Boston: Jones and Bartlett; 1998.
4. Paice J. Symptom management. In: Buchsel P, Miaskowski C, eds. Oncology nursing: assessment and clinical care. St Louis: Mosby; 1999.

5.   Doherty KM. Closing the gap in prophylactic antiemetic therapy: patient factors in calculating the emetogenic potential of chemotherapy. Clin J Oncol Nurs 1999; 3(3):113–119.

6.   Zook DJ, Yasko JM. Psychological factors: their effect on nausea and vomiting experienced by clients receiving chemotherapy. Oncol Nurs Forum 1983; 10:76–81.

7.   Liaw CC, Wang CH, Chang HK, et al Gender discrepancy observed between chemotherapy-induced emesis and hiccups. Support Care Cancer 2001; 9(6):435–441.

8.   Roila F, Tonato M, Basurto C. Antiemetic activity of high doses of metaclopramide in cisplatin-treated cancer patients: a randomised double-blind trial of the Italian Oncology Group for Clinical Research. J Clin Oncol 1988; 5:141–149.

9.   Andrykowski M, Gregg ME. Development of anticipatory nausea: a prospective analysis. J Consult Clin Psychol 1992; 53:447–454.

10. Gralla RJ, Itri LM, Pisko SE. Antiemetic efficacy of high dose metaclopramide: randomized trials with placebo and prochlorperazine in patients with chemotherapy induced nausea and vomiting. N Engl J Med 1981; 3055:905–909.

11. Roila F, Tonato M, Basurto C. Protection from nausea and vomiting in cisplatin-treated patients: high dose metaclopramide combined with methylprednisolone versus metaclopramide combined with dexamethasone and diphenhydramine: a study of the Italian Oncology Group for Clinical Research. J Clin Oncol 1989; 7:1693–1700.

12. D'Aquisto RW, Tyson LB, Gralla RJ. The influence of a chronic high alcohol intake on chemotherapy induced nausea and vomiting. Proc Am Soc Clin Oncol 1986; 5:257.

13. Royal Marsden Hospital (RMH). Drugs and Therapeutics Advisory Committee (DTAC) Prescribing Guidelines. August 2004.

14. Olver I, Paska W, Depierre A, et al. A multicentre double-blind study comparing placebo, ondansatron, and ondansatron plus dexamethasone for the control of cisplatin-induced delayed emesis. Ann Oncol 1996; 7:945–952.

15. Cooper R, Gent P. An overview of chemotherapy-induced emesis highlighting the role of lorazepam as adjuvant therapy. Int J Palliat Nurs 2002; 8(7): 331–335.

16. Musty RE, Rosti R. Effects of smoked cannabis and oral delta(9)-tetrahydrocannabinol on nausea and emesis after cancer chemotherapy: a review of state clinical trials. J Cannabis Therap 2001; 1(1):29–42.

17. Winningham ML, MacVicar MG. The effect of aerobic exercise on patient reports of nausea. Oncol Nurs Forum 1988; 15:447–450.

18. Troesch LM, Rodehaver CB, Delaney EA, et al. The influence of guided imagery on chemotherapy-related nausea and vomiting. Oncol Nurs Forum 1993; 20:1179–1185.

19. Dundee JW, Ghaly RG, Fitzpatrick KTJ, et al. Acupuncture prophylaxis of cancer chemotherapy-induced sickness. J Roy Soc Med 1989; 82:268–271.

20. Sadler C. Can acupressure relieve nausea? Nurs Times 1989; 85(51):32–34.

21. Dundee JW, Yang J. Prolongation of the antiemetic action of P6 acupuncture by acupressure in patients having cancer chemotherapy. J Roy Soc Med 1990; 83:360–362.

Chapter **17**

Gastrointestinal effects

Ramani Sitamvaram

INTRODUCTION

Chemotherapy can profoundly affect the gastro-intestinal (GI) tract and can result in a number of distressing side effects.[1] Ninety per cent of the GI crypt epithelium is made up of undifferentiated and goblet cells which are found in the small intestine. These cells are mitotically active and, as such, are vulnerable to cytotoxic attack.[2] The most common chemotherapy induced toxicities to the GI tract are:

- nausea
- vomiting
- mucositis
- oesophagitis
- diarrhoea
- constipation.

(See also Chs 18 and 19.)

DIARRHOEA

Diarrhoea has been defined as:

> An abnormal increase in the quantity, frequency and fluid content of stool and can be associated with urgency, perianal discomfort and incontinence.[3]

Diarrhoea can occur when the epithelial cells of the intestines have a rapid turnover rate and are damaged by chemotherapy, particularly antimetabolites. Chemotherapy inhibits cell replication and disrupts cell replacement. The mucosal cells become ulcerated and inflamed and produce increased amounts of mucus and the peristaltic rate is increased. This results in an increased throughput of intestinal substances.[4]

Diarrhoea is common following chemotherapy treatment (Box 17.1).

Box 17.1	Common chemotherapy agents with diarrhoea as a side effect

Capecitabine
Cisplatin
Cytosine arabinoside (cytarabine)
Cyclophosphamide
Daunorubicin
Docetaxel
Doxorubicin
5-Fluorouracil
Interferon
Irinotecan
Leucovorin
Methotrexate
Oxaliplatin
Topotecan

Severe diarrhoea in patients can induce dehydration, hypotension and neutropenic sepsis, if the granulocyte nadir occurs at the same time.[5] The degree and duration of the symptoms of diarrhoea depend on the drug, the dose schedule and the duration of treatment. (See also Ch. 48: GvHD.)

Assessment of diarrhoea and constipation

Identifying the underlying cause is essential to the successful management of both diarrhoea and constipation. The assessment should include a careful history of the patient's bowel habits, including any changes in:[6]

- frequency of bowel action
- volume, consistency and colour of stool
- presence of mucus, blood or offensive odour
- pain or discomfort on defecation
- use of medication to stimulate defecation
- dietary history
- medical history
- lifestyle changes.

Management of diarrhoea

Effective management should focus on the cause of the diarrhoea and in providing physical and psychological support for the patient. Diarrhoea can be very debilitating and distressing and patients must be encouraged to report even the mildest diarrhoea so that it can be controlled.

Nutritional status should be maintained by encouraging patients to take adequate fluids, proteins and calories.[4]

Pharmacological management may be necessary and drugs such as loperamide or codeine could be used to slow peristalsis.

If diarrhoea is persistent, it may be necessary to discontinue, delay or reduce the dose of the contributory chemotherapeutic agent.

The WHO[7] common toxicity criteria include an assessment tool for grading the severity of diarrhoea (Table 17.1).

CONSTIPATION

Constipation is defined as delayed movement of intestinal content through the bowel and is associated with dry stool, which may be difficult to pass.[8]

Constipation can be a presenting symptom of cancer or a side effect of treatment.[9] Chemotherapy agents that most commonly cause constipation are the vinca alkaloids.[2]

Symptoms of constipation

- Reduced or infrequent defecation
- Difficulty in defecation
- Hard and bulky stools
- Feeling of incomplete emptying of rectal contents.[10]

Constipation is associated with abdominal pain, feeling of bloatedness, general malaise, anorexia, restlessness, retention of urine and faecal incontinence.[10]

Table 17.1 National cancer institute common toxicity[7] criteria for grading severity of diarrhoea

	Grade 0	Grade 1	Grade 2	Grade 3	Grade 4
Number of stools	Normal	Increase of 2–3 stools per day	Increase of 4–6 stools per day	Increase of 7–9 stools per day	Greater than 10 stools per day
Symptoms	None	None	Moderate and nocturnal stools but not interfering with normal activity	Severe cramping and incontinence; interfering with daily activity	Grossly bloody diarrhoea and need for parenteral support

Management of constipation

Effective treatment is dependent on the cause. Strategies that may help include:

- making dietary and lifestyle changes
- introducing a high-fibre diet and increased fluid intake
- encouraging adequate physical activity within the limits of the patient's condition
- educating the patient on the risks and the need for early reporting of symptoms
- advising patients to take the prescribed medication
- ensuring privacy.

References

1. Holmes S. Cancer chemotherapy: a guide for practice. 2nd edn. Dorking, UK: Asset Books; 1997.
2. Fischer DS, Knobf MT, Durivae J. Cancer chemotherapy handbook: management of toxic effects of chemotherapy. 5th edn. St Louis: Mosby; 1997.
3. Cope DG. Management of chemotherapy-induced diarrhea and constipation. Nurs Clin N Am 2001; 36(4):695–707.
4. Wilkes G. Potential toxicity and nursing management in cancer chemotherapy. In: Barton-Burke M, Wilkes GM, Ingwerson K, eds. Cancer chemotherapy. A nursing process approach. 3rd edn. Boston: Jones and Bartlett; 1996.
5. Allegra C, Grem J. Antimetabolites. In: DeVita VT, Hellman S, Rosenberg SA , eds. Cancer principles & practice on oncology. 5th edn. Philadelphia: Lippincott Raven; 1997.
6. Taylor C. Constipation and diarrhoea In: Bruce L, Finlay TMD, eds. Gastroenterology. Oxford: Churchill Livingstone; 1997.
7. WHO. Handbook for cancer treatment. WHO Offset Publication No 48. Geneva: World Health Organisation; 1997.
8. Winney J. Constipation. Nurs Stand 1998; 13(11)49–56.
9. Culhane B. Constipation. In Yasko J, Ed. Guidelines for cancer care. Symptom management. Reaton VA: Reaton Pub.; 1983.
10. Maestri Banks. Assessing constipation. Nurs Times 1996; 92(21)28–30.

Chapter **18**

Mucositis

Caroline Soady

DEFINITION

Mucositis is an inflammatory reaction of the gastro-intestinal, respiratory or genitourinary mucosa, the most common sites being the oral cavity and oesophagus.[1]

Chemotherapy affects the mucosa directly through the toxic effects on rapidly dividing tissues and indirectly by myelosuppression, increasing susceptibility to infections and bleeding.[2] As a result of mucositis, systemic chemotherapy regimens may be altered, with drug doses adjusted, omitted or delayed. This can contribute to a reduced chemotherapeutic effect.[3–5] This toxicity can result in patients requiring hospitalisation and dramatically affecting overall quality of life.[6] Cytotoxic drugs that cause mucositis can be found in Table 18.1.

Generally, mucositis begins a few days after chemotherapy has been administered, peaks at a week and then slowly resolves unless complicated by infections or repeated chemotherapy administration.[7]

ORAL MUCOSITIS

Definition

Oral mucositis is defined as inflammation of the lining of the oral cavity[4] and is also known as stomatitis.[8,9]

Oral assessment

A baseline oral assessment should be performed prior to commencing chemotherapy, using an appropriate oral assessment guide: e.g. Eilers' oral assessment guide.[10] When choosing an oral assessment guide, the healthcare professional should question its ease of use, its applicability to the client population and its proven reliability and validity.[11] The oral assessment guide is

Table 18.1   Cytotoxic drugs that cause mucositis listed according to chemical groups[7, 8, 22]

Alkylating agents	Antimetabolites	Antimitotic antibiotics	Miscellaneous	Taxanes	Plant alkaloids
Ifosfamide	Cyclocytidine	Adriamycin	Cisplatin	Paclitaxel	Vinblastine
Melphalan	Cytarabine	Bleomycin	Hydroxyurea	Taxotere	Vincristine
	Floxuridine	Daunorubicin	Procarbazine		
	5-Fluorouracil	Daunomycin	Podophyllotoxins		
	6-Mercaptopurine	Dactinomycin	(Etoposide)		
	Methotrexate	Doxorubicin			
	6-Thioguanine	Mithramycin			
		Mitomycin C			
		Mitoxantrone (mitozantrone)			

then used as necessary to perform a thorough and frequent oral assessment in order to monitor oral health status, plan the appropriate intervention and evaluate the outcome. Following the work of the London Standing Conference, Cancer in the Capital Workshops, on the development of cancer nursing standards of care,[12] the oral care standard has been implemented at the Royal Marsden NHS Trust. This consists of an oral assessment guide (based on Eilers' oral assessment guide), an oral care plan and a suggested nursing and pharmacological interventions sheet (Fig. 18.1). Twenty-five years ago, Beck[13] found that there was a significant improvement in oral status when a systematic oral care protocol was used. Once mucositis is evident, a standardised assessment for evaluating the degree of mucositis should be used:[14] e.g. the World Health Organisation scoring system[15] – see Table 18.2.

A dental assessment should also be performed to establish a baseline in oral/dental status[16] and to identify complications, e.g. periodontal disease that will require treatment prior to commencing chemotherapy.[17] Patients in poor oral health at the start of treatment and those receiving inadequate oral care during treatment are at higher risk of developing mucositis.[18]

Signs and symptoms

Direct effects range from a few localised ulcerations to almost complete denudation of the oral mucosa.[5] Patients often describe the initial symptoms as a burning sensation in the mouth, which progresses to sensitivity to hot or cold and spicy or salty food,[4] resulting in pain. The clinical signs of chemotherapy-induced stomatitis include erythema, cracked lips, difficulty wearing dentures or swallowing, pain, bleeding, xerostomia, ulceration and pseudomembranous formations.[19] The buccal, labial, soft palatal mucosa, ventral surface of the tongue and floor of mouth are most commonly affected.[8] This has a devastating impact on the function

of the aerodigestive tract. The oral intake of diet and fluids is impaired, while the oropharyngeal airway can become compromised due to swelling and bleeding and a reduced gag reflex that decreases the patient's ability to protect the airway.[20] Systemic opiates may be required in combination with topical agents to provide effective pain relief to enable the patient to take adequate fluids to sustain hydration.[17] The ability to take sufficient diet and fluids orally will depend on the severity of the mucositis (see Table 18.2). In extreme situations, patients are unable to swallow even their own saliva and will require intravenous hydration,[17] total parenteral nutrition or an enteral feeding tube. (See also Ch. 19.)

The disrupted oral tissues act as a portal of entry for the systemic spread of bacterial, viral or fungal infection.[21] Extensive oral mucositis often coincides with a decrease in granulocyte counts.[22] (See also Chs 13 and 20.)

Mucositis can have a significant impact on the patient's psychological well-being, with symptoms interfering with social and sexual expression and affecting the patient's body image. Borbasi et al[23] found that while patients were prepared for acute mucositis, the longer-term problems of altered taste, difficulty swallowing, mouth dryness and associated loss of appetite caused unanticipated distress.

Combination treatment

The likelihood of a patient experiencing oral stomatitis is greatly increased where multiple and high-dose chemotherapy agents are used or chemotherapy is used in combination with radiotherapy.[17] The extent of mucositis is dependent on the previous condition of the oral cavity and the dosage, schedule and combination of the cytotoxic drugs.[11] Patients over 50 years of age have an increased incidence of mucositis, thought to be due to a physiological decline in renal function, resulting in

Name: **Hospital No:**   **Need No:**

ORAL ASSESSMENT TOOL *(Adapted from Eilers 1988)*
Assess all inpatients on admission and then as indicated by the assessment score unless patients condition changes

Date: Time:							

Voice: *Talk with the patient*
    1. Normal
    2. Deeper/raspy
    3. Difficulty							

Swallow: *Observation*
    1. Normal
    2. Pain on swallowing
    3. Unable to swallow							

Mucous Membrane: *Observe with a pen torch*
    1. Pink and moist
    2. Reddened/coated
    3. Ulceration's +/– bleeding							

Saliva: *Touch centre of tongue and floor of mouth with*
spatula and ask patient to describe saliva, using these headings.
    1. Watery
    2. Thick/ropy
    3. Absent							

Tongue: *Feel and observe with a pen torch*
    1. Pink and moist
    2. Coated/shiny +/– reddened
    3. Blistered/cracked							

Lips: *Feel and observe*
    1. Smooth, pink and moist
    2. Dry/cracked
    3. Bleeding/ulcerated							

Gums: *Gently press with tip of tongue depressor.*
    Observe with a pen torch.
    1. Pink and firm
    2. Oedematous +/– redness
    3. Spontaneous bleeding							

Teeth / Dentures: *Observe with a pen torch*
    1. Clean, no debris
    2. Localised plaque, debris
    3. Generalised plaque debris							

Nutritional status: *Ask the patient their views*
    1. Normal
    2. Soft diet
    3. Fluids only / NBM (nil by mouth)							

Analgesic requirement:
    1. None
    2. Topical analgesia
    3. Systemic analgesia							

Complications: *Observe with a pen torch*
    1. No evidence
    2. Haemorrhagic mucositis
    3. Infection (viral/fungal)							

Taste: *Ask the patient their views*
    1. Normal
    2. Impaired/changed
    3. No taste							

Self Care Assessment:
    1. Performs oral care by self
    2. Needs encouragement and education
    3. Refuses/unable to perform oral care							

Patients on High Dose Chemotherapy / Critical Care Unit or **Patients with Head & Neck cancer - please add a score of 9**							
Total Assessment Score							
Decide Intervention Level (1, 2 or 3) on assessment score (see section A overleaf)							
Assessor's Signature							

Figure 18.1   Oral assessment tool and suggested nursing and pharmacological interventions.

Patient Care Need: To maintain patient safety and comfort related to oral care

♦ Knowledge deficit about oral care
♦ Risk of oral complications associated with treatment and medical condition
♦ Patient comfort related to oral care

Anticipated Outcome:

♦ Patient will verbalise an understanding of oral care and the possible oral side-effects/complications of treatment
♦ Patients oral care will be performed and managed effectively by self or the help of a family member or nurse in order to detect and manage complications early and for patient comfort

Nursing Interventions:

A **Patient Assessment**
Assess and identify the risks of or oral complications using the oral assessment tool and decide the intervention level and frequency of assessment

Assessment Score	13–20	21–26	27–39
Intervention Level	Level 1	Level 2	Level 3
Assess	Weekly	Daily	Daily

NB For palliative care patients comfort may be the priority and the specific nursing interventions below may not be appropriate.

♦ Assess the patients oral pain to determine effectiveness of prescribed analgesia and start a pain assessment chart if appropriate
♦ Check that the patient / carer fully understands the intended care, and has received patient information leaflet if appropriate

Refer to the following Royal Marsden guidelines as appropriate
DTAC Prescribing Guidelines, Symptom Control Guidelines & the suggested nursing and pharmacological interventions by the London Cancer Standards Oral Group (modified)

B **Level 1 Interventions**

♦ Brush teeth with soft toothbrush and fluoride toothpaste **4 times daily.**
♦ If dentures are worn, remove from mouth and brush thoroughly 4 times daily. Rinse mouth with mouthwash 4 times daily. Soak overnight in fresh denture solution.
♦ Rinse with recommended mouthwash for 30 seconds after meals and before bed or 4 times daily then spit out.
♦ Avoid eating/drinking for 30 minutes after mouthwash.
♦ If mouthwash causes a "burning" sensation dilute with an equal volume of water and rinse for 1 minute or alternatives may be sought.
♦ Apply aqueous cream or yellow soft paraffin to lips to moisten (if necessary).

Level 2 Interventions (see nursing and pharmacological interventions for specific problems)

♦ **Increasing frequency of level 1 intervention to 2 – 4 hourly.**
♦ Provide with regular analgesia as required.
♦ For **signs of infection** – swab areas of localised suspicion if appropriate. Administer topical anti-fungal and/or anti-viral treatments as prescribed. Allow 30 mins between mouthwashes and anti fungal application.
♦ For **haemorrhagic mucositis** – check platelets/clotting and administer blood components as prescribed. Irrigate mouth with normal saline. Give Tranexamic acid 500mg (5 mls) diluted with 5 mls water as mouthwash. Advise on soft diet.
♦ For **dry mouth** – advise to use water or suck fresh pineapple chunks or provide with artificial saliva replacement products.

Level 3 Interventions (see nursing and pharmacological interventions for specific problems)

♦ **Increasing frequency of level 2 intervention to 1 – 2 hourly**
♦ Substitute soft toothbrush with sponge sticks
♦ Introduce treatment for specific problems as necessary for pain, ulceration, infection, dry mouth, bleeding

Patient / Carer Education:

C *Inform and discuss with the patient/carer:*
♦ How to assess the oral cavity and the frequency
♦ The availability of symptom control measures e.g. pain control, relaxation therapy
♦ The reason for using a bowl when performing oral care (not the sink) to minimize the risk of pseudomonas infection if appropriate
♦ When to report any symptoms and the importance of reporting any concerns/side-effects
♦ Smoking cessation advice if appropriate

Additional Interventions:

Instructions For Use:
♦ Date, time, sign and print name care plan when initiated, enter need number
♦ Individuals as appropriate. Date/time/sign any additional entries/interventions
♦ If need/outcome/interventions are stopped/changed or not applicable – DELETE by drawing a line through the entry, date/time/sign this deletion

Date/Time initiated: Signature: *Print Name: Job Title:*

Figure 18.1   Cont'd.

SUGGESTED NURSING AND PHARMACOLOGICAL INTERVENTIONS

These suggestions may help guide practice and offer patients and care providers acceptable choices in the management of oral care. Wherever possible, interventions are supported by evidence but in some instances there is no definitive evidence available. These interventions may offer alternative choices when first line care is not effective / acceptable. Comfort may be paramount for some palliative care patients and the nursing interventions should reflect the patients' choices / condition.

Patient Care Need	Suggested Nursing and Pharmacological Interventions
Voice	◆ Refer to Speech and Language Team. ◆ Explore alternative forms of communication.
Swallow	◆ Liaise with Speech and Language Team to confirm if a referral is appropriate e.g. if coughing after swallowing, gurgly voice or inability to swallow. ◆ Refer to the Dietitian if weight loss ≥ 10% of patient. ◆ Ensure adequate analgesia.
Taste	◆ Dietician referral, Huldij (1986). ◆ Encourage experimentation of alternative taste and flavours. In the presence of stomatitis/mucositis advise patients against spicy or citrus foods, Scannell D'Agostino (1989). ◆ Consider anti-emetics or appetite stimulants, Regnard & Fitton (1989).
Lips	◆ Offer oral ulceration and anti-inflammatory preparations as prescribed unless contraindicated e.g. Difflam, Mucaine, Sucralfate, Aspirin or Paracetamol gargle. ◆ Keep lips moisturised with lubricants i.e. yellow paraffin, aqueous cream, Loden et al (1991). ◆ Swab suspicious lesions, if positive for Herpes commence anti-viral treatment as prescribed.
Tongue	◆ Adcortyl in OraBase. ◆ Sulcrafate, Pfeffer (1990), Epstein & Wong (1994). ◆ In absence of mucositis/stomatitis, suck fresh pineapple chunks or soda bicarbonate mouthwash may reduce slough.
Saliva	◆ **Absence of saliva** – Use water to rinse mouth, Ice chips,Suck fresh pineapple chunks or Saliva replacement products. ◆ **Thick and ropey** – Regular water, Saliva replacement products, Krishnasamy (1995), Ice chips, Nebulised saline, Steam inhalations or Mucodine. ◆ **Excessive saliva** – Hyoscine, Palliative Care Formulary (1998).
Mucous Membrane & Gums	◆ If **bleeding** – check full blood count (platelets) and clotting if indicated and administer blood components as prescribed. Irrigate mouth with normal saline. Administer Tranexamic Acid 500 mg (5 mls) diluted with 5 mls water as mouthwash. Advise on soft diet. ◆ If **any suspicious areas** swab and if indicated commence anti-fungal/anti-viral/antibacterial treatment as prescribed. ◆ If **oral ulceration** – administer anti-inflammatory preparations as prescribed unless contraindicated e.g. Difflam, Mucaine, Sulcrafate, Aspirin and Paracetamol gargle, Mucilage combined with raspberry mucilage as appropriate. ◆ Offer ice chips. ◆ Encourage Chlorhexidine mouthwash – There is evidence indicating it is effective at removing plaque when used with a foam swab, Ransier et al (1995). However there is also evidence to suggest in the presence of mucositis it exacerbates symptoms and the mechanical effect of irrigating the mouth with water is as effective and more acceptable to patients, Dodd et al (1996) NB Chlorhexidine and Nystatin should not be used concurrently, Foote et al (1994).
Teeth/Dentures	◆ Encouragement and supervision of mouthcare regimen, Madeya (1996). ◆ Small soft toothbrush and fluoride toothpaste, Pearson (1996). ◆ Consider alternative approaches to plaque removal if a soft tooth brush and toothpaste cannot be tolerated i.e. pink foam sticks or a gloved finger and gauze, Krishnasamy (1995), Madeya (1996). ◆ Liaise with Dental hygienist / Dental department to confirm if a referral is appropriate, Toth et al (1996). ◆ Advise regular review by a dental surgeon, Xavier (2000).
Analgesia	◆ Assessment of oral pain and monitoring of the efficacy of analgesia, McGuire (1998). ◆ Soluble or topical analgesia e.g. Mucaine, Sucralfate. ◆ Anti inflammatory mouthwash e.g. Aspirin or Paracetamol gargles, Difflam, Feber (2000). ◆ Opiate analgesia, Trans-dermal, Intravenous or Subcutaneous preparations.
Smoking Cessation	◆ Discuss patients needs for Nicotine Replacement Therapy. ◆ Supporting advice given with written information and/or refer to a stop smoking service, if appropriate.

London Cancer Standards Oral Care Group – February 2002 Modified by Royal Marsden Hospital 2003

Figure 18.1   Cont'd.

Table 18.2 WHO criteria for grading mucositis and leukopenia by means of the nadir of the white blood cell (WBC) count[15]

Grade	Mucositis	WBC
0	Normal – no mucositis	$>3.9 \times 10^9/l$
1	Mild tissue changes (focal): white anemic changes; erythematous patches, no sensitivity; normal eating	$3.0–3.9 \times 10^9/l$
2	Mild tissue changes (focal): erythematous/ thinning mucosa; small ulceration <2 mm; slight sensitivity; normal eating	$2.0–2.9 \times 10^9/l$
3	Moderate tissue changes (focal diffuse): erythematous/ denuded/ulcerated mucosa; up to half mucosal area involved; blood clots, no active bleeding; moderate sensitivity, difficulty with eating/drinking	$1.0–1.9 \times 10^9/l$
4	Marked tissue changes (diffuse): erythematous/ denuded/ulcerated mucosa; half mucosal area or more involved; active oozing/bleeding marked pain; no eating possible	$<1.0 \times 10^9/l$

increased chemotherapy toxicity.[21] An awareness of these facts will assist the healthcare professional in devising effective and realistic oral care strategies.

Frequency of oral care
As changes in the oral cavity can occur rapidly, the frequency of assessment and care must be adapted to the individual: e.g. patients with severe mucositis should receive oral care every 2 hours.[3]

Mouth care tools
Although there are a variety of mouth care tools available, the decision on which should be used will depend on the severity of the mucositis and the presence of associated treatment complications such as thrombocytopenia. A toothbrush is the most effective tool for removing plaque and debris[3,13,24] but can be dependent on user technique.[25] Foamsticks are a suitable alternative for patients with pain and/or thrombocytopenia.[3]

Mouth care products
There are a number of products that have been found to be beneficial for the management of mucositis: a summary of these can be found in Table 18.3. However, further research is required.

Patient education

Where appropriate, patients or carers should be taught the following:

- suspected or anticipated oral complications
- which areas of the oral cavity to assess
- assessment methods and frequency
- how to use an oral assessment guide
- symptoms that must be reported back to the healthcare team
- how to contact members of the healthcare team
- the time frame in which notification should occur
- how to evaluate the effectiveness of different oral care strategies.[14]

(See also Ch. 5 for further information.)

GASTROINTESTINAL MUCOSITIS

Gastrointestinal involvement may present as epigastric burning or blood-tinged vomit or stool.[1] (See also Ch. 17 for further information.)

Table 18.3   Mouth care products

Reference	Aims	Research variables	Sample	Method	Results	Limitations	Recommendations
Anderson et al[37]	To determine efficacy of oral glutamine for patients with cancer undergoing chemotherapy	Glutamine vs glycine suspension (placebo)	24 patients (16 children and 8 adults)	Randomised, double-blind cross-over trial	Glutamine significantly reduced duration and severity of chemotherapy-associated stomatitis	Small sample size. G-CSF also given to study participants	Further studies required to determine most effective schedule, dose and form of administration of glutamine
Cascinu et al[38]	To verify the activity of cryotherapy in the prevention of 5FU-induced stomatitis	Ice chips administered 5 min prior to chemotherapy vs No intervention administered prior to chemotherapy	84 patients commencing 5FU chemotherapy	Randomised, controlled trial	Cryotherapy can reduce significantly the severity of mucositis	Small sample size	Recommend using cryotherapy for patients receiving bolus 5FU regimens
Chiara et al[31]	To assess efficacy of sucralfate gel in treatment of chemo-induced mucositis	Sucralfate gel vs placebo	40 patients	Double-blind placebo controlled, randomised pilot study	Sucralfate gel did not demonstrate a significant advantage over the placebo	Authors did not give details of placebo	Further studies are required
Dodd et al[5]	To test effectiveness of oral hygiene teaching programme in conjunction with two mouthwashes for prevention of mucositis	Type of mouthwash – chlorhexidine or sterile water. Incidence, days to onset, severity of mucositis	222 patients starting mucositis-inducing chemotherapy	Randomised, double-blind placebo controlled clinical trial	No significant differences between two mouthwashes in prevention of oral mucositis	Utilised an oral assessment guide rather than a specific mucositis rating scale	Utilise water instead of chlorhexidine
Elzawawy[26]	To investigate the ability of allopurinol mouthwash to reduce 5FU-induced oral mucositis	Allopurinol mouthwash (before and after)	18 patients who experienced 5FU-induced stomatitis in previous cycles	Comparative	Degree of stomatitis diminished in 15 out of 18 patients	Small sample size	Further controlled trials

Continued

Table 18.3   Mouth care products—cont'd.

Reference	Aims	Research variables	Sample	Method	Results	Limitations	Recommendations
Ferretti et al[34]	To evaluate a 0.12% chlorhexidine mouthrinse as prophylaxis against cytotoxic-therapy-induced damage to oral soft tissues	Type of mouthwash – chlorhexidine vs control (mouthwash without chlorhexidine)	40 inpatients receiving high-dose chemotherapy 30 outpatients receiving high-dose head and neck radiation	Prospective, double-blind randomised trial as prophylaxis	Reduction in incidence and severity of mucositis for inpatient group. A little/no reduction in mucositis observed with outpatient group	–	Chlorhexidine provides prophylaxis against oral mucositis and oral microbial pathogens in patients undergoing chemotherapy. Optimum schedules for dosages and duration of use remain to be defined
Kenny[9]	To determine the efficacy of two different oral care protocols in decreasing the incidence of stomatitis	Two oral care protocols A and B that differed on the agents used	18 haematology patients being treated with high doses of chemotherapy alone or in combination with radiotherapy	Comparative	Lower incidence of stomatitis in subjects using oral care protocol A (not statistically significant)	Small sample size. All subjects did not receive the same protocol	Agents used in both protocols appeared to be comparable; decisions on which agent to use should be based on other factors, e.g. cost, patient preference. Utilise a larger sample size: use subjects with same diagnosis and treatment modality. Compare two oral care protocols, varying only one agent
Mahood et al[27]	To test the hypothesis that oral cryotherapy results in the development of less mucositis	Oral cryotherapy	95 patients scheduled to receive first cycle of 5FU plus leucovorin	Randomised controlled trial	Cryotherapy inhibited development of 5FU-induced mucositis	–	Recommend utilising the protocol for patients receiving daily bolus of 5FU plus leucovorin
Meloni et al[28]	To evaluate the efficacy of eating ice pops during melphalan infusions	Ice pops	18 patients	Pilot study	Only 1 out of 18 developed mucositis above grade 3 WHO criteria	10 out of 18 received G-CSF during treatment	Recommend adopting this for patients having melphalan as a single agent or in combined regimens

Study	Aim	Intervention	Sample	Study type	Results		Recommendations
Okuno et al[36]	To determine whether glutamine can decrease-5FU-associated mucositis	Glutamine vs placebo	134 patients	Randomised, double-blind, placebo controlled trial	Glutamine was no more effective than the placebo	Cryotherapy also used – authors recognise this could have impact on results. (Authors felt unethical not to provide cryotherapy, as effects are well known and beneficial.) Authors did not give details of placebo	Recommend further study, with new methods to assess benefit of glutamine with cryotherapy
Porteder et al[29]	To establish whether local prostaglandin E$_2$ has any beneficial effect or not on inflammatory process and pain associated with mucositis	Prostaglandin E$_2$	10 patients who had received combined radio and chemotherapy for oral and maxillary cancer. Control group of 14 patients	Comparative	8 out of 10 patients completed treatment as scheduled; severity of mucositis was less compared to those not receiving prostaglandin	–	Recommend utilising this to help in prevention and treatment of stomatitis secondary to combined radio and chemotherapy for oral malignancies
Rocke et al[35]	To determine whether a longer duration of cryotherapy (60 min) provides additional protection than existing 30 min protocol	Ice chips	179 patients receiving first course of 5FU plus leucovorin (69 patients received both on separate cycles)	Randomised clinical trial	60 min of cryotherapy was no more beneficial than 30 min	–	Recommend continuing with 30 min of oral cryotherapy when giving IV push 5FU

Continued

Table 18.3   Mouth care products—cont'd.

Reference	Aims	Research variables	Sample	Method	Results	Limitations	Recommendations
Soloman[32]	To determine whether sucralfate would reduce pain and promote healing of oral ulcers associated with cancer therapy	Sucralfate suspension. Evaluation before and after	18 patients with chemo-induced mucositis	Pilot study	10 patients had definite responses	Small sample size	Recommend that sucralfate suspension may be effective for treatment of chemo-induced mucositis
Sprinzl et al[33]	To evaluate the potential benefit of a once daily performed mouthwash containing a solution of GM-CSF	Type of mouthwash	35 patients with head and neck cancer receiving chemo-radiotherapy	Prospective, randomised, open parallel-grouped single centre study	No superiority of GM-CSF in comparison to conventional mouthwash	–	Topical use of GM-CSF for treatment of oral mucositis induced by chemoradiation cannot be recommended for this patient group
Wadleigh et al[30]	To determine efficacy of vitamin E in treatment of chemotherapy-induced mucositis	Vitamin E vs placebo oil	18 patients	Randomised double-blind placebo controlled trial	6 out of 9 had complete resolution of lesions within 4 days, while 8 out of 9 receiving the placebo did not	–	Recommend future studies to determine whether success is due to local application or systemic absorption

References

1. Focazio B. Mucositis. Am J Nurs 1997; 97(12):48–49.
2. Fulton JS, Middleton GJ, McPhail JT. Management of oral complications. Semin Oncol Nurs 2002; 18(1):28–35.
3. Porter H. Oral care. In: Grundy M, ed. Nursing in haematological oncology. London: Harcourt; 2000:219–227.
4. Coleman S. An overview of the oral complications of adult patients with malignant haematological conditions who have undergone radiotherapy or chemotherapy. J Adv Nurs 1995; 22:1085–1091.
5. Dodd MJ, Larson PJ, Dibble SL, et al. Randomized clinical trial of chlorhexidine versus placebo for prevention of oral mucositis in patients receiving chemotherapy. Oncol Nurs Forum 1996; 23(6):921–927.
6. Dalberg J, Sorensen JB. Cryotherapy (oral cooling) as prevention of chemotherapy-induced stomatitis. A literature review. J Cancer Care 1996; 5:131–134.
7. Larson PJ, Miaskowski C, MacPhail L, et al. The PRO-SELF mouth aware program: an effective approach for reducing chemotherapy-induced mucositis. Cancer Nurs 1998; 21(4):263–268.
8. Madeya ML. Oral complications from cancer therapy: part 1 – pathophysiology and secondary complications. Oncol Nurs Forum 1996; 23(5):801–807.
9. Kenny SA. (1990) Effect of two oral care protocols on the incidence of stomatitis in haematology patients. Cancer Nurs 1990; 13(6):345–353.
10. Eilers J, Berger AM, Peterson MC. Development, testing and application of the oral assessment guide. Oncol Nurs Forum 1988; 15(3):325–330.
11. Porter H. Mouth care in cancer. Nurs Times 1994; 90(14):27–29.
12. www.nursingtimes.net/london-lscn/index.html
13. Beck S. Impact of a systematic oral care protocol on stomatitis after chemotherapy. Cancer Nurs 1979; June:185–199.
14. Madeya ML. Oral complications from cancer therapy: part 2 – nursing implications for assessment and treatment. Oncol Nurs Forum 1996; 23(5):808–819.
15. World Health Organization. Handbook for reporting results of cancer treatment. WHO: Geneva; 1979:48:195–210.
16. Toth BB, Frame RT. Dental oncology: the management of disease and treatment-related oral/dental complications associated with chemotherapy. Curr Probl Cancer 1983;10:7–35.
17. Graham KM, Pecararo DA, Ventura M, et al. Reducing the incidence of stomatitis using a quality assessment and improvement approach. Cancer Nurs 1993; 16(2):117–122.
18. Spijkervet FKL, Sonis ST. New frontiers in the management of chemotherapy-induced mucositis. Curr Opin Oncol 1998; 10(Suppl 1):S23–S27.
19. Wojtaszek C. Management of chemotherapy-induced stomatitis. Clin J Oncol Nurs 2000; 4(6):263–270.
20. Majorana A, Schubert MM, Porta F, et al. Oral complications of paediatric hematopoietic cell transplantation: diagnosis and management. Support Care Cancer 2000; 8:353–365.
21. Raber-Durlacher JE, Weijl NI, Abu Saris M, et al. Oral mucositis in patients treated with chemotherapy for solid tumors: a retrospective analysis of 150 cases. Support Care Cancer 2000; 8:366–371.
22. Beck SL. Mucositis. In: Groenwald SL, Frogge M, Goodman M, et al, eds. Cancer symptom management. Massachusetts: Jones & Bartlett; 1996:308–323.
23. Borbasi S, Cameron K, Quested B, et al. More than a sore mouth: patients' experience of oral mucositis. Oncol Nurs Forum 2002; 29(7):1051–1057.
24. Toth BB, Chambers MS, Fleming TC. Prevention and management of oral complications associated with cancer therapies: radiotherapy/chemotherapy. Texas Dental J 1996; June:23–29.
25. Pearson LS. A comparison of the ability of foam swabs and toothbrushes to remove dental plaque: implications for nursing practice. J Adv Nurs 1996; 23:62–69.
26. Elzawawy A. Treatment of 5-fluorouracil induced stomatitis by allopurinol mouthwashes. Oncology 1991; 48:282–284.
27. Mahood DJ, Dose AM, Loprinzi CL, et al. Inhibition of fluorouracil induced stomatitis by oral cryotherapy. J Clin Oncol 1991; 9(3):449–452.
28. Meloni G, Capria S, Proia A, et al. Ice pops to prevent melphalan-induced stomatitis. Lancet 1996; 347:1691–1692.
29. Porteder H, Rausch E, Kment G, et al. Local prostaglandin E2 in patients with oral malignancies undergoing chemo and radiotherapy. J Cranio-Max-Fac Surg 1988; 16:371–374.
30. Wadleigh RG, Redman RS, Graham ML, et al. Vitamin E in the treatment of chemotherapy induced mucositis. Am J Med 1992; 92:481–484.
31. Chiara S, Nobile MT, Vincenti M, et al. Sucralfate in the treatment of chemo-induced stomatitis: a double-blind, placebo-controlled pilot study. Anticancer Res 2001; 21:3707–3710.
32. Soloman MA. Oral sucralfate suspension for mucositis. N Engl J Med 1986; 315(7):459–460.
33. Sprinzl GM, Galvan O, de Vries A, et al. Local application of granulocyte-macrophage colony stimulating factor (GM-CSF) for the treatment of oral mucositis. Eur J Cancer Care 2001; 37:2003–2009.
34. Ferretti GA, Raybould TP, Brown AT, et al. Chlorhexidine prophylaxis for chemotherapy- and radiotherapy-induced stomatitis: a randomised double-blind trial. Oral Surg Oral Med Oral Pathol 1990; 69(3):331–338.
35. Rocke LK, Loprinzi CL, Lee JK, et al. A randomised clinical trial of two different durations of oral cryotherapy for prevention of 5-fluorouracil related stomatitis. Cancer 1993; 72(7):2234–2238.

36. Okuno SH, Woodhouse CO, Loprinzi CL, et al. Phase three controlled evaluation of glutamine for decreasing stomatitis in patients receiving fluorouracil (5FU) based chemotherapy. Am J Clin Oncol 1999; 22(3):258–261.

37. Anderson PM, Schroeder G, Skubitz KM. Oral glutamine reduces the duration and severity of stomatitis after cytotoxic cancer chemotherapy. Cancer 1998; 83(7):1433–1439.

38. Cascinu S, Fedeli A, Fedeli SL, et al. Oral cooling (cryotherapy), an effective treatment for the prevention of 5-fluorouracil-induced stomatitis. Eur J Cancer B Oral Oncol 1994; 30B(4):234–236.

Chapter **19**

Malnutrition

Louise Henry

INTRODUCTION

Achieving and maintaining a good nutritional status for cancer patients is often difficult. Metabolic changes affecting appetite and the utilisation of nutrients cause many patients to lose weight prior to diagnosis.[1,2] Anticancer treatments, including surgery, radiotherapy and chemotherapy, can all further reduce food intake due to the development of side effects such as taste changes, pain, mucositis and nausea and vomiting.[3] Nutrition-related problems are more common in patients with advanced disease.[4,5]

CANCER CACHEXIA

Cachexia is characterised by progressive weight loss, muscle wasting and weakness. It is usually but not always accompanied by anorexia. Cachexia differs from starvation in that individuals fail to adapt to a decrease in intake by reducing metabolic rate and trying to conserve muscle mass.[6] The incidence of cancer cachexia ranges from 30 to 80% and is dependent upon the site and type of tumour.[7]

Impact of cancer cachexia and weight loss

A presence of 5% unintentional weight loss in 1 month or 10% weight loss over 3 months is associated with a decrease in tolerance of treatment, higher mortality, morbidity and a decrease in the quality of life.[8–12] As chemotherapy dosage is based upon body surface area, thinner patients receive less chemotherapy and have a higher incidence of breaks from treatment due to toxicities.[13]

Primary cachexia
Primary cachexia is cachexia without a mechanical or functional aetiology: i.e. it is disease-related.

Aetiology It is multifactorial and the exact patho-genesis is unknown. Cachexia can be considered to occur because of three factors:[12]

1. Metabolic changes:
   - normal or raised metabolic rate
   - altered carbohydrate metabolism
   - altered fat metabolism
   - altered protein metabolism.

It is thought that a number of inflammatory cytokines (e.g. tumour necrosis factor/cachectin, interleukins 1, 2, 4 and 6, gamma interferon) secreted by cancer cells are responsible for the alterations in metabolism.[14,15]

2. Anorexia.
3. Reduced intake due to disease site: e.g. cancer of the oesophagus causing dysphagia, cancer of the larynx causing dysphagia, bowel obstruction secondary to ovarian cancer, nausea, and vomiting secondary to raised intracranial pressure etc.

Treatment of cachexia At present, there is no way of reversing the process other than the complete eradication of the tumour itself.

Secondary cachexia

Secondary cachexia is known as iatrogenic cachexia: i.e. it is treatment-related.

All cancer treatments can potentially affect nutritional status and food intake, either directly or indirectly. The nature and severity of nutrition impact symptoms[3] will depend on the drugs used, their dosage and frequency of administration. Much of the medication used in the control of symptoms, such as pain, or in the treatment of sepsis, will also affect food intake. Previous or concurrent other treatment such as surgery or radiotherapy will also affect nutritional status and in many instances exacerbate problems. Psychosocial issues will greatly affect the patient's ability to maintain his nutritional status. Depression, anxiety, economic hardship, fatigue and disability can all affect food intake.[16]

Weight loss and chemotherapy

1. Direct effects of chemotherapy agents:
   - nausea and vomiting – due to direct stimulation of centres for nausea and vomiting
   - diarrhoea/malabsorption – most chemotherapeutic agents will alter the surface of the intestinal villi
   - micronutrient imbalance – some chemotherapeutic agents will cause losses of certain minerals or other micronutrients, e.g. platinum-containing drugs can cause the loss of magnesium.

2. Indirect effects of chemotherapy agents.
   A reduction in food intake may occur as a result of the following:
   - anorexia
   - fatigue (both related to cancer cachexia and chemotherapeutic drugs)
   - taste changes
   - food aversion[17]
   - dry mouth
   - stomatitis
   - diarrhoea
   - constipation
   - infection.

Patients are likely to become more malnourished with each chemotherapy cycle unless effective nutrition support and symptom management is instigated.

Anorexia/loss of appetite
Aetiology
- Thought to be as a result of tumour-produced peptides and oligopeptides that directly affect the hypothalamic control of the appetite centre, causing a reduced appetite, changes in taste perception and feelings of early satiety.[18]
- Can be as a consequence of depression and anxiety.
- Can be as a result of social factors such as isolation, limited income and lack of access to cooking facilities, unfamiliar hospital food.
- Fatigue.
- Pain.
- As a side effect of medication, e.g. analgesia, some antibiotics.
- As a consequence of other treatment side effects such as nausea and vomiting, dry mouth, food aversions, diarrhoea, constipation.

Management The underlying cause needs to be established and intervention planned on this basis.

Pharmacological interventions Many drugs have been tried to improve appetite. These include megestrol acetate, corticosteroids, cannabinoids, hydralazine sulphate and anabolic steroids.[19,20] Their efficacy is variable, with benefits usually short term. Most are associated with undesirable side effects.

Non-pharmacological interventions The following dietary advice should be given:

- Eat small, frequent meals.
- Eat foods high in energy and protein. Try to fortify foods by adding foods such as skimmed milk powder, oil, butter, sugar and honey. Many commercial glucose polymer powders and protein supplements are available on prescription.

- Avoid 'filling up' with low energy and protein density foods (e.g. jelly, tea, coffee).
- Separating drinks from meals can decrease early satiety.
- Time meals to take advantage of when the patient's appetite is at its best – generally this is breakfast time, with a progressive decrease in appetite and intake as the day progresses.
- Aim to take nutritional supplements when appetite is poor, e.g. in the evening
- Alcohol can stimulate the appetite.[21]
- Exercise may stimulate the appetite.
- Try to eat in a pleasant environment, e.g. away from unpleasant odours, and encourage patients to eat in a day room rather than at the bedside.
- Encourage experimentation with food.
- If anorexia is persistent and accompanied by weight loss, consider enteral tube feeding.
- Social factors: referral to social services for assessment of benefit entitlement, housing issues; referral to occupational therapist for advice regarding adaptation of cooking equipment.

Nausea

Nausea does not necessarily lead to reduction in intake if patients adapt the diet as necessary. (See also Ch. 16.)

Dietary advice and other non-pharmacological measures
- Relaxation before eating.
- Avoid odours such as food cooking. Advise patient to get away from the kitchen and if possible move away from areas where food is prepared. Fresh air from an open window or a walk outside may be beneficial. Cold or room temperature foods have fewer odours than those that are cooked.
- Eat small frequent snacks/meals.
- Try sucking boiled sweets or chewing gum.
- Sucking peppermints or trying peppermint cordial.
- Try fizzy drinks (they can induce belching, which can help relieve symptoms of nausea).
- Try ginger-containing drinks or foods (ginger is traditionally thought to have antiemetic properties).

Vomiting

Persistent vomiting will lead to a reduction in nutrient intake and jeopardise nutritional status. (See also Ch. 16.)

Dietary advice and non-pharmacological management
- Encourage rest after eating.
- Eat small frequent snacks.
- See Nausea advice (above).
- Consider parenteral feeding if vomiting persistent and intractable.

Xerostomia (dry mouth)

Xerostomia may cause reduction in intake since chewing and swallowing can be more difficult. It is often associated with changes in taste perception. (See also Ch. 18.)

Dietary advice and non-pharmacological interventions
- Limited success.
- Try increasing liquids with foods, e.g. sauces and gravies, and take sips of drinks between mouthfuls of food.
- Suck on ice cubes or ice lollies. Try flavouring with citrus fruits or juices.
- Suck slices of citrus fruits.
- Avoid eating very dry foods such as bread.
- Chew chewing gum; suck boiled sweets.

Food aversions
Aetiology

Food aversions are closely associated with taste changes, nausea and vomiting and can lead to an unbalanced diet and hence malnutrition.

Management
Pharmacological interventions:
- Prophylactic use of antiemetics during and after chemotherapy administration.

Dietary advice and non-pharmacological interventions:
- Relaxation techniques to reduce anxiety.
- Advise patients to avoid consuming favourite foods and drinks prior to, during and immediately after treatment.
- Try reintroducing foods when the patient is feeling well and is not due to have treatment soon after trying the foods.
- Ask the dietitian to check diet for deficiencies/nutritional balance.

Taste changes
Aetiology
- Taste changes can be caused by circulating factors secreted by cancer cells, and can often result in nausea and, in extreme cases, vomiting.
- Chemotherapeutic agents may cause changes in taste perception.
- Exacerbated by the presence of xerostomia and mucositis.

Dietary advice and non-pharmacological management

- Concentrate on foods that are pleasant tasting.
- Encourage the patient to experiment with food (especially with foods not normally liked).

- Use condiments and sauces to disguise taste.
- Marinate meats to disguise taste. If this fails, substitute meat protein with protein from dairy foods or beans and pulses.
- Suggest alternatives to foods often affected, e.g. try hot squash or milky drinks in place of tea and coffee.
- Eat cold foods.

Stomatitis/mucositis/oesophagitis

These conditions limit the patient's physical ability to eat by affecting his ability to chew and swallow. They often affect taste perceptions. (See also Ch. 18.)

Dietary advice and non-pharmacological management
- Increase oral hygiene.
- Use a soft toothbrush.
- Avoid spicy and rough textured foods.
- Use gravies and sauces to moisten foods.
- Try ice lollies/flavoured ice cubes.
- Avoid alcohol as it can act as an irritant.
- Patients will probably require nutritional supplements.

Diarrhoea/malabsorption
Aetiology
- They can be disease-related, e.g. carcinoid syndrome.
- Drug-related damage to intestinal villi.
- Pancreatic failure, e.g. cancer of the pancreas.

Diarrhoea and malabsorption may cause rapid weight loss and anorexia. Patients can also become deficient in specific nutrients.

Dietary advice and non-pharmacological interventions
- Eat small frequent meals.
- Drink plenty of fluids to avoid becoming dehydrated.
- In extreme cases, the patient may become temporarily intolerant of dairy products.
- Patients with persistent high-volume diarrhoea may require parenteral nutrition (PN) and 'bowel rest'.

(See also Ch. 17.)

Constipation
Aetiology Analgesia, immobility, decreased oral intake and dehydration can cause early satiety and nausea/constipation.

Dietary advice and non-pharmacological interventions
- Increase fluid intake.
- Increase dietary fibre intake (although it is not recommended that pure bran is added to foods).

However, generally, this is not adequate to resolve constipation in the sick patient.
- Encourage gentle exercise.

(See also Ch. 17.)

Excessive weight gain
Aetiology Some patients, particularly those receiving hormonal therapy and high doses of corticosteroid, will experience increased appetite and weight gain.

The cause of the weight gain is unclear but is likely to be multifactorial. Possible causes include:

1. Increased food intake:
   - patients seen to increase intake to alleviate side effects of treatment such as nausea
   - to satisfy 'food cravings'.
2. Alteration in appetite controlling mechanisms/ removal of the psychological constraints on nutritional intake:
   - 'comfort eating', resulting from depression/ anxiety.
3. Decreased physical activity (secondary to fatigue or disability).

Dietary advice and non-pharmacological interventions
1. The patient should aim to maintain weight at a body mass index (BMI) of 20–25 kg/m².
2. Encourage general healthy eating advice:
   - eat 5 portions of fruit/vegetables per day
   - eat a diet low in saturated fat
   - moderate alcohol intake
   - reduce salt intake.
3. Increase exercise as tolerated (seek advice from physiotherapist)

The impact of this weight gain on future disease progression is not known.

Aim of nutrition support

The support should be to maintain or improve nutritional status while taking issues of prognosis into account. At present, it remains unclear which patients can be safely left without nutrition support and which patients benefit from nutrition support.

Assessment of nutritional status

There is no single reliable measure of nutritional status. Weight can be a useful indicator, particularly when compared to previous weights. This must be looked at in the context of a general clinical assessment to rule out oedema, large tumour bulk, etc. Food intake and appetite should also be considered.

Albumin and other plasma proteins are not reliable indicators of nutritional status as they are influenced by other factors.

Nutritional requirements

Energy and protein requirements can be calculated using standard formulae.[22,23] As these are, at best, only estimates, it is essential that the patient's progress is closely monitored. Requirements for vitamins, minerals and trace elements are thought to be as those for the general population.[24]

METHODS OF NUTRITION SUPPORT

Oral intake

Most patients prefer to eat a 'normal' diet where possible. Simple advice concerning high-energy, high-protein snacks, modified texture diets and fortifying foods is all that is needed for the majority of patients. Patients often need reassurance that it is acceptable and desirable for them to break away from the usual 'healthy eating' principle applied to the 'well' population when trying to gain weight.

Sip feeds and nutritional supplements

Wide ranges of prescribable and non-prescribable supplements are available. They are available as sweet drinks (both 'milky' type and 'non-milky' juice type), soups or puddings. Many are nutritionally complete and can be used to replace meals or in addition to meals. Most supplements benefit from being served cold or warm and may be modified in other ways to improve taste and texture.

There are also a variety of modular supplements, including glucose polymers and protein powders, that can be used to fortify foods.

The use of supplements should be carefully monitored.

Enteral tube feeding

Indication

Patients who are unable to take an adequate oral diet due to anorexia, dysphagia or mucositis. They must have a functioning gastrointestinal (GI) tract.

The choice of tube will depend on the site of the tumour, anticipated length of time of feeding, gut function, etc. A variety of tubes are available, including nasogastric tubes, gastrostomy (surgically, endoscopically placed or radiological inserted) and jejunostomy. Each type of tube is indicated in specific cases.

Contraindications

- Bowel obstruction, intractable nausea and vomiting.
- Persistent, profuse diarrhoea.
- Severe short-gut syndrome/high-output fistula.

Feeding regimen

A wide variety of commercially produced, sterile, low-lactose, gluten-free tube feeds are available. New developments include disease-specific feeds and feeds with immuno-enhancing nutrients added, e.g. glutamine, fish oils.[25] The appropriate feed can be delivered using either bolus feeding, 'gravity drip' feeding or via a dedicated feeding pump. Again, the choice of delivery route will be dependent on whether feeding is a sole source of nutrition or an adjunct to normal food intake, the ability of the patient to care for the feeding system and cost issues. Home enteral feeding is widely used in the UK.

Possible complications

1. Tube-related problems:
   - tube blockage
   - tube displacement
   - infection at tube insertion site.
2. GI disturbances:
   - nausea
   - distension
   - diarrhoea and malabsorption.

Parenteral nutrition

Parenteral nutrition is the intravenous administration of sterile, nutritionally complete solutions containing nitrogen, carbohydrate, lipid, vitamins and minerals. It can be very effective in delivering exact quantities of nutrients and has no impact on GI symptoms. Enteral feeding should always be viewed as preferable to the parenteral route and every effort should be made to use the GI tract. Failure to stimulate the GI tract can lead to marked atrophic changes in the bowel and pancreas and can contribute to the occurrence of cholestasis.[26,27] Enteral nutrition (EN) and 'standard care' (i.e. hydration/no nutrition support) are associated with a lower risk of infection than PN. However, mortality and the risk of infection tend to be increased with 'standard care' than with PN in a malnourished patient population.[28] What is not clear at present is whether it is a case of EN having fewer complications than PN or is it that EN is inherently better than PN.[28,29]

PN can be administered via central line or peripheral line.

Indication for parenteral nutrition
- GI tract is not functioning: e.g. in complete bowel obstruction.
- All methods of EN have been considered and are not possible: e.g. jejunostomy feeding.
- Complete bowel rest is required: e.g. small bowel fistula, breakdown of anastamosis, severe pancreatitis, etc.
- Total nutrient requirements cannot be met using the enteral route only, due to limited absorption/tolerance of enteral feed: e.g. radiation enteritis, severe diarrhoea, severe nausea and vomiting following chemotherapy, etc.

Contraindications for parenteral nutrition
- Well-nourished patient who is likely to resume oral intake within 7 days.
- GI tract is functioning – considering using all available routes of enteral feeding: e.g. nasogastric feeding, nasojejunal feeding, jejunostomy feeding, etc.
- Lack of vascular access.
- Patient has a very poor prognosis. (Research in oncology suggests that the benefits of PN are often outweighed by undesirable side effects and complications of PN in patients with advanced disease.[4,30])

Possible complications
- Catheter-related.
- Metabolic.
- Sepsis.
- Gut atrophy.

Home parenteral feeding is complex and expensive to provide and needs the involvement of a specialist PN feeding team. It should not be undertaken lightly.

Psychosocial impact of artificial feeding

Patients forced to rely on artificial feeding can experience depression, anxiety and stress related to problems with feeding equipment and side effects of the feeding process and body image changes.

Nutrition support in bone marrow transplant

There is a lack of definitive research in this area.[31] PN is still widely used in this population group and several studies have been published; however, the evidence for the use of PN is unclear. When considering the use of standard PN versus PN enriched with glutamine, it is likely that patients receiving the glutamine-enriched PN have a shorter hospital stay and reduced incidence of positive blood cultures (but not necessarily an overall reduction in morbidity). Despite a move throughout the UK's bone marrow transplant (BMT) centres towards the use of EN in such patients, there is an absence of evaluable evidence on the role of EN in BMT.[31]

IMMUNONUTRITION AND NOVEL SUBSTRATES

In recent years, several studies have been conducted to investigate the possible benefits of immunonutrition in patients.[32–35] At present, there is no definitive answer as to who would benefit most from such products, despite heavy promotion by their manufacturers. However, it is likely that the development of 'cancer-specific' nutritional supplements and enteral feeds will continue to be widely pursued over the next few years.

DIET AND NUTRITION AS A CURE FOR CANCER

At present, there is no evidence that a particular food or diet can cure cancer. A wide range of articles, books, internet sites and complementary or alternative therapists make unrealistic claims on the benefits of following particular diets or taking certain supplements. For the patient the information can be confusing and misleading. Many confuse the findings of epidemiological nutrition research into the aetiology of cancer with diet and the treatment of cancer. It is also difficult to extrapolate from animal nutrition research to human cancers.

Patients are often advised that the body should be 'starved' to cure the cancer or that the cancer is a toxin that can be removed by dietary 'detoxification'.[36] Advice is often to follow a vegan diet with a high fruit, vegetable and grain content, and avoid caffeine, alcohol and 'processed' foods. This is often also accompanied by the use of expensive vitamin, mineral and other supplements.

Such diets tend to be most widely used by young women and very anxious patients.[37,38] There is often a great deal of emphasis placed upon the patients taking responsibility for their own cure. The benefits in terms of returning control to the patient and promoting self-help must be balanced against the practical difficulties and financial cost of such diets, their low nutrient density, the potential for toxicities from the nutritional supplements prescribed and the feelings of guilt experienced by patients if they fail to adhere to strict regimes.[36]

References

1. Lindsey AM, Piper BF. Anorexia and weight loss, indicators of cachexia in small cell lung cancer. Nutr Cancer 1985; 7:65–76.
2. Ovesen L, Hannibal J, Mortensen EL. The interrelationship of weight loss, dietary intake and quality of life in ambulatory patients with cancer of the lung, breast, and ovary. Nutr Cancer 1993; 19:159–167.
3. Ottery FD. Supportive nutrition to prevent cachexia and improve quality of life. Semin Oncol 1995; 3:98–111.
4. Gallagher-Allred CR. Nutritional care of the terminally ill. Maryland: Aspen; 1989.
5. Strasser F. Eating-related disorders in patients with advanced cancer. Support Care Cancer 2003; 11(1):11–20.
6. Barber MD, Ross JA, Feron KC. Disordered metabolic response with cancer and its management. World J Surg 2000; 24:681–689.
7. Van Bokhirst-de van der Schuer, van Leeuwen PA, Kuik DJ, et al. The impact of nutritional status on the prognoses of patients with advanced head and neck cancer. Cancer 1999; 86(3):519–527.
8. Shils ME. Principles of nutrition support. Cancer 1979; 43:2093–2102.
9. DeWys WD, Begg C, Lavin PT, et al. Prognostic effect of weight loss prior to chemotherapy in cancer patients. Eastern Cooperative Oncology Group. Am J Med 1980; 69(4):491–497.
10. Landel AM, Hammond WG, Meguid MM. Aspects of amino acid and protein metabolism in the cancer-bearing states. Cancer 1985; 55(Suppl 1):230–237.
11. O'Gorman P, McMillan DC, McArdle CS. Impact of weight loss, appetite and the inflammatory response on quality of life in gastrointestinal cancer patients. Nutr Cancer 1998; 32(2):76–80.
12. Bosaeus I, Daneryd P, Lundholm K. Dietary intake, resting energy expenditure, weight loss and survival in cancer patients. J Nutr 2002; 132(Suppl 11): 3465S–3466S.
13. Andreyev HJ, Norman AR, Oates J, et al. Why do patients with weight loss have a worse outcome when undergoing chemotherapy for gastrointestinal malignancies? Eur J Cancer 1998; 34(4):503–509.
14. Toomey D, Redmond HP, Bouchier-Hayes D. Mechanisms mediating cancer cachexia. Cancer 1995; 76:2418–2426.
15. Tisdale MJ. Cancer cachexia, metabolic alterations and clinical manifestations. Nutrition 1997; 13:1–7.
16. Schmale AH. Psychological aspects of anorexia. Cancer 1979; 43(5):2087–2092.
17. Mattes RD, Curran WJ, Alavi J, et al. Clinical implications of learned food aversions in patients with cancer treated with chemotherapy or radiation therapy. Cancer 1992; 70(1):192–200.
18. Rossi FF, Cangiano C. Increased availability of tryptophan in brain as a common pathogenic mechanism for anorexia associated with different diseases. Nutrition 1991; 7:364–367.
19. Tchekmedyian NS, Halpert C, Ashley J, et al. Nutrition in advanced cancer, anorexia as an outcome variable and target of therapy. JPEN J Parenter Enteral Nutr 1992; 16(Suppl. 6):88S–92S.
20. Bruera E. Clinical management of anorexia and cachexia in patients with advanced cancer. Oncology 1992; 2:35–42.
21. Yeomans MR, Hails NJ, Nesic JS. Alcohol and the appetizer effect. Behav Pharmacol 1999; 10(2):151–161.
22. Schofield WN. Predicting basal metabolic rate, new standards and review of previous work. Hum Nutr Clin Nutr 1985; 39(Suppl 1):5–41.
23. Elai M. Artificial nutritional support. Med Intern 1990; 82:3392–3396.
24. Department of Health. Dietary reference values for food energy and nutrients for the Untied Kingdom. London: HMSO; 1991.
25. Barber MD, McMillan DC, Preston T, et al. Metabolic response to feeding in weight-losing pancreatic cancer patients and its modulation by a fish oil enriched nutritional supplement. Clin Sci 2000; 98(4):389–399.
26. Hughes CA, Dowling RH. Speed of onset of adaptive mucosal hypoplasia and hypofunction in the intestine of parenterally fed rats. Clin Sci 1980; 59:317–327.
27. Payne-James J, Grimble G, Silk D (eds) Artificial nutrition support in clinical practice. 2nd edn. London: GMM; 2001.
28. Braunschweig CL, Levy P, Sheean PM, et al. Enteral compared with parenteral nutrition, a meta-analysis. Am J Clin Nutr 2001; 74(4):534–542.
29. Klein S, Koretz RL. Nutrition support in patients with cancer, what do the data really show? Nutr Clin Pract 1994; 9(3):91–100.
30. MacGeer AJ, Detsky AS, O'Rourke K. Parenteral nutrition in cancer patients undergoing chemotherapy: a meta analysis. Nutrition 1990; 6(3):233–240.
31. Murray SM, Pindoria S. Nutrition support for bone marrow transplant patients. Cochrane Database Syst Rev 2002; (2):CD002920.
32. Barber MD, Ross JA, Voss AC, et al. The effect of an oral nutritional supplement enriched with fish oil on weight-loss in patients with pancreatic cancer. Br J Cancer 1999; 81(1):80–86.
33. Kemen M, Senka M, Homann HH, et al. Early postoperative enteral nutrition with arginine-omega-3 fatty acids and ribonucleic acid-supplemented diet versus placebo in cancer patients, an immunologic evaluation of impact. Crit Care Med 1995; 23(4):652–659.
34. Kenler AS, Swails WS, Driscoll DF, et al. Early enteral feeding in post surgical cancer patients. Fish oil structured lipid-based polymeric formula versus a standard polymeric formula. Ann Surg 1996; 223(3):316–333.

35. McCarter MD, Gentilini OD, Gomez ME, et al. Preoperative oral supplement with immunonutrients in cancer patients. JPEN J Parenter Enteral Nutr 1998; 22(4):206–211.

36. Cunningham RS, Herbert V. Nutrition as a component of alternative therapy. Semin Oncol Nurs 2000; 16(2):163–169.

37. Downer SM, Cody MM, McCluskey P, et al. Pursuit and practice of complementary therapies by cancer patients receiving conventional treatment. BMJ 1994; 309:86–89.

38. Sollner W, Maislinger S, DeVries A, et al. Use of complementary and alternative medicine by cancer patients is not associated with perceived distress or poor compliance with standard treatment but with active coping behaviour, a survey. Cancer 2000; 89(4):873–880.

Further reading

Bozzetti F, Cozzaglio L, Biganzoli E, et al. Quality of life and length of survival in advanced cancer patients on home parenteral nutrition. Clin Nutr 2002; 21(4):281–288.

Bozzetti F, Braga M, Gianotti L, et al. Postoperative enteral versus parenteral nutrition in malnourished patients with gastrointestinal cancer, a randomised multicentre trial. Lancet 2001; 358(9292):1487–1492.

Expert Group on Vitamins and Minerals. Safe upper levels for vitamins and minerals. Food Standards Agency UK; 2003.

Chapter **20**

Leucopenia and neutropenia

Shelley Dolan

GENERAL INFORMATION

Leucocytes (white blood cells) are far less numerous than red blood cells and account for less than 1% of the blood volume. There are, on average, 4000–11 000 white blood cells (WBCs) per cubic millimetre of blood. Leucocytes can be grouped into two main categories: those with membrane-contained cytoplasmic granules, called granulocytes; and those without granules, known as agranulocytes.

The granulocytes are further subdivided into the following cells:

- Neutrophils, the most numerous of the WBCs, account for about half of the WBC population and are about twice the size of red blood cells (RBCs). Neutrophils take 6–9 days to develop and last from 6 hours to a few days.
- Eosinophils account for 1–4% of WBCs and are similar in size to the neutrophils. Eosinophils take 6–9 days to develop and last for 8–12 days.
- Basophils, the rarest WBC, account for only 0.5% of the WBC population and are the same size or slightly smaller than neutrophils. Basophils take 3–7 days to develop and last a few hours to a few days.

The agranulocytes can also be further subdivided into the following cells:

- Lymphocytes, the second most numerous WBC in the blood, are smaller than other WBCs. Lymphocytes take days to weeks to develop and last for hours to years.
- Monocytes account for 4–8% of WBCs and are the largest of the WBCs. Monocytes take 2–3 days to develop and last for months.[1]

THE PRODUCTION AND DEVELOPMENT OF LEUCOCYTES

Leucocytes are formed in the bone marrow, originally from a single stem cell, the haemocytoblast, but then quickly divide into either a myeloid or a lymphoid stem cell. The granulocytes are derived from the myeloid stem cell and the agranulocytes from the lymphoid stem cell.

The development of the neutrophil is as follows (see Fig. 20.1 for other WBCs):

Haemocytoblast → Myeloid stem cell → Myeloblast → Promyelocyte → Neutrophilic myelocyte → Neutrophilic band cell → Neutrophil

Leucopoiesis is the production of leucocytes and, like erythropoiesis, is under hormonal control. The hormones responsible for leucopoiesis are cytokines and can be divided into the interleukins and the colony-stimulating factors. These hormones are mainly produced by the macrophages and the T lymphocytes. The cytokines are released as a response to a complex network of chemical triggers involved in the immune response of the body to infection.[1]

THE FUNCTION OF THE LEUCOCYTES

Leucocytes are essential elements in the body's protection against disease. White blood cells protect the body from damage by bacteria, viruses, parasites, toxins and tumour cells.

Neutrophils are the most numerous of the WBCs and account for more than half of the whole WBC population.[1] The neutrophils are therefore the mainstay of the body's fight against bacterial infection and are therefore described in greater detail below.

Neutrophils are active phagocytic cells that are drawn to areas of inflammation. They concentrate on bacteria and some fungi, which they then ingest and destroy.

Neutrophils have granules that contain peroxidases and other hydrolytic enzymes and are called lysosomes. They also have other smaller granules that contain proteins called defensins. This bacterial destruction is initiated by a process called respiratory burst. In this process, oxygen is actively metabolised to produce potent substances such as bleach and hydrogen peroxide and defensin-mediated lysis takes place.[1]

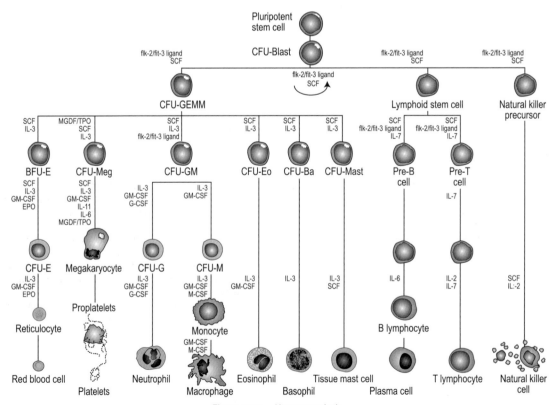

Figure 20.1 Haematopoiesis.

THE CAUSES OF NEUTROPENIA

The major causes of neutropenia in the patient with cancer can be divided into two main groups: either those associated with decreased production or with increased destruction.[2]

Causes of decreased production of neutrophils:

- drug-induced (chemotherapy and other drug treatments)
- primary marrow failure (leukaemias, myelodysplastic syndrome)
- infection
- malnutrition.

Causes of increased destruction or consumption of neutrophils:

- sepsis
- autoimmune processes
- hypersplenism.

Drug-induced neutropenia can be further subdivided into two pathways: the first where the drug reduces cell replication due to its toxicity (anticancer chemotherapy); and the second where the neutropenia is thought to be immunologically mediated and this can be caused by a large number of drugs. The second type of drug-induced neutropenia is more common in women, older patients and those with an allergy profile.[2]

THE EFFECTS AND TREATMENT OF LEUCOPENIA AND NEUTROPENIA

While the patient has a reduced WBC count, he is at a much greater risk from infection. The degree of his vulnerability will depend on the extent and the length of time taken for the WBCs to recover.[6]

Severe neutropenia, which is defined as fewer than 500 neutrophils/μl of blood, can last for 2–4 weeks in the patient who has received marrow ablative high-dose chemotherapy.[3]

THE TREATMENT OF LEUCOPENIA AND NEUTROPENIA

Much of the essential care of a patient who is severely leucopenic will depend on active protection and prevention of infection, early detection and aggressive management of any infection.

The cause of the neutropenia (where not related to high-dose chemotherapy as above) needs to be identified and treated where possible.

The use of replacement granulocyte transfusions, although more popular in the 1970s and 1980s, has declined in the last decade and seems to be associated with several toxicities, including severe pulmonary complications.[4]

Much more popular over the last two decades has been the use of myeloid growth factors, known as colony-stimulating factors. Granulocyte colony-stimulating factor or G-CSF has been shown in several studies to shorten the period of neutropenia.[7]

References

1. Marieb EN (ed.). Human anatomy and physiology. 5th edn. Santa Fe: Benjamin-Cummings; 2001:650–676.
2. Groeger JS. Critical care of the cancer patient. St Louis: Mosby Year Book; 1991:86–103.
3. Whedon MB, Wujcik D. Blood and marrow stem cell transplantation: principles, practice and nursing insights. Boston: Jones and Bartlett; 1997:205–220.
4. Wright DG, Robichaud KJ, Pizzo PA. Lethal pulmonary reactions associated with the use of amphotericin B and leukocyte transfusions. N Engl J Med 1981; 304:1185–1189.
5. Morstyn G, Campbell L, Souza LM. Effect of granulocyte colony stimulating factor on neutropenia induced by cytotoxic chemotherapy. Lancet 1988; 1:667–672.
6. Meza L, Baselga J, Holmes FA, et al. Incidence of febrile neutropenia (FN) is directly related to duration of severe neutropenia (DSN) after myelosuppressive chemotherapy. Proc Am Soc Clin Oncol 2002:2556; Abs 2840.
7. Knoop T. Myelosuppression related to the treatment of cancer. Oncology Supportive Care 2003; 1(3):6–19.

Chapter 21

Anaemia

Shelley Dolan

GENERAL INFORMATION

Anaemia is a disturbance in erythrokinetics that results in a haemoglobin concentration below the expected normal for the age and sex of the patient.[1] The cause of this is a decrease in erythrocytes (red blood cells) and therefore of haemoglobin. Anaemia can be due to decreased production of erythrocytes, an increased destruction or a combination of the two.

In health, there are 4–6 million erythrocytes per mm^3 (µl) of blood (Table 21.1). Their development takes 5–7 days and they last for 100–120 days in the blood.

ERYTHROCYTES AND THEIR FUNCTION

Erythrocytes (red blood cells) are small cells with a diameter of about 7.5 µm and are shaped like biconcave discs. Mature erythrocytes have a plasma membrane but no nucleus or organelles. The structure of an erythrocyte gives it flexibility so that it can twist, turn and become cup shaped as it is carried along through capillaries with very small diameters.[2]

The function of erythrocytes is to transport oxygen and carbon dioxide. Their small size and biconcave shape means that they have a large surface area, which is ideal for gas exchange. Each erythrocyte carries about 250 million haemoglobin molecules. Haemoglobin is composed of the protein globin, which is bound to the red haem pigment. Globin is made up of four polypeptide chains (two alpha and two beta) and four haem groups. At the centre of each of these haem groups is an atom of iron. Each atom of iron can combine reversibly with one molecule of oxygen.[2]

The erythrocytes take up the oxygen in the lungs and then move in the blood supply towards the tissues. In the tissues this process is reversed and the

Table 21.1 Normal blood values

Red cells	Normal values in men	Normal values in women
Haemoglobin	13.3–16.7 g/dl	11.8–14.8 g/dl
Haematocrit	40–54%	35–47%
Red blood cell count	$4.3–5.7 \times 10^9/l$	$3.9–5.0 \times 10^9/l$

erythrocytes give up their oxygen. About 20% of the carbon dioxide transported by the blood is combined with the globin in the erythrocytes. The remainder of the carbon dioxide is collected from the tissues and moved to the lungs to be excreted from the body.

ERYTHROCYTE PRODUCTION – HAEMATOPOIESIS

The erythrocytes are formed in the red bone marrow of the bones. The haematopoietic pathway of the erythrocyte is shown in Figure 21.1.

This haematopoietic pathway from stem cell to reticulocyte takes 3–5 days. The reticulocytes, rich with haemoglobin, are then released into the blood supply and within 2 days become fully mature erythrocytes. In healthy people, reticulocytes will account for 1–2% of all erythrocytes and are therefore used clinically as an estimate of the rate of erythrocyte production.

The hormone erythropoietin (EPO) provides the direct stimulus for erythrocyte production. A basal level of EPO constantly circulates in the blood to ensure erythrocyte production. The stimulus for more EPO production is a drop in blood oxygen levels. EPO is produced mainly in the kidneys and a small percentage by the liver.

CAUSES OF ANAEMIA

There are many causes of anaemia in the patient with cancer, as shown in Table 21.2. Anaemia is usually described using a pathophysiological classification or a morphological classification, as shown in Table 21.3. Anaemia is also divided into absolute or relative anaemia. Relative anaemia is where there is a normal erythrocyte count but an abnormal blood volume. Absolute anaemia is where there is an abnormal erythrocyte count, and this is the most common type in patients with cancer.[1]

Relative anaemia

- Macroglobulinaemia.
- Splenomegaly.

Absolute anaemia

Decreased production of erythrocytes
- Primary marrow failure (leukaemia, myeloma, lymphoma).
- Drug-induced (anticancer chemotherapy and other drugs).
- Substrate deficiencies (iron, vitamin B_{12}).
- Metastatic tumour with bone marrow infiltration.
- Immune deficiency (red cell aplasia, chronic lymphocytic leukaemia).
- Chronic disease states (renal or hepatic failure).
- Acute or chronic infection.
- Endocrine malfunction.

Increased destruction or loss of erythrocytes
- Haemorrhage.
- Phlebotomy (especially in acute conditions).
- Intrinsic abnormalities (membrane/globin defects).

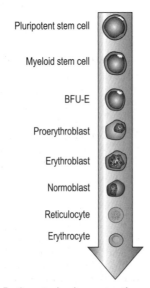

Pluripotent stem cell

Myeloid stem cell

BFU-E

Proerythroblast

Erythroblast

Normoblast

Reticulocyte

Erythrocyte

Figure 21.1 Erythrocyte development pathway.

Table 21.2 Pathophysiological classification

Decreased production	Destruction or increased loss
Bone marrow failure	Acute haemorrhage
Bone marrow suppression	Chronic haemorrhage
Haematinic deficiency anaemia	Haemolysis

Table 21.3   Morphological classification

Description	MCV	MCHC	Blood film
Normocytic, normochromic	Normal	Normal	Size and colour normal
Macrocytic	Increased	Normal	Larger red cells, colour normal
Microcytic, hypochromic	Decreased	Decreased	Small, pale red cells
Normocytic, hyperchromic	Normal	Increased	Normal size, darker colour

MCV, mean cell volume; MCHC, mean corpuscular haemoglobin concentration.
Source: adapted from Rubin and Faber.[3]

- Extrinsic effects – haemolysis secondary to chemotherapy, radiotherapy, infection, antibody reactions.
- Hypersplenism.

THE EFFECTS OF ANAEMIA AND ITS TREATMENT

The patient with anaemia becomes progressively fatigued and dyspnoeic during exertion. Other effects are headaches, dizziness and irritability. If the patient is severely anaemic, tachyarrhythmias, tachypnoea and hypotension can occur.[4,9]

The treatment of anaemia in the patient with cancer will involve correcting the cause of the anaemia as well as supportive treatment with blood transfusions:[1]

- Following marrow ablative chemotherapy, patients will need to be supported with transfusions until their marrow recovers.
- In the case of haemorrhage, any overt bleeding points will need to be identified and treated where possible with endoscopy, surgery or direct pressure.

Table 21.4   Drug treatment of haemorrhage

Drug	Action
Tranexamic acid[6]	Inhibits fibrinolysis by impairing fibrin dissolution
Aprotinin[6]	A proteolytic enzyme inhibitor that acts on plasmin and kallikrein

During these procedures, the patient will need to be supported with clotting factors and platelet transfusions where relevant. Pharmacological agents are also relevant, such as treatment with tranexamic acid or infusions of aprotinin (Table 21.4).[5]

- Autoimmune anaemia will be treated according to the type of antibody. Warm antibody haemolytic anaemia will be treated with glucocorticoid therapy. Patients may go on to require a splenectomy. Cold antibody haemolytic anaemia may respond to drug therapy such as chlorambucil or cyclophosphamide. Plasmaphoresis may also be used to give temporary respite by reducing the antibody reactions.[1]

REPLACEMENT TRANSFUSIONS

The preferred choice of replacement therapy will be packed red cells administered intravenously.[1] Research continues to be conducted about the optimum haemoglobin level and the level necessary to transfuse, but generally blood should be administered if there is any evidence of shock, oxygen transfer problems or overt bleeding.[5]

There are risks associated with blood transfusion about which the general public are increasingly aware. It is therefore essential that patients are informed about risks and receive information, verbal and written, about blood transfusion safety. Every hospital has a Blood Transfusion Committee that will monitor blood transfusion safety, ensuring that national safety guidelines are followed.[7,8,10] (See also Ch. 60.)

References

1. Groeger JS. Critical care of the cancer patient. St Louis: Mosby Year Book; 1991:88–92.
2. Marieb EN (ed.). Human anatomy and physiology. 5th edn. Santa Fe: Benjamin-Cummings; 2001:653–660.
3. Rubin E, Faber JL. Pathology. Philadelphia: JB Lippincott; 1988.
4. Whedon MB, Wujcik D. Blood and marrow stem cell transplantation: principles, practice and nursing insights. Boston: Jones and Bartlett; 1997:205–219.
5. Dolan S. Haemorrhagic problems. In: Grundy M, ed. Nursing in haematological oncology. London: Baillière Tindall; 2000:201–211.

6.   British National Formulary. In: BNF No 47, March 2004. London: British Medical Association and Royal Pharmaceutical Society of Great Britain; 2004.

7.   Department of Health. Review of blood products. Committee on Safety of Medicines. London: Department of Health; 1998.

8.   BCSH. Guidelines for the clinical use of red cell transfusions. British Journal of Haematology 2001; 113:24–31.

9.   Ludwig H, Strasser K. Symptomatology of anemia. Seminars in Oncology 2001; 28(2 Suppl 8):7–14.

10.   Mcclelland B. Handbook of transfusion medicine. HMSO: London; 2001.

Chapter **22**

Thrombocytopenia

Shelley Dolan

GENERAL INFORMATION

Thrombocytopenia is the term used to denote a low platelet count. The normal platelet count is 250 000–500 000 cells/mm^3 (µl) of blood. A platelet count of fewer than 50 000 platelets/mm^3 of blood is usually used to define thrombocytopenia.[1]

Platelets are formed in the bone marrow and are responsible, together with several other agents, for the clotting of the blood.

Thrombocytopenia causes spontaneous bleeding from small blood vessels throughout the body. Severe thrombocytopenia, or when coupled with other clotting disorders, can cause major bleeding and significant morbidity or death.[2]

HAEMATOPOIESIS

The developmental pathway of the platelet is as shown in Figure 22.1 and takes 4–5 days to develop.

The life span of a platelet is 5–10 days.

HAEMOSTASIS

Platelets play two key roles in the clotting of the blood:

- They form a haemostatic plug that temporarily seals a hole in a vessel wall. This is known as platelet adherence.
- As they break down, platelets liberate several chemicals that promote further clotting.[3]

Thrombocytopenia will occur as the result of any condition that suppresses or destroys the bone marrow, which includes malignancies affecting the bone marrow such as leukaemia or other cancers that have metastasised into the bone marrow, or the effects of

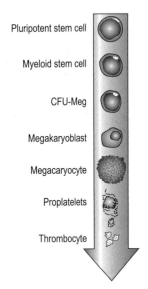

Pluripotent stem cell

Myeloid stem cell

CFU-Meg

Megakaryoblast

Megacaryocyte

Proplatelets

Thrombocyte

Figure 22.1   Thrombocyte development pathway.

ionising radiation or drugs.[3] Thrombocytopenia can also be due to the side effects of certain drugs such as heparin and Persantin (dipyridamole).[4,5]

TREATMENT OPTIONS FOR THROMBOCYTOPENIA

The treatment options will depend to some extent on the cause of the thrombocytopenia. If the cause is newly diagnosed bone marrow malignancy, such as acute lymphoblastic leukaemia, the optimum therapy will be to treat the cause and commence anticancer chemotherapy. Even in this scenario, the patient will need supportive therapy to increase the platelet count. Platelets are replaced using a platelet transfusion.

Platelet transfusions

There are four types of platelet transfusions:

1. The type most commonly used is 'pool platelets'. This is where the unit of platelets has been derived from 6 units of blood pooled to make 1 unit of platelets. The blood used is derived from anonymous donors and prepared in the central blood transfusion centres.
2. The next type are single donor platelets, again obtained from the blood transfusion centre, but this time taken from one single anonymous donor.
3. The third type is 'matched unrelated donor' platelets. These are obtained from the blood transfusion centre, having been matched to the individual patient.
4. Finally, a cancer centre may place a member of their patient's family on an aphoresis system and, where there is a match, obtain related donor platelets.

The choice of platelet source depends very much on the clinical situation. As a general rule, all patients are treated with type 1 pool platelets. However, where the patient is in the midst of their acute therapy, such as a stem cell transplant, and they have severe thrombocytopenia and do not achieve a reasonable increment with pool platelets, their team may go on to request single donor or matched unrelated donor (MUD) platelets. MUD platelets will usually only be used in an emergency situation and this is only possible when there are family members who are a 'match' and who consent to donate platelets.

Decision to transfuse with platelets

Generally, patients who are acutely ill will have platelets transfused when their platelet count has fallen below 50 000. However, all transplant units should have agreed unit guidelines for the management of platelet transfusions.

In the non-acute setting where a patient has a chronically low platelet count and is not receiving any invasive therapy, lower platelet counts may be accepted.[6,7]

If any patient who has a low platelet count is to undergo invasive therapy, e.g. a lumbar puncture or insertion of a skin-tunnelled catheter, a platelet transfusion should be given prior to the procedure.

Finally, some patients never recover the ability to manufacture platelets and are thus supported in the community or from their local hospital with regular platelet transfusions.[6,7]

References

1. Marieb EN (ed.). Human anatomy and physiology. 5th edn. Santa Fe: Benjamin-Cummings; 2001.
2. Dolan S. Haemorrhagic problems. In: Grundy M, ed. Nursing in haematological oncology. London: Baillière Tindall; 2000:201–211.
3. Groeger JS. Critical care of the cancer patient. St Louis: Mosby Year Book; 1991.
4. Betrosian AP, Theodossiades G, Lambroulis G, et al. (2003) Heparin-induced thrombocytopenia with pulmonary embolism and disseminated intravascular coagulation associated with low-molecular-weight heparin. Am J Med Sci. 2003; 325(1):45–47.
5. Hibbard AB, Medina PJ, Vesely SK. Reports of drug-induced thrombocytopenia, Ann Intern Med 2003; 138(3):239.
6. Whedon MB, Wujcik D. Blood and marrow stem cell transplantation: principles, practice and nursing insights. Boston: Jones and Bartlett; 1997:205–219.
7. National Blood Service. Guidelines for the management of platelet transfusion refractoriness. UK: NBS; 2002.

Chapter 23

Alopecia

Lisa Dougherty

INTRODUCTION

Alopecia is the partial or total loss of hair. Chemotherapy-induced alopecia is the temporary loss of all body hair, which includes the hair on the head, eyelashes, eyebrows, pubic hair and body hair.

CHEMOTHERAPY DRUGS THAT CAUSE ALOPECIA

The following drugs cause complete hair loss:

- dactinomycin
- daunorubicin
- docetaxel
- doxorubicin
- epirubicin
- etoposide
- paclitaxel

The following drugs cause partial hair loss but may cause complete loss if given in high doses or in combination with the drugs above:

- cyclophosphamide
- 5-fluorouracil
- mitoxantrone (mitozantrone)
- vinca alkaloids

THE PATIENT'S PERSPECTIVE

Alopecia has been identified as the most distressing side effect of cancer chemotherapy.[1-4] It has been identified as such a devastating prospect that some patients may refuse to accept treatment.[1,4] Hair loss can also result in changes to the patient's body image[5,6] that may not be improved by the regrowth of hair.[7] Those patients who have relapsed undergoing chemotherapy that causes alopecia may find the loss of hair to be more devastating for the second time.[8]

PREVENTION

Two main techniques have been tested to prevent chemotherapy-induced hair loss: scalp tourniquets and scalp cooling.

Scalp tourniquets

This method works by minimising the contact of the drug with hair follicles, by occluding the superficial blood vessels supplying the scalp by using pressure.[9] Some found this method effective but others reported this method to be time-consuming, uncomfortable and ineffective.[10]

Scalp cooling

Scalp cooling has an advantage over scalp tourniquet in that it inhibits the cellular uptake of a drug, which is temperature-dependent.[11] Scalp hypothermia (scalp temperature of 22°C)[12] produces changes in the scalp circulation by causing vasoconstriction of superficial vessels (Fig. 23.1). Decreased blood flow to the scalp reduces the amount of the drug reaching the hair follicles and thus minimises damage to the scalp hair.[10,13] Scalp cooling has been successfully used to reduce or prevent hair loss with the following drugs:

1. doxorubicin[14–17]
2. epirubicin[18,19]
3. taxanes.[20,21]

Scalp cooling should not be offered to:

- patients with haematological disease, unless the consultant feels it is appropriate on grounds of quality of life[22]
- patients receiving drugs that cause hair loss where there is no research or evidence as to the effectiveness
- patients who have already received a first course of chemotherapy that may induce hair loss, but who were not offered or declined scalp cooling.

The potential risk of scalp metastases, albeit remote,[23–26] should be addressed and discussed with the patient.[27,28]

Types of scalp cooling systems

There are many types of scalp cooling systems.

Caps

- Home-made caps formed from hot/cold gel packs and moulded onto a wig stand to make shape.[15,29]
- Commercial caps, e.g. Chemocap (a cryogel cap; Fig. 23.2).[20,21,27,30]

Scalp cooling machines

- A thermocirculator system with a reliable temperature control where coolant is pumped between two layers of a lightweight cap.[31]
- The use of refrigerated air passed over the patient's scalp via a hair-drying helmet.[19,32]
- An electrically cooled cap.[23]

The success of all these methods in preventing hair loss varies and the amount of hair loss experienced by the patient is dependent on a number of factors:

1. Involvement of the liver with metastatic disease as the disease leads to elevated plasma levels of doxorubicin over a longer period of time.[17]
2. Inadequate cooling.[29]

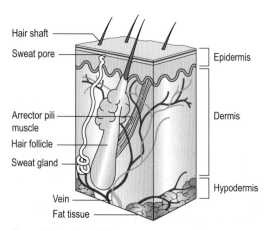

Figure 23.1 Hair follicle.

Labels: Hair shaft, Sweat pore, Arrector pili muscle, Hair follicle, Sweat gland, Vein, Fat tissue, Epidermis, Dermis, Hypodermis

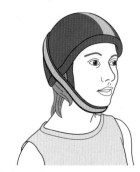

Figure 23.2 Scalp cooling cap.

3. When anthracyclines are used in combination with other drugs that cause alopecia. Success is improved when single agent doxorubicin is used (80%), whereas adding other alopecia-causing drugs reduces success to 50–60%.[14,33]

Research shows that scalp cooling can be very distressing.[34] Dougherty found that 50% of patients who underwent scalp cooling found it to be worthwhile and 70% would undergo the procedure again in order to prevent hair loss.[35] Patients have reported adverse effects during and following treatment, such as headaches, claustrophobia and 'ice phobias'.[34]

More recently, biological methods of preventing chemotherapy-induced hair loss have focused on promoting hair growth or protecting hair follicles.[28] (See also Ch. 30.)

SUPPORTING THE PATIENT

The nurse's role is to support and provide choices and information.[3,28] Being able to talk about how they feel may be helpful for many patients, and understanding the meaning and level of importance of hair to each individual is a useful interaction.[36] It is useful to inform patients that:

- Information about how to care for their hair is important as it may help to reduce loss. Patients should be advised to use a wide-toothed comb or a soft hairbrush but encouraged to brush or comb their hair daily.
- As chemotherapy causes hair to become dry and brittle, they should use a mild shampoo with a neutral pH and hair should be washed only one or twice a week, with tepid water.
- They should avoid the use of hot hair dryers or heated rollers as well as hair dyes, perms and anything that will further dry out their hair.

- They may notice scalp tenderness just prior to hair loss and that the loss may be gradual or it may be sudden.
- Hair loss may start within a couple of days of beginning treatment or may not occur for some weeks. It is often difficult to predict when this will happen and it is very individual.
- Where hair loss does occur, they should pay attention to care of the scalp and protect it from excess heat and cold. Patients should be advised to use a sunblocking cream or to cover their head with a hat or light scarf when out in the sun. They can use a mild moisturiser if the scalp becomes dry or tender.

ADAPTATION TO HAIR LOSS

It is important to ensure that, if a patient fails to retain hair or decides not to undergo scalp cooling, adequate time is spent helping the patient to adapt to the hair loss physically, psychologically and socially.[3] This can be achieved by ensuring that all patients who may lose their hair see the surgical appliance officer as soon as possible, in order to obtain a wig that can be matched to the patient's desired hairstyle and colour. Advice can be given on hair care and various ideas of hats, turbans and scarves, and reinforced with a hair care information booklet. It is important to stress to the patient that their hair will always grow back and will be a reasonable length, 3–5 cm within 3–4 months. Remind patients that their hair may grow back slightly differently: e.g. a different shade or colour, curlier than before or very straight. However, it will eventually go back to the original colour and style and it appears to grow back in better condition.

References

1. Tierney AJ. Preventing chemotherapy-induced alopecia in cancer patients: is scalp cooling worthwhile? J Adv Nurs 1987; 12:303–310.
2. Carr K. How I survived the fall out. You magazine, Mail on Sunday 1998; 10 May:61–67.
3. Pickard-Holley S. The symptom experience of alopecia. Semin Oncol Nurs 1995; 11(4):235–238.
4. Williams J, Wood C, Cunningham-Warburton P. A narrative study of chemotherapy induced alopecia. Oncol Nurs Forum 1999; 26(9):1463–1468.
5. Wagner L, Bye MG. Body image and patients experiencing alopecia as a result of cancer chemotherapy. Cancer Nurs 1979; 2:365–369.
6. Baxley KO, Erdman LK, Henry EB, et al. Alopecia: effect on cancer patients' body image. Cancer Nurs 1984; 7(6):499–503.
7. Munstedt K, Manthey N, Sachesse H, et al. Changes in self-concept and body image during alopecia induced cancer chemotherapy. Support Care Cancer 1997; 5:139–143.
8. Gallagher J. Women's experiences of hair loss associated with chemotherapy – longitudinal perspective. Proceedings of 9th International Conference in Cancer Nursing 1996:52.
9. Maxwell MB. Scalp tourniquets for chemotherapy-induced alopecia. Am J Nurs 1980; 5:900–902.

10. Parker R. The effectiveness of scalp hypothermia in preventing cyclophosphamide induced alopecia. Oncol Nurs Forum 1987; 146:49–53.

11. Dean JC, Salmon SE, Griffith KS, et al. Prevention of doxorubicin-induced hair loss with scalp hypothermia. N Engl J Med 1979; 301:1427–1429.

12. Bulow J, Friberg L, Gaardsting O, et al. Frontal sub-cutaneous blood flow and epi- and subcutaneous temperatures during scalp cooling in normal man. Scand J Clin Lab Invest 1985; 45:505–508.

13. Kennedy M, Packard R, Grant M. The effects of using Chemocap on occurrence of chemotherapy-induced alopecia. Oncol Nurs Forum 1983; 10(1):19–24.

14. Middleton J, Franks D, Buchanan RB. Failure of scalp hypothermia to prevent hair loss when cyclophos-phamide is added to doxorubicin and vincristine. Cancer Treatment Reports 1985; 694:373–375.

15. David JA, Speechley V. Scalp cooling to prevent alopecia. Nurs Times 1987; 32(83):36–37.

16. Gregory RP, Cooke T, Middleton J, et al. Prevention of doxorubicin induced alopecia by scalp hypothermia: relation to degree of cooling. Br Med J 1982; 284:1674.

17. Satterwhite B, Zimm S. The use of scalp hypothermia in the prevention of doxorubicin-induced hair loss. Cancer 1984; 54:34–37.

18. Robinson MH, Jones AC, Durrant KD. Effectiveness of scalp cooling in reducing alopecia caused by epiru-bicin treatment of advanced breast cancer. Cancer Treat Rep 1987; 71:913–914.

19. Adams L, Lawson N, Maxted KJ, et al. The prevention of hair loss from chemotherapy by the use of cold air scalp cooling. Eur J Cancer Care 1992; 15:16–18.

20. Le Menager M, Genouville C, Bessa EH, et al. Docetaxel induced alopecia can be prevented. Lancet 1995; 346:371–372.

21. LeMenager M, Le Comte S, Bonneterre ME, et al. Effectiveness of cold cap in the prevention of docetaxel induced alopecia. Eur J Cancer 1997; 33(2):297–300.

22. Purohit OP, Coleman RT, Steers JM, et al. A six-week chemotherapy regimen for relapsed lymphoma efficacy results and the influence of scalp cooling. Ann Oncol 1992; 3(Suppl 5):126.

23. Ron IG, Kalmus Y, Kalmus Z, et al. Scalp cooling in the prevention of alopecia in patients receiving depilating chemotherapy. Support Care Cancer 1997; 5:136–138.

24. Witman G, Cadman E, Chen M, et al. Misuse of scalp hypothermia. Cancer Treat Rep 1981; 65(5–6):507–508.

25. Tollenaar RAEM, Liefes GJ, Replaer van Driel OJ, et al. Scalp cooling has no place in the prevention of alopecia in adjuvant chemotherapy in breast cancer. Eur J Cancer 1994; 30A(10):1448–1453.

26. Crowe M, Kendrick M, Woods S. Is scalp cooling a procedure that should be offered to patients receiving alopecia induced chemotherapy for solid tumours. Proceedings of 10th International Conference of Cancer Nursing, Jerusalem, 1998:64.

27. Peck HJ, Mitchell H, Stewart AL. Evaluating the efficacy of scalp cooling using penguin cold caps. Eur J Cancer Care 2000; 4(4):246–248.

28. Batchelor D. Hair and cancer chemotherapy. Eur J Cancer Care 2001; 10:147 –163.

29. Hunt J, Anderson JE, Smith IE. Scalp hypothermia to prevent Adriamycin-induced hair loss. Cancer Nurs 1982; 51:25–31.

30. Wilson C. The ice cap that could help save your hair. Daily Mail 1994; September 20:36–37.

31. Guy R, Parker H, Shah S, et al. Scalp cooling by thermocirculator. Lancet 1982; 1(8278):937–938.

32. Symonds RP, McCormick CV. Adriamycin alopecia prevented by cold air scalp cooling. Am J Clin Oncol 1986; 95:454–457.

33. Tierney AJ, Taylor J. Chemotherapy-induced hair loss. Nurs Standard 1991; 538:29–31.

34. Tierney AJ, Taylor J, Jose Closs S. A study to inform nursing support of patients coping with chemotherapy for breast cancer. Report prepared for the Scottish Home and Health Department; 1989.

35. Dougherty L. Scalp cooling to prevent hair loss in chemotherapy. Prof Nurse 1996; 118:1–3.

36. Freedman TG. Social and cultural dimensions of hair loss in women treated for breast cancer. Cancer Nurs 1994; 174:334–341.

Chapter **24**

Renal effects and tumour lysis

Shelley Dolan

THE FUNCTION OF THE KIDNEYS IN HEALTH

The primary function of the kidneys is to filter nearly 200 litres of fluid every 24 hours from the circulating blood. This filtration includes ridding the body of unwanted toxins and waste material and returning to the blood substances that are required. The kidneys also produce various substances such as the enzyme renin, which regulates blood pressure and kidney function, and the hormone erythropoietin, which stimulates red cell production. The kidneys have a role in gluconeogenesis during prolonged fasting, and they metabolise vitamin D to its active form.[1]

CAUSES OF RENAL FAILURE IN THE CANCER PATIENT

Renal hypoperfusion

This is caused by:

- dehydration
- bleeding
- gastrointestinal (GI) losses
- diuretic therapy
- decreased intake of fluid.

Obstruction to outflow

This is caused by:

- primary tumour invasion of the kidney, ureters or bladder.
- lymphoma, pelvic tumours
- retroperitoneal metastases
- blood clots
- calculi or stones.

Acute parenchymal failure

This is caused by:

- tumour invasion – leukaemia, lymphoma
- tumour lysis syndrome (TLS)
- nephrotoxic chemotherapy, e.g. high-dose methotrexate, melphalan, cisplatin, gallium nitrate, streptozocin, mitomycin, ciclosporin, plicamycin or ifosfamide[2]
- radiation nephritis
- hyperviscosity syndrome
- hypercalcaemia
- multiple myeloma
- severe sepsis
- disseminated intravascular coagulation
- nephrotoxic drugs – antimicrobials, non-steroidal anti-inflammatory drugs, radiographic contrast media.

RENAL EFFECTS ASSOCIATED WITH ANTICANCER CHEMOTHERAPY

The kidneys are at risk from the chemotherapy itself but also from several other factors. It is important to note that most cancer patients who present with acute renal failure (ARF) have multiple causes.[2] Therefore, when aiming to protect the patient, all possible renal threats should be considered. It is an essential part of care to monitor renal function prior to, during and after cancer chemotherapy in order to try and preserve renal function.

Renal protective therapy

All cancer patients receiving chemotherapy are at risk from developing renal effects. It is therefore important for clinicians to be aware of the contributory factors that place a patient in a high-risk position.

Patient management to avoid renal complications should include:

- the monitoring of fluid balance
- the monitoring of serum biochemistry
- a protective environment
- serum antibiotic levels and
- haemodynamic parameters.

If the patient is at risk of developing TLS or sepsis, then the following warning signs should be recognised, and then protective action and increased monitoring should be instituted immediately:

- any early signs of renal impairment, such as oliguria or a urine output of less than 0.5 ml/kg/h
- prolonged hypotension
- a rising serum urea, creatinine, sodium or potassium.

Protection for the kidneys consists of trying to return the blood pressure to the patient's previous 'normal' level using fluid replacement and if necessary inotropic therapy. Ensuring that the patient does not become intravascularly depleted can be difficult if the patient becomes septic or has 'capillary leak syndrome'. Meticulous avoidance of toxic drug levels using forced diuresis following nephrotoxic chemotherapy such as melphalan or delaying anti-microbials until the serum level is appropriate are also used. Ensuring that the patient is intravascularly hydrated and the use of renal protective agents such as allopurinol is also part of many chemotherapy regimes.

TUMOUR LYSIS SYNDROME

Where the patient is thought to be at risk from TLS, clinicians need to identify the patient before chemotherapy treatment in order that the patient can be monitored closely. There will also need to be referral and discussion with the clinicians in the environment where renal replacement therapy will be provided if this becomes necessary.

TLS is a syndrome that can occur following the administration of chemotherapy or radiotherapy for bulky disease or high white cell count disease. Therefore, TLS is most commonly seen following the treatment of lymphoma, teratoma or high white cell count leukaemia. The damage to the kidneys is caused by the release of intracellular products into the circulation following the rapid breakdown of malignant cells. The patient develops hyperuricaemia, hyperphosphataemia, hyperkalaemia and hypocalcaemia.[3] In any patient who has pre-existing renal disease TLS is more likely to be severe. As the syndrome develops, the rising serum potassium can cause life-threatening cardiac arrhythmias.[4]

Management of TLS

The treatment of TLS is based on its prevention by identifying high-risk patients and then ensuring the following:

- accurate and frequent monitoring of fluid and electrolyte balance
- optimum hydration and the maintenance of a urine output of at least 3 litres/24 hours
- if the urine output falls, commencing inotropes or diuretic therapy
- allopurinol oral or intravenously, 500 mg/m² daily, to control hyperuricaemia
- acetazolamide 250 mg intravenously to increase the excretion of uric acid through the kidneys

- the use of a urolytic enzyme – e.g. SR29142 is currently being studied.[5]

If, despite the above measures, severe TLS develops, initial rises in potassium may be controlled with calcium gluconate or the administration of a dextrose and insulin infusion. However, if the patient's urine output can no longer be maintained in the presence of rapidly worsening metabolic balance, renal replacement therapy will have to be instituted immediately. The dialytic method of choice for TLS is a continuous filtration method to compensate for the continuing lysis of cells. The method most commonly used in the cancer setting is continuous veno-venous haemodiafiltration (CVVHDF) therapy.

CONCLUSION

If the cancer patient develops acute renal failure, overall recovery will depend on the cause and whether any other organ is affected. If the kidneys are affected following severe sepsis or in the presence of respiratory failure, the mortality rates are very high, rising to 85–95%, depending on the stage of the cancer. Renal protective therapy is therefore essential in the management of the cancer patient receiving chemotherapy.

References

1. Marieb EN (ed.). Human anatomy and physiology. 5th edn. Santa Fe: Benjamin-Cummings; 2001:1003–1039.
2. Groeger JS. Critical care of the cancer patient. St Louis: Mosby Year Book; 1991:150–164.
3. Akasheh MS, Chang CP, Vesole DH. Acute tumour lysis syndrome: a case in AL amyloidosis. Br J Haematol 1999; 107(2):387.
4. Fassas AB, Desikan KR, Siegel D, et al. Tumour lysis syndrome complicating high dose treatment in patients with multiple myeloma. Br J Haematol 1999; 105(4):938–941.
5. Mahmoud HH, Leverger G, Patte C, et al. Advances in the management of malignancy – associated hyperuricaemia. Br J Cancer 1998; 77(4):18–20.

Chapter **25**

Electrolyte abnormalities

Shelley Dolan

GENERAL INFORMATION

Cancer patients are particularly susceptible to a variety of electrolyte abnormalities. Many abnormalities are those associated with chronic disease, malnutrition and organ failure but patients who are receiving anticancer chemotherapy are additionally at risk.

Anticancer chemotherapy has many side effects: e.g. gastrointestinal (GI) toxicity, which severely affects the fluid and electrolyte balance of the body.

Drug therapy can also directly affect electrolytes. An obvious example of this is in the systemic treatment of severe fungal infections, where amphotericin B, the drug most widely used until the last 2–3 years, causes depletion of serum potassium.

ELECTROLYTE BALANCE IN HEALTH

The electrolytes include salts, acids and bases, but when thinking about electrolyte balance and toxicities the term refers to the balance of salts in the body.

The salts contain minerals that are essential for neuromuscular function, membrane permeability and many other cellular functions, and for secretory function. It is the salts that also have a direct effect on the movement of fluids in the body. Many salts are important to cellular activity but, for clinical purposes, the ones that will be examined more closely are sodium, potassium, calcium and magnesium.

Salts are ingested in food and fluids, and small amounts are generated through metabolic activity. Salts are excreted from the body in sweat, urine and faeces. Large losses from the body occur with GI losses, vomiting or diarrhoea, severe bleeds, and covert losses through leaky capillaries and 'third spacing', e.g. due to a paralytic ileus.[1]

Salts are regulated by renal mechanisms, which are in turn controlled by various hormonal controls, e.g. aldosterone. Each of the major salts will now be explored, but it is important to recognise that their functions are co-dependent and in clinical practice they should never be viewed in isolation.

SODIUM

Sodium has the most important role in regulating both the extracellular fluid (ECF) and water distribution in the body. Sodium salts represent 90–95% of all solutes in the ECF and account for about 280 mOsm of the total solute concentration (300 mOsm) (Box 25.1). The normal serum concentration of sodium is 136–145 mEq/L (Table 25.1), and it is thus the most plentiful cation in the ECF and the one that exerts the most significant osmotic pressure.

The control of sodium and water in the body are linked to the blood pressure and volume. Sodium is therefore affected by many neural and hormonal agents, including aldosterone, antidiuretic hormone (ADH), atrial natriuretic peptide (ANP), oestrogens, progesterone and glucocorticosteroids.

Hypernatraemia

With sodium concentration levels above 145 mEq/L, hypernatraemia is caused by either dehydration, excess sodium intake or renal failure. Clinically, hypernatraemia is very dangerous and will cause central nervous system dehydration, which will lead to confusion, lethargy, fitting and, finally, unconsciousness and death.

In the cancer patient who is receiving many toxic drugs, both anticancer and antimicrobial therapy, a rising sodium concentration should be noted and measures taken immediately to reduce intravenous ingestion of sodium and to protect renal function. It should be noted that many intravenous preparations of antimicrobials contain high amounts of sodium.

Box 25.1   Osmolality
The osmolality of a solution refers to the number of solute particles dissolved in one litre of water. It is also reflected in the ability of the solution to cause osmosis, and to alter certain physical properties of the solvent, e.g. boiling and freezing points[1]

Table 25.1   Normal values for electrolyte concentrations

Electrolyte	Normal value (mEq/L)
Potassium	3.5–5.3
Sodium	136–145
Magnesium	0.79–1.05
Calcium	4.5–4.8

Hyponatraemia

With ECF levels below 130 mEq/L, hyponatraemia is caused by excessive losses from the body, renal disease, excess ADH secretion and deficiency of aldosterone (Addison's disease). Clinically, hyponatraemia, especially if of sudden onset, is very dangerous and will lead to cerebral oedema, confusion, irritability, and fitting, fluid overload and heart failure.

In the cancer patient who is receiving chemotherapy, GI losses can be profound, with some agents causing losses in diarrhoea or vomiting of several litres per day. There may also be covert losses, particularly with sequestration of fluid in the abdomen and third spacing, as a result of GI toxicity. Adrenocorticotrophic hormone (ACTH) deficiency can also cause severe hyponatraemia and should therefore be excluded.[2]

Where there is severe dehydration, the patient will require rehydration, together with careful sodium replacement. In extreme cases where there is cerebral oedema, the patient may require potent diuretic therapy such as with mannitol. There is no absolute evidence that rapid correction of serum sodium can cause further cardiac failure or central pontine myelinolysis (a non-inflammatory demyelination of the central basis pontis), but in clinical practice sodium replacement is managed conservatively over a 24–48 hour period.[3,4]

Patients with severe sodium imbalance, either hyper- or hyponatraemia, will need to be managed in an area where full cardiac, pressure and neurological monitoring is possible.[5]

POTASSIUM

The normal range of potassium is 3.5–5.3 mEq/L.

Hyperkalaemia

Hyperkalaemia is caused primarily by renal failure, but it can also be caused by a deficit in aldosterone, overinfusion of intravenous potassium and burns or severe tissue injuries.[1]

Clinically, hyperkalaemia can lead to nausea, vomiting, diarrhoea, cardiac arrhythmias leading to cardiac arrest, skeletal muscle weakness and flaccid paralysis.

In the patient receiving anticancer chemotherapy, the most common cause for hyperkalaemia is renal failure. Cancer patients are at risk from renal failure from several causes (see Ch. 24). Tumour lysis syndrome (TLS) is a cause of acute renal failure associated with chemotherapy or radiotherapy that causes a rapid rise in potassium.[6]

The treatment of hyperkalaemia is dependent on careful monitoring of serum potassium, especially where there is a high risk of abnormality. The renal failure should be reversed where possible, while the patient is treated with either calcium gluconate or insulin to reduce the serum potassium. It should be noted that these agents will only bring about a temporary change if the cause of the renal failure is still present. The patient may therefore require renal replacement therapy such as haemodialysis or, where there are acute changes such as with TLS, a continuous method of renal filtration. If the hyperkalaemia has precipitated a cardiac arrest, the peri-arrest treatment is intravenous calcium gluconate 10 ml followed by assessment of potassium level.[7]

Hypokalaemia

Hypokalaemia is caused primarily by GI losses, but also by malnutrition, Cushing's disease, hyperaldosteronism, diuretic therapy and antifungal agents.[1]

Clinically, low serum potassium can lead to cardiac arrhythmias, muscular weakness, hypoventilation and mental confusion.

As stated previously, the cancer patient undergoing chemotherapy is exquisitely sensitive to GI toxicity and should therefore be recognised as being at high risk. Any patient who is neutropenic, and therefore at risk of infection, will need to be carefully monitored if commencing therapy with either intravenous amphotericin B or the aminoglycosides.[6] Potassium levels should be carefully monitored and appropriate replacement undertaken as soon as possible. For many patients, oral potassium therapy is very hard to take either because of severe nausea, oral toxicity or because the preparations are unpalatable. For patients in the acute phase of therapy, intravenous potassium replacement should be the therapy of choice.

MAGNESIUM

The normal range of magnesium is 0.79–1.05 mEq/L of blood.

Hypermagnesaemia

Hypermagnesaemia is rare and is caused by either a deficiency of aldosterone or an excess of magnesium intake (antacids). Clinically, the patient would become lethargic, have impaired CNS function, which could lead on to coma, and respiratory depression.

Hypomagnesaemia

Hypomagnesaemia occurs more often and is due to GI losses, following surgical correction of hyperparathyroidism, malnutrition, diuretic therapy and alcoholism.[1] Clinically, a low magnesium will cause increased neuromuscular excitability, fitting and cardiac arrhythmia.

Again, the cancer patient is particularly at risk of developing a low serum magnesium as the result of GI losses, particularly from the lower GI tract.[8] Hypomagnesaemia is also related to certain drugs that are commonly used while patients are receiving chemotherapy, such as aminoglycosides, platinum compounds, amphotericin, ciclosporin, steroids and diuretics.[6]

It is important to remember that hypomagnesaemia will be accompanied by hypocalcaemia and hypokalaemia, and magnesium replacement will be essential to correct the other electrolytes.

The treatment of hypomagnesaemia is to treat the cause where possible and to replace the magnesium either enterally or parenterally. In patients with normal renal function, 16–32 mEq/L of magnesium can be given over 4–6 hours. Frequent assessment of magnesium levels should be made.

CALCIUM

The normal range of calcium is 4.5–4.8 mEq/L.

Hypercalcaemia

Hypercalcaemia is the most common metabolic emergency seen in cancer patients. It is thought that hypercalcaemia will occur in 10–20% of all cancer patients at some stage of their disease.[9] There are many causes of hypercalcaemia, the most common being neoplastic disease itself, particularly lung or breast cancer, myeloma or lymphoma. The most likely cause of hypercalcaemia with these tumours is the secretion of tumour products that affect calcium metabolism.[10] However, it is important, especially in the patient who is receiving chemotherapy, to ensure that there is not another or concurrent cause, e.g. acute or chronic renal failure, hyperparathyroidism, immobilisation-induced hypercalcaemia or adrenal insufficiency.[6]

Clinically, the symptoms of hypercalcaemia will be vomiting, altered mental status, acute abdomen, cardiac arrhythmias, cardiac arrest and death.

The treatment of hypercalcaemia long term is concentrated on identifying the cause and reversing or reducing the tumour burden. However, hypercalcaemia commonly occurs in patients with advanced disease or those who are acutely ill and already receiving optimum therapy.

In moderate hypercalcaemia, as judged by the serum calcium (<14 mg/dl) and relatively unsymptomatic patient, the following measures should be instituted:

1. Saline hydration and diuresis.

If normal levels of calcium, not sustained add:

2. Glucocorticosteroids.
3. Calcitonin.
4. Bisphosphanate intravenously.

In life-threatening hypercalcaemia (>14 mg/dl) and severe symptoms:

1. Saline hydration and diuresis and diuretics plus calcitonin.
2. If insufficient response in 12–24 hours, add more potent drug, depending on chemotherapy options and renal status.

3. Plicamycin.
4. A second-generation bisphosphonate: e.g. zoledronic acid.[11,12]
5. Gallium nitrate infusion.[6]

Hypocalcaemia

Hypocalcaemia is not as common in cancer patients as hypercalcaemia. In many instances of apparent hypocalcaemia, the patient's albumin is severely depleted and the patient's serum calcium is lowered. However, in this situation the patient's ionic calcium level remains stable and the patient will be asymptomatic. True hypocalcaemia is most commonly associated with hypomagnesaemia and will require correction of the magnesium before the calcium is corrected. Rarely, hypocalcaemia is seen as a result of TLS, or after a massive blood transfusion.

The symptoms associated with hypocalcaemia are tingling of the fingers, tremors, tetany, fitting and cardiac arrhythmias.[1]

The treatment of hypocalcaemia will be dependent on the causes mentioned above and will usually consist of replacing magnesium and enteral calcium supplementation.

References

1. Marieb EN (ed.). Human anatomy and physiology. 5th edn. Santa Fe: Benjamin-Cummings; 2001:1047–1054.
2. Yamamoto T, Fukuyama J, Kabayama Y, et al. Dual facets of hyponatraemia and arginine vasopressin in patients with ACTH deficiency. Clin Endocrinol (Oxf) 1998; 49(6):785–792.
3. Ayus JC, Krothapalli RK, Arieff AI. Changing concepts in treatment of severe symptomatic hyponatraemia. Rapid correction and possible relation to central pontine myelinosis. Am J Med 1985; 78:897–902.
4. Filippella M, Cappabianca P, Cavallo LM, et al. Very delayed hyponatremia after surgery and radiotherapy for a pituitary macroadenoma. J Endocrinol Invest 2002; 25(2):163–168.
5. Oh TE. Intensive care manual. Sydney: Butterworths; 1995:505–511.
6. Groeger JS. Critical care of the cancer patient. St Louis: Mosby Year Book; 1991:141–162.
7. Resuscitation Council. Advanced life support. 2001.
8. Agus ZS, Wasserstein A, Goldfarb S. Disorders of calcium and magnesium homeostasis. Am J Med 1982; 72:473–488.
9. Lin JT. Bony pathology in the cancer patient. J Womens Health (Larchmt) 2002; 11(8):691–702.
10. Moseley JM, Kubota M, Diefenbach-Jagger H. Parathyroid hormone related protein purified from a human lung cancer cell line. Natl Acad Sci 1987; 84:5048–5052.
11. Rosen L, Harland SJ, Oosterlinck W. Broad clinical activity of zoledronic acid in osteolytic to osteoblastic bone lesions in patients with a broad range of solid tumors. Am J Clin Oncol 2002; 25(6 Suppl 1):S19–24. Review.
12. Lipton A, Small E, Saad F, et al. The new bisphosphonate, Zometa (zoledronic acid), decreases skeletal complications in both osteolytic and osteoblastic lesions: a comparison to pamidronate. Cancer Invest 2002; 20 (Suppl 2):45–54.

Chapter **26**

Skin and nail changes

Lisa Wolf

INTRODUCTION

The integumentary system (skin) is one of the largest organs of the body. The three main functions of the skin are protection, temperature control and sensation.[1]

Chemotherapy can induce alterations of the integumentary system, which may be:

- Generalised, due to the destruction of the basal cells of the epidermis
- Localised, due to cellular alterations at the site of chemotherapy administration or along the veins used.[2]

(See also Chs 10 and 48.)

DRUGS THAT CAUSE SKIN AND NAIL CHANGES

Drugs that can cause skin and nail changes are listed in Box 26.1.

SKIN REACTIONS ASSOCIATED WITH SPECIFIC CHEMOTHERAPY DRUGS

Skin reactions associated with specific chemotherapy drugs will now be considered.[3–9]

Transient erythema/urticaria

Cutaneous reaction
Transient erythema/urticaria may be generalised or localised at the site of chemotherapy.

Pathophysiology
The exact mechanism of transient erythema/urticaria is unknown; it may be a vascular reaction. It usually occurs within a few hours and then gradually disappears.

Box 26.1   Examples of common cytotoxic drugs that cause skin and nail changes

Asparaginase
Bleomycin
Busulfan
Cytarabine
Dactinomycin
Doxorubicin
Epirubicin
Etoposide
5-Fluorouracil
Hydroxyurea
Methotrexate
Mitomycin C
Mitroxantrone (mitrozantrone)
Streptozocin

Assessment
Perform skin assessment. Transient erythema or urticaria is more common with doxorubicin and bleomycin.

Patient education
Warn patient of this possibility and provide reassurance.

Hyperpigmentation

Cutaneous reaction
Hyperpigmentation can affect the nail beds, oral mucosa or the skin surfaces along the veins used for drug administration, in particular with 5-fluorouracil (5-FU).

Pathophysiology
Hyperpigmentation is thought to be due to a variation in the amount and distribution of melanin and the direct stimulation of the melanocyte. It is believed that 5-FU causes endothelial fragility, which results in the drug escaping into the tissues, causing hyperpigmentation of the overlying skin. Hyperpigmentation occurs within a few weeks post-chemotherapy administration and is usually temporary, subsiding within a few months and may eventually resolve.

Assessment
Hyperpigmentation is seen more commonly in dark-skinned people and those receiving alkylating agents and the antitumour antibiotics.

Patient education
The patients should be advised to:

- avoid exposure to the sun
- use protective sunscreens

- wear protective clothing, such as long sleeves and wide-brimmed hats.

Photosensitivity

Cutaneous reaction
Photosensitivity is characterised by an exaggerated sunburn with urticaria and stinging.

Pathophysiology
This is as a result of cytotoxic drugs that also have radiosensitising properties and the cutaneous reaction is thought to occur via a phototoxic mechanism involving UVB light.

Assessment
Perform skin assessment. Photosensitivity is common with doxorubicin, bleomycin, 5-FU and methotrexate.

Patient education
The patients should be advised to:

- avoid exposure to the sun
- use protective sunscreens
- wear protective clothing, such as long sleeves and wide-brimmed hats.

Radiation recall

Cutaneous reaction
Such reactions are manifested by erythema, blisters, hyperpigmentation, oedema, vesicle formation, exfoliation and sometimes ulcer formation.

Pathophysiology
The administration of specific chemotherapy drugs may result in an inflammatory reaction in tissue that has previously been irradiated. Such reactions can occur in the lungs, skin, gastrointestinal tract and heart. Enhancement reaction occurs if chemotherapy is given within a week of irradiation and recall reactions may happen within weeks, months or even years following treatment.

Assessment
Perform skin assessment. Radiation recall is common with doxorubicin and dactinomycin.

Patient education
Patients should be made aware of:

- the possibility of radiation recall
- the importance of reporting any changes in their skin
- cleansing and moisturising skin to maintain skin integrity

- protecting from sun exposure
- avoiding restrictive clothing
- avoiding extremes in temperature.

Nail changes

Cutaneous reaction

Nail changes include hyperpigmentation, discoloration, onycholysis (partial separation of nail plate from nail bed), transverse banding and Beau's lines (nail grooving). The nail may become thickened and brittle.

Pathophysiology

Nail changes are thought to be due to chemotherapeutic toxicity of the nail matrix.

Assessment

Assess condition of nails prior to commencing chemotherapy.

Patient education

Patients need to be educated about potential effects, reassured that they are temporary and advised to use nail polish if they so wish.

Palmar/plantar syndrome – acral erythema

Cutaneous reaction

Initially, the patient experiences burning, swelling, tingling and erythema of the palm, fingers and soles of the feet that can progress to blistering and desquamation of the affected area. It can be associated with sensory impairment or paraesthesia. The syndrome is progressive and usually causes a treatment break.

Pathophysiology

The exact mechanism is unknown. It may be a vascular reaction.

Assessment

Perform skin assessment. Plantar/palmar syndrome is common with high-dose cytarabine, methotrexate, 5-FU, hydroxyurea and etoposide.

Patient education

The patient should be advised to:

- avoid extremes of temperature
- use an emollient cream
- take prescribed pyridoxine as this may help to minimise the syndrome.[10]

References

1. Mortimer PS. Management of skin problems. Medical aspects. In: Doyle D, Hanks GWC, MacDonald N, eds. Oxford textbook of palliative medicine. 2nd edn. Oxford: Oxford University Press; 1998:617–627.
2. Brager BL, Yasko J. Care of the client receiving chemotherapy. Virginia: Reston Publishing Company; 1984.
3. Barton MB, Wilkes GM, Ingwersen KC. Cancer chemotherapy care plans. 2nd edn. London: Jones & Bartlett; 1998.
4. Barton MB, Wilkes GM, Ingwersen KC. Cancer chemotherpy. A nursing process approach. 2nd edn. London: Jones & Bartlett; 1991.
5. Baquiran DC, Gallagher J. Lippincott's cancer chemotherapy handbook. New York: Lippincott; 1998.
6. DeSpain JD. Dermatological toxicity. In: Perry MC, ed. The chemotherapy source book. Baltimore: Williams & Wilkins; 1992:531–547.
7. Holmes S. Cancer chemotherapy. A guide for practice. Surrey: Asset Books; 1997.
8. Tenenbaum L. Cancer chemotherapy and biotherapy. 2nd edn. Philadelphia: WB Saunders; 1994.
9. Otto SE. Oncology nursing. 3rd edn. St Louis: Mosby; 1997.
10. Vukelja SJ, Lombardo FA, James WD, et al. Pyridoxine for the palmar-plantar erythrodysesthesia syndrome. Ann Intern Med 1989; 111(8):688–689.

Chapter **27**

Chemotherapy–induced neurological toxicities

Rachel Merien–Bennett

INTRODUCTION

Chemotherapy-induced neurotoxicity can occur as the result of direct or indirect damage to the central nervous system (CNS), peripheral nervous system or any combination of these.[1] It is essential that a distinction is made between the two components of the nervous system. The brain and the spinal cord make up the CNS. This is responsible for the neurological functions of mental status, level of consciousness, motor power, sensory function, cerebellar function and cranial nerve function. The peripheral nervous system consists of peripheral nerves, which are primarily responsible for sensing pain, temperature and sensation. The particular area of the nervous system affected determines which neurological deficit exists.[2]

Neurological toxicity remains a major complication for patients undergoing chemotherapy. Its clinical presentation varies considerably, and it can therefore be difficult to confirm the diagnosis.

GENERAL NEUROTOXICITY EFFECTS

Symptoms of neurotoxicity may include cerebellar effects (tremor, loss of balance and fine motor movements), peripheral neuropathy, confusion, somnolence and auditory and visual impairment.[3] Neurotoxicity is usually temporary, resolving once treatment is completed, although at times permanent neurological deficits may result.[1]

THE BLOOD–BRAIN BARRIER

The blood–brain barrier is a critical component of the nervous system that determines whether a chemotherapy agent is able to reach the nervous system.

The blood–brain barrier blocks certain chemotherapy agents from entering the nervous system at the cellular level.[4] This barrier, however, is different around the peripheral nerves than in the CNS. This explains why certain chemotherapy agents (e.g. vincristine) affect the peripheral nerves and not the CNS. Chemotherapy will only have neurotoxic effects if it is able to cross the blood–brain barrier.[5] (See also Ch. 45.)

Potentiating factors

The route of administration can also affect the occurrence and severity of neurotoxicity; e.g. drugs given intrathecally may exhibit neurotoxic effects that are not manifested when given intravenously.[4] Similarly, the actual dosage level can also influence neurotoxic effects. Such effects can also be exacerbated by concurrent radiotherapy to the CNS.[6]

Other factors

Abnormalities in neurological function may of course be related to factors other than chemotherapy. These include the primary tumour or secondary deposits, which may involve the nervous system. Metabolic or electrolyte imbalances may also cause neurological disturbance. Similarly, concurrent medical diseases may be manifested through neurological deficits.[7] These factors may be difficult to differentiate from chemotherapy-induced neurotoxicity. Careful assessment is therefore required. (See also Ch. 53.)

ASSESSMENT AND MANAGEMENT

Treatment for most chemotherapy-associated neurotoxicities is limited. The focus of care should be on early recognition of neurotoxicity and careful monitoring of patients at high risk of toxicity. Astute neurological assessment is critical in patients receiving potentially neurotoxic agents.[8] Recommendations for assessing neurological function vary according to the purpose of the assessment. Effective communication skills and up-to-date knowledge are essential requirements for carrying out a comprehensive assessment.

There are several reports of agents that either block the development of certain chemotherapy-induced neurotoxicities or help reverse the toxicity. However, the mechanisms of action for these drugs are largely unknown.[9] Methylene blue, for example, can be administered intravenously or by mouth to act as an effective antidote to ifosfamide encephalopathy.[10] It may also be effective when given prophylactically. Agents such as amifostine and adrenocorticotrophic hormone (ACTH) analogues have also been advocated as potentially neuroprotective, although such agents

might be considered in patients with chemoresponsive disease for whom only a neurotoxic agent is effective. Their role needs to be further defined, and current evidence is insufficient to recommend their routine use.[11] Significant neurotoxicity will usually dictate a reduction in chemotherapy dosage, drug withdrawal or substitution with an alternative agent.

Table 27.1 summarises the neurotoxic effects of certain chemotherapy agents.[12] (See also Neurotoxicity section in Ch. 48.)

Table 27.1 Neurological effects of chemotherapy agents

Chemotherapy agent	Neurological effect
Asparaginase (SC)	Lethargy, depression, drowsiness, coma
Carboplatin	Otological (deafness)
Cladribine	Paraesthesia (tingling), dizziness
Cisplatin	Peripheral neuropathy, otological
Cytarabine	Cerebellar dysfunction, peripheral neuropathy
Docetaxel	Paraesthesia, asthenia (lack of strength), mild myalgia (muscular pain)
Fludarabine	Weakness, visual disturbances
Etoposide	Peripheral neuropathy
5-Fluorouracil	Ataxia (loss of coordination)
Hydroxyurea (oral)	Seizure, hallucinations
Ifosfamide	Lethargy, disorientation, confusion, dizziness
Methotrexate (IV)	Dizziness, blurred vision
Methotrexate (IT)	Chemical arachnoiditis (inflammation of membrane, headaches, back or shoulder pain, fever). Paresis (partial paralysis, usually transient, nerve palsies and cerebellar dysfunction. Chronic leukoencephalopathy irritability, dementia, somnolence, coma)[3]
Paclitaxel	Sensory peripheral neuropathy (numbness, tingling, burning)
Procarbazine (oral)	Headaches, depression, insomnia, ataxia, dizziness, neuropathy
Raltitrexed (Tomudex)	Arthralgia, asthenia (reversible)
Vinblastine	Peripheral neuritis
Vincristine	Peripheral neuritis
Vindesine	Commutative neurotoxicity
Vinorelbine	Peripheral neuropathy

SC, subcutaneous; IV, intravenous; IT, intrathecal.

References

1. Groenwald S, Hansen Frogge M, Goodman M, et al. Cancer nursing: principles and practice. 4th edn. Boston: Jones and Bartlett; 1997.

2. Armstrong T, Rust D, Kohtz J. Neurologic, pulmonary and cutaneous toxicities of high dose chemotherapy. Oncol Nurs Forum 1997; 24(1) Suppl: 23–33.

3. Holden S, Felde G. Nursing care of patients experiencing cisplatin related peripheral neuropathy. Oncol Nurs Forum 1987; 14:13–17.

4. Cline MJ, Haskel CM. Cancer chemotherapy. Philadelphia: WB Saunders; 1980.

5. Holmes S. Cancer chemotherapy. A guide for practice. Surrey: Asset Books; 1997.

6. Kaplan R, Wiernik P. Neurotoxicity of antineoplastic drugs. Semin Oncol 1982; 9:103–130.

7. Wilson J, Marsarryk T. Neurological emergencies in the cancer patient. Semin Oncol 1989; 16:490–503.

8. Cameron J. Ifosfamide neurotoxicity: a challenge for nurses, a potential nightmare for patients. Cancer Nurs 1993; 16(1):40–46.

9. Gilbert M. Neurologic complications. In: Abeloff M, Armatige J, Lichter A, et al., eds. Clinical oncology. 2nd edn. Edinburgh: Churchill Livingstone; 2000:1000–1020.

10. Kupfer A, Aeschlimann C, Cerny T. Methylene blue and the neurotoxic mechanisms of ifosfamide encephalopathy. Eur J Clin Pharmacol 1996; 50(4):249–259.

11. Hensley ML. American Society of Clinical Oncology Clinical Practice Guidelines for the use of chemotherapy and radiotherapy protectants. J Clin Oncol 1999; 17:3333–3355.

12. Eli Lilly Co. Cytotoxic chemotherapy – guidelines to the preparation and administration of cytotoxic drugs for the nursing care of patients. 5th edn. Basingstoke: Eli Lilly Oncology; 1997.

Chapter **28**

Cardiac effects

Shelley Dolan

GENERAL INFORMATION

The primary function of the heart is to pump the blood around the body to provide adequate perfusion to the organs of the body. The heart does this by contracting the muscular walls of the left ventricle, which then causes blood to be ejected through the aortic valve into the aorta. With each contraction, the ventricle ejects approximately 70 ml of blood (in an adult): this is called the stroke volume. The heart contracts in healthy adults at a rate of about 70/min: therefore, every minute 70×70 or 4900 ml of blood is ejected from the heart.

There are many causes of cardiac injury in the cancer patient, from direct infiltration of metastases to infections and drug toxicity (see below).

CAUSES OF CARDIAC DAMAGE IN PATIENTS WITH CANCER

- Primary cardiac tumours.
- Metastatic infiltration.
- Bacterial infections.
- Cardiac tamponade/pericardial effusions.
- Infusion of cryopreserved stem cells (dimethyl sulfoxide has been shown to be cardiotoxic in susceptible patients[1]).
- Fungal infections.
- Graft versus host disease (GvHD).
- Chemotherapy-induced toxicity.
- Radiation-induced toxicity.
- Viral infections.[2]

We now explore the effects on the heart of anticancer chemotherapy. The effects are divided up into acute and then chronic effects.

ACUTE CARDIAC TOXICITIES

Acute toxicity following the administration of anthracycline therapy

The damage caused to the heart by doxorubicin is from a combination of:

- mitochondrial changes
- cellular degeneration
- a loss of myocardial fibrils.

Although doxorubicin causes acute toxicities, chronic changes such as fibrotic damage are also common.[2] There are three major manifestations of this anthracycline-induced toxicity, with no specific treatment other than supporting of the cardiovascular system. Research is continuing in the use of cardioprotective agents that allow anthracycline therapy to be used at a higher dose without causing cardiotoxicity. The cardioprotective agents currently in use are dexrazoxane and amifostine; other strategies that have been explored are the increased intake of dietary glutamine and the use of the antioxidant probucol.[3]

Conduction and rhythm disturbances

Conduction and rhythm disturbances are the most commonly seen problems. The incidence of electrocardiograph (ECG) disturbance is estimated at up to 40% and is higher in any patient with previously abnormal ECG recordings.[4] These abnormalities include:

- ST and T wave changes
- sinus tachycardia
- atrial and ventricular ectopics
- supraventricular tachycardia
- ventricular tachycardia
- complete heart block.

The abnormalities may occur either during infusion or after treatment with anthracycline.[5] Most of the ECG changes are transient, with conduction abnormalities returning to normal within a few days to 2 months.[4] Research continues to establish minimally invasive techniques, such as serial blood troponins and natriuretic peptides, for monitoring the patient during their chemotherapy for cardiotoxicity.[6]

Left ventricular dysfunction

Left ventricular dysfunction is less common than ECG changes. In various studies this complication has been shown to occur in older patients and in those who have previous underlying cardiac disease.[7] However, this complication can be seen at any age and may be associated with low-dose anthracycline administration in cumulative doses.[8] Most incidences of left ventricular dysfunction respond to standard medical management and patients show some clinical recovery within

72–96 hours. It may take weeks to months for full cardiac recovery to be demonstrated on echocardiographic imaging.[4]

Myopericarditis

Myopericarditis is a rare complication that seems to happen in a younger age range of patients who have previously healthy cardiac function. This toxicity usually presents within days, but can begin 3–4 weeks following administration of anthracycline. Patients show the signs of pericarditis as well as left ventricular dysfunction, with either a temporary illness or in some cases rapid deterioration and death.[4]

Acute toxicity with high–dose cyclophosphamide

Cyclophosphamide is used at high dose in some patients with solid tumours but more commonly in the transplant setting. Most transplant centres use cyclophosphamide, an alkylating agent, in their pre-transplant conditioning at doses of 50–60 mg/kg/day. It is at these doses that cardiac complications can occur. The risks may be greater if the patient has been pre-treated with other cardiotoxic agents such as total body irradiation (TBI), high-dose ara-C (cytabarine) or 6-tioguanine.

The cardiac complications caused by cyclophosphamide are haemorrhagic myocardial necrosis, serosanguineous pericardial effusions, fibrinous pericarditis and a thickening of the left ventricular wall.[2]

The clinical picture associated with cyclophosphamide toxicity is severe and usually occurs 1–10 days following its administration.

The symptoms are associated with pulmonary oedema, cardiomegaly, poor peripheral circulation and generalised oedema. The condition may worsen in the presence of sepsis and, at its worse, progresses to cardiac tamponade and death.[9]

As with anthracycline toxicity, there is no specific treatment for cyclophosphamide toxicity other than the supportive care directed at reducing cardiac load and work and, occasionally, the use of a pericardio-peritoneal window in patients with recurrent pericardial effusions.[2]

CHRONIC TOXICITIES

Chronic toxicity is the most common form of doxorubicin toxicity and is manifested by chronic dilated cardiomyopathy. This cardiomyopathy usually develops late in the chemotherapy cycle or shortly after the end of the course.[10,11] This chronic toxicity is significantly attenuated by the chelation of iron. Chronic cardiomyopathy has also been identified in the survivors of childhood cancer who have been treated previously with doxorubicin.[11]

References

1. Zennhausern R, Tobler A, Leoncini L, et al. Fatal cardiac arrhythmia after infusion of dimethyl sulfoxide-cryopreserved hematopoietic stem cells in a patient with severe primary cardiac amyloidosis and end-stage renal failure. Ann Hematol 2000; 79(9):523–526.

2. Whedon MB, Wujcik D. Blood and marrow stem cell transplantation. Boston: Jones and Bartlett 1997:287–288.

3. Nelson MA, Frishman WH, Seiter K, et al. Cardiovascular considerations with anthracycline use in patients with cancer. Heart Dis 2001; 3(3):157–168.

4. Groeger JS. Critical care of the cancer patient. St Louis: Mosby Year Book; 1991:69–76.

5. Von Herbay A, Dorken B, Mall G, et al. Cardiac damage in autologous bone marrow transplant patients: an autopsy study. Klinische Wochenschrift 1988; 66:1175–1181.

6. Sparano JA, Brown DL, Wolff AC. Predicting cancer therapy-induced cardiotoxicity: the role of troponins and other markers. Drug Saf 2002; 25(5):301–311.

7. Bristow M, Thompson PD, Martin RD. Early anthracycline cardiotoxicity. Am J Med 1978; 65:823.

8. Singer JW, Narahara KA, Ritchie JL. Time and dose dependent changes in ejection fraction determined by radionuclide angiography after anthracycline therapy. Cancer Treat Rep 1978; 62:945.

9. Goldberg MA, Antin JH, Guinan EC, et al. Cyclophosphamide cardiotoxicity: an analysis of dosing as a risk factor. Blood 1986; 68(5):1114–1118.

10. Lefrak EA, Pitha J, Rosenheim S. A clinicopathologic analysis of Adriamycin cardiotoxicity. Cancer 1973; 32:302.

11. Ferrans VJ, Clark JR, Zhang J, et al. Pathogenesis and prevention of doxorubicin cardiomyopathy. Tsitologiia 1997; 39(10):928–937.

Chapter **29**

Pulmonary effects

Moira Stephens

INTRODUCTION

Cancer chemotherapy-induced pulmonary toxicity may become clinically evident weeks, months or years after treatment, and has several common features:

- dyspnoea
- dry cough
- progressive worsening of symptoms with a poor prognosis for recovery.

PULMONARY EFFECTS OF CYTOTOXIC DRUGS

Cancer chemotherapeutic drugs that may affect pulmonary function may be broadly put into three groups, as shown in Table 29.1.

In addition, there are reports in the literature that mitomycin, in combination with vinca alkaloids, and

Table 29.1   Cytotoxic drugs with pulmonary effects[1,2]

Hypersensitive pulmonary reaction	Non-cardiogenic pulmonary oedema	Chronic pneumonitis/ pulmonary fibrosis
Bleomycin	Cyclophosphamide	Bleomycin
6-Mercaptopurine	Cytarabine	Busulfan
Methotrexate	Ifosfamide	Carmustine
Mitomycin	Methotrexate	Cyclophosphamide
Procarbazine		Fludarabine
		Ifosfamide
		Methotrexate
		Mitomycin

gemcitabine, in combination with docetaxol, as well as the latter two agents being used alone, cause pulmonary toxicity.[3–5]

Acute hypersensitivity pulmonary reaction

The pathology of this reaction is of a desquamative interstitial pneumonitis or an eosinophilic pneumonitis.

Non–cardiogenic pulmonary oedema

This complication tends to occur within days of the beginning of treatment and is most commonly associated with cytarabine, methotrexate and cyclophosphamide.

Chronic pneumonitis/pulmonary fibrosis

The clinical manifestations of dry cough, dyspnoea and rales usually occur months after a critical cumulative dose of the drug responsible is reached or exceeded, which in bleomycin is 400 units and carmustine is >1500 mg/m² in adults and >750 mg/m² in children.

The radiographic findings in pneumonitis or fibrosis demonstrate an interstitial pneumonitis with a reticular or nodular pattern. Pulmonary function tests demonstrate restrictive ventilatory defect with hypoxia, hypocapnia and chronic hyperventilation.[6]

Of the chemotherapy agents, bleomycin has been reported as a clinical cause of pulmonary toxicity in 40% of cases.[7]

PATHOPHYSIOLOGY

The function of the lungs is to oxygenate the blood and to remove carbon dioxide. In order to achieve this, ventilation of the lungs is performed by the respiratory muscles under control of the respiratory centre in the brain. Alteration in pCO_2 is the most important factor in respiratory control in health. The sensitivity of the medullary chemoreceptor to pCO_2 can be reset either upwards in prolonged ventilatory failure, such as pulmonary fibrosis or pneumonitis, or downwards when a patient is placed on a mechanical ventilator. In pulmonary fibrosis, the patient becomes dependent on hypoxic drive to maintain ventilation, and administration of oxygen to these patients can then lead to ventilatory failure and death.

The lung tissue itself must overcome its own inertia and stiffness and an inability to do this, such as may be caused by the effect of some chemotherapy agents, can lead to respiratory failure.

Factors that may increase the risk and severity and aggravate pulmonary toxicity are:

- prior or simultaneous radiotherapy[6]
- hypersensitivity to the chemotherapy agent[2]

- simultaneous or subsequent oxygen therapy
- high doses of pulmonary toxic chemotherapy or combinations of them[7]
- renal insufficiency
- cisplatin[6]
- pulmonary infections[7]
- children are more at risk than adolescents or adults for the development of chronic respiratory damage.[6]

MANAGEMENT OF PULMONARY EFFECTS

- Assessment of patient's pulmonary function prior to receiving pulmonary toxic chemotherapy agents may be of help in deciding on treatment regimes for individual patients, especially if combination radiotherapy is planned.
- Follow-up of patients may include chest x-ray and pulmonary lung function tests in asymptomatic patients.
- Lung biopsy may be indicated to differentiate chronic fibrosis from lung metastasis.
- Patient and healthcare worker's awareness of the risks of general anaesthesia in patients with pulmonary toxicity.
- Management of dyspnoea.

Management of dyspnoea

Management of dyspnoea[8–14] can be broadly summarised into two categories: pharmacological interventions and non-pharmacological interventions.

Pharmacological interventions
- Bronchodilators.
- Corticosteroids.
- Expectorants.
- Oxygen therapy (role of oxygen not clearly established).
- Opioids – oral, subcutaneous, intravenous routes (nebulised route not clearly established).
- Methylxanthine drugs – aminophylline and theophylline.
- Antibiotics (for symptomatic relief).
- Benzodiazepines.
- Nebulised saline.

Non-pharmacological interventions
- Breathing exercise and positioning techniques.
- Fatigue management.
- Relaxation techniques.
- Acupuncture.
- Moving air, such as from a fan or open window.

References

1. Rosenow EC, Limper AH. Drug-induced pulmonary disease. Semin Respir Infect 1995;10:86–95.
2. Helman DL Jr, Byrd JC, Ales NC, et al. Fludarabine-related pulmonary toxicity: a distinct clinical entity in chronic lymphoproliferative syndromes. Chest 2002; 122(3):785–790.
3. Dunsford ML, Mead GM, Bateman AC, et al. Severe pulmonary toxicity in patients treated with a combination of docetaxel and gemcitabine for metastatic transitional cell carcinoma. Ann Oncol 1999; 10(8):943–947.
4. Kris MG, Pablo D, Gralla RJ, et al. Dyspnea following vinblastine or vindesine administration in patients receiving mitomycin plus vinca alkaloid combination therapy. Cancer Treat Rep 1984; 68(7–8):1029–1031.
5. Rivera MP, Kris MG, Gralla RJ, et al. Syndrome of acute dyspnea related to combined mitomycin plus vinca alkaloid chemotherapy. Am J Clin Oncol 1995; 18(3):245–250.
6. Lanzowsky P. Manual of pediatric hematology and oncology. 3rd edn. San Diego: Academic Press; 2000.
7. Stover DE. Pulmonary toxicity. In: DeVita VT, Hellman SH, Rosenberg SA, eds. Cancer; principles and practice of oncology. 4th edn. Philadelphia: Lippincott; 1993:2362–2370.
8. Bruera E, Macmillan K, Pither J, et al. Effects of morphine on the dyspnea of terminal cancer patients. J Pain Symptom Manage 1990; 5:341–344.
9. Bredin M. Relax and breath information. Booklet and CDrom. Institute of Cancer Research, Macmillan Cancer Relief.
10. Zeppetella G: Nebulized morphine in the palliation of dyspnea. Palliat Med 1997; 11:267–275.
11. Argyropoulou P, Patakas D, Koukou A, et al. Buspirone effect on breathlessness and exercise performance in patients with chronic obstructive pulmonary disease. Respiration 1993; 60:216–220.
12. Booth S, Kelly MJ, Cox NP, et al. Does oxygen help dyspnea in patients with cancer? Am Rev Respir Crit Care Med 1996; 153:1515–1518.
13. Corner J, Plant H, A'Hern R, et al. Non-pharmacological intervention for breathlessness in lung cancer. Palliat Med 1996; 10:299–305.
14. Filshie J, Penn K, Ashley S, et al. Acupuncture for the relief of cancer-related breathlessness. Palliat Med 1996; 10:145–150.

Chapter **30**

Hepatic effects

Lisa Wolf

INTRODUCTION

The liver is the largest intra-abdominal organ and is the focal point of intermediary metabolism and energy production.[1] Its functions include the conjugation and excretion of steroid hormones, the detoxification of drugs and the conversion of fat-soluble waste products to water-soluble substances for excretion by the kidneys.[1] Hepatocytes perform many synthetic and catabolic functions, with many clinical features of liver disease resulting from derangement of these processes.

In general, the liver is able to withstand damage when drugs are metabolised, as the hepatocytes have a slow mitotic rate and are therefore less susceptible to cytotoxic drug effects.[2] The hepatic artery carries cytotoxic agents to the liver from the bloodstream when they are given intravenously and the portal vein does so from oral drugs via the intestinal tract. Metabolism by the liver is the main route of elimination for many drugs, including chemotherapy drugs. Hepatotoxicity is caused by a direct toxic effect to the liver when drugs are metabolised.

HEPATOTOXICITY

Damage to the liver occurs in several forms:[3,4]

- veno-occlusive disease (VOD)
- chronic hepatic fibrosis
- hepatocellular necrosis
- fatty changes
- cholestasis
- hepatocellular dysfunction.

(See also Ch. 48 for VOD.)

Chemotherapy used in very high doses, such as that used with autologous bone marrow transplantation, and combination chemotherapy may also produce hepatotoxicity. Abdominal radiotherapy, combined with chemotherapeutic drugs such as vincristine and doxorubicin, can induce severe hepatic injury. (See also Ch. 48 for GvDH liver toxicity and Ch. 1.)

Signs and symptoms

Possible signs and symptoms of hepatotoxicity are:

- jaundice
- ascites
- right upper quadrant abdominal pain and tenderness with hepatomegaly
- malaise
- fatigue
- anorexia
- nausea.

Before the onset of jaundice, the patient may notice darkening of the urine and lightening of stool colour. This is caused by failure of the liver cells to excrete conjugated bilirubin. The patient's urine should be tested for bilirubin if any signs and symptoms are reported or noticed.[5]

Hepatotoxic drugs

Certain cytotoxic agents have been implicated as hepatotoxins (Box 30.1).

Assessment

The patient's hepatic function must be assessed in terms of baseline liver function tests (LFTs) prior

---

Box 30.1   Examples of hepatotoxic drugs
Asparaginase
Azathioprine
Carmustine
Chlorambucil
Cisplatin (dose-related)
Doxorubicin
Etoposide
6-Mercaptopurine
Methotrexate
Mitomycin C
Streptozocin

---

to initiating treatment. If these LFTs are abnormal, then known hepatotoxic drugs should be avoided. Abnormal liver function can also increase the toxicity of any drug. (See also Ch. 8.)

Patient risk factors must be identified:[6,7]

- pre-existing liver disease
- tumour involvement (primary or secondary)
- previous or concurrent irradiation of the liver
- immunosuppression (hepatic infections, viral hepatitis)
- graft versus host disease (see also Ch. 48)
- transfusion of blood products
- excessive alcohol intake
- identification of concurrent administration of hepatotoxic drugs, e.g. certain anaesthetic agents, phenothiazines.

Management

1. Monitoring of hepatic function prior to subsequent drug administration to ascertain the development of hepatic dysfunction.[4,5] Biochemical changes that may occur are altered levels of the following indicators (normal adult values and ranges given):

   - alanine transaminase (ALT)   <40 U/L
   - alkaline phosphatase (AP)   24–110 U/L
   - gamma-glutamyl   male <54 U/L;
     transferase (GGT)   female <35 U/L
   - bilirubin   <17 μmol/L
   - aspartate transaminase (AST)   10–42 U/L
   - lactate dehydrogenase (LDH)   180–325 U/L.

2. Drug withdrawal, dose modifications and/or intermittent dosing schedules should be considered in the light of abnormal LFTs (see Ch.1). The aetiology of abnormal LFTs must be defined and all possible factors considered. In certain circumstances, a liver biopsy may be required.[4,8,9] The distinction between a disease-induced abnormality and a drug-induced abnormality may alter the patient's management in that drugs suspected of causing toxicity may be discontinued. However, a reduction in the dose of the toxic agent may be sufficient to reverse hepatic damage, enabling planned treatment to be continued.

3. The patient needs to be informed as to what signs and symptoms to be aware of and the importance of reporting these promptly. These include signs of jaundice, tenderness over the liver area, urine and stool colour changes, fatigue, anorexia and nausea.

References

1. Epstein O, Perkin GD, de Bono DP, et al. Clinical examination. London: Mosby; 1997.

2. Brager BL, Yasko J. Care of the client receiving chemotherapy. Virginia: Reston Publishing Company; 1984.

3. Baquiran DC, Gallagher J. Lippincott's cancer chemotherapy handbook. New York: Lippincott; 1998.

4. Perry MC. Hepatotoxicity of chemotherapeutic agents. In: Perry MC, ed. The chemotherapy source book. Baltimore: Williams & Wilkins; 1992.

5. Otto SE. Oncology nursing. 3rd edn. St Louis: Mosby; 1997.

6. Barton MB, Wilkes GM, Ingwersen KC. Cancer chemotherapy. A nursing process approach. 2nd edn. London: Jones & Bartlett; 1991.

7. Barton MB, Wilkes GM, Ingwersen KC. Cancer chemotherapy care plans. 2nd edn. London: Jones & Bartlett; 1998.

8. Holmes S. Cancer chemotherapy. A guide for practice. Surrey: Asset Books; 1997.

9. Tenenbaum L. Cancer chemotherapy and biotherapy. 2nd edn. Philadelphia: WB Saunders; 1994.

Chapter **31**

The effects of chemotherapy on wound healing

Wayne Naylor

OVERVIEW OF WOUND HEALING

Under normal circumstances, wounds heal by progressing through a series of different but overlapping phases. Healing begins with haemostasis (Fig. 31.1), which occurs as soon as a wound is created and results in the formation of a fibrin and platelet 'plug' that seals the wound. Haemostasis is followed by the inflammatory phase (Fig. 31.2) when local blood vessels dilate and the wound is infiltrated by neutrophils and macrophages, which remove foreign bodies, including bacteria, and non-viable tissue. The characteristic inflammatory signs of heat, redness and oedema are present during this phase. Proliferation (Fig. 31.3) occurs next and in this phase new tissue is formed, including granulation and epithelial tissue, to repair the wound defect. Finally, in a phase called maturation (Fig. 31.4), the new tissue is remodelled to form a scar.[1] The whole process is controlled and maintained by the release of growth factors and cytokines, which are predominantly produced by macrophages.[2,3] Wound healing may be influenced by a number of factors, one of these being chemotherapeutic agents. These agents include cytotoxic, steroid and immunosuppressant drugs. (See also Ch. 20.)

EFFECT OF CHEMOTHERAPY ON WOUND HEALING

The administration of cytotoxic chemotherapy as an adjuvant treatment to surgery has been shown to reduce the strength of healed surgical wounds and increase postoperative wound complications.[4] This is thought to be due to an inhibition of fibroblast action in the healing wound, and hence a suppression of protein synthesis (i.e. collagen).[4–6] Many cytotoxic drugs

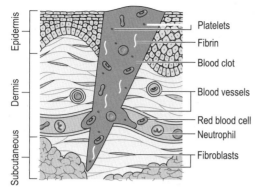

Figure 31.1   Haemostasis in a wound. (© Wayne Naylor, 2000.)

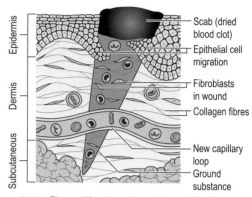

Figure 31.3   The proliferative phase of wound healing. (© Wayne Naylor, 2000.)

also have an immunosuppressive action that may inhibit the inflammatory response in the early stages of wound healing.[6] It has also been suggested that the general debilitation caused by profound nutritional deficiencies, as a side effect of intensive chemotherapy regimes, may significantly affect wound healing in this patient group.[5] In the case of fungating wounds, cytotoxic chemotherapy may have a beneficial effect by destroying malignant cells and therefore decreasing the size of the wound.[7–9] This in turn will help to relieve wound symptoms by reducing pressure on nerves and blood or lymph vessels, reducing exudate production and the tendency of the wound to bleed, and in some cases may allow the wound to heal. (See also Ch. 19.)

STEROIDS AND WOUND HEALING

Steroids may affect wound healing by suppressing the action of fibroblasts in the healing wound.[10] These

cells are primarily responsible for the production of collagen and ground substance, the basic scaffolding of the skin. As steroids have an anti-inflammatory effect, the inflammatory phase of healing may be arrested and the potential for wound infection increased.[5] Steroids may also affect the function of macrophages, impair the formation of new blood vessels and inhibit wound contraction. Administering oral or topical vitamin A has been shown to counteract the effects of steroids. Although the exact method by which vitamin A works is not known, the effect may be due to its enhancing effects on the immune system.[5,11]

IMMUNOSUPPRESSANTS AND WOUND HEALING

Immunosuppressants have a profound effect on wound healing by inhibiting the immune response. This reduces the activity of neutrophils and

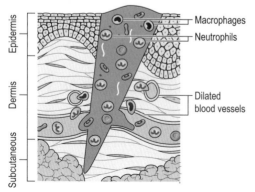

Figure 31.2   The inflammatory phase of wound healing. (© Wayne Naylor, 2000.)

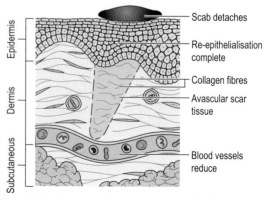

Figure 31.4   The maturation phase of wound healing. (© Wayne Naylor, 2000.)

macrophages, thereby increasing the risk of wound infection and delaying the removal of dead tissue and foreign bodies through phagocytosis.[11] The impairment of macrophages may also prevent the wound from moving forwards through the other phases of healing. (See also Ch. 13.)

References

1. Naylor W, Laverty D, Mallett J. The Royal Marsden Hospital handbook of wound management in cancer care. Oxford: Blackwell Science; 2001.
2. Flanagan M. The physiology of wound healing. J Wound Care 2000; 9(6):299–300.
3. Silver IA. The physiology of wound healing. J Wound Care 1994; 3(2):106–109.
4. Bland KI, Palin WE, van Fraunhofer A et al. Experimental and clinical observations of the effects of cytotoxic chemotherapeutic drugs on wound healing. Ann Surg 1984; 199(6):782–789.
5. Stadelmann WK, Digenis AG, Tobin GR. Impediments to wound healing. Am J Surg 1998; 176(Suppl 2A):39S–47S.
6. Lotti T, Rodofili C, Benci M et al. Wound-healing problems associated with cancers. J Wound Care 1998; 7(2):81–84.
7. Miller C. Management of skin problems: nursing aspects. In: Doyle D, Hanks GWC, MacDonald N, eds. Oxford textbook of palliative medicine. 2nd edn. Oxford: Oxford University Press; 1998:642–656.
8. Haisfield-Wolfe ME, Rund C. Malignant cutaneous wounds: a management protocol. Ostomy/Wound Management 1997; 43(1):56–66.
9. Hallett A. Fungating wounds. Nurs Times 1995; 91(39):81–85.
10. Moore P, Foster L. Acute surgical wound care 2: the wound healing process. Br J Nurs 1998; 7(19):1183–1187.
11. Cutting K. Factors affecting wound healing. Nurs Stand 1994; 8(50):33–36.

Chapter **32**

Loss of fertility

Moira Stephens

INTRODUCTION

Infertility can be defined as the inability of a woman to conceive or of a man to produce viable sperm.

A number of chemotherapy agents affect fertility in both males and females to varying degrees. Chemotherapy can sometimes cause premature ovarian failure in women who have not already been through a natural menopause (iatrogenic menopause). (See also Ch. 33)

Certain classes of chemotherapy, such as alkylating agents, are more likely to induce permanent infertility than other cytotoxic agents (Table 32.1).[1]

EFFECT OF CHEMOTHERAPY ON MALE FERTILITY

Both mature and immature testes are at risk.[3] The testes are extremely sensitive to chemotherapy and spermatogenesis is affected more frequently than testosterone production. The germinal cells within the seminiferous tubules are directly affected. Testicular biopsies in patients treated by chemotherapy show aplasia of the germinal epithelium with normal Sertoli's and Leydig's cells, which is reflected in a reduced sperm count and normal testosterone levels.[4]

Clinical manifestations of gonadal dysfunction affecting fertility in men are:

- testicular germ cell aplasia
- reduced testicular volume
- azoospermia
- oligospermia
- atrophic seminiferous tubules.

Table 32.1   Risk of infertility and chemotherapy agents.[2]

Male	Female
Definite infertility	*Definite infertility*
Busulfan	Busulfan
Chlorambucil	Cyclophosphamide
Cyclophosphamide	L-Phenylalanine
Nitrogen mustard	Nitrogen mustard
Nitrosoureas	
Procarbazine	
Probable infertility	*Probable infertility*
Cisplatin	Etoposide
Cytarabine	
Doxorubicin	
Etoposide	
Vinblastine	
Unlikely infertility	*Unlikely infertility*
Methotrexate	Methotrexate
6-Mercaptopurine	6-Mercaptopurine
Vincristine	
Fertility risk unknown	*Fertility risk unknown*
Bleomycin	Bleomycin
	Cisplatin
	Cytarabine
	Doxorubicin
	Nitrosoureas
	Vinca alkaloids

Recovery of fertility depends on a number of factors, including:

- age at treatment
- the nature of the drugs
- the cumulative total of doses
- duration of drug administration
- underlying disease and irradiation.

Late recovery of spermatogenesis up to 14 years post treatment has been reported,[5] although this is rare.

EFFECT OF CHEMOTHERAPY ON FEMALE FERTILITY

Following chemotherapy, the process of follicular growth and the maturation of oocytes are affected, which results in ovarian fibrosis and follicular destruction. This is manifested clinically by menstrual irregularity and amenorrhoea, increased levels of follicle-stimulating hormone (FSH) and luteinising hormone (LH), together with reduced levels of oestradiol. This results in menopausal symptoms and sexual dysfunction. Chemotherapy also causes damage to the uterine endometrium, which may lose the ability to proliferate in response to hormonal stimulation. This may affect embryo implantation and the ability to carry a pregnancy to full term.[6]

Prepubertal ovaries are more resistant than post-pubertal ovaries to damage by alkylating agents.[7] The most important risk factor for ovarian failure is age at treatment; recovery of gonadal function is often reported in younger women, but few pregnancies are reported.

Recovery of fertility depends on a number of factors, including:

- age at treatment and pubertal status
- the nature of the drugs
- the cumulative total of doses
- duration of drug administration
- underlying disease and disease status
- pretreatment fertility status
- irradiation.

(See also Chs 33 and 48.)

MANAGEMENT OF LOSS OF FERTILITY

A variety of options, with varying, but mainly limited, success rates, may be available to both men and women.

Men

Semen cryopreservation

Semen cryopreservation is offered to men prior to initial chemotherapy treatment, except in the case of immediate life-threatening disease or complications of disease. Cryopreserved sperm may later be thawed and injected into the cervix or uterus at the time of ovulation; this has a 25% fertilisation rate, although is rarely actually used.[8] When the quantity of sperm available is small, in vitro fertilisation (IVF) techniques are generally recommended.[8]

Intrauterine insemination

Intrauterine insemination (IUI) involves the preparation of the semen sample so that higher concentrations of the most motile sperms are selected and injected through the cervix around the time of ovulation.

Intracytoplasmic insemination

Intracytoplasmic insemination (ICSI) is a type of IVF where one sperm is injected directly into one egg to fertilise it, which is useful when severe problems exist with sperm quality or quantity.[8]

Donor insemination

Donor insemination is widely available and may be considered when the man has been sterilised by treatment and cryopreserved sperm are unavailable.[8] The donors are unknown to the couple and have been thoroughly screened for infection. Usually a donor is chosen who has similar physical characteristics to the male partner.

Women

Oocyte cryopreservation

Oocyte cryopreservation has so far yielded disappointing results. The oocytes are arrested in meiosis; the chromosomes are, at this point, resting on the spindle and this is very sensitive to ice crystals, leading to problems with thawing. The procedure requires surgical intervention and may delay curative treatment.

Ovarian cryopreservation

Ovarian cryopreservation has been undertaken fairly successfully with lambs but there have been no human successes to date.

In vitro fertilisation

IVF techniques may be used for women with functioning ovaries. Oocyte production is stimulated by hormonal manipulation and harvested under ultrasonic guidance. The harvested ova are mixed with stored or fresh sperm samples in a test tube. The resulting embryos are placed into the female and any excess embryos can be stored frozen. It is possible to obtain donor sperm, oocytes or embryos.[8]

Oocyte donation

Oocyte donation may be considered in the presence of ovarian failure. Donated oocytes must be obtained and fertilised. Because of the ovarian failure, it is necessary to administer exogenous endocrine support to the mother in early pregnancy. In later pregnancy, the placenta produces sufficient hormones to maintain the pregnancy.[8]

Adoption

Adoption may also be considered.

Management of infertility begins at diagnosis and with consideration being given to the various interventions available and with specialist gynaecological advice being sought. Emotional support and information must be given to both the patient and their partners, as infertility has long-term physical, psychological and emotional consequences and the prospect of infertility may influence a patient's decision to undertake curative treatment.

LEGISLATION IN THE UK

The Human Fertilisation and Embryology Authority (HFEA), set up in the UK in 1991, ensures that all UK treatment clinics offering IVF or donor insemination (DI), or storing eggs, sperm or embryos, conform to high medical and professional standards and are inspected regularly.

The HFEA also licenses and monitors all human embryo research, supervising controlled research for the benefit of humankind.

All of the HFEA's policy and licensing decisions are taken by the HFEA's 21 members, who are appointed by UK health ministers in line with the 'Nolan' principles. Members are selected not as representatives of any particular group or organisation, but because of their personal knowledge and expertise. To enable a wide spectrum of interests and views to be heard, more than half of the HFEA's membership must come from disciplines other than medicine or human embryo research.

USEFUL CONTACTS: WEBSITE LINKS

United Kingdom links

The Human Fertilisation and Embryology Authority (HFEA)
A statutory body which regulates, licenses and collects data on fertility treatments such as IVF and donor insemination, as well as human embryo research, in the UK: www.hfea.gov.uk

British Infertility Counselling Association (BICA)
BICA is the only professional association for infertility counsellors and counselling in the UK. BICA aims to encourage and facilitate its members to provide the highest standards of counselling support to people affected by impaired fertility: www.bica.net/

CARE – Centres for Assisted Reproduction
CARE has one of the most experienced teams of fertility treatment specialists in the world.
CARE offers various types of support for patients at all stages of the treatment cycle, from answering initial questions to support after the completion of the cycle: www.carefertility.com

Infertility Network UK
It provides high-quality support and information to those suffering from infertility in Great Britain: www.infertilitynetworkuk.com

United States links

Advanced Reproductive Care, Inc. (ARC)
Advanced Reproductive Care, Inc., is dedicated to the advancement of reproductive health, education and research.
It comprises a national network of physicians specialising in infertility treatment: www.arcfertility.com/

The American Fertility Association (AFA)

Advice from experts and support from friends that can help you to build the family you want.

Join the AFA and receive information, referral lists, resources and support: www.americaninfertility.org/

Cornell Institute for Reproductive Medicine

Center for Male Reproductive Medicine and Microsurgery.

The Cornell's website provides information and advice about many aspects of male infertility: www.maleinfertility.com/

Early Menopause.com

A website and support community for women who are experiencing early menopause.

An explanation of early menopause, frequently asked questions, symptoms, HRT and more: www.earlymenopause.com/

FertilityPlus

Information written by patients for patients.

A non-profit website for patient information on trying to conceive. www.fertilityplus.org/

References

1. Wang C, Ng PR, Chan TK. Effect of combination chemotherapy on pituitary-gonadal function in patients with lymphoma and leukaemia. Cancer 1980; 45:2030–2037.
2. Gradisher WJ, Schilisky RL. Ovarian function following radiation and chemotherapy for cancer. Semin Oncol 1989; 16(5):425–436.
3. Shalet SM, Hann IM, Lendon M, et al. Testicular function after combination chemotherapy in childhood for acute lymphoblastic leukaemia. Arch Dis Child 1981; 56:275–278.
4. Fairley FK, Barrie JU, Johnson W. Sterility and testicular atrophy related to cyclophosphamide therapy. Lancet 1972; I:568–569.
5. Watson AR, Rance CP, Bain J. Long term effects of cyclophosphamide on testicular function. Br Med J 1985; 291:1457–1460.
6. Apperley J, Reddy N. Mechanism and management of treatment related gonadal failure in recipients of high dose chemoradiotherapy. Blood Rev 1995; 19:93–116.
7. Lanzowsky P. Manual of pediatric hematology and oncology. 3rd edn. San Diego: Academic Press; 2000.
8. Joint Council for Clinical Oncology. Management of gonadal toxicity resulting from the treatment of adult cancer. London: Royal College of Physicians;1998.

Chapter **33**

The menopause and hormone replacement therapy

Karen Handscomb

INTRODUCTION

The menopause is normally a natural event that occurs between the ages of 45 and 55 due to a fall in the level of oestrogen. The ovarian follicles become resistant to the effects of the follicle-stimulating hormone (FSH) and the luteinising hormone (LH). As a response to this, there is a fall in oestrogen and progesterone and a rise in FSH and LH. It is vital that the oncology team address the issue of the menopause as part of the process of informed consent, as it has a direct bearing on a woman's quality of life long after cancer treatment has been completed.

EARLY MENOPAUSE

Chemotherapeutic agents can sometimes cause premature ovarian failure in women who have not already been through a natural menopause (iatrogenic menopause).

Premature ovarian failure is dependent on:

1. the type of drug given
2. the dose that is given
3. if drugs are given in combination
4. a woman's age – there is increased risk of the ovaries failing if the woman is over 35
5. previous gynaecological problems.

It is important that all women who go through an early menopause are given hormone replacement therapy (HRT) until the age when a natural menopause would have occurred (usually 50).

Where there are uncertainties as to whether the menopause has occurred, FSH, LH and oestrogen levels can be taken and the woman asked if she has developed any symptoms. Sometimes a bone density scan is useful to show any signs of oesteoporosis[1] – the most rapid loss occurs immediately after the menopause and then slows down. The interactive Menopause Decision Tree is a useful tool and can be found at the website given in the Useful Contacts section.

THE SYMPTOMS OF THE MENOPAUSE

Menopausal symptoms will be unpredictable: there is no indication about how severe they will be or which symptoms a woman may develop. There is a quagmire of taboos, cultural variances and societal meanings associated with the menopause.

The timing of an early menopause is also variable. Anecdotally, women who have had their ovaries removed prior to the menopause often report severe symptoms almost immediately and this should pro-actively be taken into consideration as part of their plan of care.

In other women their ovarian function may fluctuate over time and the menopause may start earlier than they might have expected without cancer treatment. Conway[2] suggests that if a woman has not had a period for 6 months the diagnosis of a premature menopause is secure.

As you will notice from Table 33.1, the symptoms of the menopause can also be attributed to cancer and its treatment. This may cause additional anxiety for the woman and her family, and skilled listening and information-giving is essential at this time.

Table 33.1   Menopausal symptoms

Type	Symptoms	Early, intermediate or late onset
Psychological	Depression	Early
	Short-term memory loss	Early
	Impatience	Early
Physiological	Tiredness and lethargy	Early
	Hot flushes	Early
	Night sweats	Early
	Dizziness	Early
	Hair and skin dryer and more brittle	Intermediate
	Nausea	Early
	Palpitations	Early
	Difficulty sleeping	Early
	Vaginal dryness	Intermediate
	Incontinence	Intermediate
	Oesteoporosis	Long term
	Heart disease	Long term

HORMONE REPLACEMENT THERAPY

The hormones in HRT work in exactly the same way as a woman's ovaries and mimic the monthly cycle. It is usual to give both oestrogen and progestogen (synthetic progesterone), although if a woman has had a hysterectomy progestogen is not given.

If the woman has a loss of libido, testosterone may also need to be included.

HRT can be given in either:

- a tablet taken every day
- a patch, which is changed twice a week
- a vaginal ring, which is changed every 3 months
- a pessary or tablet inserted into the vagina
- a gel applied to the skin daily
- an implant placed under the skin which is replaced every 6–9 months.

It is important that women taking HRT are reviewed for the first visit at 3 months and then 6 monthly in a skilled and informed way. This can be separately from their oncology follow-up, particularly as information is often conflicting, incomplete and confusing.[3]

ALTERNATIVES TO HORMONE REPLACEMENT THERAPY

There are also many alternatives to HRT that treat symptoms as they arise, either through non-hormonal medical treatments or complementary therapies. Some complementary therapies such as acupuncture are becoming increasingly available for menopausal symptoms.

Many women do not wish to consider taking HRT, wish to stop taking HRT or have been advised not to take HRT for a variety of reasons after a cancer diagnosis. It is important that they are aware of the consequences of the more silent changes, such as osteoporosis.[1]

CONFLICTING ADVICE

Answering questions around the menopause and HRT is skilled and relies on an extensive knowledge base, often from professionals outside of the cancer care team.[4] Women choose to take HRT for a variety of reasons and the issues are different for them all. They are sometimes confused by conflicting information in the media and a lack of consensus within the medical community.

Cancer Research UK's excellent website helps to present and make sense of the news (see Useful Contacts section).

This time provides an ideal opportunity to discuss with women lifestyle changes such as breast awareness and nutritional changes that will have potential long-term benefits and maximise their quality of life[5] and this time also provides women the benefits of talking with others in the same situation (see Daisy Network in Useful Contacts section).

USEFUL CONTACTS

The Amarant Trust

Provides independent information and education on the menopause: www.amarantmenopausetrust.org.uk

Cancer Research

Cancer Research UK's excellent website helps to present and make sense of the news and can be found at: www.cancerresearchuk.org

Menopause Decision Tree

The interactive Menopause Decision Tree is a useful tool and can be found at: www.menopausematters.co.uk.

Women's Health Concern

Charity providing information and advice on a range of women's health issues: www.womens-health-concern.org

The British Menopause Society

Organisation for healthcare professionals interested in menopause.
Telephone: 01628 890199

The Daisy Network

Support organisation for women who have undergone an early menopause: www.daisynetwork.org.uk

Menopause Matters

Patient information about the menopause and treatment: www.menopausematters.co.uk

References

1. Lobo RS. Benefits and risks of oestrogen replacement therapy. Am J Obstet Gynecol 1995; 173:982–989.
2. Conway GS. In: Singer D, Hunter M, eds. Premature menopause: a multidisciplinary approach. London: Whurr; 2000.
3. Mahon SM, Williams M. Information needs regarding menopause: results from a survey of women receiving cancer prevention and detection services. Cancer Nurs 2000; 23(3):176–185.
4. Woodward L. The menopause: how nurses can help. NTPlus 2000; 96(42):11–13.
5. Lee SJ (ed.). The Sheffield Protocol for management of the menopause and the prevention and treatment of oesteoporosis. The Sheffield Protocol; 2000. (Obtainable at Osteoporosis 2000, 47 Wilkinson St, Sheffield S10 2GB.)

Chapter 34

Cancer–related fatigue

Jackie Edwards

GENERAL INFORMATION

Cancer-related fatigue (CRF) is the most frequently reported[1,2] yet untreated symptom in cancer care today.[3] The idiosyncratic, multidimensional and multifactorial nature within the patient's expression of the symptom are major hurdles in gaining a true picture.[4] Words such as tiredness, overwhelming, unpleasant, exhausted, lethargy, listless and disinterested are drawn from the literature on health,[5] and myasthenia, stress, cachexia from the literature relating to ill health.[6] This illustrates the problem of semantics, in that each patient could have different meanings and means of expression of their experience, and the professionals' different understandings may vary enormously. To date, theories and mechanisms of CRF are unclear. Interrelated and compounding factors have been attributed to the existence of other symptoms that have made it difficult to isolate the causative factors of CRF,[7,8] if indeed there are separate origins within the symptom experience. Without specification of the exact meaning of CRF, it has been associated with other symptoms such as pain, nausea, vomiting, breathlessness and somatic or psychological conditions.[9] Guidelines for practice have been developed but to date there are no universally accepted assessment scales for use within clinical practice.

DEFINITION

Although there is no widely accepted definition of CRF, one account that illustrates degrees of debilitation and impact upon the quality of life individuals can experience is that:

> Fatigue is a subjective, unpleasant symptom which incorporates total body feelings ranging from tiredness to exhaustion creating an unrelenting

overall condition which interferes with individuals' ability to function to their normal capacity.[10]

The recognition of fatigue as a symptom incorporating assessment of the physical, social, emotional and spiritual dimensions is a priority for healthcare professionals caring for patients given the highly subjective, multidimensional factors.

AETIOLOGY

The prevalence of fatigue is estimated to be between 25 and 75% of patients who are receiving or are immediately post cancer treatment.[11] The causative factors behind the phenomena during chemotherapy are not clearly understood. It is unlikely that fatigue is the result of one factor alone: rather, interrelated factors are proposed. Numerous associated variables are believed to be significant in the clinical manifestation of the symptom. These include disease-related, treatment-related, demographic, psychological, physical, social and behavioural variables.[7,11,12] The relationship between variables is as yet unclear. In addition, fatigue appears to become more problematic for patients with advanced cancer.[13,14] There appears to be some points in time when CRF is present and most problematic. The pattern of fatigue can be variable. In some individuals it has been found to occur at its worst in the early afternoon or evening, in others the peak can be during certain days of chemotherapy cycles[15] or immediately following a course of chemotherapy.[16–19]

Box 34.1   Guidelines for the assessment of the patient with cancer–related fatigue[21]

Patient history:

- Onset of tiredness (this will identify whether the experience has been acute or chronic in nature)
- Duration
- Severity
- Daily pattern
- Course over time
- Exacerbating factors and associated distress.

Description of fatigue–related phenomena:

- This should include the words used by the patient to describe their experience.

Physical examination

Review of laboratory and imaging studies:

- This will assist in identifying hypotheses pathogenesis.

Box 34.2   Patient educational materials

Useful information and services available to patients, their families, friends and healthcare staff:
CancerBACUP www.cancerbacup.org.uk provide a patient booklet and video on fatigue.

Box 34.3   Interventions: areas of care to consider

Non–pharmaceutical strategies:

- An individualised holistic approach to assessment, planning, implementation and evaluation of care so that the patient's understanding and meaning of CRF can be explored, and preferred strategies for coping can be adopted.
- Provision of information in relation to the nature and experience of fatigue.[22]
- An awareness of potential for experience at any point during treatment from both inpatient/outpatient and community perspectives.
- Haemoglobin level maintained above 9.0 g/dl in adults and 8.0 g/dl in children (see also Ch. 21)
- Rest, relaxation periods interspersed activity devised to patients likes/dislikes.[22,23]
- Encourage nutritionally balanced diet and fluids.[22]
- Relief of additional symptoms.[22]
- Exercise such as taking a low-impact aerobic class, daily walks.[24,25]
- Rehabilitation programmes such as 'beating fatigue' – assessment/monitoring, education, coaching in the management of fatigue.[26]

Pharmaceutical strategies:

- Although evidence is scant, erythropoietin (a haematological growth factor that regulates the proliferation, maturation and differentiation of red blood cells) has been reported as improving energy levels in cancer patients during treatment.[26,27]
- Many professionals recommend glucocorticoids as a pharmaceutical treatment for CRF,[1,27] but it is unclear whether steroids are of any benefit.
- The potential role of levocarnitine supplementation for treating CRF in non-anaemic patients is under investigation in patients who experience loss of caratine in the urine following administration of ifosfamide and cisplatin.[28]

APPROACHES IN EVALUATION AND MANAGEMENT OF CANCER-RELATED FATIGUE

All patients will have experienced fatigue prior to the cancer diagnosis as a naturally occurring phenomenon following excessive exertion and/or mental concentration. For many people fatigue is the first presenting symptom of cancer. Existing self-selected mechanisms for management, such as diets (high-energy drinks, stimulants such as caffeine), or relaxation techniques, e.g. massage, are commonly adopted in the general population, and patients will bring with them their own ways of management. A comprehensive individualised patient assessment will be required; this assessment incorporates both subjective and objective parameters. A guide to assessment is provided in Box 34.1. Three questions are proposed in gaining an overview of the patient's experience of fatigue:[20]

1. Are you experiencing fatigue?
2. If yes, how severe has it been, on average, during the past week, using a 0–10 number scale?
3. How is the fatigue interfering with your ability to function?

Providing explanations and information of appropriate self-care strategies, such as planning the day around treatments, avoiding energetic activities or stress 24 hours prior to treatment, can be an important part of management for many individuals. Useful patient educational materials are available to assist patients and their carers in gaining an understanding of the phenomena they are experiencing (Box 34.2). Ideally, this information should be provided before the patient begins chemotherapy to enable the personal development of coping strategies. There is now a growing body of knowledge on the role of interventions to reduce and manage CRF. Interventions that can be considered are given in Box 34.3.

References

1. Vogelzang NJ, Breitbart W, Cella D, et al. Patient, caregiver, and oncologist perceptions of cancer-related fatigue: results of a tripart assessment survey. The Fatigue Coalition. Semi Hematol 1997; 34(3:Suppl 2):12.
2. Stone P, Richardson A, Ream E, et al. Cancer-related fatigue: inevitable, unimportant and untreatable? Results of a multi-centre patient survey. Cancer Fatigue Forum. Ann Oncol 2000; 11(8):971–975.
3. Curt GA. Fatigue in cancer. BMJ 2001; 322(7302):1560.
4. Winningham ML, Nail LM, Burke MB, et al. Fatigue and the cancer experience: the state of the knowledge. Oncol Nurs Forum 1994; 21(1):23–36.
5. Fu M, LeMone P, McDaniel RW, et al. A multivariate validation of the defining characteristics of fatigue. Nurs Diag 2001; 12(1):15–27.
6. Winningham ML. The puzzle of fatigue: How do you nail pudding to the wall. In: Winningham ML, Barton-Burke M, eds. Fatigue in cancer. London: Jones and Bartlett; 2000:3–29.
7. Piper BF, Lindsey AM, Dodd MJ. Fatigue mechanisms in cancer patients: developing nursing theory. Oncol Nurs Forum 1987; 14(6):17–23.
8. Piper BF, Dibble SL, Dodd MJ, et al. The revised Piper Fatigue Scale: psychometric evaluation in women with breast cancer. Oncol Nurs Forum 1998; 25(4):677–684.
9. Smets EM, Garssen B, Schuster-Uitterhoeve AL, et al. Fatigue in cancer patients. Br J Cancer 1993; 68(2):220–224.
10. Ream E, Richardson A. Fatigue in patients with cancer and chronic obstructive airways disease: a phenomenological enquiry. Int J Nurs Stud 1997; 34(1):44–53.
11. Servaes P, Verhagen C, Bleijenberg G. Fatigue in cancer patients during and after treatment: prevalence,

correlates and interventions. Eur J Cancer 2002; 38(1):27–43.
12. Hockenberry-Eaton M, Hinds PS. Fatigue in children and adolescents with cancer: evolution of a program of study. Semin Oncol Nurs 2000; 16(4):261–272.
13. Richardson A, Ream E. Research and development. Fatigue in patients receiving chemotherapy for advanced cancer. Int J Palliat Nurs 1996; 2(4):199–204.
14. Krishnasamy M. Fatigue in advanced cancer – meaning before measurement? Int J Nurs Stud 2000; 37(5):401–414.
15. Richardson A, Ream E, Wilson-Barnett J. Fatigue in patients receiving chemotherapy: patterns of change.[Erratum appears in Cancer Nurs 1998; 21(3):195]. Cancer Nurs 1998; 21(1):17–30.
16. Richardson A, Ream E. The experience of fatigue and other symptoms in patients receiving chemotherapy. Eur J Cancer Care 1996; 5(2:Suppl):30.
17. Jacobsen PB, Hann DM, Azzarello LM, et al. Fatigue in women receiving adjuvant chemotherapy for breast cancer: characteristics, course, and correlates. J Pain Symptom Manage 1999;(4):233–242.
18. Schwartz AL, Nail LM, Chen S, et al. Fatigue patterns observed in patients receiving chemotherapy and radiotherapy. Cancer Invest 2000; 18(1):11–19.
19. Sitzia J, Hughes J, Sobrido L. A study of patients' experiences of side-effects associated with chemotherapy: pilot stage report. Int J Nurs Stud 1995; (6):580–600.
20. Piper BF. The groopman article reviewed. Oncology 1998; 12:345–346.
21. Portney RK, Itri LM. Cancer-related fatigue: guidelines for evaluation and management. In: Marty MPS, ed.

Fatigue and cancer; scientific update 5. London: Elsevier; 2001:17–32.

22. Skalla KA, Lacasse C. Patient education for fatigue. Oncol Nurs Forum 1992; 19(10):1537–1541.

23. Dimeo FC, Stieglitz RD, Novelli-Fischer U, et al. Effects of physical activity on the fatigue and psychologic status of cancer patients during chemotherapy. Cancer 1999; 85(10):2273–2277.

24. Yarbro CH. Interventions for fatigue. Eur J Cancer Care 1996; 5(2:Suppl):8.

25. Porock D, Kristjanson LJ, Tinnelly K, et al. An exercise intervention for advanced cancer patients experiencing fatigue: a pilot study. J Palliat Care 2000; 16(3):30–36.

26. Ream E, Richardson A, Alexander-Dann C. Facilitating patients' coping with fatigue during chemotherapy-pilot outcomes. Cancer Nurs 2002; 25(4):300–308.

27. Stone P, Richardson A, Ream E, et al. Cancer-related fatigue: inevitable, unimportant and untreatable? Results of a multi-centre patient survey. Cancer Fatigue Forum. Ann Oncol 2000; 11(8):971–975.

28. Graziano F, Bisonni R, Catalano V, et al. Potential role of levocarnitine supplementation for the treatment of chemotherapy-induced fatigue in non-anaemic cancer patients. Br J Cancer 2002; 86(12):1854–1857.

SECTION 3

Management of cancer

SECTION CONTENTS

Treatment for cancer is usually organised and delivered by teams who specialise in the site of origin or histological type. This section is based around the contributions of teams like this. The bulk of each section is made up of a medical perspective of the cancer and treatment type. In general they will cover background, diagnosis and investigations and a brief overview of chemotherapy treatment. The overview of treatment should be seen as a brief summary, as it would be impossible to cover all current patient problems encountered and all of the treatment possibilities and bases of evidence. There are some references to other types of treatment, e.g. surgery or radiotherapy, in many of the chapters, as it is often impossible to ignore the previous or future treatment options for a patient who presents for chemotherapy.

In addition, each chapter also contains a patient management section written by a specialist nurse. These chapters tend to concentrate on themes that are exemplars or unique to that patient group. For example, the nurse writing the gynaecology chapter has examined fertility and body image and the sarcoma nursing chapter covers the issues of young adult patients and rehabilitation. Many of the issues covered in one chapter will also be applicable to patients with other types of cancer, so it is worthwhile to look at these chapters as covering important aspects of the patient's cancer journey through treatment.

Chapter **35**

Chemotherapy in childhood cancer

Editors: Jackie Edwards, Tom Devine and Louise Soanes

Contributors: Maggie Breen, Patsy Caunter, Shirley Langham, Jane Mashru and Ross Pinkerton

INTRODUCTION

The major differences within the management of children receiving chemotherapy compared to adults are to be found in the six themes of this chapter:

1. the network of care for the child/teenager with cancer
2. aetiology and pathology of childhood cancers
3. chemotherapy administration in childhood cancer
4. supportive care of the child following chemotherapy
5. the role of chemotherapy in palliative care
6. the late effects of chemotherapy.

THE NETWORK OF CARE FOR THE CHILD/TEENAGER WITH CANCER

Compared to adults, cancer in children is rare. It will affect approximately 1 child in 10 000 per year under the age of 16 years. It is currently the commonest cause of non-accident-related deaths in Europe and the USA, with around 500 deaths per year in the United Kingdom (UK).[1] In the UK, paediatric cancer services are generally based in regional children's cancer centres that are members of the United Kingdom Children's Cancer Study Group (UKCCSG). This approach has proven effective in improving mortality and morbidity rates.[2] The UKCCSG carries out cooperative national and international clinical trials, the primary aims of which are the introduction of innovative drug regimens, the collection of scientific data and the recording of children's pathways of care.[3] Balanced against the benefits of centralised care there is also a recognition of the burden to continuing family life by having to travel lengthy distances to receive treatment and supportive care.[4] Therefore, a model of sharing parts of the treatment and supportive care with health-care professionals nearer to or in the patient's home has been established.[5,6] This system of care is of particular relevance for children with acute lymphoblastic leukaemia (ALL), as the majority of chemotherapy can safely be delivered within an outpatient or home setting.

AETIOLOGY AND PATHOLOGY OF CHILDHOOD CANCERS

Children's cancers can be divided into three broad groups:

- leukaemia/lymphoma
- central nervous system tumours
- other solid tumours.

With many tumours in children, the high degree of chemo- and radiosensitivity has led to impressive cure rates, including those with non-localised disease at presentation, such as metastatic nephroblastoma, hepatoblastoma and malignant germ cell tumours. There remain, however, a number of tumours in which, despite initially high response rates, relapse is common and the majority of children die from their disease. It is beyond the remit of this section to give an in-depth overview of individual childhood cancers; however, a brief outline of childhood cancer can be found in Table 35.1. This is followed by a short description of the common investigational procedures a child is likely to undergo in order to obtain an accurate diagnosis; lastly, there is a short overview on how chemotherapy is used to treat particular childhood cancers.

Accurate diagnosis, classification, staging and baseline measurements are all prerequisites before treatment of childhood cancer can begin.[7] Biological tumour markers are also required with certain childhood cancers to assist in accurate diagnosis (Table 35.2), forecast prognosis (Table 35.3), planning treatment and assessing response to treatment.[8] In this way, more intensive treatment is directed to those with poor prognostic indicators while limiting drug toxicity to those with standard or good prognostic indicators.

To undergo the many investigations necessary to collect this information (Table 35.4), many younger patients will require heavy sedation or general anaesthetic – e.g. during tissue collection, bone marrow aspiration and cerebrospinal fluid sampling – to ensure that physical and psychological distress to the patient and family is minimised. The provision of prompt and ready access to paediatric anaesthesia is a vital component, as are the fundamentals of information-giving and the use of play therapists to promote the use of

relaxation and distraction techniques to reduce anxiety and pain.

Leukaemias and lymphomas

Leukaemias and lymphomas are curable with chemotherapy alone in the majority of cases. Radiation therapy may be used selectively: e.g. cranial irradiation for relapsed ALL and localised radiation for some forms of recurrent non-Hodgkin's lymphoma (NHL). Radiotherapy may also be used in Hodgkin's disease (HD).

Acute lymphoblastic leukaemia
Induction therapy to achieve a remission (defined as less than 5% blast cells in bone marrow) is achieved using a combination of intravenous (IV) vincristine, oral dexamethasone, intramuscular (IM) asparaginase and, in higher risk cases, IV daunorubicin. Complete remission is achieved in over 90% of patients, who then go on to receive a series of consolidation blocks of chemotherapy. Consolidation blocks include combinations of IV etoposide, IV cytarabine, oral 6-tioguanine, IV cyclophosphamide and, in higher risk cases, moderately high-dose IV methotrexate. This is followed by a 2–3-year period of continuing chemotherapy (maintenance therapy), comprising oral 6-mercaptopurine or 6-tioguanine and/or oral weekly methotrexate, with monthly IV vincristine given with a 5-day pulses of oral dexamethasone.

Non-Hodgkin's lymphoma
There are two main types of NHL: B lineage and T lineage. T-cell lymphoma frequently presents as a mediastinal mass with or without bone marrow involvement. It is treated in the same way as ALL. B NHL may present as localised nodal disease, commonly in the abdomen or nasopharynx, which may often involve bone marrow and the central nervous system (CNS). This is treated with high-dose pulsed chemotherapy given every 3 weeks for a 4–6-month period. Combination regimens include IV cyclophosphamide, IV vincristine, IV doxorubicin and oral prednisolone, combined with high-dose IV methotrexate with IV folinic acid rescue, following methotrexate completion. Failure to administer folinic acid correctly could result in extreme methotrexate toxicity and compromise prognosis. Methotrexate is alternated with blocks of IV cytarabine combined with IV etoposide or high-dose IV methotrexate.

Acute myeloid leukaemia
Acute myeloid leukaemia (AML) is treated over a relatively short period with intensive chemotherapy, usually 4–5 courses. Currently in the UK courses

Table 35.1   Childhood cancers and approaches to treatment

Diagnosis	Definition	Chemotherapy	IT therapy	Surgery	Radiotherapy	Haemopoietic stem cell transplant
Acute lymphoblastic leukaemia (ALL)	A malignancy in the cells along the lymphoid path of haemopoietic maturation and differentiation	X	X			High risk or relapsed
Non-Hodgkin's lymphoma (NHL)	Cancer of the lymphoid system	X	X			High risk or relapsed
Acute myeloid leukaemia (AML)	A malignancy in the cells along the myeloid path of haemopoietic maturation and differentiation	X	X			High risk or relapsed
Hodgkin's disease	Cancer of the lymphoid system	X		X		High risk or relapsed
CNS tumours	The most common tumours of childhood: the two main types are gliomas and medulloblastomas	X		X	X	
Retinoblastoma	A malignancy arising from embryonic retinal cells			X	X	
Soft tissue sarcomas	A group of tumours (rhabdomyosarcoma is the most common soft tissue sarcoma in childhood) with a common origin in the mesenchyme (cells that normally mature into muscle, fat, fibrous tissue, bone and cartilage)	X		X	X	Autologous
Osteosarcoma	A malignant tumour of the bone tumour the most common primary sites are long bones	X		X	X	
Ewing's sarcoma	Although often classified as a bone tumour this tumour can occur in the soft tissues approximating bone	X		X	X	
Neuroblastoma	Malignant tumours arising from the primordial neural crest cells that develop into the sympathetic system	X		X	X	Autologous
Wilms' tumour	The most common malignant renal tumour in childhood	X		X	X	
Germ cell tumours	Germ cells develop in the human embryo at 4 weeks gestation and migrate to the pelvis or scrotal sac: hence, germ cell tumours can occur in the gonads or tissues along the path of migration	X		X	X	
Liver tumour	Hepatoblastoma and hepatocellular carcinoma are the primary cancers of childhood	X		X		

Table 35.2   Tumour markers in childhood cancers

Tumour marker	Cancer
Serum alpha fetaprotein (AFP)	Malignant germ cell tumours
	Hepatoblastoma
Beta-hCG	Malignant germ cell tumours
Urinary catecholamines,	Neuroblastoma
vanillylmandelic acid (VMA)	
and homovanillic acid (HVA)	

consist of:

- IV fludarabine, cytosine, GCSF idarubicin (ADE or FLAG-ida)
- IV mitoxantrone (mitozantrone) and ara-c (MIDAC)
- IV amsacrine, cytarabine, and etoposide (MACE)
- IV cytarabine, IM asparaginase (CLASP).

Once used widely, allogeneic bone marrow transplantation (sibling or unrelated donor) is reserved for patients with high-risk cytogenetic factors, e.g. Philadelphia-positive ALL, or slow response to initial chemotherapy.

CNS-directed therapy for leukaemia or non-Hodgkin's lymphoma

Cranial irradiation has now largely been replaced by the prophylactic use of intrathecal (IT) chemotherapy, with, in some cases, the addition of high-dose IV methotrexate. In relapsed or high-risk ALL patients, IT cytarabine and IT dexamethasone may be combined with IT methotrexate. The risk of CNS disease is less in AML and, therefore, the number of treatment lumbar punctures is fewer. Conversely, in advanced Burkitt's lymphoma, the risk is greater and, therefore, intrathecal chemotherapy is included.

Hodgkin's lymphoma

In the current UK protocol, radiotherapy has largely been replaced by the use of combination chemotherapy. A regimen of alternating oral chlorambucil, IV vinblastine, oral procarbazine and oral prednisolone (CHLVPP) with IV doxorubicin, bleomycin, vincristine and dacarbazine (ABVD) is given for a total of 4–6 courses, depending on the stage of the disease at the time of diagnosis. Radiotherapy is reserved for

Table 35.3   Prognostic markers for children's cancers

Prognostic marker	Cancer
N-myc amplification	Neuroblastoma
Ph+ (Philadelphia chromosome)	C-all

Table 35.4   Diagnostic imaging

Imaging technique	Used for
X-ray films	Diagnosis and reassessment:
	• leukaemias
	• lymphomas
	• CNS tumours
	• solid tumours
Computed tomography (CT) scan	Diagnosis and reassessment:
	• lymphomas
	• CNS tumours
	• solid tumours
Magnetic resonance imaging (MRI)	Diagnosis and reassessment:
	• CNS tumours
	• solid tumours
Meta-iodobenzylguanidine (MIBG)	Diagnosis and reassessment of neuroblastoma
Ultrasound scanning (USS)	Diagnosis and reassessment:
	• lymphomas
	• solid tumours
Technetium bone scans	Assessment of tumours that can metastasise to bone

biopsy-proven residual disease at completion of chemotherapy.

CNS tumours

Medulloblastoma/primitive neuroectodermal tumour

Chemotherapy is given either prior to standard radiotherapy or following radiotherapy. Preoperatively, more intensive chemotherapy can be given, as following cranio-spinal irradiation the risk of severe myelosuppression is much increased. In the current SIOP/UKCCSG primitive neuroectodermal tumour (PNET) III protocol preoperative chemotherapy comprises combinations of IV vincristine, cyclophosphamide and carboplatin and IV vincristine, cyclophosphamide and etoposide given for a total of 4 courses over 14 weeks. Post-radiation chemotherapy, if indicated, comprises 7 courses of IV vincristine, cisplatin and oral CCNU (lomustine) given over 6 weeks.

Low-grade glioma

Chemotherapy is increasingly used in the management of low-grade glioma, either to avoid the use of radiation altogether or to delay its use in the younger child, in an attempt to limit the neurological sequelae of radiation. The current protocol combines weekly IV vincristine for 10 weeks, with 3-weekly IV carboplatin, then 4-weekly combinations of IV carboplatin and vincristine for up to 12 months. This is most frequently used in optic pathway glioma, but may also be used in other sites where complete resection is not feasible.

High-grade glioma

No single or combined chemotherapy regimen is of clear benefit in high-grade glioma, but with unresectable tumours a combination of oral procarbazine, CNNU and IV vincristine has been given in addition to standard radiotherapy. Oral temozolomide may also have a role in palliation following relapse.

Germ cell tumours

Malignant germ cell tumours (GCT) in the CNS may be pure germinoma or a mixed teratoma: the latter may be secreting or non-secreting. The role of chemotherapy in pure germinoma remains controversial, as cure rates are exceeding 90% at 5 years with radiotherapy alone. In current protocols, chemotherapy is used to reduce the dosage or extent of radiation therapy. In which case a combination of IV ifosfamide, carboplatin and etoposide is used.

Similar cisplatinum-based chemotherapy regimens are used in secreting GCT, where cerebospinal fluid (CSF) or plasma levels of alpha fetoprotein (AFP) and/or beta human chorionic gonadotrophin (β-hCG) act as a marker for diagnosis and tumour response.

Solid tumours

Retinoblastoma

This tumour is highly curable with a combination of surgery and conservative irradiation strategies. In children with more advanced disease, the role of chemotherapy regimens such as IV vincristine, carboplatin and etoposide is being investigated.

Soft tissue sarcomas

The most common soft tissue sarcoma in childhood is rhabdomyosarcoma, either embryonal or alveolar subtype. Less commonly, synovial sarcoma, soft tissue Ewing's sarcoma and fibrosarcoma are seen.

Standard chemotherapy for rhabdomyosarcoma comprises IV vincristine, dactinomycin with ifosfamide (IVA) or cyclophosphamide. These are currently given for a total of eight 3-weekly cycles, with the addition of radiation therapy if indicated. IV ifosfamide has not been shown to be superior to cyclophosphamide in North American studies where a more aggressive approach to local radiation to achieve local control is used. At present, ifosfamide remains in use in the European SIOP regimens. A current randomised study is evaluating the potential benefit of the addition of IV etoposide, epirubicin and carboplatin to the standard IVA regimen in rhabdomyosarcoma. A similar treatment approach using IVA is used to treat soft tissue Ewing's sarcoma. The role of chemotherapy in synovial sarcoma or other low-grade sarcomas remains unclear. There is no evidence that adjuvant treatment is of benefit, but IVA may be used to try and facilitate surgery in an extensive tumour.

Osteosarcoma

Standard chemotherapy given prior to definitive limb-sparing surgery comprises IV doxorubicin combined with cisplatin. This appears to be as effective as the more complex Rosen regimen, where IV bleomycin, cyclophosphamide, dactinomycin and high-dose IV methotrexate are used in addition.

Ewing's sarcoma

The standard regimen comprises IV ifosfamide, doxorubicin and vincristine. Recent randomised European trials showed the addition of IV etoposide to IVA was of no benefit. The current randomised trial evaluates the potential role of high-dose therapy using oral busulfan and high-dose IV melphalan in poor-risk patients.

Neuroblastoma

The standard regimen combines IV vincristine, cisplatin, etoposide and cyclophosphamide (OPEC). Variations on this regimen have been evaluated, with increased doses, such as in the Kushner regimen, where high-dose IV platinum is combined with etoposide and high-dose IV cyclophosphamide combined with doxorubicin. In rapid COJEC, carboplatin is alternated with cisplatin in a high-dose intense regimen, where chemotherapy is given every 10 days. The latter protocol appeared to be superior to standard OPEC in the ENSG V randomised trial and is now part of the current European study for high-risk patients. The use of high-dose IV melphalan alone has been shown to improve outcome in patients with advanced disease and the current trial compares oral busulfan and IV melphalan with high-dose IV carboplatin, etoposide and melphalan.

In advanced disease, oral *cis*-retinoic acid has been shown to be of benefit in patients who achieve a complete remission. This is given orally for a total of 6 courses at the end of treatment.

Treatment decisions are based on both clinical stage and the biology of the tumour. In the absence of poor biological risk factors, a more conservative approach can be used in localised disease, where surgery alone, even in bulky tumours, is usually adequate. The outcome in infants under 1 year of age is also favourable and for these patients less-intensive chemotherapy may be used.

Wilms' tumours

Standard combinations in Wilms' tumour include IV vincristine, dactinomycin and doxorubicin. These are given in protocols ranging from the use of IV vincristine alone for localised, initially resected, disease, to intensive AVA (dactinomycin, vincristine and Adriamycin) with all three combined for those with metastatic disease.

Extracranial germ cell tumours

Germ cell tumours, usually affecting the gonads or mediastinum, are treated with combinations of IV carboplatin, etoposide and bleomycin. More intensive regimens, adding IV ifosfamide and doxorubicin, have been used but do not appear to be superior. Treatment duration is guided by the tumour markers, either β-hCG or AFP.

Liver tumours

Liver tumours in children are mainly hepatoblastoma, although hepatocellular carcinoma may occur. The standard chemotherapy regimen is PLADO, comprising IV platinum and doxorubicin. Under current investigation is the role of IV cisplatin as a single agent in patients with localised tumours and also a more intensive version of PLADO, combining IV carboplatin and cisplatin.

THE ROLE OF CHEMOTHERAPY IN CHILDHOOD CANCER

Chemotherapy is the primary treatment modality used to cure many childhood cancers.[9,10] Chemotherapy is used in several different ways and in combination with radiation and surgery. All chemotherapy should be given in accordance with local policies and procedures; the basis of good practice is safety and patient comfort. Nurses giving chemotherapy must ensure they are familiar with the treatment protocol and the needs of the patient and family.[11] The most common routes of chemotherapy administration in children are intravenous, oral and intrathecal: the principles of the safe administration of chemotherapy are discussed elsewhere in this book. In this section the specific needs of children/adolescents will be discussed. The parameters for the administration of each chemotherapy are defined within each specific treatment protocol, and all nurses involved in the administration of chemotherapy must ensure they have the knowledge and competence to undertake this task.

Three areas are worth highlighting:

- The dose of chemotherapy is based on the child's surface area, using a combination of a child's height/ length and weight, and therefore careful monitoring for fluctuations in the child's weight throughout treatment must take place to ensure the correct dose is administered. The fluid requirement (Box 35.1) that accompanies nephrotoxic chemotherapeutic

---

> **Box 35.1   Calculation of a child's fluid requirements**
>
> - To maintain normal hydration – 2 L/m^2 or 83 ml/kg/day
>   Additional fluids would be required when a significant increase in insensible loss occurs: e.g. due to high fever or persistent diarrhoea
> - To hyperhydrate – 3 L/m^2 or 125 ml/kg/day
> - To promote the prompt excretion of nephrotoxic drugs or to reduce the risk of tumour lysis syndrome

agents is also calculated from the child's body weight.[11]

- At the start of a treatment protocol, potential measures to preserve fertility should be addressed with the child and family. For postpubescent male patients, cryopreservation of semen should be offered.[12–14] In girls of all ages, treatment is still in the experimental stage and therefore not yet widely available.[12]
- With over 65% of children with cancer now being cured, the long-term sequelae of chemotherapy in children are an important consideration at the start of treatment. For this reason, baseline endocrine investigations, where long-term sequelae are predicted, are performed.

Chemotherapy administered in childhood cancers

Three areas of care are key to the safe administration of chemotherapy to children:

- assessment
- route of administration
- setting.

Assessment before chemotherapy administration

Assessment forms an integral aspect in the care of a child receiving chemotherapy. Assessment must incorporate the physical, psychological (especially the child's cognitive development) and the social contexts of child and family life. The child and family should be involved, insofar as they wish to be, in planning care. Prior to the administration of chemotherapy the following should considered:

1. The child's diagnosis and treatment protocol.
2. Differential full blood count.
3. Other baseline parameters: e.g. renal function, urea and electrolytes, liver function tests.
4. Body surface area (height and weight).
5. The child's clinical condition: consider the child's vital signs and pre-existing conditions.

6. The child and parents are made aware of the clinical profile of the chemotherapy they are to receive: e.g. name of agents, potential side effects, length of treatment, symptom recognition/management strategies.

7. Anticipated side-effects include:

- nausea and vomiting – use of the appropriate antiemetic prior to chemotherapy can minimise the chance of this occurring.

- dehydration – to ensure adequate hydration, especially when the child is at high risk of tumour lysis syndrome during induction chemotherapy for ALL and T-cell lymphoma where there is rapid cell breakdown, high rates of IV fluids, hyperhydration, is administered.

Routes of chemotherapy administration

The three routes for administration of chemotherapy in common use are:

- intravenous
- oral
- intrathecal.

Intravenous administration of chemotherapy

Intravenous chemotherapy for children is routinely delivered via a central venous access device (CVAD). These have greatly contributed to the management of childhood cancer, reducing a child's exposure to repeated venous cannulation with its associated psychological trauma.[15] They also allow for chemotherapy to be administered safely outside the hospital environment and for complex IV supportive care to be provided following high-dose chemotherapy, e.g. blood products, parenteral nutrition, IV antibiotics and other supportive IV drugs.[6]

Oral administration of chemotherapy

Following several clinical trials and subsequent modifications to treatment protocols, the current belief is that a prolonged oral treatment phase is beneficial in maintaining long-term remission in childhood ALL.[16] The practice of individual dose adjustment of oral chemotherapy has also become a feature of recent trials, and is likely to remain so as the metabolism of thiopurines is better understood.[16,17]

The use of oral cytotoxic drugs differs substantially from that in adults due to the limitations inherent for children in their ability to swallow capsules or tablets whole.[18] The problem is further compounded by the fact that liquid preparations of cytotoxic drugs are rarely available and doses based on the child's body surface area or weight often dictate that whole capsules or tablets be divided. The resulting risk of contamination

from crushing or cutting tablets is a potential hazard. Tablets are formulated with a protective coat to protect the handler from unwarranted exposure. Crushing and breaking tablets disrupts this protective coating. If unavoidable, to minimise this, use an enclosed tablet crusher, a pill cutter or dispersible tablets. Capsules should never be opened by nursing staff or parents on the ward or at home as the contents are easily lost into the atmosphere, posing risks of inhalation to all and inaccurate dosing for the child.[11] To prevent this occurrence, the capsule should be opened in the pharmacy department under controlled conditions or, when feasible, prescribing adjusted to avoid the need for opening the capsule.

Over time, with the assistance of play therapists, even small children have been helped to master the technique of swallowing tablets or capsules. They should always be discouraged from crunching tablets, as particles may lodge between their teeth and cause stomatitis; for this reason, children should be encouraged to drink copiously following oral chemotherapy.[11]

Intrathecal administration of chemotherapy

Some of the commonest types of cancer found in children – in particular, leukaemia and lymphoma – have the ability to penetrate the CNS and circulate in the CSF. Therefore, this group of children are given prophylactic, therapeutic IT chemotherapy via a lumbar puncture (LP). Following a series of tragic incidents around the world in which the intravenous drug vincristine was injected in error intrathecally with fatal consequences, there are now national statutory requirements that must be followed.[19]

In the UK, young children commonly undergo LPs under a short general anaesthetic. For older children and adolescents, it may be possible to employ self-distraction or relaxation strategies together with an appropriate local anaesthesia. Such an approach may also be useful for younger children who find undergoing a general anaesthetic distressing. Whichever approach is taken, carrying out an LP on a child with cancer requires a multiprofessional approach involving the combined skills of play therapists, nurses, anaesthetists, operating department assistants (ODAs), paediatricians and the child and his family.

CHEMOTHERAPY MANAGEMENT WITHIN A MODEL OF SHARED CARE

The diagnosis of specific cancers has implication for where children receive care. Currently, the role of the paediatric oncology centre (POC) is to confirm a diagnosis, prescribe, administer, guide and support the child and family through complex treatment regimens. Children with ALL and with solid tumours requiring less intense treatment can receive much of their care in their local paediatric oncology shared care unit (POSCU) or in the home given by children's community nurses (CCNs). As yet, a uniform pattern of care has not been formalised. The current structure and level of shared care are shown in Table 35.5.

The growth of day care and home care services has resulted in significant benefits for families and service providers alike, including:[11]

- Psychological trauma associated with repeated and prolonged periods of hospitalisation for children is kept to a minimum.[20]
- Reduced risk of infection from resistant hospital microbiological flora.[21]
- Potential disruption to family routines is reduced. For example, children frequently able to attend school during treatments and the parents able to work if treatments are scheduled outside these hours.[11]
- Home care enhances a family's sense of normality, which in turn is conducive to the child's well-being.[22]

Supportive care, such as management of febrile neutropenic episodes, thrombocytopenia and anaemia, can frequently be provided by the POSCU. Many POSCUs now administer a limited number of outpatient chemotherapies to children who are on established treatment regimens, particularly maintenance chemotherapy for ALL.[23] A smaller number have the resources to offer more complex day case or inpatient chemotherapy, with the explicit agreement of the POC.

Frequent, accurate and comprehensive two-way communication between POSCU and the POC is an essential requirement, specifically relating to adjustments to doses, and the detection, investigation and management of toxicity. The prompt and complete return of clinical trial data is of particular importance when joint aspects of children's cancer treatment are shared.

Supportive care of the child following chemotherapy

Physical symptoms experienced by children as a consequence of chemotherapy are similar to those experienced by adults. Difference relates to intensity of treatment approaches and children's ability to absorb, distribute, metabolise and eliminate drugs. Only those strategies that differ from adult cancer management will be discussed. Tables 35.6A and B give an overview of childhood cancer symptoms and the specific management each requires, and include:

- neutropenia
- thrombocytopenia
- anaemia
- nausea and vomiting
- mucositis
- diarrhoea
- constipation
- anorexia, cachexia, malnutrition.

(Text continued on p. 261)

Table 35.5   Shared care

	Inpatient care	Outpatient care
POC	Assessment, diagnosis, establishment of treatment protocol	Care that can be given as an outpatient but requires specialist services available at the POC
	Full management of complex treatment regimens	Complex chemotherapy regimens: e.g. neuroblastoma
POSCU Minimum level	Management of febrile neutropenia Treatment directed by POC	Biochemical, haematological and bacteriological evaluation
POSCU Intermediate level	Local paediatrician responsible for care Frequent discussions with POC No inpatient chemotherapy Management of febrile neutropenia	Local paediatrician responsible for care Frequent discussions with POC Mainly bolus chemotherapy e.g. vincristine
POSCU Maximum level	Local team manage care with some support from as required POC	Local paediatrician responsible for care
	Limited in-patient chemotherapy	Chemotherapy IV bolus and stipulated short infusions: e.g. doxorubicin
Home	Not applicable	Blood sampling At present, single bolus dose chemotherapy: e.g. cytarabine

POC, paediatric oncology centre; POSCU, paediatric oncology shared care unit.

Table 35.6A Symptoms and their management: neutropenia; thrombocytopenia; and anaemia

Symptom	Neutropenia	Thrombocytopenia	Anaemia
Definition and pathophysiology	Neutrophil count less than 1×10^9/L. Severe neutropenia: neutrophil count less than 0.5×10^9/L. Infection is a major complication in neutropenia following chemotherapy. Three categories of patient based upon risk factors: 1. Febrile non-neutropenia 2. Low-risk febrile neutropenia = look well, no documented site of infection or any high risk comorbidities, anticipated to have fewer than 7 days of neutropenia remaining. 3. High-risk neutropenia = prolonged neutropenia >7 days, recurrent, new infection, uncontrolled malignancy, clearly defined infection, clinically unstable, mucositis[1]	A platelet count <100×10^9/L. Usual cause reduced megakaryocytes accompanying replacement of bone marrow by disease or aplasia secondary to chemotherapy[2]	A haemoglobin <10×10^9/L. Diminished erythrocyte production. A common symptom in children following chemotherapy. It has been estimated that 80% will experience this symptom, secondary to chemotherapy regardless of the tumour type.[3] Usual rate of decline in child's haemoglobin concentration is 0.8–1.0 g/dl per week (i.e. 1/120th of the total red cell mass per day). Reductions more rapid than this indicate bleeding or haemolysis.[2]
Assessment	Patients in all risk categories require that a careful history and physical examination occurs. Assess for fever over 38°C, skin integrity, abdominal pain, cough, tachypnoea, stomatitis, perianal fissures, CAVD exit site	Assess for bleeding bruising, petechiae, purpura. Monitor blood counts weekly; more frequently if the child is symptomatic. Blood counts are required if an intramuscular injection, insertion of nasogastric tube for feeding, surgery is predicted and prior to lumber punctures to ensure platelet count is sufficient	The following influence the criteria for a blood transfusion based on a low Hb: <ul><li>bone marrow disease</li><li>chemotherapy agents</li><li>religious belief of child and parents</li><li>age of the child.</li></ul> Most children who are mildly anaemic remain asymptomatic; however, assess for fatigue, tachycardia, dyspnoea, pallor

Continued

Table 35.6A Symptoms and their management: neutropenia; thrombocytopenia; and anaemia—cont'd

Symptom	Neutropenia	Thrombocytopenia	Anaemia
Care guidelines	If the child is febrile and neutropenic, IV antibiotics (according to local policy) are imperative. Recognize subtle signs of infection and impending septic shock. Education of parents and child in the prevention of infection and the actions to be taken if the child becomes febrile at home. In nonneutropenia febrile patients, low-risk patients, outpatient IV. Antibiotic therapy is possible followed by oral antibiotics. Refer to POC for outpatient IV, antibiotic policy. The major problem in administration of outpatient antibiotic therapy is the limited number of antimicrobial agents suitable for such use.[4,5] Children receiving chemotherapy which cause prolonged neutropenia or severe neutropenia are at increased risk of bacterial or fungal infection and may be given granulocyte colony-stimulating factor (G-CSF).	There is no reason to restrict the active inquiring child from social activities such as play. Platelet transfusion should be given dependent upon local policy, but consider: • Symptoms of bleeding (petechiae, purpura or spontaneous bruising). • The need to undertake invasive procedures: e.g. lumbar puncture. • Persistent fever with a platelet count of <20 × 10⁹/L. • Asymptomatic child but platelet count <10 × 10⁹/L. • Hypertensive children should have their platelet count maintained at >50 × 10⁹/L. • Girls who have reached their menarche/receiving highly myelosuppressive treatments are at high risk of bleeding.[6] Administration of oestrogen to stop their menstrual cycle is required until their platelet count has reached 50 × 10⁹/L unsupported on the completion of treatment. • Teenage boys who wish to shave should use an electric razor rather than wet shave.[11]	Educate parents/the child to recognise the early signs of anaemia: i.e. pallor, fatigue, reluctance to participate in energetic play activities, irritability. Late signs may include dyspnoea, tachypnoea, dizziness, headache, and tachycardia. There is limited information on the role of recombinant human erythropoietin (EPO) from anaemia caused by defective EPO production in the body following chemotherapy. It may be of benefit in reducing the requirement for blood transfusions.[7,8] It is not current practice to administer EPO products in the UK. Current guidelines for administration of packed cells are: • less than 1 year old with Hb ≤ 7 g/l • 1–12 years old Hb ≤ 8.0 g/l • 13–19 years old Hb ≤ 9.0 g/l.

Table 35.6B Symptoms and their management: nausea and vomiting; mucositis; diarrhoea; constipation: and anorexia, cachexia and malnutrition

Symptom	Nausea and vomiting	Mucositis	Diarrhoea	Constipation	Anorexia, cachexia, malnutrition
Definition and pathophysiology	Nausea: the recognition of the need to vomit. Vomiting: the forceful expulsion of the gastric contents. Chemotherapeutic agents can stimulate the chemoreceptor trigger zone in the medullary lateral reticular formation of the brain.[9] A distressing side effect for children during cancer treatment.[10] Anxiety: anticipatory nausea and vomiting is a conditioned response to the anticipation of chemotherapy administration. This is more likely to occur if initial chemotherapy induced nausea and vomiting is poorly controlled.[11]	Inflammation of the oral mucosa. A common and distressing side effect in children following chemotherapy.[10,12]	Abnormal increase in the quantity frequency, or liquidity of stools. Common pathogens: • *Clostridium difficile* • *Cryptosporidium.* Chemotherapy agents: • dactinomycin • cisplatin • daunorubicin • tioguanine.	A decrease in the normal frequency of stool production. Constipation is a common symptom in children with cancer.[12]	Reduced intake of fluid and food resulting in total weight loss. Frequent consequence of childhood cancer treatments. Between 6 and 50% of children with cancer experience malnutrition during treatment.[13]
Contributing factors	Symptoms vary in onset, intensity and duration. Time: can be acute (less than 24 hours after the administration of chemotherapy) or delayed (more than 24 hours after the administration), depending on the type of chemotherapy.[9] Children with a previous history of nausea and vomiting, i.e. motion sickness, may be at increased risk of chemotherapy-induced nausea and vomiting.[14]	Mucositis is more prevalent in children receiving high-dose chemotherapy. Following peripheral blood stem cell transplant (PBSCT), mucositis occurs in 100% of patients.[15,16] Types of chemotherapy: • doxorubicin • cytarabine • daunorubicin • melphalan • methotrexate. Physical trauma and/or thrombocytopenia: may lead to bleeding and further mucosal damage.		Multiple interrelated factors can induce constipation. Constipation has been categorised in children into primary, secondary and iatrogenic factors.[18] Primary: poor dietary intake of fibre, reduced fluid intake, lack of physical mobility and exercise, lack of privacy when toileting. Secondary (pathological): spinal cord compression, intestinal obstruction,	Causes can be multifactorial; decreased ingestion of food is frequently a direct result from treatment aggravated by nausea and vomiting.[19] The extent of the problem will relate to type, stage and location of the cancer, and the intensity of treatment.[13] Regular nursing assessments should be carried out at diagnosis and during treatment. Culture: incorporate the family's cultural and

Continued

Table 35.6B Symptoms and their management: nausea and vomiting; mucositis; diarrhoea; constipation: and anorexia, cachexia and malnutrition—cont'd

Symptom	Nausea and vomiting	Mucositis	Diarrhoea	Constipation	Anorexia, cachexia, malnutrition
		Neutropenia and/or poor dental hygiene: may lead to secondary infection.[17]		electrolyte imbalance. Iatrogenic (medical interventions): drugs, e.g analgesia and vinca alkaloids.	religious beliefs within the assessment and management of nutrition. Developmental stage: the normal food fads of childhood should be taken into consideration. The interaction of the side effects of chemotherapy – i.e. nausea/vomiting, anorexia, mucositis and alteration in taste – must be considered.[11] Corticosteroids can increase appetite and cause food fads for short periods and create a false sense of the child's overall nutritional status.
Care guidelines	Staff should be aware of the emetogenic potential of each chemotherapy regimen and administer the appropriate prophylactic antiemetics. Reassess the child and individualise the antiemetic plan to take account of the child's needs and wishes. Consider the use of non-pharmacological interventions, e.g. distraction therapy,[20] particularly with older children. 5-Hydroxytryptamine (5–HT₃) antagonists have improved control of nausea and vomiting in children.[9] Prophylactic measures before intrathecal chemotherapy can	The assessment of a child's mouth and the management of mucositis is best carried out using a recognised oral assessment guide (OAG) and a relevant treatment algorithm.[23] The use of a soft toothbrush and chlorhexidine or saline mouthwashes has proven beneficial.[24] Prophylactic use of oral glutamine may minimise mucositis in children receiving chemotherapy.[25] Adequate analgesia to control pain and enhance compliance and comfort with oral hygiene regimen is paramount.[26]	Frequent loose stools can, if uncorrected, lead to severe dehydration and fluid and electrolyte imbalance in children, particularly in the young where diarrhoea can rapidly account for a significant loss of body fluid. Monitor fluid and electrolytes balance and body weight at least daily if a child has diarrhoea. Intravenous fluid replacement may be necessary if the child cannot maintain oral	Encourage a diet with sufficient fibre and adequate fluid intake. Consider prophylactic aperient use in certain chemotherapy protocols and prolonged analgesia where constipation is highly likely. Encourage the child to return to daily social activities, e.g. play, to be independently mobile. Avoid rectal suppositories in children who are neutropenic due to the risk of causing systemic sepsis as a result of pathogens entering the systemic system via	All patients should be assessed at diagnosis. Assessment should include weight, serum albumin, dietary history and a current record of food intake, treatment strategies and tumour type.[27,28] Intervention strategy must be considered in the light of each child's quality of life. Many children, in particular teenagers, dislike the option of a nasogastric tube due to its cosmetic appearance, and non-compliance can be problematic.

minimise severe vomiting.[21] Prophylactic prescribing and administration of antiemetics according to antiemetic potential of chemotherapy drugs should occur. Dexamethazone alongside a 5-HT$_3$ antagonist is a useful adjuvant in controlling severe emesis.[22] Antiemetics should be continued on discharged patients until nausea or vomiting has subsided or the anticipated antiemetic potential has ceased.

intake or is dehydrated.[39] It is equally important to regularly review fluid management for, as the diarrhoea subsides, fluid overload may supersede the risk of dehydration. Antispasmodic drugs may help relieve pain from abdominal cramps.[11] Diarrhoea may lead to breakdown of perianal region and increase the risk of opportunistic infections.[11] Children who wear nappies are at greater risk of perianal breakdown; therefore, frequent nappy changes with appropriate skin care is vital to minimise the risk of skin breakdown.

damage to the mucosal barrier.[11] Ensure the child's privacy and dignity is maintained at all times.

The family, mothers in particular, feel that maintaining nutritional needs is the aspect of the child's care that they should be able to maintain and control. Providing information on strategies to promote healthy eating habits during chemotherapy is important. Early referral to a paediatric dietician should be a routine part of a child's treatment for cancer.[27] Education of the family/child is important to manage the child's nutritional needs during treatment. Provision of facilities so that families can cater for a child's cultural and religious needs maintains parental involvement in care and encourages normal eating habits. Enteral feeding for the management of children where weight loss is experienced or can be predicted. This strategy can be safe and cost-effective.[29] Home nasogastric feeding is recommended in patients who are malnourished due to poor appetite and can be managed by the family with appropriate support.[19]

Continued

Table 35.6B Symptoms and their management: nausea and vomiting; mucositis; diarrhoea; constipation: and anorexia, cachexia and malnutrition—cont'd

Symptom	Nausea and vomiting	Mucositis	Diarrhoea	Constipation	Anorexia, cachexia, malnutrition
					There is evidence to suggest that enteral feeding is superior to parenteral feeding as enteral feeding maintains the structural and functional integrity of the gastrointestinal (GI) tract, decreases the risk of bacterial infection and improves patient outcomes.[30] Children who are unable to tolerate a nasogastric tube, and for certain high-intensity chemotherapy regimens, a gastrostomy should be considered. Parenteral feeding should be reserved for children where using the GI tract is inadvisable due to either surgery, severe infection, severe mucositis, stomatitis or the radiation field.[17] Total parenteral nutrition can support a child's nutritional needs during a persistent fever by increasing whole body protein turnover and reducing the likelihood of mucositis and gut toxicity.[19]

Only the most frequent supportive care interventions required of a POSCU are discussed in more detail:

- neutropenia
- CVAD line infections
- *Pneumocystis carinii* pneumonia (PCP)
- varicella
- childhood infections and immunisations.

The role of supportive care in reducing treatment-related mortality is now recognised as a vital component of care.[16,17] This includes the prevention, early detection and management of childhood infections within the community setting, following administration of chemotherapy that results in reduced immunity.

Neutropenia

Mortality during treatment for childhood cancer relates to the patient's underlying disease, its treatment, the hospital environment or the breakdown of the body's natural defence barriers.[24] The most vulnerable sites of infection in the immunocompromised child are the skin, oral mucosa, respiratory tract, digestive tract, sinuses and perianal area.[24] Early detection and treatment in children is essential to prevent life-threatening septicaemia. Physical isolation on admission to POSCU, due to the uncontrollable nature of general paediatric ward infectious referrals, is essential. Sepsis as a result of treatment-related neutropenia is one of the most common causes of non-disease-related death during treatment in childhood cancer.[25]

CVAD infections

Nearly all children receiving chemotherapy will have a CVAD inserted: either a permanent skin-tunnelled catheter, an implantable port or a temporary peripherally inserted central catheter (PICC). In the past 20 years CVADs have revolutionised the treatment approach to childhood cancer chemotherapy. However, permanent skin-tunnelled catheters are a potential site and port of infection, especially in the immunocompromised child. CVAD-related infection is defined as the isolation of a single organism – the common organism being coagulated negative staphylococcus.[26] The prevention or early recognition of such infections is a key role of nurses caring for a child with cancer, as they are the staff member who most frequently uses and helps care for the device.

Pneumocystis carinii pneumonia

Pneumocystis carinii pneumonia (PCP) is more common in children receiving high-dose chemotherapy; however, children with ALL are at significant risk of PCP due to immunosuppression that results from prolonged treatment.[27] To minimise the risk of PCP, prophylactic oral co-trimoxazole is currently scheduled on two consecutive days each week for the entire duration of treatment. Any immunocompromised patient experiencing a dry persistent cough, pyrexia, dyspnoea or tachypnoea should immediately be referred to the POC for medical assessment and potential management of PCP.[27] It should be borne in mind that co-trimoxazole can cause myelosuppression in some ALL patients, thereby compromising optimum use of maintenance chemotherapy (S Mellor pers comm 2000). In such instances prophylactic inhaled pentamidine can be substituted, in accordance with national guidelines.[28]

Varicella infections

Chickenpox is only ever acquired through direct contact with a contagious person. The incubation period for chickenpox is up to 3 weeks, but it is contagious for 48 hours before a rash appears.

In immunocompromised children, chickenpox (varicella) and shingles (herpes zoster) carries significant morbidity for patients during treatment and up to 6–12 months following treatment. Primary infection of patients with a lymphocyte count below 0.5×10^9 /L is associated with a high risk of visceral dissemination to lung, liver and brain in the absence of antiviral therapy.[27] A universal policy when chickenpox contact occurs and varicella zoster immunoglobulin (VZIG) is required is contained in guidelines drawn up by the Royal College of Paediatrics & Child Health (Table 35.7).

The risk of contact with chickenpox and measles at school is relatively high. Pupils and parents in the child's school need to be aware that they must contact the school if their child develops chickenpox. If the child with cancer has been in contact with this child in the 48 hours prior to chickenpox, they must contact the POC.

Shingles is caused by the same virus, which has lain dormant and can become reactivated when immunity is impaired. Shingles is infectious only when the rash is present and is less contagious if the rash is covered with clothing. For all children with cancer who develop chickenpox or shingles, hospitalisation is recommended to monitor the patient's clinical condition and institute antiviral measures promptly should they become necessary.

Measles

Measles infection in the immunocompromised patient can result in high mortality and morbidity.[27]

Table 35.7   Chickenpox contact and use of varicella-zoster immunoglobulin (VZIG)

Definition of significant exposure to varicella–zoster:

Index case	Timing of exposure	Duration of exposure
Clinical chickenpox and disseminated zoster (incubation period 14–21 days from contact). Infectious period 48 hours before rash and until all vesicles are dry	48 hours before rash until all lesions have crusted	Contact in same room for 15 min. Face to face contact
Shingles or localised zoster	Day of onset of rash until all lesions have crusted	Contact in same room for 15 min. Face to face contact

Criteria for giving VZIG?

- All immunocompromised children who have not had chicken pox or are known to be VZV IgG negative or equivocal
- Immunocompromised children known to be VZV IgG positive should have their VZV IgG re-tested as close to the date of exposure as possible (no later than 7 days from contact). If this is negative or equivocal, VZIG IgG should be given
- Children undergoing BMT who have received multiple blood transfusions or immunoglobulin may have acquired VZ antibody passively; these patients do not need VZIG if antibody is detected at the time of exposure
- Children who cannot receive an intramuscular injection should be given intravenous normal immunoglobulin
- Children who have received VZIG should be isolated for up to 28 days after exposure, to protect susceptible patients and staff
- Aciclovir prohylaxis should start at day 10 of contact for 4 weeks for patients who are particularly high risk: e.g. conditioning for BMT or surgery within 4 weeks
- The child and family should be informed that VZIG will not prevent acquiring chicken pox but should reduce the morbidity and provide a degree of protection for up to 3 weeks

Source: adapted from Royal College of Paediatrics and Child Health.[31]
IgG = immunoglobulin G.

The introduction of the measles, mumps and rubella (MMR) vaccine in 1988 has been successful in reducing the incidence of measles within the general population,[29] although caution is still needed particularly in areas where uptake of the MMR vaccination is becoming an increasing cause for concern. If a child comes into contact with measles and has not had the MMR vaccine, they will require an intramuscular (IM) injection of human normal immunoglobulin as soon as possible, ideally within 48 hours of a confirmed contact.[30]

Immunisations

Although the aforementioned childhood infectious diseases are a cause of concern in the immunocompromised patient, contact with mumps or rubella is of little significance.[5] However, it is important to emphasise the need for siblings to be vaccinated to reduce opportunistic spread of infectious diseases within a household. Inactivated polio vaccine (IPV) should be used for siblings, as the live oral polio vaccine (OPV) poses a cross-infection risk to the immunocompromised child.[30] Guidelines for immunisation during and following standard treatment, and following intensive chemotherapy regimens allogeneic haemopoietic stem cell transplant required/rescue (HSCT), have been provided by the Royal College of Paediatrics and Child Health.[31] The current guidelines are being followed by

all regional children's cancer centres within the UK (Box 35.2).

THE ROLE OF CHEMOTHERAPY IN PALLIATIVE CARE

'The time at which potentially curative treatment is abandoned is a very personal decision between the doctor, family and as often as possible, the child'.[32] Once the clinical decision – that cure is no longer possible – has been reached, a further decision has to be taken: whether to move straight to symptom control, which may include oral chemotherapy, or to enter the child in a phase I or phase II clinical trial.

Oral chemotherapy

Single-agent oral cytotoxic drugs have been shown to be highly effective in producing both short-term regression and stable disease in children where cure is no longer possible. Oral etoposide and cyclophosphamide have been shown to provide significant symptom relief and so contribute to the child's quality of life (QOL).[32] Regimens are designed to minimise the risk of toxicity, such as nausea and vomiting, myelosuppression and mucositis, and the accompanying need for hospitalisation or further invasive procedures.

Box 35.2   Guidelines for immunisations in children following chemotherapy

Immunisations during and until 6 months following completion of standard treatment

All children who are immunocompromised must not receive live vaccines during cancer treatments and for the following 6 months after cessation of treatment. This will include MMR (measles, mumps and rubella) vaccine, oral polio vaccine (OPV), bacille Calmette-Guérin (BCG), oral typhoid and yellow fever. Inactivated polio vaccine (IPV) can be administered in place of OPV.

Influenza vaccine is recommended annually in the autumn for all patients receiving chemotherapy, and for those still within 6 months of completion of chemotherapy.

Immunisations 6 months and later following completing for treatment

At 6 months following completion of treatment, administer an additional booster of diphtheria, tetanus, acellular pertussis, IPV, Hib, meningococcal and MMR vaccines. Subsequent routine booster doses (e.g. pre-school) will not be necessary if they are scheduled to be given within 1 year of this additional dose.

If patient has previously had BCG, and is considered to be in a high-risk group for tuberculosis, check tuberculin test and, if negative, revaccinate. If patient has not previously had BCG, immunise according to local policy. Ensure that the primary health care team is informed.

Varicella zoster is not routinely administered.

HLA-identical sibling donor allogenic or syngeneic haemopoietic stem cell transplant

At 12 months post-HSCT (haemopoietic stem cell transplant), administer:

- diphtheria, tetanus, acellular pertussis – 3 doses at monthly intervals
- IPV – 3 doses at monthly intervals
- Hib – 3 doses at monthly intervals
- meningoc – 3 doses at monthly intervals.

At 15 months post-HSCT, administer:

- pneumococcal vaccine – give conjugate vaccine initially, followed by polysaccharide vaccine once the child is 24 months post-HSCT. If child under 24 months of age, give 3 doses of conjugate vaccine at monthly intervals (note: polysaccharide vaccine to follow 1 year later).

At 18 months and 24 months post-HSCT, administer:

- MMR (at least 12 months off all immunosuppressive treatment). These 2 doses should usually be given with a minimum 6 month interval, but the second dose can be given 4 weeks after the first in the event of a local measles outbreak.

At 24 months post-HSCT, administer:

- Polysaccharide pneumococcal vaccine – 1 dose.

Every autumn, administer:

- Influenza vaccine (for as long as the patient remains clinically immunocompromised or is considered to be at increased risk from influenza virus infection).

Any other allogenic HSCT

Re-immunisation schedule as above, but starting and continuing 6 months later (i.e. starting at 18 months post-HSCT).

Re-immunisation of autologous HSCT recipients

Re-immunisation programme commences 1 year after an autologous HSCT.

Otherwise, the schedule is identical to that for HLA-identical sibling donor allogenic or syngeneic HSCT (see above).

Source: Royal College of Paediatrics and Child Health.[31]

Children's participation in investigational therapies

Children are, as with adults, offered entry into a phase I or phase II clinical trial only when curative therapy is deemed no longer possible. Entering a child into such trials raises a number of ethical issues: not least, the possibility of creating unrealistic hopes of cure, especially amongst parents. On the other hand, excluding children from entry into early clinical trials could lead, at best, to a 'delayed availability of a potential active agent and, at worst to unavailability of a potentially beneficial agent, if it fails to demonstrate activity in adult cancer'.[33]

Maximising the child's involvement in the decision to participate in a phase I or phase II clinical trial cannot be overemphasised, including providing opportunities to explore the impact participation in a trial might have upon symptom control, the progress of the disease and the scenario of death. The decision ultimately to enter a child into a clinical trial 'must not be influenced by the inevitable desperation of the family to do something in the face of a hopeless situation. The performance status of the child and the extent of the disease must provide some likelihood of at least short-term benefit'.[32] (See also Chs 6 and 9.)

Phase I clinical trials

The controversial first clinical stage (a phase I trial) primary end point is to establish the dose-limiting toxicity (DLT) of a new drug and determine the maximum tolerated dose (MTD). The MTD is defined as the dose level immediately below the dose level at which DLT was experienced. The compound is trialled in as few patients as necessary, usually 3 patients per cohort, at a given dose level. Only when tolerability and reversibility of toxicity has been established for a level are a further 3 patients recruited to a subsequent level until the primary end point of the trial is established. Entry into phase I clinical trials is highly controversial, especially the early dose levels of a phase I trial, which are unlikely to be of direct therapeutic benefit to the participants. It should be noted, however, that paediatric clinical trials generally follow those in adults with starting doses of 60% the adult MTD and it is therefore not unreasonable to expect some antitumour activity even at the earlier dose levels.

Furthermore, not infrequently significant symptomatic benefit can be achieved in such studies even in the absence of a clear objective response.[32]

Phase II clinical trials

Phase II clinical trials investigate compounds, at the MTD established in a phase I trial, to gain information on the efficacy in achieving tumour response. The design of a phase II trial is immensely important; end points should be clearly defined and measurable. A strict inclusion and exclusion criteria is operated, not only to protect vulnerable patients from unwarranted inclusion but also to guard against jeopardising the study findings by either incorrectly declaring a drug effective (false-positive error) or declaring an active drug ineffective (false-negative error).

Care of the child and family receiving investigational therapy

Presently, the guidelines for the ethical and scientific conduct of clinical trials involving human subjects are laid out in the good clinical practice (GCP) guidelines agreed in 1997.[34] The guidelines are currently being developed into European directives that are set to become law in countries in the European Union in 2004. In the United Kingdom, phase I and phase II clinical trials are only carried out in a UKCCSG-designated POC. Protocols are devised by the New Agents Group (NAG), a subgroup of the UKCCSG. The clinicians from POC working in the centres where phase I and phase II clinical trials are undertaken are able to take active participation in protocol development. When designing protocols, care is taken to minimise the burden placed upon the child and family, while at the same time ensuring sound scientific principles are followed. As far as possible the protocol should be strictly adhered to in order to ensure the child has the maximum chance of benefit and is valuable in relation to the study end points.

At the POC, experienced medical, nursing and pharmaceutical staff are on hand to guide and support the child and family through the trial. The research nurse is pivotal in ensuring the smooth running of the trial. Liaising with other clinical research personnel, the specialist symptom control team, the local hospital and home care team is essential if the disruption to family life is to be minimised at a time when the need to maximise the child's and family's quality of life is of the utmost importance. The research nurse, together with the child and family, has to devise a person-centred protocol which takes account of the individual needs of the child and family and at the same time ensures that the requirements of the trial and the safety of the child is not compromised.

THE LATE EFFECTS OF CHEMOTHERAPY

The number of childhood cancer survivors, currently thought to be 1 in 1000 young adults, has increased over the last 30 years with the introduction of multimodal therapies of chemotherapy, radiotherapy and surgery.[35–37] Children are considered to be cured of their disease and therefore long-term survivors when disease-free for 5 years and at least 2 years off treatment.[36] It has been predicted that there will be 5000 new childhood cancer survivors worldwide each year.[36]

Long-term side effects of chemotherapy

The long-term side effects of chemotherapy are dependent on the dose received and the combination of drugs used. Side effects are exacerbated by the addition of radiotherapy and/or surgery.[38] Children undergoing a bone marrow transplant (BMT) receive high-dose chemotherapy, with or without total body irradiation (TBI) pretransplant, and as a consequence can suffer severe long-term side effects affecting many body systems.[39]

In 1995 the UKCCSG established guidelines to ensure that the provision of care for the long-term follow-up of childhood cancer survivors is consistent and comprehensive across the UK.[40] Children require assessment in long-term follow-up clinics once treatment has been completed, and visits to the clinic should be at least annually throughout childhood and into adulthood.

Non-endocrine late effects of chemotherapy

Neurological dysfunction

Cranial irradiation causes neurological dysfunction, as outlined in Table 35.8.[37,41] Similar, but less severe, neurological dysfunction is seen after IT chemotherapy with methotrexate[36,38] and high-dose IV methotrexate.[35] Problems usually become apparent 2–5 years after treatment.[36] Children under 5 years of age are at particular risk of CNS impairment following cranial irradiation and IT methotrexate due to the increased vulnerability of the still-developing brain.

Hearing loss

Cisplatin is the main chemotherapeutic agent that causes hearing loss. The effects (which are dose-related and inversely related to age) are bilateral, irreversible and usually affect high-frequency sounds.[38]

Cataracts

About 12% of children who receive chemotherapy with TBI and BMT are at risk of developing cataracts, with high doses of radiation causing more damage. Children treated with chemotherapy alone do not appear to be at risk.[42] Treatment with steroids over a prolonged period can also cause cataracts.[39]

Cardiac failure

Anthracyclines (doxorubicin and daunorubicin) are cardiotoxic and can cause late-onset cardiac failure,

with severe cases requiring heart transplants.[43] Other chemotherapy agents (see Table 35.11) can cause both acute and long-term cardiac problems.[35,36,38] Cumulative doses of anthracyclines above 228 mg/m^2 can cause abnormalities visible on echocardiography,[35] including myocardial dysfunction and arrhythmias.[36] Patients often have no obvious symptoms of cardiac failure at rest but should take care when undertaking strenuous exercise,[35] and particular care also needs to be taken during times of increased cardiac stress, including pregnancy and anaesthesia.[36,38]

Lungs

The side effects are usually related to the dose of chemotherapy given: bleomycin, in particular, can cause pulmonary toxicity at doses as low as 60 mg/m^2.[35,36]

Patients receiving combination therapy, including high-dose chemotherapy, whole lung irradiation and TBI, are also at risk.[35,38] Health professionals, parents and patients should be particularly aware that treatment with bleomycin poses a significant risk of respiratory failure during anaesthesia.[36,38]

Renal failure

Children treated with dactinomycin and doxorubicin in conjunction with abdominal radiotherapy for treatment of Wilms' tumour are at increased risk of long-term renal damage. Dactinomycin and doxorubicin act as radiosensitisers, increasing the effects of radiotherapy.[35]

Liver failure

Long-term liver damage can be caused by daily low-dose methotrexate and 6-mercaptourine, drugs used to treat ALL.[36] Patients are often asymptomatic[35] and liver function tests and liver size can remain normal until liver fibrosis and cirrhosis develop.[38]

Second malignancy

An estimated 3–12% of children treated for cancer develop a second malignancy within 20 years of the initial diagnosis.[35]

Psychological effects

Coping with an illness such as childhood cancer can cause psychological problems (see Table 35.8); however, it is recognised that most adult survivors of childhood cancer appear to make a good psychological recovery.[44,45]

Endocrine late-effects of chemotherapy

Gonadal failure

The chemotherapy agents discussed in Table 35.9 affect rapidly dividing cells such as those found in the

Table 35.8 Non-endocrine late effects and long-term follow-up guidelines

Non-endocrine late effects	Treatment responsible	Long-term follow-up guidelines
Neurological dysfunction: 1. Memory disturbance 2. Seizures 3. Motor difficulties 4. IQ deficits 5. Multiple endocrine abnormalities Seizures + cerebellar symptoms[31]	Cranial irradiation Ciclosporin A (used to treat GvHD)	Psychological assessment Educational statement
High-frequency hearing loss possibly affecting language development and school performance	Cisplatin	Hearing assessment at end of treatment ENT referral if necessary
Cataracts	Cranial irradiation Total body irradiation (TBI) Prolonged steroid treatment	Annual eye check in clinic Ophthalmology referral once cataracts suspected
Left ventricular failure Congestive heart failure Coronary artery disease Cardiac arrhythmias Sudden death[32]	Anthracyclines: 1. Doxorubicin 2. Daunorubicin Cyclophosphamide (high-dose) Mitoxantrone (mitozantrone) High-dose radiotherapy (40 Gy) to heart area	Chest X-ray, ECG and echocardiogram at end of treatment Echocardiogram 5 yearly Referral to cardiac specialist if necessary
Interstitial pneumonitis Pulmonary fibrosis	Bleomycin BCNU/ CCNU Busulfan Cyclophosphamide Methotrexate Melphalan Vinblastine High-dose chemotherapy + lung irradiation + TBI	If symptomatic: 1. Chest X-ray 2. Lung function tests Referral to respiratory specialist Health education about regular exercise and dangers of smoking Care during anaesthesia
Acute renal toxicity (related to dose and length of treatment): e.g. >50 mg/m^2 50–75% of children will have problems[33,34]	Cisplatin Cyclophosphamide Ifosfamide	Glomerular filtration rate (GFR) at end of treatment Then annual: 1. Urea, electrolyte and creatinine measurements
Fibrosis of bladder wall Haemorrhagic cystitis Atypical bladder epithelium Renal tubular necrosis Invasive carcinoma of bladder (rare)	Cyclophosphamide	2. GFR and renal ultrasound 3. BP 4. Early morning urine for creatinine/ protein ratio
Liver impairment (rarely liver failure)	Methotrexate 6-mercaptopurine	Liver function tests at end of treatment Advice about alcohol intake where appropriate
Second malignancy	Radiotherapy Chemotherapy, including high doses of alkylating agents Genetic predisposition for malignancy Previous history of Hodgkin's disease[34] Previous history of ovarian cancer History of familial retinoblastoma	Health education: 1. Healthy eating 2. Adequate exercise 3. Avoidance of smoking 4. Use of skin protection in sunlight Information about risk of second malignancy
Psychological problems[35]	Anxiety Fearfulness School phobia Emotional difficulties	Psychological support available to child and family through initial treatment and long-term follow-up

Table 35.9   Gonadal failure

Chemotherapy agent	Side effect – males	Side effect – females
Alkylating agents, including: cyclophosphamide procarbazine	Damage to germinal epithilium & Sertoli cells can cause poor/absent sperm production. Cyclophosphamide in total doses above 11 g can cause azoospermia. Some patients show a slow recovery in sperm counts many years after treatment. Leydig cells are not damaged by cyclophosphamide; thus, the development of secondary sexual characteristics occurs as normal through puberty.[33,36] 50% of prepubertal boys who receive cyclophosphamide and TBI for BMT will develop small testes and raised basal FSH levels, indicative of testicular damage. Occasional damage to Leydig cells and production of testosterone	Ovarian failure Prepubertal girls appear to be less affected than postpubertal women.[37] High-dose cyclophosphamide and TBI increase risk of ovarian failure.[32,33] Chemotherapy can reduce availability of eggs, thereby inducing early menopause[33]
MOPP (nitrogen mustard, vincristine, procarbazine and prednisone)	Azoospermia/subfertility	
ABVD (doxorubicin, bleomycin, vinblastine and dacarbazine) chemotherapy	Less toxic than MOPP but can cause transient azoospermia[32]	
Radiotherapy to ovaries, spine, brain		Radiotherapy, more so than chemotherapy, appears to affect the gonads in females

Table 35.10   Long-term follow-up guidelines for chemotherapy related endocrine late effects

Endocrine problem	Long-term follow-up guidelines
Gonadal failure	*Referral to a paediatric endocrinologist for:* Annual monitoring of growth and pubertal staging using the Tanner scoring system[38] during puberty Luteinising hormone (LH), follicle-stimulating hormone (FSH), testosterone (m) and oestrogen (f) checked annually Testosterone/oestrogen replacement to induce puberty and maintain secondary sexual characteristics if gonadal failure evident In girls, use of hormone replacement therapy (HRT) to induce menstruation Pubertal and adult women – detailed history of menstrual cycle Advice about appropriate use of contraception Information to girls about the potential risk of early menopause and implications for fertility in adulthood Referral to a fertility specialist as soon as couples want to start planning to conceive.
Growth failure	*Referral to a paediatric endocrinologist for:* 6/12 or annual measurements of height, sitting height and leg length (to determine annual growth velocity and to check upper and lower body proportions) Pituitary function testing for growth hormone deficiency if growth velocity falls below average for the age of the child Treatment with growth hormone, if growth hormone deficiency/insufficiency present.

Table 35.11 Summary of chemotherapy long-term effects

Cytotoxic agent	Cardiac	Endocrine growth	Endocrine fertility	Renal	Respiratory	Neurological	Hearing	Liver	Second malignancy
Actinomycin D								×	
BCNU			×	×	×				×
Bleomycin					×			×	
Busulfan		×	×		×				×
Carboplatin			×	×			×		
CCNU			×	×	×				
Chlorambucil			×						×
Cisplatin			×	×			×		×
Cyclophosphamide	×	×	×	× (bladder)	×				×
Cytarabine			×			×			
Dacarbazine			×						
Dactinomycin				×					
Daunorubicin	×								
Doxorubicin	×			×	×				
Epirubicin	×								
Idarubicin	×								
Ifosfamide			×	×		×			
Methotrexate				×	×			×	×
Melphalan			×	×	×				×
Mitoxantrone (mitozantrone)	×								
Chlormethine (mustine)			×	×					
Procarbazine			×		×				
Vinblastine			×						
Vincristine			×			×			
Etoposide			×						×
6-mercaptopurine								×	

gonads, and thus can cause problems with pubertal development and fertility.[38,43]

Preserving fertility

Sperm banking should be offered to teenagers or older males who have reached mature pubertal status at diagnosis and should be done if possible before cancer treatment commences.

At present, routine methods for preserving fertility in females are not available. Cryopreservation of ovarian tissue in females is still experimental; however, it is anticipated that future technology will make it possible to extract ovacytes from the cryopreserved tissue. This technique is not widely available and is usually only carried out in experienced research centres. Table 35.10 gives long-term follow-up guidelines for patients with gonadal failure.

Growth failure

Growth failure can occur during any chronic childhood illness, and treatment for childhood cancer is no exception. With chemotherapy treatment alone, however, long-term growth problems would not be expected. Some degree of growth failure can be seen after intense chemotherapy regimens.[43] Treatment with cyclophosphamide and busulfan, used as conditioning for BMT, can cause growth hormone insufficiency (inadequate levels of growth hormone are produced by the pituitary gland).[39] Table 35.10 gives long-term follow-up guidelines for patients with growth failure.

CONCLUSION

Long-term follow-up of survivors of childhood cancer ensures that accurate data about the late effects of cancer treatment are collected. Table 35.11 provides a summary of the late effects seen with chemotherapy treatment. This is a process that benefits both existing and future survivors of childhood cancer.[37] Current survivors are able to access appropriate healthcare support and treatment when required, and regular monitoring and collection of data enable future treatment regimens to be adjusted, with the aim of achieving cure, but minimising long-term side effects. It is important that the cost of cure be balanced against the risks associated with long-term effects of treatment.[36]

References – text

1. Terracini B, Coebergh JW, Gatta G, et al. Childhood cancer survival in Europe: an overview. Eur J Cancer 2001; 37(6):810–816.
2. Stiller CR. Centralisation of treatment and survival rates for cancer. Arch Dis Child 1988; 63:23–30.
3. Hollis R. Childhood cancer into the 21st century. Paediatr Nurs 1997; 9(3):12–15.
4. Muir KR, Parkes SE, Boon R, et al. Shared care in paediatric oncology. J Cancer Care 1992; 1(1):15–17.
5. Patel N, Sepion B, Williams J. Development of a shared care programme for children with cancer. J Cancer Nurs 1997; 1(3):147–150.
6. Edwards J, Breen M. Intravenous chemotherapy for children at home. Cancer Nurs Pract 2002; 1(5):26–29.
7. Groenwald SL, Hansen Frogge M, Goodman M, et al. Cancer nursing. Principles and practice. 4th edn. London: Jones and Bartlett; 1997.
8. Kellie SJ. Serum markers in tumour diagnosis and treatment. In: Pinkerton CR, Plowman PN, eds. Paediatric oncology. Clinical practice and controversies. London: Chapman and Hall Medical; 1997:108–135.
9. Balis FM, Holcenberg JS, Blaney SM. General principles of chemotherapy. In: Pizzo PA, Poplack DG, eds. Principles and practice of pediatric oncology. London: Lippincott, Williams and Wilkins; 2002:237–308.
10. Alcoser PW, Rodgers C. Treatment strategies in childhood cancer. J Pediatr Nurs 2003; 18(2):103–112.
11. Hooker L, Palmer S. Administration of chemotherapy. In: Gibson F, Evans M, eds. Paediatric oncology. Acute nursing care. London: Whurr; 1999:22–58.
12. Wallace WH, Thomson AB. Preservation of fertility in children treated for cancer. Arch Dis Child 2003; 88(6):493–496.
13. Bahadur G, Ling KL, Hart R, et al. Semen quality and cryopreservation in adolescent cancer patients. Hum Reprod 2002; 17(12):3157–3161.
14. Bahadur G, Ling KL, Hart R, et al. Semen production in adolescent cancer patients. Hum Reprod 2002; 17(10):2654–2656.
15. Hollis R, Denton S, Dixon G. General surgery. In: Gibson F, Evans M, eds. Paediatric oncology. Acute nursing care. London: Whurr; 1999:277–317.
16. Chessells JM. Recent advances in management of acute leukaemia. Arch Dis Child 2000; 82:438–442.
17. Lampert F, Henze G. Acute lymphoblastic leukaemia. In: Pinkerton CR, Plowman PN, edis. Paediatric oncology, clinical practice and controversies. London: Chapman and Hall Medical: 1997:258–277.
18. Bleyer WA, Danielson MG. Oral cancer chemotherapy in pediatric patients. Obstacles and potential for development and utilisation. Drugs 1999; 58(3):133–140.
19. Health Service Circular. Safe administration of intrathecal chemotherapy. 022. 2001. London: Department of Health; 2001.
20. Muller DJ, Harris PJ, Wattley L. Nursing children, psychology research and practice. London: Harper and Row; 1986.
21. Campbell S, Glasper EA. Children's nursing. London: Mosby; 1995.

22. While AE. An evaluation of a paediatric home care scheme. J Adv Nurs 1991; 16:1413–1421.

23. Chessells JM. Maintenance treatment and shared care in lymphoblastic leukaemia. Arch Dis Child 1993; 73:368–373.

24. Wujcik D. Infection control in oncology patients. Nurs Clin N Am 1993; 28(3):639–650.

25. Wetzel RC, Tobin JR. Shock. In: Rogers MC, ed. Textbook of pediatric intensive care. Baltimore: Williams and Wilkins; 1992:563–613.

26. Mays CL. Central venous catheters. The Children's Hospital Oakland. Hematology/oncology handbook. St Louis: Mosby, 2002:14–144.

27. Lowis SP, Oakhill A. Management of acute complications of therapy. In: Pinkerton CR, Plowman PN, eds. London: Chapman Hall Medical; 1997:677–705.

28. Health and Safety Executive. Control of Substances Hazardous to Health Regulations. London: HMSO; 1999.

29. Hargrave DR, Hann II, Richards SM, et al. Progressive reduction in treatment-related deaths in Medical Research Council Childhood Lymphoblastic Leukaemia Trials from 1980 to 1997 (UKALL VIII, X and XI). Br J Haematol 2001; 112(2):293–299.

30. Salisbury D, Begg N. Immunisations against infectious diseases. London: The Stationary Office; 1996.

31. Immunisations of the immunocompromised child: Best Practice Statement. London: Royal College of Paediatrics and Child Health; 2002.

32. Pinkerton CR. In: Devine T, ed. Oral chemotherapy in palliative care. 2001.

33. Devine T. Presenting a case for involving children with a terminal illness in clinical trials. Int J Palliat Nurs 2001; 7(4):162,164,166–170. 2001; 7(10):482–484.

34. International Conference on Harmonisation for the Registration of Pharmaceuticals for Human Use. Good practice guidelines: Consolidation Guidelines. Ottawa: Health Canada Publications; 1997.

35. Deelatt CA, Lampkin BC. Long-term survivors of childhood cancer: evaluation and identification of sequelae of treatment. CA-A Cancer J Clin 1992; 42(5):263–282.

36. Hobbie W, Ruccione K, Moore I. Late effects in long-term survivors. In: Foley GV, Fochtman D, Hardin Mooney K, eds. Nursing care of the child with cancer. London: WB Saunders; 1993:466–496.

37. Hawkins M, Stevens M. The long term survivors. Br Med Bull 1996; 52(4):898–923.

38. Chesterfield P. Late effects of chemotherapy. In: Gibson F, Evans M, eds. Paediatric oncology. Acute nursing care. London: Whurr; 1999:144–153.

39. Niethammer D, Mayer E. Long-term survivors: an overview on late effects, sequelae and second neoplasms. Bone Marrow Transplant 1998; 21(s2):s61–s63.

40. Kissen GDN, Wallace WHB. The United Kingdom Children's Cancer Study Group, Late Effects Group: long term follow-up therapy based guidelines. Milton Keynes: Pharmacia and Upjohn; 2000.

41. Cohen A, Roselle R, Mecca S. Endocrine late effects in children who underwent bone marrow transplantation: review. Bone Marrow Transplant 1998; 21(s2):s64–s67.

42. Leung W, Hudson M, Strickland D. Late effects of treatment in survivors of childhood acute myeloid leukaemia. J Clin Oncol 2000; 18(18):3273–3279.

43. Wallace, H. Late endocrine effects of cancer treatment in childhood. Reading: Colloid House Medical Publications; 1994.

44. Kazak AE. Psychological issues in childhood cancer survivors. J Assoc Pediatr Oncol Nurs 1989; 6(1):15–16.

45. Makipernaa A. Long-term quality of life and psychological coping after treatment of solid tumours in childhood. Acta Paediatrica Scand 1989; 78:728–735.

References – tables

1. Freifeld AC, Walsh TJ, Pizzo PA. Infectious complications in the pediatric cancer patient. In: Pizzo PA, Poplack DG, eds. Principles and practice of pediatric oncology. Philadelphia: Lippincott-Raven; 1997:1069–1114.

2. Buchanan GR. Hematologic supportive care of the pediatric cancer patient. In: Pizzo PA, Poplack DG, eds. Principles and practice of pediatric oncology. Philadelphia: Lippincott-Raven; 1997:1051–1068.

3. Michon J. Incidence of anemia in pediatric cancer patients in Europe: results of a large, international survey. Med Pediatr Oncol 2002; 39(4):448–450.

4. Aquino VM, Tkaczewski I, Buchanan GR. Early discharge of low-risk febrile neutropenic children and adolescents with cancer. Clin Infect Dis 1997; 25(1):74–78.

5. Oppenheim BA, Anderson H. Management of febrile neutropenia in low risk cancer patients. Thorax 2000; 55(Suppl 9): 63–69.

6. Bevan JA, Maloney KW, Hillery CA, et al. Bleeding disorders: a common cause of menorrhagia in adolescents. J Pediatr 2001; 138(6):856–861.

7. Varan A, Buyukpamukcu M, Kutluk T, et al. Recombinant human erythropoietin treatment for chemotherapy-related anemia in children. Pediatrics 1999; 103(2):E16.

8. Buyukpamukcu M, Varan A, Kutluk T, et al. Is epoetin alfa a treatment option for chemotherapy-related anemia in children? Med Pediatr Oncol 2002; 39(4):455–458.

9. Sallan SE, Billett AL. Management of nausea and vomiting. In: Pizzo PA, Poplack DG, eds. Principles and practice of pediatric oncology. Philadelphia: Lippincott-Raven; 1997: 1201–1208.

10. Hedstrom M, Haglund K, Skolin I, et al. Distressing events for children and adolescents with cancer: child,

parent, and nurse perceptions. J Pediatr Oncol Nurs 2003; 20(3):120–132.

11. Selwood K, Gibson F, Evans M. Side effects of chemotherapy. In: Gibson F, Evans M, eds. Paediatric oncology. Acute nursing care. London: Whurr; 1999:59–128.

12. Collins JJ, Brynes ME, Dunkel IJ, et al. The measurement of symptoms in children with cancer. J Pain Sympt Manage 2000; 19(5):363–373.

13. Andrassy RJ, Chwals WJ. Nutritional support of the pediatric oncology patient. Nutrition 1998; 14(1):124–129.

14. Gibson F, Face S, Hayden S, Morgan N. Nursing management of chemotherapy-induced nausea and vomiting in children. Current prescribing and administration practice – is it being used to its full potential? Eur J Oncol Nurs 2000;4(4):252–255.

15. Bennett-Rees N, Soanes L. Complications of bone marrow transplant. In: Gibson F, Evans M, eds. Paediatric oncology. Acute nursing care. London: Whurr; 1999:225–240.

16. Spijkervet FK, Sonis ST. New frontiers in the management of chemotherapy-induced mucositis. Curr Opin Oncol 1998; 10(Suppl 7):S23–27.

17. Bryant R. Managing side effects of childhood cancer. J Pediatr Nurs 2003; 18(2):113–125.

18. Aitken TJ. Gastrointestinal manifestations in the child with cancer. J Pediatr Oncol Nurs 1992; 9(3):99–109.

19. Alexander RH, Rickard KA, Godshall B. Nutritional supportive care. In: Pizzo PA, Poplack DG, eds. Principles and practice of pediatric oncology. Philadelphia: Lippincott-Raven; 1997:1167–1181.

20. Schneider SM, Workman ML. Virtual reality as a distraction intervention for older children receiving chemotherapy. Pediatr Nurs 2000; 26(6):593–597.

21. Parker RI, Prakash D, Mahan RA, et al. Randomized, double-blind, crossover, placebo-controlled trial of intravenous ondansetron for the prevention of intrathecal chemotherapy-induced vomiting in children. J Pediatr Hematol/Oncol 2001; 23(9):578–581.

22. White L, Daly SA, McKenna CJ, et al. A comparison of oral ondansetron syrup or intravenous ondansetron loading dose regimens given in combination with dexamethasone for the prevention of nausea and emesis in pediatric and adolescent patients receiving moderately/highly emetogenic chemotherapy. Pediatr Hematol Oncol 2000; 17(6):445–455.

23. Nelson W, Gibson F, Hayden S, et al. Using action research in paediatric oncology to develop an oral care algorithm. Eur J Oncol Nurs 2001; 5(3):180–189.

24. Kennedy L, Diamond J. Assessment and management of chemotherapy-induced mucositis in children. J Pediatr Oncol Nurs 1997; 14(3):164–174.

25. Anderson PM, Schroeder G, Skubitz KM. Oral glutamine reduces the duration and severity of stomatitis after cytotoxic cancer chemotherapy. Cancer 1998; 83(7):1433–1439.

26. Collins JJ, Geake J, Grier HE, et al. Patient-controlled analgesia for mucositis pain in children: a three-period crossover study comparing morphine and hydromorphone. J Pediatr 1996; 129(5):722–728.

27. Bowman LC, Williams R, Sanders M, et al. Algorithm for nutritional support: experience of the metabolic and infusion support service of St. Jude Children's Research Hospital. Int J Cancer 1998; 11:76–80.

28. Han-Markey T. Nutritional considerations in pediatric oncology. Semin Oncol Nurs 2000; 16(2):146–151.

29. der Broeder E, Lippens RJJ, van't Hof MA, et al. Effects of naso-gastric tube feeding on the nutritional status of children with cancer. Eur J Clin Nutr 1998; 52:494–499.

30. DeSwarte-Wallace J, Firouzbakhsh S, Finklestein JZ. Using research to change practice: enteral feedings for pediatric oncology patients. J Pediatr Oncol Nurs 2001; 18(5):217–223.

31. Niethammer D, Mayer E. Long-term survivors: an overview on late effects, sequelae and second neoplasms. Bone Marrow Transplant 1998; 21(s2):s61–s63.

32. Deelatt CA, Lampkin BC. Long-term survivors of childhood cancer: evaluation and identification of sequelae of treatment. CA-A Cancer J Clin 1992; 42(5):263–282.

33. Hobbie W, Ruccione K, Moore I. Late effects in long-term survivors. In: Foley GV, Fochtman D, Hardin Mooney K, eds. Nursing care of the child with cancer. London: WB Saunders; 1993:466–496.

34. Chesterfield P. Late effects of chemotherapy. In: Gibson F, Evans M, eds. Paediatric oncology. Acute nursing care. London: Whurr; 1999:144–153.

35. Allen L, Zigler E. Psychological adjustment of seriously ill children. J Am Acad Child Psychiatr 1986; 25(5):708–712.

36. Wallace, H. Late endocrine effects of cancer treatment in childhood. Reading: Colloid House Medical Publications; 1994.

37. Lanzkowsky P. Manual of pediatric hematology and oncology. 3rd edn. California: Academic Press; 2000.

38. Buckler J. A reference manual of growth and development. 2nd edn. Oxford: Blackwell Science; 1997.

39. Panzarrella C, Rasco Baggott C, Comeau M, et al. Management of disease and treatment-related complications. In: Rasco Baggott C, Paterson Kelly K, Fochtman D, et al., Vol eds. Nursing care of children and adolescents with cancer/ Association of Pediatric Oncology Nurses. 3rd edn. Philadelphia: WB Saunders; 2002.

Chapter **36**

Systemic therapy for breast cancer

CHAPTER CONTENTS

MEDICAL CARE FOR PATIENTS WITH BREAST CANCER

Stephen RD Johnston

GENERAL INFORMATION

Breast cancer affects one in 12 women in the UK and causes about 21 000 deaths per year. Prevalence is about five times higher, with over 100 000 women living with breast cancer at any one time. Of the 15 000 new cases of breast cancer per annum in the UK, the majority will present with primary early operable disease.[1]

The risk of breast cancer increases with age, doubling every 10 years up to the menopause. The cause of breast cancer in the majority of women is unknown. Risk factors include:

- early age at menarche
- older age at menopause
- older age at birth of first child
- family history
- previous benign pathological features on breast biopsy (i.e. atypical hyperplasia)
- excess alcohol intake
- radiation exposure to developing breast tissue
- oral contraceptive use
- postmenopausal hormone replacement therapy
- obesity.

The relative risk of developing breast cancer in different countries varies up to fivefold. Only approximately 5% of breast cancers can be attributed to mutations in the genes BRCA1 and BRCA2.[2]

Diagnosis

The majority of women present with a palpable lump in the breast that is either detected by themselves, or by a healthcare professional during a physical examination. Alternatively, breast cancer may be detected through screening mammography that is offered to the age group in the population with the highest incidence (age 50–65 years old). A diagnosis of breast cancer is confirmed through a 'triple assessment', which involves:

- clinical examination
- radiological assessment by mammogram or ultrasound
- cytological or histological confirmation by taking a fine-needle aspirate or biopsy from the suspicious area in the breast.

The primary management of breast cancer involves surgery for the majority of women. This may be curative in many instances, and it yields important further information about the individual cancer, which helps to determine an individual's prognosis. In addition, accurate staging and pathological assessment of the primary tumour influences whether subsequent treatment with radiotherapy, chemotherapy or endocrine therapy is required.

Definitions and staging information

In general, there are two types of breast cancer: invasive and non-invasive. Non-invasive ductal carcinoma in-situ (DCIS) or lobular carcinoma in-situ (LCIS) are tumours characterised by the presence of malignant cells in the breast ducts or lobules, but with no evidence that they breach the basement membrane which normally surrounds the epithelial cells within the normal breast ducts and lobules. This condition is most frequently detected by screening mammography, although in some women it may present as a palpable lump in the breast.

Invasive breast cancer involves the presence of malignant cells that have breached the basement membrane. Tumours arise from the epithelial cells that line either the ducts or lobules within the breast, giving rise to invasive ductal cancer (approximately 80–85% cases) or invasive lobular cancer (approximately 15–20%). Clinically, women with invasive breast cancer are separated into three main groups: those with early operable breast cancer, locally advanced disease or metastatic breast cancer.

Early operable breast cancer
Primary 'early operable' breast cancer is the presence of malignant disease that is confined to the breast (and/or axillary nodes) and which is of a size and in a position to render a potentially curative surgical procedure possible (this does not include locally advanced

disease or inflammatory breast cancers – see below). These can be further divided into those with tumours greater than 4 cm or multifocal cancers that are usually treated surgically by mastectomy, and those with tumours less than 4 cm or unifocal cancers that can be treated by breast conserving surgery (wide local excision or lumpectomy).

Although staging investigations will have found no metastatic disease at the time of diagnosis, these women are at risk of either local or distant recurrence. This risk is highest through the first 5 years, but still remains up to 15–20 years after surgery. While attempts have been made to establish an individual's risk of recurrence from various different prognostic factors, in clinical practice the following provide the most significant information:

- tumour size
- axillary node status
- oestrogen receptor (ER) status

In addition, high pathological grade (i.e. grade III poorly differentiated tumours) together with the presence of lymphovascular invasion are tumour factors associated with an increased risk of recurrence. Those with node-positive disease have a 50–60% chance of relapsing within 5 years, whereas for those with node-negative disease the risk is only 30–35%. Adjuvant systemic therapy is given to patients deemed to be at higher risk in order to eliminate micrometastatic disease remaining after surgery, thereby increasing the chance of cure.

Locally advanced breast cancer
Locally advanced breast cancer is formally defined according to the TNM staging system[3] as disease presentation with evidence (clinical or histopathological) of skin and/or chest wall involvement (ulceration or fixation), and/or axillary nodes matted together by tumour extension. Thus, it includes T4 a–d; N2 disease, but the absence of metastases (M0), i.e. stage IIIB. On a practical level patients are described as having 'locally advanced' breast cancer if they present with a primary breast cancer which is deemed unsuitable for primary surgery due to either:

- large size and fixation of tumour to underlying muscle or superficial skin
- local ulceration of tumour
- fixed loco-regional disease in the axilla
- presentation with inflammatory breast cancer.

Metastatic breast cancer
Women develop 'metastatic' breast cancer when there is either spread or recurrence of secondary tumours at

distant sites, including bone, liver, lung or soft tissue, and this is no longer treatable by surgery. Secondary tumours may develop despite adjuvant systemic drug therapy (where the aim was to eliminate micrometa-static disease following primary surgical treatment for early breast cancer). Once the disease has spread from the breast to form secondary sites of metastases, the condition is deemed incurable. However, very effective treatments can be given that may offer long periods of remission and good health in metastatic disease. The natural history of breast cancer is such that many patients, particularly those with slow-growing hormone-sensitive breast cancer, can live with their disease, which may be deemed more of a chronic condition.

TREATMENT OVERVIEW

Surgery and radiotherapy

The primary management of early operable breast cancer involves initial surgery (either breast conserv-ing surgery or mastectomy), followed by radiotherapy either to the breast (i.e. following wide local excision) or chest wall (i.e. after mastectomy). The aim of com-bined loco-regional treatment with surgery and radio-therapy is to remove the primary breast cancer and reduce as much as possible the risk of local recurrence within the breast or on the chest wall. The role of sur-gery to the axilla is to accurately stage the patient's tumour by determining whether there has been any spread to axillary lymph nodes, and also if there is axillary involvement to treat that disease by surgical removal. Following a full axillary dissection, additional radiotherapy to the axilla is not routinely given because it substantially increases the risk of subsequent arm lymphoedema (over 30%). However, depending on the extent of node involvement and risk of further regional recurrence, radiotherapy treatment fields may extend to include the supraclavicular fossa and/or internal mammary chain.

Systemic therapy

Early operable breast cancer

The use and role of systemic drugs in breast cancer therapy depends on the clinical stage of the disease. For women with early operable breast cancer, systemic drugs (either chemotherapy or endocrine therapy, or the combination of both) are used to further reduce the risk of recurrence, in particular the risk of metastatic recurrence (secondary tumours) at distant sites. These drug treatments may be given in the adjuvant setting (i.e. following initial primary surgical therapy), or for large primary cancers in the neoadjuvant setting

(i.e. before surgery is undertaken). The aim of systemic drug treatment in the adjuvant or neoadjuvant setting is to enhance the chance of cure by eliminating any cells (micrometastatic disease) that may exist at the time of diagnosis. As discussed below, there is clear evidence that both adjuvant systemic chemotherapy and adjuvant endocrine therapy (tamoxifen or ovarian ablation) can further reduce the risk of breast cancer recurrence and improve overall survival. Indeed, the wider use of such therapies in the UK since the mid 1980s has almost certainly accounted for the significant and consistent fall in breast cancer mortality which has been observed since 1990.[4]

Locally advanced breast cancer

For women with locally advanced breast cancer that cannot be managed by initial surgery, treatment may involve either radical radiotherapy to the breast, or alter-natively initial systemic-drugs (usually chemotherapy and/or endocrine therapy, depending on the oestrogen receptor status). Because women with locally advanced breast cancer have a much higher risk of recurrent disease within the breast, if there is successful tumour shrinkage following systemic drug therapy, the patient may be offered surgery and/or radiotherapy with the aim of increasing the chance of local control within the breast.

Metastatic breast cancer

For metastatic breast cancer, the main role of systemic drug treatment is to palliate symptoms of advanced disease through the effective control of tumour growth. Drugs are more likely to be used when patients have activation of their disease, with the aim of inducing a remission or stabilisation of the tumour, and consequently improving the patient's quality of life. Treatments tend to be used in sequence, and patients may initially benefit from endocrine therapy if they have an oestrogen receptor-positive (ER+ve) cancer before chemotherapy is considered. Equally, the management of bone metastases has been signifi-cantly enhanced by the use of bisphosphonates to treat hypercalcaemia, control bone pain and, more recently, to reduce the incidence of subsequent frac-tures and prevent the progression of disease activity within the bone. There is an increasing use of adju-vant endocrine and cytotoxic systemic therapies in early breast cancer. The interval since completion of such treatment and the development of metastases (disease-free interval) is an increasingly important factor in determining whether metastatic disease is likely to be resistant to further systemic therapy, and which treatment options may be successful in the advanced setting.[5]

SYSTEMIC ADJUVANT THERAPY FOR EARLY BREAST CANCER

The aim of systemic adjuvant therapy is to reduce the risk of breast cancer recurrence, which for some patients may translate into an increased chance of cure and long-term survival free of breast cancer. The evidence that such therapy is effective has come from large randomised controlled trials (RCTs) of adjuvant therapy in early operable breast cancer. The data from these trials have been analysed in world overviews or meta-analyses and, as such, these describe the beneficial effects of adjuvant systemic therapy for patients with early breast cancer. This benefit is expressed either as the proportional reduction in the annual odds of recurrence or death (i.e. the odds ratio or hazard ratio), or as an absolute improvement in either the 5- or 10-year recurrence-free survival or overall survival. Any percentage improvement in survival is generally much less than the impact on recurrence.

The currently available treatments for systemic adjuvant therapy in early operable breast cancer include one of the following four options:

- combination chemotherapy, which involves two or more cytotoxic drugs given intravenously every 3–4 weeks for between 4 and 6 months.
- tamoxifen, a non-steroidal antioestrogen taken as daily oral endocrine therapy for between 2 and 5 years
- ovarian ablation, which may involve surgical bilateral ovariectomy, radiation-induced oophorectomy or medical suppression of ovarian function with LHRH (luteinising hormone releasing hormone) agonists as endocrine therapy for premenopausal women
- sequential chemo–endocrine therapy
- aromatase inhibitors.

The decision to use systemic adjuvant therapy, and more importantly of which option to use, is made primarily on the presence or absence of one or more adverse pathological features in the primary breast cancer. The five most important pathological features relate to:

- tumour size
- axillary nodal involvement
- histological grade
- lymphovascular invasion
- oestrogen receptor status.

In many circumstances where ER+ve tumours are associated with nodal involvement and/or lymphovascular invasion, sequential chemo–endocrine therapy is administered. Age, menopausal status and general fitness are also patient-related factors that are considered in decisions about systemic adjuvant therapy. For example, in premenopausal women the option of ovarian ablation also exists either as an alternative to chemotherapy in some circumstances, or as the optimal endocrine treatment, perhaps in conjunction with tamoxifen. Likewise, the benefit of chemotherapy is somewhat less in women aged over 70 years old than in those aged 30–35 years old. Finally, it is increasingly common that the patient's own perspective of benefit vs harm impacts on what degree of risk reduction they would accept 6 months of cytotoxic chemotherapy for.

Combination chemotherapy in early breast cancer

Systemic adjuvant chemotherapy can produce a significant reduction in risk of recurrence and improvement in overall survival for a wide range of women with early breast cancer. The benefit appears to be independent of axillary nodal or menopausal status, although the absolute improvements are greater in those with node-positive disease. Most evidence of benefit comes from studies in women under 50 years old, but women aged 50–69 years old have also been shown to benefit from combination chemotherapy, although the degree of absolute benefit and tolerability of treatment may be somewhat less than in younger patients.

Absolute benefit of adjuvant chemotherapy – overview meta-analysis

A systematic review of 47 RCTs has compared the outcome in terms of recurrence and overall survival in over 18 000 women with early breast cancer randomised to either administration of combination chemotherapy or no chemotherapy.[6] For women aged under 50 years old, there was a highly significant proportional reduction in recurrence (35 ± 4%, two-sided significance $p < 0.00001$) and all cause-related death (27 ± 5%, $p < 0.00001$). For women aged 50–69 years old, a smaller but still significant proportional reductions in recurrence (20 ± 8%, $p < 0.00001$) and death (11 ± 3%, $p = 0.001$) was seen. Proportional reductions were similar for women with node-negative and node-positive disease, and the 10-year survival according to nodal status and age together with the improvement in absolute survival with adjuvant combination chemotherapy is summarised in Table 36.1.

Toxicity of adjuvant chemotherapy

In general terms, the toxicities of combination chemotherapy may include:

- nausea and vomiting
- alopecia

Table 36.1 10-year survival with combination chemotherapy vs placebo, according to nodal status and age

	Control	Chemotherapy	Absolute benefit	SD	Significance (two-sided)
Age <50 years old:					
Node +ve	41.4%	53.8%	+12.4%	2.4	$p < 0.00001$
Node −ve	71.9%	77.6%	+5.7%	2.1	$p = 0.02$
Age 50–69 years old:					
Node +ve	46.3%	48.6%	+2.3%	1.3	$p = 0.002$
Node −ve	64.8%	71.2%	+6.4%	2.3	$p = 0.005$

- bone marrow suppression
- fatigue and
- gastrointestinal disturbances.

These side effects are usually mild, short term and fully reversible. Prolonged chemotherapy is much more likely to be associated with lethargy and haematological toxicity (anaemia and neutropenia), whereas anthracycline regimens will invariably induce complete alopecia. Fertility and ovarian function may be permanently affected by chemotherapy, especially in women aged over 40 years old, although for some patients with hormone-dependent cancer this could contribute to the adjuvant benefit derived (see Ovarian ablation section below). Long-term risks following chemotherapy may include induction of second cancers (especially haematological malignancies, although the risk is very low) and cardiac impairment with cumulative anthracycline dosages. Provided the cumulative dose of doxorubicin does not exceed 400 mg/m^2, the risk of congestive heart failure is <1%.

Which is the optimal adjuvant chemotherapy regimen?

There is no clear consensus on which is the optimal 'standard' adjuvant chemotherapy regimen for early breast cancer, although there may be benefits for some drugs or regimens in certain patients. The most widely used regimen in clinical trials was CMF (cyclophosphamide, methotrexate and 5-fluorouracil or 5-FU). Directly randomised comparisons of 'more' vs 'less' prolonged polychemotherapy have failed to show any additional survival advantage in using more than a few months chemotherapy. A systematic review of 11 RCTs involving 6104 patients compared longer regimens (which doubled the length of chemotherapy from between 4 and 6 months to between 8 and 12 months) vs shorter chemotherapy regimens and showed no additional benefit.[6] Likewise, increasing either the total dose or the dose intensity of any one of the drugs has not been shown to improve outcome. Several RCTs have failed to show significant improvement from enhanced-dose regimens,[7] whereas others have

demonstrated reduced efficacy approaching untreated controls when suboptimal doses are used.[8]

A systematic review of 11 trials involving 5942 patients[6] compared various anthracycline-containing regimens (i.e. AC, FEC, CAF) which include either of the drugs doxorubicin (Adriamycin) or 4-epi-doxorubicin (epirubicin) vs the standard CMF regimen. This showed a significant ($p = 0.006$) reduction in recurrence rates for anthracycline regimens, with a modest but significant improvement in 5-year survival (69% to 72%; $p = 0.02$). However, the absolute benefits of these regimens must be balanced against their toxicity for individual patient groups: for example, in older patients. Alternating sequences of cytotoxic agents may prove an effective way of circumventing acquired drug resistance and thus enhancing the efficacy of a regimen, such as the Milan regimen of single agent anthracycline followed by standard CMF chemotherapy.[9]

New drugs and delivery strategies New and highly active cytotoxic agents such as the taxanes are currently being examined with anthracyclines either in combination or sequence. Preliminary results with paclitaxel (Taxol) given for 4 cycles after conventional doxorubicin/cyclophosphamide (AC) have suggested a significant further improvement in disease-free and overall survival. However, there remains no consensus regarding the role of taxanes as adjuvant chemotherapy in breast cancer, especially as one other similar trial appears to show no benefit.[10] Several current trials continue to address this issue.

There is no evidence from RCTs that high-dose chemotherapy with haematological support (bone marrow transplantation or peripheral stem cell support) in patients with high-risk early breast cancer (i.e. >10 positive lymph nodes).[11] With some studies reporting evidence of treatment-related mortality for high-dose therapy without any evidence that breast cancer mortality is improved, this treatment is not recommended as standard therapy even for high-risk patients, unless in the context of a clinical trial.

Finally, delivering chemotherapy every 2 weeks with haematological growth factor support may be more effective than conventional 3 week therapy, and ongoing trails continue to assess this as a better delivery strategy.

Tamoxifen

In postmenopausal patients, adjuvant tamoxifen taken for up to 5 years can significantly reduce the annual odds of recurrence and death. An overview meta-analysis has provided evidence that benefit is seen only in those with ER+ve tumours and that this occurs irrespective of age, menopausal status, nodal involvement or the addition of chemotherapy. Five years of therapy with tamoxifen is significantly better than shorter durations, but the available evidence shows no benefit associated with prolonging treatment beyond 5 years. Tamoxifen carries a slightly increased risk of endometrial cancer, but has no overall effect on non-breast cancer mortality.

Absolute benefit of adjuvant tamoxifen – overview meta-analysis

A systematic review of 55 RCTs in 37 000 women with early breast cancer has compared the benefit of adjuvant tamoxifen vs placebo.[12] For women aged >50 years old, who are usually postmenopausal, tamoxifen reduced the annual odds of recurrence by 29%, and of death from any cause by 20%. Five years of adjuvant tamoxifen had an equally substantial effect on recurrence and long-term survival in all age groups (Table 36.2).

This implies that for women with ER+ve tumours, adjuvant tamoxifen has a highly significant effect, irrespective of age or menopausal status. Likewise, benefit was found in women irrespective of axillary nodal status.

Women with ER+ve tumours benefited most from treatment with tamoxifen, emphasising the importance of oestrogen receptor measurement in the assessment of primary breast carcinomas. The proportional reduction in recurrence for women with ER+ve tumours was $50 \pm 4\%$, compared with $6 \pm 11\%$ for those with oestrogen receptor-negative (ER–ve) tumours. For women with completely ER–ve disease, the overall benefits of adjuvant tamoxifen remain a matter

Table 36.2	Absolute benefit of adjuvant tamoxifen
Age (years old)	Proportional reduction in recurrence
<50	$45 \pm 8\%$
50–59	$37 \pm 6\%$
60–69	$54 \pm 5\%$
>70	$54 \pm 13\%$

for research, although they may still derive other preventative benefits, as there is a $47 \pm 9\%$ reduction ($p < 0.00001$) in contralateral breast cancer rate for those who took tamoxifen for 5 years.

Optimal duration of adjuvant tamoxifen

The proportional reduction in recurrence was significantly greater with increasing duration of adjuvant tamoxifen ($p < 0.00001$). This corresponded with a $26 \pm 4\%$ proportional reduction in death for 5 years of tamoxifen, compared with only $12 \pm 3\%$ for 1 year of tamoxifen usage. For those who took 5 years of tamoxifen, the absolute improvement in 10-year survival is shown in Table 36.3. These findings were confirmed by an RCT comparing 5 years vs 2 years of adjuvant tamoxifen.[13]

The benefits and risks of prolonged therapy beyond 5 years are unclear. In the largest trial[14] in the systematic review,[12] 1153 patients who had completed 5 years of tamoxifen were randomised to either placebo or 5 more years of tamoxifen. Disease-free survival after 4 years further follow-up was greater for those switched to placebo rather than those who continued tamoxifen (92% vs 86%, $p = 0.003$), although this did not impact on overall survival. Other studies have shown no detriment in continuing tamoxifen beyond 5 years, but equally have failed to demonstrate any further improvement.[15] Two major international trials of tamoxifen duration are in progress (aTTom and ATLAS), although because of concerns regarding long-term toxicity with tamoxifen (see below) and in the absence of further definitive data, current practice has been to recommend tamoxifen for 5 years outside the setting of a clinical trial.

Long-term risks with adjuvant tamoxifen

Tamoxifen is associated with a small but statistically significant increased risk of endometrial cancer. The systematic review found an increased hazard ratio of 2.58 ± 0.35 for any duration of tamoxifen usage.[12] For 5 years of tamoxifen, this resulted in a cumulative risk over 10 years of 2 endometrial cancer-related deaths (95% CI 0–4) per 1000 women.[16] There was no evidence of an increased incidence of other cancers.

Bone loss in premenopausal women (1.4% bone loss per annum) does occur with tamoxifen,[17] although in postmenopausal women tamoxifen has bone-protective effects because of the drug's partial agonist effects on that tissue.[18] Mixed effects on cardiovascular risk are seen with tamoxifen, with a significant reduction in low-density lipoprotein cholesterol, associated with a reduced incidence of myocardial infarction in some studies, but an increased risk of thrombosis, which may correlate with 1 extra death per 5000 women years of tamoxifen attributed to

Table 36.3 10-year survival in treated (tamoxifen for 5 years) vs control patients

	Control	Tamoxifen	Absolute benefit	SD	Significance (two-sided)
Node +ve	50.5%	61.4%	+10.9%	2.5	$p < 0.00001$
Node –ve	73.3%	78.9%	+5.6%	1.3	$p < 0.00001$

pulmonary embolus. However, no statistical increase was seen in other non-breast cancer-related mortality (i.e. cardiac or vascular) with tamoxifen usage in the overview analysis,[12] and in general the drug is perceived to be extremely safe.

Summary

For women with ER+ve early operable breast cancer, the substantial benefits from tamoxifen in reducing breast cancer mortality in the adjuvant setting significantly outweigh any small increased risk from any long-term toxicities. The widespread use of tamoxifen may be the major reason for the improved mortality from the disease.[19] The risk–benefit ratio may vary amongst different patient groups, with the current overview suggesting that ER–ve patients derive little improvement in survival from tamoxifen. Even in ER+ve patients, the benefit of reducing breast cancer mortality could be offset with prolonged therapy beyond 5 years (by the emergence of drug-resistant breast cancer and adverse effects on the endometrium), and thus results of long-term adjuvant tamoxifen trials are awaited.

Ovarian ablation

For women aged under 50 years old with early breast cancer, it has been shown that ablation of functioning ovaries (either by irradiation or surgery) significantly improves long-term survival. This benefit may occur in the absence of adjuvant chemotherapy. A systematic review of 12 trials ($n = 2102$) with at least 15 years follow-up in premenopausal women compared ovarian ablation by irradiation or surgery with no ablation.[20] There was a significant improvement in both 10-year recurrence-free survival (45% vs 39%, $p = 0.0007$) and overall survival (52.4% vs 46.1%, $p = 0.001$). The benefit was independent of axillary nodal status. There is no good evidence on the long-term effects on the body of ovarian ablation. Concerns exist about the late sequelae, especially the effect on bone mineral density and cardiovascular risk. The acute side effects are usually menopausal symptoms such as hot flushes, mood disturbance and vaginal dryness.

In the five trials that compared ovarian ablation and chemotherapy vs chemotherapy alone, the absolute benefit of ablation was smaller than in trials of ovarian ablation alone. This may be explained by the fact that cytotoxic chemotherapy may itself suppress ovarian function in premenopausal women, making the effect of ovarian ablation difficult to detect in such combined trials. When only premenopausal women were considered in the absence of chemotherapy, there was a 27% proportional improvement in recurrence-free survival. Several RCTs in progress are addressing the role of gonadotrophin-releasing hormone analogues (LHRH agonists) such as goserelin (Zoladex), which are delivered by depot subcutaneous injections monthly, and induce a medical oophorectomy. The advantage of this approach is that treatment is reversible, which allows preservation of fertility in younger women with oestrogen receptor-positive tumours. Early results suggest that in ER+ve premenopausal women, the effects of goserelin (administered for 2–3 years) are at least as good as CMF chemotherapy. Furthermore, an ECOG trial showed that the addition of goserelin to anthracycline chemotherapy in women who were still premenopausal following chemotherapy led to a further significant improvement in overall survival. At least two of the trials (UK and Sweden) are addressing the role of these drugs alone or in combination with tamoxifen as adjuvant endocrine therapy for premenopausal women.

Adjuvant aromatase inhibitors

A large randomised trial has recently reported that, for postmenopausal women, the aromatase inhibitor anastrozole (which induces maximal oestrogen suppression) may be a more effective and better-tolerated treatment option than tamoxifen.[21] In the trial of 9366 patients, preliminary results after a median of 33 months follow-up have shown a significant improvement in 3-year disease-free survival of 89.4% for anastrozole compared with 87.4% for tamoxifen (hazard ratio 0.83, 95% CI 0.71–0.96, $p = 0.013$). While further follow-up of this trial is needed to see if survival is improved, the side-effect profile was better for anastrozole. Incidence of endometrial cancer ($p = 0.02$), less vaginal bleeding and discharge ($p < 0.0001$), cerebrovascular events ($p = 0.0006$), hot flushes ($p < 0.0001$) and venous thromboembolic events ($p = 0.0006$) were all significantly reduced. However, anastrozole was associated with more musculoskeletal events and a higher incidence of fractures (p <0.0001), raising concerns about the potential long-term effects on bone mineral density. These preliminary results are very encouraging, and for the first time offer an alternative endocrine therapy for postmenopausal women in situations where there may be concerns about the potential risks of tamoxifen.

More recently, trials have suggested that switching to aromatase inhibitors after 2–3 years of tamoxifen may be superior to 5 years of tamoxifen alone. Likewise, extended adjuvant therapy beyond 5 years of tamoxifen with letrazole has proved superior to placebo, with significant improvement in overall disease-free survival (hazard ratio 0.57, 95% CI 0.43–0.75, p=0.00008)[22] and for node-positive patients an improvement in overall survival (hazard ratio 0.61, 95% CI 0.38–0.97, p=0.04).

Summary

There no longer appears to be limited subgroups of patients who should or should not receive adjuvant chemotherapy, as potential exists for some degree of benefit from adjuvant systemic therapy for most women. The information on the benefit of 5 years of tamoxifen is now very clear for women with ER+ve breast cancer, and it is likely that this occurs independent of chemotherapy. Finally, radiotherapy, which has always been deemed important after breast conserving surgery in reducing the local recurrence rate, may also impact on survival from systemic relapse. RCTs have shown that in premenopausal women with high-risk disease, the addition of radiotherapy to CMF chemotherapy following mastectomy improved survival from 34% to 48%.[23] While different treatment modalities may each have an impact on outcome in the adjuvant setting, the side effects of each treatment need to be weighed against the absolute quantitative benefit for a given individual patient. It remains difficult to give general recommendations of treatment for patient groups, and decisions must continue to be made on an individual patient basis in consultation with an experienced oncologist.

SYSTEMIC THERAPY FOR LOCALLY ADVANCED/METASTATIC BREAST CANCER

The role of systemic therapy in locally advanced breast cancer that is inoperable is to cause tumour shrinkage and improve the chances of local control within the breast. The goal of treatment for women with metastatic breast cancer is often considered palliative, although again this is achieved by controlling tumour growth and inducing a remission. Both endocrine therapy and chemotherapy are used as systemic therapies in both groups of patients to induce tumour regression. As such, these treatments (in conjunction with supportive care measures) relieve tumour-related symptoms, either within the breast in those with locally advanced disease, or in specific sites of secondary disease such as the lungs, liver or bone. In addition, bisphosphonates represent a specific systemic therapy option for the management of bone metastases, while the first biological therapy for advanced breast cancer has recently been introduced.

The choice of initial systemic treatment, in particular whether endocrine or chemotherapy is used first, is based on a variety of clinical factors (see Table 36.4). The decision for an individual patient and clinician of which specific drug or regimen to use (either alone or in combination) is dependent on several factors. These include prior therapies received in the adjuvant and/or metastatic setting in association with the response and progression-free interval,[5] together with the likelihood of benefit from any proposed therapy balanced against a given drug's side effects and tolerability profile for that patient. Until the recent introduction of some of the new therapies, it had been considered by many that systemic drug treatments for advanced breast cancer were likely to have a very minimal impact on overall survival. However, the significant gains in efficacy seen with new hormone, cytotoxic and biological therapies have already produced evidence that these drugs may significantly improve tumour response rates and quality of life and also impact on patient survival, even in metastatic disease.

Endocrine therapy

Approximately two-thirds of human breast carcinomas express oestrogen receptors (ERs) and thus may be dependent on oestrogen for their growth. Routine immunohistochemical assays on paraffin-embedded tissue that can be performed retrospectively on the excised primary tumour mean that this information should now be available for all breast cancer patients. For these patients, endocrine treatment options when they develop locally advanced or metastatic breast cancer include tamoxifen, aromatase inhibitors for postmenopausal women, LHRH agonists for premenopausal women, and progestins.

Tamoxifen

Tamoxifen is an oral, non-steroidal, competitive ER antagonist that has been the first-line endocrine agent of choice for hormone-sensitive metastatic disease.[24] The likelihood of responding to tamoxifen is maximal in those with ER+ve disease (60–70%) with a median duration of response of 12–15 months.[25–27] Tamoxifen is well tolerated in women with advanced breast cancer: less than 3% of women discontinue tamoxifen as a result of toxicity, and reported adverse effects include minor gastrointestinal upset (8%), hot flushes (27%), and menstrual disturbance in premenopausal women (13%).[28] For those with bone metastases, tumour flare may occur in <5% who are treated with tamoxifen, and this can result in increased pain or symptomatic hypercalcaemia.

A key problem in advanced breast cancer is that most women (>90%) who initially respond to tamoxifen subsequently relapse and develop acquired resistance. However, it is clear that in these cases their tumours can remain endocrine-sensitive and respond to further hormonal interventions.[29] However, an emerging scenario is that most patients have already received tamoxifen in the adjuvant setting and often relapse with metastatic disease while still taking tamoxifen. For these patients, therapies with aromatase inhibitors or LHRH agonists are used.

Aromatase inhibitors

Aromatase inhibitors reduce serum oestrogen levels in postmenopausal women by preventing the conversion of adrenal androgens (androstenedione and testosterone) into oestradiol (E1) and oestrone (E2) in peripheral tissues such as fat, muscle and liver. This is the major source of postmenopausal circulating oestrogens, whereas in premenopausal women oestrogens are synthesised in the ovary. Aromatase inhibitors are indicated only for postmenopausal women to prevent the peripheral conversion of androgens into oestrogens and, on their own, they are not effective in reducing the much higher levels of circulating oestrone and oestradiol seen in premenopausal women.

The first-generation non-steroidal aromatase inhibitor for the treatment of endocrine-sensitive postmenopausal breast cancer was aminoglutethimide, but its major problem was the lack of specificity for the aromatase enzyme and the fact that it inhibited the adrenal synthesis of both glucocorticoids and mineralocorticoids (which required concomitant use of hydrocortisone). Within the last 5 years, third-generation potent oral aromatase inhibitors have entered the clinic, including the non-steroidal inhibitors anastrozole (Arimidex), letrozole (Femara), together with the steroidal aromatase inactivator exemestane (Aromasin). These drugs are 2–3 orders of magnitude more potent than aminoglutethimide and are highly selective for the aromatase enzyme without affecting mineralocorticoid or glucocorticoid synthesis.

In the metastatic second-line setting following failure on tamoxifen, phase III trials have been conducted in over 2000 women and have demonstrated clinical superiority for aromatase inhibitors over megestrol acetate as second-line therapy. An analysis of two randomised phase III trials of 764 patients treated with either anastrozole or megestrol acetate as second-line therapy after tamoxifen failure demonstrated equivalent efficacy in terms of objective response rates (10.3% and 7.9%, respectively) and disease stabilisation for 6 months (25.1% and 26.1 %, respectively), although better tolerability was shown for anastrozole.[30] A subsequent analysis following a median of 31 months follow-up showed a significant improvement in overall survival for anastrozole (hazard ratio 0.78, $p = 0.02$).[31] For letrozole, improvements were seen in objective tumour response rate (hazard ratio 1.82, $p = 0.04$) and time to treatment failure compared with megestrol acetate, although no impact on survival was detected.[32] In the recently reported trial with exemestane, duration of response, time to disease progression and overall survival were all significantly better than megestrol acetate.[33] These improvements in clinical end points, together with their consistent superior tolerability profile over megestrol acetate (i.e. reduced weight gain and thromboembolic events), have defined aromatase inhibitors as the standard endocrine treatment in advanced breast cancer for postmenopausal women following tamoxifen failure.

Recently, trials have asked whether aromatase inhibitors should challenge tamoxifen as the first-line endocrine agent of choice. The great potential of these studies is to see whether complete oestrogen blockade provided by these drugs provides greater control of hormone-sensitive breast cancer than tamoxifen, thus circumventing the problem of acquired tamoxifen resistance.[29] Published data in one trial with anastrozole compared with tamoxifen as first-line therapy in ER+ve breast cancer showed that anastrozole significantly

Table 36.4	Clinical factors determining choice of endocrine versus cytotoxic therapy for metastatic disease

- Patient factors
  - Age and performance status
  - Severity and nature of symptoms
  - Prior systemic therapies in adjuvant setting

- Disease factors
  - Tumour biology (ER status, HER2)
  - Duration of treatment-free interval
  - Dominant site disease (visceral versus soft tissue/bone)

prolonged the time to disease progression from 5.6 to 11.1 months ($p = 0.005$),[34] although in a larger trial no difference was found between the treatments.[35] Likewise, data have shown a significantly higher response rate (30% vs 20%, $p < 0.001$) and prolonged time to disease progression (median 9 months vs 6 months, $p < 0.0001$) than tamoxifen in a prospective randomised first-line endocrine therapy trial in over 900 patients,[36] whereas higher response rates were seen with exemestane than tamoxifen.[37] It remains to be seen in metastatic disease whether these benefits for aromatase inhibitors will translate into substantial gains in survival over tamoxifen.

Luteinising hormone–releasing hormone agonists

While tamoxifen is also active in premenopausal women with ER+ve breast cancer, tamoxifen-induced stimulation of the pituitary–ovarian axis can result in significantly elevated plasma oestradiol levels, which in theory at least could compete with tamoxifen for binding to oestrogen receptors. Previously, the alternative endocrine treatment for premenopausal women involved surgical ablative therapy by ovariectomy. Only two relatively small clinical trials have compared tamoxifen and ovariectomy for premenopausal women with metastatic breast; they showed no major differences in results.[38,39]

Subsequently, LHRH analogues such as buserelin (Suprefact) and goserelin (Zoladex) were shown to be effective in premenopausal metastatic breast cancer. These drugs act in premenopausal women to medically suppress ovarian function by inducing a fall in secretion of the pituitary gonadotrophin luteinising hormone (LH) and follicle-stimulating hormone (FSH). As such, these drugs have induced objective response rates of 38% (>50% if ER+ve) in over 400 women in a series of small phase II studies in advanced premenopausal breast cancer. Subsequent randomised clinical trials showed that LHRH agonists produced similar clinical benefit to bilateral oophorecetomy in terms of both control of the disease and overall survival, but without the need for surgical intervention.[40,41]

In clinical practice, medical ovarian ablation with LHRH agonists is usually reserved as treatment for premenopausal women with ER+ve metastatic breast cancer following failure of tamoxifen (which had often been given in the adjuvant setting). Recently, studies in premenopausal women have examined combined endocrine therapy in an attempt to induce 'complete oestrogen blockade', with suppression of plasma oestradiol by LHRH agonists and blockade of ER by tamoxifen. These trials have suggested that combined treatment may be a more effective first-line endocrine therapy in premenopausal women than either tamoxifen

or LHRH agonists alone.[42,43] A recent meta-analysis of the only four randomised trials confirmed that LHRH agonists plus tamoxifen significantly improved both progression-free survival (hazard ratio 0.70, $p = 0.0003$) and overall survival (hazard ratio 0.78, $p = 0.02$) compared with LHRH agonists alone.[44] As such, this combined therapy may become the new standard of care for hormone-sensitive (ER+ve) premenopausal advanced breast cancer.

Chemotherapy

First-line chemotherapy for patients with locally advanced/metastatic breast cancer achieves an objective tumour response in 40–60% patients, with a median response duration of 6–12 months. It is well established that patients who achieve an objective response (complete or partial remission) are more likely to have significant relief of their symptoms with an improvement in their performance status.[4,45] A small fraction of patients achieve complete remission, which may remain for an extended length of time.[46] Although there are no randomised data in metastatic breast cancer of first-line chemotherapy compared with best supportive care to demonstrate the impact of chemotherapy on survival, retrospective studies have shown that chemotherapy is probably associated with a modest 9–12 months gain in survival.[47]

Second-line chemotherapy may be considered for patients who fail to respond to first-line therapies or who relapse following an initial response. The likelihood of response is often somewhat less (15–30%), with median duration of response of approximately 4–9 months, although this is higher if patients had a good response to initial first-line therapy and/or have a prolonged interval (over 12 months) since completion of their prior therapy. Third- and fourth-line chemotherapy may be considered in some patients of good performance status in whom chemosensitivity has been demonstrated previously.

A number of active cytotoxic drugs have proven activity as single agents in breast cancer. In general, these drugs have been used in established combinations that have been shown to give higher response rates, presumably due to each drug's different mode of action, which increases the chance of avoiding drug resistance to a given single agent. More recently, the newer drugs that are used as second- or third-line therapy have been given as single agents.

Anthracyclines

Doxorubicin (Adriamycin) is an anthracycline that is considered one of the most active cytotoxic drugs in breast cancer, with response rates of 40% when given as a first-line single agent. Anthracycline combinations such as CAF (cyclophosphamide, doxorubicin, 5-FU) or AC (doxorubicin and cyclophosphamide) are widely used in view of their higher first-line response rates (50–60%) than single agent therapy. The main side effects of these drugs are alopecia, myelosuppression and potential risk of cardiac toxicity when a total lifetime cumulative dose of >550 mg/m^2 is reached. With the increasing use of adjuvant anthracycline-based chemotherapy, especially in premenopausal women, more patients will have received combination chemotherapy by the time metastatic disease develops, which may influence the likelihood of response to further treatment.[48] An increasing problem is a subgroup of patients with good performance status who have failed an anthracycline-based combination, either as first-line therapy for metastatic disease or having relapsed within a few months of adjuvant chemotherapy, in whom the response rates to further conventional chemotherapy are generally poor (<20–30%) with median durations of response of only 3–6 months.[49]

Taxanes

In patients with relapsed advanced breast cancer, especially following prior anthracycline-based chemotherapy, cytotoxic drugs such as the taxanes have shown significant efficacy compared with previously available second-line options.[50] Paclitaxel (Taxol) and docetaxel (Taxotere) are cytotoxic agents that promote the formation of stable microtubules within thecell, which then resist depolymerisation during cell division. As such, this induces cell death and this different mode of cytotoxic action means that these drugs may be active in tumours that have developed resistance to other classical cytotoxic agents such as the anthracyclines.

Several randomised phase III trials have looked at the efficacy of taxanes as second-line therapy, especially in those with anthracycline-resistant disease. For docetaxel, a significantly higher response rate was observed compared with either mitomycin/vinblastine[51] or methotrexate/5-FU,[52] with an associated increase in time to progression and, in one trial, significantly improved overall survival. In a third study, superior response rates were seen for docetaxel compared with vinorelbine/5-FU, although the difference was not significant.[53] Paclitaxel has been compared with mitomycin as second-line therapy in a small randomised phase II study,[54] whereas a randomised study of two doses of paclitaxel was performed in patients who had failed prior chemotherapy.[55] On the basis of these randomised clinical trial data to date, in June 2000 the National Institute for Clinical Excellence in

the UK recommended the use of taxanes as single agent therapy in advanced breast cancer where initial cytotoxic chemotherapy has failed.[56]

In first-line therapy for patients with advanced breast cancer who have not received an anthracycline previously, randomised trials have shown superior clinical efficacy for docetaxel compared with doxorubicin,[57] although this was not seen in two studies which compared paclitaxel with doxorubicin.[58,59] In untreated patients as first-line chemotherapy, paclitaxel was equivalent to conventional CMFP chemotherapy, although on multivariate analysis improved survival was seen.[60]

As taxanes appear to be non-cross-resistant with anthracyclines, trials were set up to determine the efficacy and tolerability of taxanes in combination with anthracyclines as first-line therapy, although there are concerns about the potential combined haematological or cardiac toxicities. The combination of docetaxel and doxorubicin (AT) was significantly more active than AC in a prospective first-line chemotherapy trial in429 women with a higher response rate (60% vs 47%, p = 0.012). Haematological toxicity in terms of grade 3/4 neutropenia was higher (96% vs 87%), with an associated significantly higher incidence of febrile neutropenia (33% vs 10%).[61] In contrast, the current published data on the randomised trials comparing doxorubicin and paclitaxel vs AC,[62] or epirubicin and paclitaxel (ET) vs epirubicin and cyclophosphamide (EC),[63,64] have failed to show any significant clinical advantage in favour of the taxane combination. It remains to be proven, therefore, whether there are any real clinical advantages to using taxanes in combinations with anthracyclines as first-line therapy, rather than reserving their use as single agents for relapsed disease, especially for patients resistant or refractory to anthracyclines.

Capecitabine

Progress has been made in developing oral derivatives of 5-FU such as capecitabine (Xeloda), which is a prodrug activated into 5-FU within the tumour. One study looked at 162 patients, of whom all had specifically shown resistance to paclitaxel, and 91% had received prior anthracyclines and 82% prior 5-FU.[65] Such patients are becoming an increasing number in routine clinical practice, given the activity and wider use of anthracyclines/taxanes in the adjuvant/first-line setting. Patients with breast cancer that recurs after these treatments often remain relatively fit, but until now limited treatment options have been available. The trial showed an objective tumour response rate of 20% with capecitabine, with a median duration of response of 8.1 months and median survival of 12.8 months. These results are clinically very significant for these heavily pretreated patients. Minimising side effects is clearly very important in the advanced breast cancer setting, and the favourable safety profile of capecitabine makes it an important option for these patients. The most common treatment-related side effects observed in phase II monotherapy studies were hand-foot syndrome, diarrhoea and nausea (1,2). Most of these were mild, with grade 3/4 severity occurring in only 10–22%, 14–16% and 4–9%, respectively. Myelosuppression and alopecia are very rare.

In terms of published randomised studies, a first-line study of 95 women aged >55 years old with untreated metastatic breast cancer compared capecitabine vs CMF, and demonstrated a higher response rate (30% vs 16%).[66] Survival in this small study was similar between the two groups. The second randomised study (511 patients) compared the combination of capecitabine and docetaxel vs docetaxel alone in women with anthracycline pretreated metastatic breast cancer.[67] The combination was significantly more effective than docetaxel alone (the previously accepted gold standard for anthracycline pretreated breast cancer). Improvements were seen in tumour response rate (42% vs 30%, $p = 0.006$), time to disease progression (median 6.2 vs 4.1 months, $p = 0.0001$) and, importantly, in overall survival (median 14.5 vs 11.5 months, $p = 0.0126$). These represent very significant further improvements upon docetaxel alone, and support preclinical data, which originally implied synergy between capecitabine and docetaxel.

New chemotherapy drugs/other regimens

There is evidence that several other cytotoxic chemotherapy agents are active in metastatic breast cancer, which may be beneficial to those who have already received anthracyclines or taxanes, either as adjuvant or first-line therapy. For example, vinorelbine (Navelbine) is a third-generation vinca alkaloid that prevents microtubulin polymerisation and has reduced neurotoxicity compared with either vincristine or vinblastine. As a single agent, the drug is very well tolerated, although myelosuppression can be the dose-limiting toxicity, and in a randomised trial in patients who had failed prior anthracyclines the response rate to vinorelbine was significantly higher than melphalan. However, when vinorelbine was combined with doxorubicin as first-line therapy in patients who had not received prior anthracyclines, the combination was no more effective than doxorubicin alone.[68] As a second-line therapy, including in patients who have failed anthracycline-based therapy, much interest has focused on recent reports that vinorelbine in combination with either

5-day or continuous infusional 5-FU appears to be a very active and well-tolerated therapy.

Other combinations that are often used in advanced breast cancer include mitoxantrone (mitozantrone) and methotrexate (MM), mitomycin C with vinblastine (MV), cisplatin/carboplatin-based regimens or the original 'gold standard' combination of cyclophosphamide, methotrexate and 5-FU (CMF) if patients have not been exposed to these drugs before. Although these regimens are generally well tolerated in advanced breast cancer, their likelihood of activity in inducing tumour responses is considered by many to be less than either anthracycline-based therapies, the taxanes or other the more recent new drug combinations outlined above. Other cytotoxic drugs such as gemcitabine, ifosfamide and topoisomerase inhibitors such as etoposide and topotecan have been examined in advanced breast cancer but are not considered standard therapeutic options for these patients as single agents. Recent trials have suggested that gemcitabine and paclitaxel may be more effective than paclitaxel alone as first-line therapy.

High-dose chemotherapy

Increasing the dose of conventional chemotherapy regimens up to two-fold has been associated with enhanced response rates, but to date has not impacted on time to progression or overall survival in advanced disease. At the same time, it is recognised that inadequate doses of chemotherapy produce an inadequate outcome. Peripheral blood stem cell harvesting has allowed high-dose chemotherapy (i.e. greater than five-fold increases in dose intensity) to be delivered, with the hope that if response rates could be enhanced further by delivery of maximally tolerated dose-intensified chemotherapy, then perhaps survival may be improved. Although numerous phase II trials reported on the high response rates which could be achieved with this approach using various drug combinations, patient selection has always been a confounding factor in interpreting the true efficacy of this approach.[69] Two large randomised trials in metastatic breast cancer have both failed to show any advantage for high-dose chemotherapy compared with conventional-dose regimens[70,71] and, as such, the treatment is not recommended for metastatic breast cancer outside the context of clinical trials.

Bisphosphonates

Up to 50% of women who develop metastatic breast cancer present with bone metastases, sometimes as their only site of disease. Many of these patients have indolent disease and, as such, can survive for many years. Bisphosphonates are bone-specific palliative agents that inhibit tumour-related osteoclast-induced bone resorption associated with breast cancer metastases. In patients with predominantly lytic bone metastases, they have been shown to significantly improve quality of life by treating hypercalcaemia, reducing bone pain and requirements for radiotherapy, and preventing skeletal complications through reducing the incidence of pathological fractures or spinal cord compression.

There have been four randomised double-blind placebo-controlled trials in breast cancer patients with bone metastases. Intravenous pamidronate (Aredia) given at a dose of 90 mg as a 2-hour infusion every month for 12 cycles was compared against placebo infusion in conjunction with chemo–endocrine therapy in 382 women with at least one lytic bone lesion.[72] The median time to the first skeletal complication was significantly longer in those given pamidronate (13.1 vs 7.0 months, p = 0.005), and overall fewer patients developed such complications (43% vs 56%, p = 0.008). Similar results were seen in 372 patients with advanced breast cancer with lytic bone metastases who were treated with endocrine therapy alone with or without pamidronate. In a recent combined update of both trials the addition of bisphosphonate therapy was shown to be significantly superior to anticancer therapy alone (endocrine and/or chemotherapy) in preventing skeletal complications and palliating symptoms from bone metastases.[74] Similar results have been demonstrated with pamidronate in a third trial in 295 patients.[75] In the final study of 173 patients, oral clodronate (Bonefos), 1600 mg daily, was compared with placebo tablets.[76] There was a significant reduction in the number of hypercalcaemic episodes (28 vs 52, p <0.01) and the incidence of vertebral fractures (84 vs 124 per 100 patient years, p <0.025). However, in all four studies there was no impact on overall survival.

Both drugs (pamidronate and clodronate) are well tolerated, and for patients with symptomatic bone metastases (i.e. generalised sites of bone pain, or pain despite radiotherapy) or significant lytic disease, it is recommended practice to initiate intravenous-based therapy (pamidronate or clodronate) for up to 6 months. In asymptomatic patients, including for example those hormone negative or resistant patients with bone-only sites of metastatic disease, together with those suitable for prolonged maintenance treatment, oral-based therapy with clodronate may be used. A few (<10%) patients may experience some gastrointestinal disturbance with clodronate. It is clear that bisphosphonates are a useful and effective palliative treatment for bone disease, and clear guidelines have now been issued in the UK by the British Association of Surgical Oncologists[77] and in the US by the American Society for Clinical Oncology for their routine use in women with metastatic breast cancer. More recently, intravenous zoledrenate (Zometa) and oral ibandronate (Bondronat) have also become available.

Biological therapies

The major limitation of conventional endocrine and chemotherapy in metastatic disease is that most tumours become resistant. Biological therapies offer a novel approach that may circumvent drug resistance. Trastuzumab (Herceptin) is a humanised monoclonal antibody directed against the cell surface growth factor receptor c-erbB2 (also known as HER-2) which is overexpressed in 25–30% breast cancers.[78] Such tumours are thought to be resistant to both endocrine and conventional chemotherapies, and Herceptin either given alone or in conjunction with conventional therapy offers an opportunity to modulate aberrant growth factor activity in patients with resistant disease. In patients with HER-2-positive tumours, trastuzumab administered as a weekly intravenous infusion produced response rates of up to 35% as first-line therapy for metastatic breast cancer.[79] In a randomised phase III trial in 469 women with HER-2-positive metastatic breast cancer,[80] the addition of trastuzumab to taxane or anthracycline-based chemotherapy significantly enhanced both response rates (62% vs 36%) and time to disease progression (8.6 vs 5.5 months). This is important, as HER-2-positive tumours have been deemed relatively resistant to certain chemotherapy regimens. One problem is the increased incidence of cardiac toxicity, in particular when given in combination with anthracyclines. Most important, the addition of trastuzumab to chemotherapy has shown a significant improvement in overall survival (median 25.1 vs 20.3 months, p = 0.046).

As such, trastuzumab represents the first example of the new generation of targeted biological therapies for advanced breast cancer to successfully enter clinical practice, and other novel drugs are in development which target various components of the internal signal transduction pathway. Clinical trials are determining whether these new drugs are active and may further enhance the response to conventional endocrine and chemotherapy options.

Summary

The systemic treatment of metastatic or locally advanced breast cancer involves utilising the most appropriate and correct sequence of therapies to gain the maximum benefit from each modality. Endocrine therapy represents the mainstay of first-line treatment of postmenopausal women with ER and/or PgR+ve metastatic breast cancer who do not have life-threatening visceral involvement. The role of chemotherapy is as first-line treatment for women in whom rapid tumour control is required (such as those with symptomatic or extensive visceral involvement), or for women with ER and/or PgR–ve or hormone refractory metastatic breast cancer. Several new therapies have entered routine clinical use in the last 5–10 years (i.e. third-generation aromatase inhibitors, taxanes, bisphosphonates) based on well-conducted randomised controlled clinical trials which have demonstrated that these provide a significant incremental improvement in the treatment for these patients. Nevertheless, the problem of drug resistance persists, although as a result of the expanded biological understanding of tumour development and progression, new biological therapies such as trastuzumab are now entering the clinic. Several more of these drugs are in development, and it is expected that these treatments (alone or in combination with existing drugs) may further improve on current therapies.

NURSING CARE FOR PATIENTS WITH BREAST CANCER

Sheila Small

INTRODUCTION

The nature and extent of supportive care for women having systemic treatment for breast cancer will vary according to the individual. Factors such as age, stage of the disease, general health, individual coping styles and the availability of social support networks may all influence the nature of supportive care which may be required.

CHEMOTHERAPY

Side effects

During patient assessment it is important to review the patient's general health status. This will include attention to nutrition and sleep, wound healing and correction of any infection or anaemia. Assessment of psychological status and psychosocial support is also important because this may influence coping styles. The principles of care for a patient receiving adjuvant chemotherapy for breast cancer are the same as for any patient receiving systemic chemotherapy. Treatment is usually given on an outpatient basis, but patients may require supportive care for specific physical-related symptoms. Some patients may experience nausea or nausea and associated vomiting. This most commonly occurs within 2–4 days of treatment. It is important that patients understand the importance of antiemetic treatments that are prescribed to cover this period. Myelosuppression occurs within 7–10 days and patients are reminded of the importance of reporting signs of infection or bleeding at this stage. Some patients may experience mucositis, and it is important that patients are advised of effective mouth-care and oral hygiene at this stage. (See also Chs 16 and 18.)

Impact on femininity

Specific symptoms such as hair loss and amenorrhoea may have a significant impact on the woman's femininity and body image. Effects of treatment may not always be visually apparent but may cause particular distress. For example some women may experience cessation of periods, which may result in premature menopause and subsequent infertility.[81,82] This may be a particularly distressing prospect for women of child-bearing age. It may also highlight issues relating to survivorship and parenting. Some women may require counselling to help deal with the issues that this may present. It may be appropriate for women to be referred to a fertility specialist who can counsel women in the specific issues relating to fertility treatments and cancer care. (See also Chs 23, 32 and 33.)

Lifestyle changes

In addition to physical symptoms, many women undergoing chemotherapy may have to face a number of lifestyle changes. They may need more support with practical help in caring for a family or they may need advice relating to welfare services if an income is affected. It is important that nurses can identify these needs and refer patients to appropriate agencies for help or advice. Effective multiprofessional working is essential in providing supportive care.

ENDOCRINE

It is estimated that as many as 70% of women under the age of 65 having adjuvant treatment for breast cancer will experience menopausal symptoms.[83] Nurses need to be able to assess the extent of these symptoms and the affect they are having on the patient's quality of life.[84,85] Table 36.5 illustrates some commonly reported

Table 36.5   Common problems associated with endocrine therapies

Problem	Advice
Hot flushes/night sweats	Wear thin layers of clothing Avoid trigger factors (alcohol, spicy foods, caffeine) Consider dietary supplements: the efficacy of dietary supplements for the management of hot flushes is still being evaluated. Supplements include soya,[86] vitamin E,[87] evening primrose oil,[88] and homeopathic remedies[89] Refer to physician for consideration of medication to include vasodilators and beta-blockers[90] and the use of hormone replacement therapy[91]
Weight gain	Examine lifestyle changes which may be attributed to weight gain Encourage regular exercise Refer to dietician for dietary advice
Dry vagina	Encourage woman to discuss feelings and expressions of intimacy with her partner Suggest extending foreplay to increase lubrication Lubricant gels such as K-Y, Senselle and Replens may help[92]
Vaginal bleeding	Establish type and frequency of bleeding to determine if this may be a menstrual bleed Check if the patient has omitted to take her drugs regularly as some hormone therapies can cause breakthrough or withdrawal bleeding Vaginal bleeding which does not represent a period or a withdrawal bleeding should be reported to a doctor and a referral to a gynaecologist is advised
Mood alterations	Patients may report feeling more forgetful and tearful. This is often exacerbated due to sleep disturbances, often caused by night sweats. It may be appropriate to assess for signs of anxiety and depression or refer to a counsellor to identify coping skills for management of mood swings and alterations

menopausal symptoms together with some useful strategies for coping with these problems.

TAXANES

Patients receiving taxanes may have advanced disease, so the supportive care needs to include symptomatic control of the disease as well as the effects of treatment. Patients with metastatic disease may experience more marked fatigue and it is important that the nurse can offer strategies to help the patient manage this condition.[93] There may be more frequent hospital admissions for patients and the role of primary care services and especially palliative care nurses may need to be discussed. Effective modes of communication between cancer centres and primary care services are essential at this stage.

BISPHOSPHONATES

These drugs are generally well tolerated with minimum side effects. However, the importance of hydration and fluid intake needs to be discussed with patients. It is also important to discuss the potential for tumour flare-up pain, as this may cause alarm for patients.

PSYCHOLOGICAL SUPPORT

In addition to the physical effects of treatment, psychological support should be available to allow patients to identify their coping styles and to be able to communicate fears or anxieties in relation to their treatment. Patients may be presented with choices and asked to make decisions relating to benefits of treatment vs potential side effects. This warrants clear communication and information-giving strategies so that patients may feel able to participate and make informed decisions regarding their treatment.

The supportive care of patients receiving systemic treatment for breast cancer needs to be holistic and patient-focused. The effects of systemic therapy may not present in isolation and may be exacerbated by the effects of other adjuvant treatments. These effects may significantly influence well-being and quality of life, which needs to be addressed in planning supportive care as well as measuring the effectiveness of treatment outcomes.

References

1. Cancer Research Campaign. Breast Cancer Factsheet. London: CRC; 1996.

2. Easton D, Ford D. Breast and ovarian cancer incidence in BRCA-1 mutation carriers. Am J Hum Genet 1995; 56:265–271.

3. UICC International Union against Cancer. In: Sobin LH, Wittekind CH, eds. TNM classification of malignant tumours, 5th edn. New York: Wiley–Liss; 1997.

4. Baum M, Priestman T, West RR, et al. A comparison of subjective responses in a trial comparing endocrine with cytotoxic treatment in advanced carcinoma of the breast. In: Mouridsen HT, Palshof T, eds. Breast cancer experimental and clinical methods. London: Pergamon Press; 1980:223–228.

5. Rubens RD, Bajetta E, Bonneterre J, et al. Treatment of relapse of breast cancer after adjuvant systemic therapy. Eur J Cancer 1994; 30A:106–111.

6. Early Breast Cancer Trialists' Group. Polychemotherapy for early breast cancer: an overview of the randomised trials. Lancet 1998; 352:930–942.

7. Fisher B, Anderson S, Wickerham DL, et al. Increased intensification and total dose of cyclophosphamide in a doxorubicin-cyclophosphamide regimen for the treatment of primary breast cancer: findings from National Surgical Adjuvant Breast and Bowel Project B-22. J Clin Oncol 1997; 15:1858–1869.

8. Wood WC, Budman DR, Korzun AH, et al. Dose and dose intensity of adjuvant chemotherapy for stage II, node-positive breast carcinoma. N Engl J Med 1994; 330:1253–1259.

9. Bonadonna G, Zambeti M, Valagussa P, et al. Sequential or alternating doxorubicin and CMF regimens in breast cancer with more than three positive nodes. JAMA 1995; 273:542–547.

10. National Cancer Institute. Consensus Statement about the role of adjuvant taxanes in early breast cancer. 2000. Online. Available: www.nci.org

11. Rodenhuis S, Richel DJ, van der Wall E, et al. Randomised trial of high-dose chemotherapy and haemopoietic progenitor-cell support in operable breast cancer with extensive axillary lymph-node involvement. Lancet 1998; 352:515–521.

12. Early Breast Cancer Trialists' Group. Tamoxifen for early breast cancer; an overview of the randomised trials. Lancet 1998; 351:1451–1467.

13. Swedish Breast Cancer Group. Randomised trial of two versus five years of adjuvant tamoxifen for post-menopausal early stage breast cancer. J Natl Cancer Inst 1996; 88:1543–1549.

14. Fisher B, Dignam J, Bryant J, et al. Five versus more than five years of tamoxifen therapy for breast cancer patients with negative lymph nodes and estrogen receptor-positive tumours. J Natl Cancer Inst 1996; 88:1529–1542.

15. Stewart HJ, Forrest AP, Everington D, et al. Randomised comparison of 5 years of adjuvant tamoxifen with continuous therapy for operable breast cancer. Br J Cancer 1996; 74:297–299.

16. Fisher B, Costantino JP, Redmond CK, et al. Endometrial cancer in tamoxifen-treated breast cancer patients: findings from the NSABP B-14. J Natl Cancer Inst 1994; 86:527–537.

17. Powles TJ, Hickish T, Kanis JA, et al. Effect of tamoxifen on bone mineral density measured by dual-energy X-ray absorptiometry in healthy premenopausal and postmenopausal women. J Clin Oncol 1996; 14:78–84.

18. Love RD, Barden HS, Mazess RB, et al. Effect of tamoxifen on lumbar spine bone mineral density in post-menopausal women after five years. Arch Int Med 1994; 154:2585–2588.

19. Beral V, Hermon C, Reeves G, et al. Sudden fall in breast cancer death rates in England and Wales. Lancet 1995; 345:1642–1643.

20. Early Breast Cancer Trialists' Group. Ovarian ablation in early breast cancer; overview of the randomised trials. Lancet 1996; 348:1189–1196.

21. ATAC Trialists Group. Anastrozole alone or in combination with tamoxifen versus tamoxifen alone for adjuvant treatment of postmenopausal women with early breast cancer: first results of the ATAC randomised trial. Lancet 2002; 359:2131–2139.

22. Goss PE, Ingle JN, Silvana M et al. A randomized trial of letrozole in postmenopausal women after five years of tamoxifen therapy for early-stage breast cancer. N Engl J Med 2003; 349(19):1793–1802.

23. Overgaard M, Hansen PS, Overgaard J, et al. Postoperative radiotherapy in high-risk premenopausal women with breast cancer who receive adjuvant chemotherapy. N Engl J Med 1997; 337:949–955.

24. Jackson IM, Litherland S, Wakeling AE. Tamoxifen and other antioestrogens. In: Powles TJ, Smith, IE, eds. Medical management of breast cancer. London: Martin Duritz; 1991:51–59.

25. McGuire WL. Hormone receptors; their role in predicting prognosis and response to endocrine therapy. Semin Oncol 1978; 5:428–433.

26. Mouridsen HT, Ellemann K, Mattsson W, et al. Therapeutic effect of tamoxifen versus tamoxifen combined with medroxyprogesterone acetate in advanced breast cancer in postmenopausal women. Cancer Treat Rep 1997; 63:171–175.

27. Kuss JT, Muss HB, Hoen H, et al. Tamoxifen as initial endocrine therapy for metastatic breast cancer: long term follow-up of two Piedmont Oncology Association (POA) trials. Breast Cancer Res Treat 1997; 42:265–274.

28. Litherland S, Jackson IM. Antioestrogens in the management of hormone-dependent cancer. Cancer Treat Rep 1988; 15:183–194.

29. Johnston SRD. Acquired tamoxifen resistance in human breast cancer – potential mechanisms and

clinical implications. Anti-Cancer Drugs 1997; 8(10):911–930.

30. Buzdar A, Jonat W, Howell A, et al. Anastrozole, a potent and selective aromatase inhibitor, versus megesterol acetate in post-menopausal women with advanced breast cancer; results of overview analysis of two phase III trials. J Clin Oncol 1996; 14:2000–2011.

31. Buzdar A, Jonat W, Howell A, et al. Anastrozole versus megestrol acetate in the treatment of postmenopausal women with advanced breast carcinoma: results of a survival update based on a combined analysis of data from two mature phase III trials. Cancer 1998; 83:1142–1152.

32. Dombernowsky P, Smith IE, Falkson G, et al. Letrozole, a new oral aromatase inhibitor for advanced breast cancer: double-blind randomised trial showing a dose effect and improved efficacy and tolerability compared with megestrol acetate. J Clin Oncol 1998; 16:453–461.

33. Kaufmann M, Bajetta E, Dirix LY, et al. Exemestane is superior to megestrol acetate after tamoxifen failure in postmenopausal women with advanced breast cancer: Results of a phase III randomized double-blind trial. J Clin Oncol 2000; 18(7):1399–1411.

34. Nabholtz JM, Buzdar A., Pollak M, et al. Anastrozole is superior to tamoxifen as first-line therapy for advanced breast cancer in postmenopausal women: results of a North American multicentre randomised trial. J Clin Oncol 2000; 18:3758–3767.

35. Bonneterre J, Thurlimann B, Robertson JFR, et al. Anastrozole versus tamoxifen as first-line therapy for advanced breast cancer in 668 postmenopausal women: results of the tamoxifen or arimidex randomised group efficacy and tolerability study. J Clin Oncol 2000; 18:3748–3757.

36. Mouridsen H, Gershanovich M, Sun Y, et al. Phase III study of Letrozole versus tamoxifen as first-line therapy of advanced breast cancer in postmenopausal women: analysis of survival and update of efficacy from the International Letrozole Breast Cancer Group. J Clin Oncol 2003; 21:2101–2109.

37. Paridaens R, Dirix LY, Beex L, et al. Exemestane is active and well tolerated as first-line hormonal therapy of metastatic breast cancer patients; results of a randomised phase II trial. Proc Am Soc Clin Oncol 2000; 19:83a(A316).

38. Ingle JN, Krook JE, Green SJ, et al. Randomised trial of bilateral oophorectomy versus tamoxifen in pre-menopausal women with metastatic breast cancer. J Clin Oncol 1986; 4:178–185.

39. Buchanan RB, Blamey RW, Durrant KR, et al. A randomised comparison of bilateral oophorectomy versus tamoxifen in premenopausal patient with advanced breast cancer. J Clin Oncol 1986; 4:1326–1330.

40. Boccardo F, Rubagotti A, Perrotta A, et al. Ovarian ablation versus goserelin with or without tamoxifen in pre-perimenopausal patients with advanced breast cancer; results of a multicentric Italian study. Ann Oncol 1994; 5:337–342.

41. Taylor CW, Green S, Dalton WS, et al. Multicenter randomised clinical trial of goserelin versus surgical ovariectomy in premenopausal patients with receptor-positive metastatic breast cancer. J Clin Oncol 1998; 16:994–999.

42. Jonat W, Kaufmann M, Blamey RW, et al. A randomised study to compare the effect of the luteinising releasing hormone (LHRH) analogue goserelin with or without tamoxifen in pre- and peri-menopausal patients with advanced breast cancer. Eur J Cancer 1995; 31:137–142.

43. Klijn JGN, Beex L, Mauriac L, et al. Combined treatment with buserelin and tamoxifen in premenopausal metastatic breast cancer; a randomised study. J Natl Cancer Inst 2000; 92:903–911.

44. Klijn JGN, Blamey RW, Boccardo F, et al. Combined tamoxifen and luteinising hormone-releasing hormone (LHRH) agonist versus LHRH agonist alone in premenopausal advanced breast cancer; a meta-analysis of four randomised trials. J Clin Oncol 2001; 19:343–353.

45. Geels P, Eisenhauer E, Bezjak A, et al. Palliative effects of chemotherapy: objective tumour response is associated with symptom improvement in metastatic breast cancer. J Clin Oncol 2000; 18:2395–2405.

46. Greenberg AC, Hortobagyi GN, Smith TL, et al. Long-term follow-up of patients with complete remission following combination chemotherapy for metastatic breast cancer. J Clin Oncol 1997; 14:2197–2205.

47. Cold S, Jensen NV, Brincker H, et al. The influence of chemotherapy on survival after recurrence in breast cancer: a population based study of patients treated in the 1950s, 1960s, and 1970s. Eur J Cancer 1993; 29:1146–1152.

48. Houston SJ, Richards MA, Bentley AE, et al. The influence of adjuvant chemotherapy on outcome after relapse for patients with breast cancer. Eur J Cancer 1993; 29A:1513–1518.

49. Buzdar AU, Hortobagyi GN, Prye D, et al. Second-line chemotherapy for metastatic breast cancer including quality of life issues. The Breast 1996; 5:312–317.

50. Vermoken JB, Ten Bokkel Huinick WW. Chemotherapy for advanced breast cancer: the place of active new drugs. The Breast 1996; 5:304–311.

51. Nabholtz JM, Senn HJ, Beswoda WR, et al. Prospective randomised trial of docetaxel versus mitomycin plus vinblastine in patients with metastatic breast cancer progressing despite previous anthracycline-containing chemotherapy. J Clin Oncol 1999; 17:1413–1424.

52. Sjostrom J, Blomqvist C, Mouridsen H, et al. Docetaxel compared with sequential methorexate and 5-fluorouracil in advanced breast cancer after anthracycline failure: a randomised phase III study with cross-over on progression by the Scandinavian Breast Cancer Group. Eur J Cancer 1999; 35:1194–1201.

53. Bonneterre J, Roche H, Monnier A, et al. Taxotere versus 5-FU and Navelbine as second-line chemotherapy in patients with metastatic breast cancer. Proc Am Soc Clin Oncol 1997; 16:A564.

54. Dieras V, Marty M, Tubiana N, et al. Phase II randomised study of paclitaxel versus mitomycin in advanced breast cancer. Semin Oncol 1995; 22:33–39.

55. Nabholtz JM, Gelman K, Bontenbal M, et al. Multicenter, randomised comparative study of two doses of paclitaxel in patients with metastatic breast cancer. J Clin Oncol 1996; 14:1858–1867.

56. National Institute for Clinical Excellence. Technology Appraisal Guidance No. 6 – guidance on the use of taxanes for breast cancer. National Institute for Clinical Excellence – June 2000. Online. Available: www.nice.org.uk

57. Chan S, Friedrichs K, Noel D, et al. Prospective randomised phase III trial of docetaxel versus doxorubicin in patients with metastatic breast cancer. J Clin Oncol 1999; 17:2341–2354.

58. Sledge GWJ, Neuberg D, Bernardo P, et al. Phase III trial of doxorubicin, paclitaxel and the combination of doxorubicin and paclitaxel as front-line therapy for metastatic breast cancer; an intergroup trial (E1193). J Clin Oncol 2003; 21:588–592

59. Paridaens R, Bigganzoli L, Bruning P, et al. Paclitaxel versus doxorubicin as first-line single agent chemotherapy for metastatic breast cancer; a European Organisation for Research and Treatment of Cancer randomised study with cross-over. J Clin Oncol 2000; 18:724–733.

60. Bishop JF, Dewar J, Toner GC, et al. Paclitaxel improves outcome compared with CMFP combination chemotherapy as front-line therapy in untreated metastatic breast cancer. J Clin Oncol 1999; 17:2355.

61. Nabholtz JM, Falkson C, Campos D, et al. Docetaxel and doxorubicin compared with doxorubicin and cyclophosphamide as first-line chemotherapy for metastatic breast cancer: results of a randomised, multicenter, phase III trial. J Clin Oncol 2003; 21:968–975.

62. Biganzoli L, Cufer T, Brunning P, et al. Doxorubicin and paclitaxel versus doxorubicin and cyclophosphamide as first-line chemotherapy in metastatic breast cancer: the European Organisation for Research and Treatment of Cancer 10961 multicenter phase III trial. J Clin Oncol 2002; 20–3114–3121.

63. Luck H, Thomsenn C, Utch M, et al. Multicentre phase III study in first-line treatment of advanced metastatic breast cancer; epirubicin/paclitaxel (ET) versus epirubicin/cyclophosphamide (EC) – a study of the AGO Breast Cancer Group. Proc Am Soc Clin Oncol 2000; 19:73A.

64. Carmichael J. UKCCR trial of epirubicin and cyclophosphamide versus epirubicin and taxol in the first-line treatment of women with metastatic breast cancer. Proc Am Soc Clin Oncol 2001; 20:22A.

65. Blum JL, Jones SE, Buzdar AU, et al. Multicenter phase II study of capecitabine in paclitaxel-refractory metastatic breast cancer. J Clin Oncol 1999; 17:485–493.

66. O'Shaughnessy JA, Blum J, Moiseyenko V, et al. Randomised, open-label, phase II trial of oral capecitabine (Xeloda) vs. a reference arm of intravenous CMF (cyclophosphamide, methotrexate and 5-fluorouracil) as first-line therapy for advanced/metastatic breast cancer. Ann Oncol 2001; 12:1247–1254.

67. O'Shaughnessy J, Miles D, Vukelja S, et al. Superior survival with capecitabine plus docetaxel combination therapy in anthracycline-pretreated patients with advanced breast cancer: phase III trial results. J Clin Oncol 2002; 20:2812–2823.

68. Norris B, Pritchard KI, James K, et al. (2000) Phase III comparative study of vinorelbine combined with doxorubicin versus doxorubicin alone in disseminated metastatic/recurrent breast cancer: National Cancer Institute of Canada Clinical Trials Group Study MA8. J Clin Oncol 2000; 18:2385–2394.

69. Rahman ZU, Frye DK, Buzdar AU, et al. Impact of selection process on response rate and long-term survival of potential high-dose chemotherapy candidates treated with standard-dose doxorubicin-containing chemotherapy in patients with metastatic breast cancer. J Clin Oncol 1997; 15:3171–3177.

70. Stadtmauer EA, O'Neill A, Goldstein LJ, et al. Conventional-dose chemotherapy compared with high-dose chemotherapy plus autologous haematopoetic stem cell transplant group. N Engl J Med 2000; 342:1069–1076.

71. Lotz JP, Cure H, Janvier M, et al. High-dose chemotherapy with haemapoietic transplantation for metastatic breast cancer; results of the French protocol PEGASE 04. Proc Am Soc Clin Oncol 1999; 18:43a.

72. Hortobagyi GN, Theriault RL, Porter L, et al. Efficacy of pamidronate in reducing skeletal complications in patients with breast cancer and lytic bone metastases. N Engl J Med 1996; 335:1785–1791.

74. Lipton A, Theriault RL, Hortabagyi GN, et al. Pamidronate prevents skeletal complications and is effective palliative treatment in women with breast carcinoma and osteolytic bone metastases. Cancer 2000; 88:1082–1090.

75. Conte PF, Latrielle J, Mauriac L, et al. Delay in progression of bone metastases in breast cancer patients treated with intravenous pamidronate: results from a multinational randomised controlled trial. J Clin Oncol 1996; 14:2552–2559.

76. Paterson AH, Powles TJ, Kanis JA, et al. Double-blind controlled trial of oral clodronate in patients with bone metastases from breast cancer. J Clin Oncol 1993; 11:59–65.

77. Breast Speciality Group of the British Association of Surgical Oncology (BASO). The management of metastatic bone disease in the United Kingdom. Eur J Surg Oncol 1999; 25:3–23.

78. Slamon DJ, Clark GM, Wong SG, et al. Human breast cancer: correlation of relapse and survival with amplification of the HER-2/neu oncogene. Science 1987; 235:177–182.

79. Vogel CL, Cobleigh M, Tripathy D, et al. First-line, non-hormonal, treatment of women with HER-2 overexpressing metastatic breast cancer with Herceptin

(trastuzumab, humanised anti-HER2 antibody). Proc Am Soc Clin Oncol 2000; 19:71a (A275).

80. Slamon D, Leyland-Jones B, Shak S, et al. Use of chemotherapy plus a monoclonal antibody against HER-2 for metastatic breast cancer that overexpresses HER2. N Engl J Med 2001; 344:783–792.

81. Rogers M, Kristjansin L. The impact on sexual functioning of chemotherapy-induced menopause on women with breast cancer. Cancer Nurs 2002; 25(1):57–65.

82. Ganz P, Rowland J, Desmon K, et al. Life after breast cancer: understanding women's health related quality of life and sexual functioning. J Clin Oncol 1998; 16(2):501–514.

83. Canney P, Hatton MQF. The prevalence of menopausal symptoms in patients treated for breast cancer. Clin Oncol 1994; 6:297–299.

84. Fenlon D. Menopause: a problem for breast cancer patients. Eur J Cancer Care 1995; 4:166–172.

85. MacPhail G. Menopause as an issue for women with breast cancer. Cancer Nurs 1999; 22(2):164–171.

86. VanPatten CL, Olivotto IA, Chambers CK, et al. Effects of soy phytoestrogens on hot flashes in postmenopausal women with breast cancer: a randomized control trial. J Clin Oncol 2002; 20(6):1449–1555.

87. Barton D, Loprinzi C, Quella S, et al. Prospective evaluation of vitamin E for hot flushes in breast cancer survivors. J Clin Oncol 1998; 16(2):495–500.

88. Chenoy R, Hussain S, Tayob Y, et al. Effect of oral gamolenic acid from evening primrose oil on menopausal flushing. BMJ 1994; 308:501–503.

89. The use of herbal and botanical therapies in menopause. Journal Watch Women's Health 2001; (703):11.

90. Notelovitz M. The non-hormonal management of the menopause. In: Studd J, Whitehead MI, eds. The menopause. Oxford: Blackwell Science; 1998:102–115.

91. Marsden J, Sacks N. Hormone replacement therapy and breast cancer. Endocrine Related Cancer 1997; 4:269–279.

92. Loprinzi CL, Abu-Ghazelah S, Sloan JA. Phase III randomized double-blind study to evaluate the efficacy of a polycarbophil-based vaginal moisturizer in women with breast cancer. J Clin Oncol 1997; 15(3):969–973.

93. Ream E, Richardson A. From theory to practice: designing interventions to reduce fatigue in patients with cancer. Oncol Nurs Forum 1999; 26(8): 1295–1303.

Further Reading

Blum JL, Dieras V, LoRusso PM, et al. Multicenter phase II study of capecitabine in taxane-pretreated metastatic breast carcinoma patients. Cancer 2001; 92:1759–1768.

Miles DW, Towlson KE, Graham R, et al. A randomised phase II study of sialyl-Tn and DETOX-B adjuvant with or without cyclophosphamide pretreatment for the active specific immunotherapy of breast cancer. Br J Cancer 1996; 74:1292–1296.

Powles TJ. Adjuvant therapy for early breast cancer: a time to refine. J Natl Cancer Inst 1997; 89:1652–1653.

Tomiak E, Verma S, Levine M, et al. Use of capecitabine in stage IV breast cancer: an evidence summary. Curr Oncol 2000; 7:84–90.

Chapter 37

Lung cancer

CHAPTER CONTENTS

MEDICAL CARE FOR PATIENTS WITH LUNG CANCER

Caroline Archer and Mary ER O'Brien

INCIDENCE

Lung cancer is a major global health problem. Approximately 500 000 new cases of lung cancer are diagnosed annually. In the UK, lung cancer accounts for 15% of all malignancies, with 38 000 new cases presenting each year. It is the most common cancer amongst males in the UK.[1] The incidence of lung cancer is now falling, probably as a reflection of changing smoking habits within the population.[2] The fall in lung cancer incidence, however, is principally amongst men, and there appears to be an increase in the incidence of lung cancer in women. The 1999 statistics for the UK have shown slightly more deaths from lung cancer amongst women than from breast cancer, traditionally the biggest cancer killer of women.[3] This is predominantly due to the rise in diagnosis of adenocarcinoma, a type of lung cancer less related to smoking, and also improvements in treatment of breast cancer. Mortality from breast cancer has fallen rapidly in recent years, unlike lung cancer, where sadly there has been little change in the mortality figures.

HISTOLOGICAL CLASSIFICATION

There are two main types of lung cancer: small cell lung cancer (SCLC) and non-small cell lung cancer (NSCLC). Approximately 75–80% of presenting cases are NSCLC and 20–25% are SCLC.

Small cell lung cancer

SCLC may have neuroendocrine features, as it is thought to arise from cells derived from the neural crest, but separate neuroendocrine tumours may also arise in the lungs, such as malignant carcinoid tumours.

Non–small cell lung cancer

NSCLC is subdivided into several histological types:

- squamous cell carcinomas
- adenocarcinomas
- bronchioalveolar carcinoma, a well-differentiated adenocarcinoma with a particular intra-alveolar distribution
- undifferentiated and
- large cell carcinomas.

The commonest subgroup within the UK is squamous cell carcinoma. Overall, the differences within the groups are small and all subgroups of NSCLC are generally treated in the same way, and are therefore grouped together.

Mesothelioma

Mesothelioma is a rare malignancy of serosal surfaces, commonly affecting the pleura and linked to previous asbestos exposure, particularly crocidolite (blue asbestos). There is an approximately 20-year latency between asbestos exposure and the development of the disease. The incidence is rising in the UK and Europe. The increase is predicted to peak in 2020, and then fall due to controls now in place regarding asbestos use.[4]

Mesotheliomas can be divided into three main histological types:

- epithelial
- sarcomatous and
- mixed.[5]

The epithelial type is the most common, probably occurring in about two-thirds of cases, and the sarcomatous type is less common but is associated with a more aggressive pattern of disease.[6]

AETIOLOGY

It has long been established that the major risk factor in lung cancer development is smoking, although some lung cancers are not related to smoking, such as alveolar cell carcinoma (only 1% of lung cancers) and adenocarcinoma. The risk of lung cancer is greater with increasing numbers of cigarettes smoked, but the duration of smoking is a stronger risk factor than daily intake. Smoking cessation is associated with a steady lung cancer risk reduction, so that in those who have stopped smoking for 10 or more years, the risk of developing lung cancer becomes similar to a lifelong non-smoker.[7] Ninety per cent of patients who develop lung cancer are, or have been, smokers.

Other exogenous carcinogens may predispose to lung cancer, such as:

- asbestos
- radiation
- arsenic
- mustard and radon gas
- chromium and nickel.[8,9]

Although there are strong environmental factors leading to lung cancer development, individuals differ in their sensitivities to these agents. Increasing evidence suggests that genetic factors may also play a role in lung cancer development. Several case–control studies have shown an association between lung cancer and family history despite the confounding factors such as common smoking habits.[10] Lung cancer is also associated with known cancer predisposition genes; adenocarcinoma of the lung is seen with increased frequency in Li-Fraumeni syndrome (see also Chs 42 and 44) and those with a retinoblastoma gene mutation have an increased risk of several cancers, including lung cancer.[11]

CLINICAL PRESENTATION

Some patients with lung cancer present without symptoms when a chest X-ray is performed for other reasons (e.g. preoperatively or for a general medical examination) but the majority of lung cancer patients are symptomatic at presentation. A list of common presenting symptoms and signs are listed in Box 37.1. SCLC, in particular, may be associated with biochemical abnormalities, and there are also a wide range of paraneoplastic syndromes that can be associated with lung cancer, the commonest being endocrine phenomenon such as hyponatraemia (low blood sodium) due to the syndrome of inappropriate antidiuretic hormone (SIADH).

Mesotheliomas tend to present more insidiously, with non-specific symptoms of slowly progressive disease. The commonest symptoms are dyspnoea, often due to a pleural effusion, and chest pain, due to the presence of the tumour on the pleural surface or invading the chest wall. Involvement of the pericardial surface can cause a pericardial effusion.

ASSESSMENT

Initial assessment of patients with suspected lung cancer is via the general practitioner's surgery. A GP may request a chest X-ray; blood tests, including electrolytes; and liver function tests. If a cough is productive,

Box 37.1   Clinical presentation of lung cancer

Common presenting signs or symptoms:

- Persistent cough
- Chest pain
- Haemoptysis
- Continual or non-resolving chest infections
- Weight loss and anorexia
- Fatigue
- Shortness of breath
- Confusion (possibly due to low sodium, high calcium or cerebral metastases)
- Bronchorrhoea (with bronchioalveolar carcinoma)
- Clubbing and hypertrophic pulmonary osteoarthropathy (HPOA)
- Superior vena cava (SVC) obstruction
- Hoarse voice

Rare presenting signs or symptoms:

- Ear pain
- Chest wall deformity
- Swelling of breast (lymphatic obstruction can occur in mesothelioma)
- Dysphagia
- Wheeze
- Bone pain

sputum analysis may be performed. Further investigations are usually hospital-based, after referral to a chest physician.

A histological or cytological diagnosis is required, and this is often made at bronchoscopy, either by direct tumour biopsy, bronchial brushings or washings of the bronchial tree. Depending on the position of the tumour, a computed tomography (CT)-guided lung biopsy may be performed. A fine needle aspirate (FNA) can be taken of any palpable lymphadenopathy, and pleural fluid, if present, can be sent for cytological examination. Blood tests performed should include a full blood count, urea and electrolytes, liver function tests, calcium and lactate dehydrogenase (LDH). A CT scan of the thorax and upper abdomen (to include liver and adrenal glands) is mandatory in all patients with lung cancer to stage the disease. Other scans, such as a CT brain or a bone scan, may be performed if symptoms indicate possible malignant involvement. As brain metastases are more common in SCLC, some centres routinely perform a CT scan of the brain in those with limited disease. A CT brain scan may also be performed on those patients with NSCLC, particularly adenocarcinomas prior to surgical resection. The presence of cerebral or any metastases would alter the

prognosis, and a potentially curative surgical resection would not be possible.

STAGING AND PROGNOSIS

The staging of lung cancer patients is usually made on CT scan. Mediastinoscopy may also be required to confirm nodal status for those with potentially operable disease. The use of positron emission tomography (PET) in addition to CT can increase the sensitivity of mediastinal node detection. In a recent prospective study with histological confirmation, the detection rate of mediastinal nodes with PET was 91%, compared with 75% for CT alone.[12] Staging in both SCLC and NSCLC is very important, as treatment is dictated by the stage of the disease at presentation.

Small cell lung cancer

The staging of SCLC is relatively simple in that the disease is classed as limited or extensive. Limited disease is that confined to the thorax, mediastinum and supraclavicular nodes, which could potentially be encompassed in a radiotherapy field. Extensive disease is that outside this definition, with metastases outside the thorax. Even those presenting with limited disease have a relatively poor prognosis, with a 5-year survival of 15–20%. Only 5% of those with extensive disease at presentation are alive at 5 years. The median survival for untreated disease is approximately 3 months. Factors at presentation associated with a poor prognosis include:

- extensive disease
- poor performance status
- high plasma LDH
- high alkaline phosphatase
- and low plasma sodium.[13]

These can be combined into a scoring system, such as the 'Manchester Score', which can be used to stratify patients for study entry.[14]

Non–small cell lung cancer

NSCLC staging is based on the tumour–node–metastases (TNM) staging system, which was modified in 1997.[15,16] The classification is listed in full in Box 37.2. Five-year survival figures show a range from 60% for stage I to only 1% for stage IV disease (Table 37.1).

Mesothelioma

There have been several staging systems suggested for mesothelioma, mainly based on surgical experiences. The most common system is based on a TNM system

---

Box 37.2   TNM classifcation for non-small cell lung cancer (NSCLC) (1997)

Tx   Tumour cannot be assessed, but tumour proven by the presence of malignant cells in sputum or bronchial washings but not visualised by imaging or bronchoscopy

T0   No evidence of primary tumour

Tis   Carcinoma in situ

T1   Tumour 3 cm or less surrounded by lung or visceral pleura, without bronchoscopic evidence of invasion more proximal than the lobar bronchus

T2   Tumour measuring more than 3 cm, or;
   • extension to the visceral pleura,
   • atelectases,
   • obstructive pneumopathy of <one lung
   • main/principal bronchus tumour more than 2 cm from carina

T3   Tumour of any size that is:
   • directly extending into chest wall, mediastinal pleura, pericardium, diaphragm, mediastinal fat or phrenic nerve
   • at the apex
   • in the main or principal bronchus <2 cm from the carina
   • atelectases or obstructive pueumopathy of one entire lung

T4   Tumour of any size with:
   • macroscopic or histological extension into the mediastinum, heart, large vessels, trachea (or compression), oesophagus (or compression) carina, vertebral body
   • malignant pleural or pericardial effusion
   • recurrent laryngeal nerve involvement
   • metastatic pleural involvement (ipsilateral)
   • multiple nodules in the same lobe

N0   No regional lymph node metastases
N1   Ipsilateral peribronchial and/or hilar nodes
N2   Ipsilateral mediastinal and/or subcarinal nodes
N3   Contralateral mediastinal, contralateral hilar, contralateral scalene, or supraclavicular nodes (either side)

M0   No distant metastases
M1   Distant metastases present

---

and requires thoracoscopic staging.[17] Very few patients in this country are considered for surgery or have thorocoscopic procedures, and therefore complicated staging systems are rarely used in practice. Treatment

is palliative and based on symptom control. Figures for survival are variable, but in the UK survival from the time of diagnosis is approximately 7–12 months, with less than 5% alive at 5 years.

SCREENING

Lung cancer has characteristics that would fit well with a screening programme. The disease is common, can be detected on chest imaging prior to the development of symptoms and has a clear high-risk population. Lung cancer detected at an earlier stage, when it is operable, also carries a much better prognosis.

Chest X-rays and/or sputum cytology were used in early studies in the 1970s and four randomised trials failed to show a benefit.[18–21] These studies, however, had their faults. Some used sputum cytology, some chest X-rays and one study was underpowered and would only have been able to detect a large difference in mortality reduction. As a result of these initial studies, screening in lung cancer was felt not to beneficial.

Table 37.1   Five-year survival for non-small cell lung cancer (NSCLC)

Stage survival		Five-year
Stage Ia	T1 N0	60%
Stage Ib	T2 N0	38%
Stage IIa	T1 N1	34%
Stage IIb	T2 N1, T3 N0	22%
Stage IIIa	T3N1	13%
	T1–3N2	9%
Stage IIIb	T4 N0–2	7%
	T1–4 N3	3%
Stage IV	M1	1%

Recently, however, there have been new studies evaluating CT scanning as a screening tool. A Japanese study in 5483 smoking and non-smoking volunteers evaluated low-dose spiral CT scan and chest X-ray, compared with chest X-ray alone. Sputum cytology was also performed for the heavy smokers in both groups: 19 of the study patients were found to have lung cancer on CT scanning with a mean tumour size of 17 mm (6–47 mm); 16 of the patients were stage I; only one of these cancers was seen on X-ray, although 3 patients had abnormalities on X-ray which were thought to be benign. The detection rate for CT was therefore greater than with X-ray, but still low at 0.48%; however, the study included non-smokers.[22]

The Early Lung Cancer Action Project (ELCAP) has reported similar experiences with helical low-dose CT. The prevalence rate of malignant disease detected by CT scan was 2.7%, compared with 0.7% for chest X-ray.[23] There were 27 cancers detected by CT and, again, these were mainly early cancers, most under 1 cm, and all but one was operable. However, the study detected abnormalities that needed further follow-up in 233 patients (23% of the study population), most of which were benign, and this obviously has health economic implications. A randomised study in the UK is being planned.

TREATMENT

All patients diagnosed with lung cancer should be discussed in a multidisciplinary team, from which treatment decisions are made. A multidisciplinary team should ideally include a thoracic surgeon, chest physician, medical oncologist, clinical oncologist, radiologist and a palliative care specialist nurse or physician.

Small cell lung cancer

Initial treatment for patients presenting with limited or extensive disease should be chemotherapy.

SCLC is the most aggressive form of lung cancer that is likely to be disseminated at diagnosis. The results of local treatments alone, such as surgery or radiotherapy, are therefore very poor.[24] These cancers grow rapidly and treatment with chemotherapy should be commenced early after diagnosis. Two or three drug combinations are usually better than single agent therapy. Regimens commonly used are a combination of a platinum agent (cisplatin or carboplatin) and etoposide (Table 37.2). Response rates are in the order of 60–90%, with 45–75% achieving a complete response.

Limited disease

Standard therapy for non-bulky limited SCLC is combined modality, combination chemotherapy and radiotherapy with

Table 37.2 Chemotherapy regimens commonly used for small cell lung cancer (SCLC)

Chemotherapy regimen	Drugs
CE	Carboplatin and etoposide
PE	Cisplatin and etoposide
ACE	Adriamycin, cyclophosphamide and etoposide
VICE	Ifosphosphamide, carboplatin and etoposide
CAV	Cyclophosphamide, carboplatin and etoposide
PE/CAV	Alternating PE/CAV

prophylactic cranial irradiation for those achieving a good response after chemotherapy.

There are some long-term survivors following initial treatment of limited disease SCLC, and therefore the initial intent of treatment is curative. The 3-year survival with chemotherapy alone is around 10%, but the addition of radiotherapy following a partial or complete response to initial chemotherapy improves overall survival by 5% at 3 years.[25] Optimal treatment therefore usually involves 4–6 cycles of combination chemotherapy to induce a partial or complete remission followed by radical thoracic radiotherapy.

One of the commonest sites for first relapse is the brain, often without relapse elsewhere. In patients in complete remission after initial chemotherapy, regardless of the use of thoracic radiotherapy, prophylactic cranial irradiation (PCI) has been shown to improve overall survival by 5.4% at 3 years (from 15.3% to 20.7%) and reduces the risk of cerebral metastases from 58% to 33%.[26] Prospective studies have also shown that PCI produces no significant deterioration in neuropsychological function.[27]

Concurrent chemoradiation and intensive chemotherapy
Concurrent use of chemotherapy and radiotherapy at the same time rather than sequential treatment has improved the treatment of other solid tumours such as oesophageal and rectal tumours and is being explored in limited disease SCLC. The use of thoracic radiotherapy, often with the first cycle of chemotherapy, has been tested by many institutions, mainly in non-randomised studies. One randomised study has compared radiotherapy (40 Gy in 15 fractions) given with either the first or last cycle of chemotherapy. A significant improvement in progression-free and overall survival was seen with initial radiotherapy

($p = 0.036$ and $p = 0.008$, respectively), although the complete response rate was similar in both arms.[28] This may be promising, but concurrent chemoradiation can be more toxic than sequential treatment and therefore patients should be of good performance status before commencing treatment.

In limited disease SCLC more intensive chemotherapy regimens may be beneficial and are being investigated. There is some evidence that by increasing the dose intensity of chemotherapy one can improve survival, with acceptable toxicity.[29] As with chemoradiation, patients need to be carefully selected for more intensive treatments to avoid unacceptable toxicity and study entry is often limited to a small patient group. Other areas under investigation are maintenance schedules, new drug combinations, vaccine treatment and radiotherapy schedules and timing.

Extensive disease

Patients with extensive disease are incurable and treatment is with palliative intent. Most patients will be treated with combination chemotherapy and, although overall response rates are in the order of 70–80%, complete remission rates in extensive disease are only 20–30%.

Combination chemotherapy regimens are similar to that used in limited disease (Table 37.2). Patients are often more symptomatic and of poorer performance status and may not tolerate chemotherapy very well. In the elderly or those with poor performance status, less-intense chemotherapy regimens have been tried, including oral etoposide. However, several prospective randomised trials of oral etoposide compared to combination chemotherapy have shown an advantage to combination chemotherapy, with no significant difference in toxicity.[30,31] Patients should be given combination chemotherapy where possible.

In general, these patients are not suitable for radical radiotherapy approaches and radiotherapy can be given at a later date to palliate symptoms. Good links with a palliative care service are essential from early after diagnosis. (See also Chs 1 and 2.)

Relapsed disease

Patients who relapse after initial treatment have very poor outcome, regardless of the original stage at presentation. Those who initially responded to treatment and relapse after 6 months can be retreated with combination chemotherapy, either the same or an alternative regimen. The response rates, however, are considerably lower. Drugs used in second-line treatment are oral etoposide, CE, EP, ACE, or topotecan. Patients who have primary resistant disease are unlikely to respond to further chemotherapy.

Radiotherapy can be used to palliate symptoms, such as bone pain and also within the thorax, if not previously used. Those who retain a good performance status should be considered for clinical trials, either phase I or II.

Non-small cell lung cancer: stage I and stage II disease

Optimal treatment for stage I and II disease is surgical resection with neoadjuvant chemotherapy given within a clinical trial or radical radiotherapy given with chemotherapy.

Surgery

Patients presenting with early stage disease, stage I and II (T1–2, N0–1) should be considered for surgery and discussed with a thoracic surgeon. Patients need to be of good performance status, have no serious concurrent medical problems and have adequate lung function, usually a forced expiratory volume (FEV$_1$) of over 1.5 litres. Surgery may involve lobectomy or complete pneumonectomy, depending on the position of the tumour.

Radical radiotherapy

Some patients who are ineligible for surgery may be considered for radical radiotherapy, although this is also contraindicated in those with poor lung function. More intensive radical radiotherapy protocols may improve survival in those considered for radical radiotherapy treatments. CHART (continuous hyperfractionated accelerated radiotherapy) involves radiotherapy fractions of 1.5 Gy given 3 times a day. This means completing 54 Gy in only 12 days, with radiotherapy treatments given over the weekend. In a study comparing this form of accelerated radiotherapy to 60 Gy given over 6 weeks, a reduction in the relative risk of death of 24% was seen: hazard ratio 0.76 (95% CI 0.63–0.92), $p = 0.004$.[32] This regimen, however, has practical implications, with evening and weekend radiographer staffing, and therefore a modification of the CHART regime is being investigated, CHARTWELL.

Adjuvant chemotherapy treatments

Adjuvant chemotherapy should be discussed in all patients suitable for this following complete surgical resection.
Adjuvant radiotherapy is not recommended following complete surgical resection.

Chemotherapy after surgical resection (adjuvant chemotherapy) has shown benefit in other solid tumours such as breast and colon cancer. The role of adjuvant chemotherapy in lung cancer has become clearer in recent months following the presentation of the results of the largest trial using cisplatin-based chemotherapy.[84] Prior to this, none of the smaller randomised phase III trials had shown benefit to adjuvant chemotherapy individually, but a meta-analysis of 8 trials involving 1394 patients showed an absolute benefit of 5% at 5 years with platinum-based chemotherapy in addition to surgery, $p = 0.08$.[33] This same meta-analysis showed that chemotherapy given before or after radical radiotherapy prolonged survival by 2–4% at 5 years. The role of chemotherapy with radical radiotherapy is another area of rapid evolution. The most recent data on the use of radiotherapy given concurrently with chemotherapy compared to sequential treatment suggests a 9% survival gain at 4 years.[85] Where possible, patients should be entered into prospective randomised trials of adjuvant and neoadjuvant chemotherapy.

Adjuvant radiotherapy

A meta-analysis has been undertaken, looking at the role of adjuvant radiotherapy following complete surgical resection in node-positive disease. Data on 2128 patients participating in 9 randomised trials of adjuvant radiotherapy actually showed a poorer survival in those patients who had adjuvant radiotherapy compared to surgery alone, with a hazard ratio of 1.21 (95% CI 1.08–1.34), $p = 0.001$, an absolute difference of 7% at 2 years.[34] Subgroup analysis showed that the detriment was seen principally in those with stage I and II disease. Changing radiotherapy techniques may make this data less applicable to clinical practice today, but postoperative radiotherapy is not currently recommended for patients after complete surgical resection.

Non-small cell lung cancer stage IIIA (T3N1, T1–3N2)

Patients with stage IIIA disease should be considered for combination chemotherapy and then assessed for radical local treatment, either radiotherapy or surgery, and preferably as part of a randomised clinical trial.

In this group of patients, some will have potentially operable disease, and a few may be cured by surgery alone.[35–37] However, the majority have disease too extensive to be removed surgically, or will be unfit for surgery due to poor performance status, general ill health or impaired lung function.

A review of the literature on outcome after operative treatment for N2 disease showed a 5-year survival ranging from 6 to 35%. Those patients with a lower T-stage tumour, squamous cell histology and minimal N2 disease, defined as one positive lower group excluding subcarinal adenopathy, had a better outcome.[38] In view of the heterogeneity in this group, good

patient selection for radical modality treatments is essential and the identification of prognostic factors can help to guide that process.

Mediastinoscopy can identify and biopsy involved nodes and therefore most patients suitable for radical treatments should undergo the procedure for suspected N2 disease on CT scanning. PET scanning can improve the accuracy of CT staging, but is not widely available. PET and CT scanning have been shown to be significantly better than CT alone for the detection of N2/N3 disease.[39]

Preoperative (neoadjuvant) chemotherapy

The role of neoadjuvant is developing following recent publications in early-stage lung cancer and will change more after the completion of the ongoing national and international trials. Preoperative chemotherapy has been studied in stage IIIa disease in an attempt to 'down-stage' the tumour prior to surgical resection. Inoperable or bulky tumours may respond to chemotherapy to allow a surgical resection. Early phase II studies showed good response rates to induction chemotherapy and led to randomised studies.

A randomised trial of 3 cycles of MIC (mitomycin, ifosfamide and cisplatin), followed by surgery, showed an improved disease-free and overall survival to preoperative MIC (20 vs 5 months and 26 vs 8 months, respectively, $p < 0.001$).[40] Updated data still show the median survival advantage to preoperative chemotherapy (22 vs 10 months, $p = 0.005$).[41] A median survival advantage was seen to 3 cycles of pre- and postoperative CEP (cyclophosphamide, etoposide and cisplatin) compared to surgery alone.[42] Updated, this shows a median survival advantage of 7 months (21 vs 14 months, $p = 0.056$).[43] Both of these small studies were stopped early due to the survival advantage.

A further, larger study of 355 patients with stage I–IIIa NSCLC has also shown a benefit to preoperative chemotherapy using 2 cycles of MIC. Approximately half the patients had stage IIIa disease. There was an increased disease-free survival for the chemotherapy arm compared to the surgery alone arm of 13.8% over 3 years, $p = 0.033$ and the overall survival figures were better with preoperative chemotherapy, but non-significant.[44] The benefit seemed to be principally in stage I and II patients rather than stage IIIa. Patients with stage IIIa disease should be considered for pre-operative chemotherapy as part of a clinical trial.

Non-small cell lung cancer stage IIIB and stage IV

Patients with stage IIIB and stage IV disease have a very poor prognosis. The 5-year survival is under 10%. Those with stage IV disease have a 5-year survival of only 1%, and median survival of 4–6 months without treatment. Any treatment is palliative, i.e. for symptom relief and disease control, although in some patients treatment may prolong survival by months. Links with palliative care services are essential early after the diagnosis.

Chemotherapy

Palliative treatment with a cisplatin-containing combination or single agent non-platinum chemotherapy should be considered in all patients with good performance status.

Chemotherapy for advanced NSCLC has been shown to improve survival in those with good performance status, and more importantly has demonstrated improved quality of life compared with best supportive care (no chemotherapy). The meta-analysis of 8 trials (778 patients) of cisplatin-based chemotherapy vs best supportive care showed a significant survival advantage to the chemotherapy arm. The hazard ratio was 0.73, p <0.0001, translating to a modest increase in median survival of 6 weeks and an absolute survival benefit of 10% at 1 year. At least 50% of the patients treated achieved symptom control and quality of life was maintained.[33]

There have been further studies comparing best supportive care and chemotherapy using MIC, MVP (mitomycin C, vinblastine and cisplatin) or IEP (ifosfamide, etoposide and cisplatin). These have confirmed the survival advantage to combination platinum-containing chemotherapy with improved quality of life.[45,46] Newer agents, gemcitabine, vinorelbine, docetaxel and paclitaxel, have also shown activity in lung cancer with a survival advantage compared to best supportive care of a similar magnitude to that seen with cisplatin combinations.[33,47–49]

Therefore, the evidence supports the use of palliative chemotherapy in those with a good performance status of 0–2. The principles of palliative treatment are to balance toxicity against benefit, and patients should be evaluated before each cycle of treatment to ensure continued response and controlled toxicity. In this way palliative chemotherapy can be effective at symptom control and improving quality of life. Factors associated with a poor outcome in advanced disease are:

- lack of response to chemotherapy
- poor performance status
- pretreatment weight loss and
- an elevated LDH.[50]

One of the most important factors in the use of chemotherapy in this group is performance status. In our own experience side effects and the risk of toxic death increased with poor performance status and this was independent of the age of the patient.[51,52]

MVP and MIC   Most agents and combinations have shown modest objective response rates of around 30% but several studies have shown that around 70% of patients report symptomatic benefit despite not gaining a formal response.[46,53,54] The Royal Marsden study demonstrated a response rate of 21% to MVP, but 75% of patients had a complete or significant improvement of at least one of their tumour-related symptoms, translating to an overall symptom response rate of 67%.[54] The symptomatic improvement was seen after 1 course of chemotherapy in 61% and after 2 courses in 96% of responding patients. A similar symptomatic benefit and response rate was seen with 3 and 6 cycles of MVP, but there was significantly less toxicity with 3 courses.[55] Generally, this means that benefits of chemotherapy can be seen early and excessive toxicity can be avoided. (See also Chs 7 and 14.)

Vinorelbine   In the UK, MVP and MIC have been the most common regimens used, but there has been increasing use of the newer agents alone or in combinations. Vinorelbine has shown efficacy and good tolerability as a single agent when given to an elderly population (over 70 years old), producing a significant improvement in median survival, 21 weeks to 28 weeks, $p = 0.03$. The combination of cisplatin and vinorelbine has also been shown to be superior to cisplatin alone, with an improved median survival of 8 vs 6 months, $p = 0.0018$.[56] The combination has shown superiority to vinorelbine alone.[57] However, those patients with a performance status of 2 had more toxicity and less benefit from vinorelbine/cisplatin compared to vinorelbine alone.[58]

There have been two randomised studies comparing cisplatin/vinorelbine to UK-type cisplatin combinations. An Italian study showed no significant difference in response rate, time to progression or overall survival to cisplatin/vinorelbine compared with a mitomycin, vindesine and cisplatin combination.[59] A further Portuguese study has reported an interim analysis of a phase III trial comparing MVP vs vinorelbine/cisplatin vs 2 gemcitabine/cisplatin regimens, which has shown superior activity to vinorelbine and gemcitabine doublets compared to MVP, but further follow-up is needed with survival data.[60]

Cisplatin/vinorelbine may be considered as an alternative to MVP or MIC for those with good performance status. Single agent vinorelbine is an outpatient schedule with a good side-effect profile suitable for palliation in the elderly or those with a performance status of 2, or where cisplatin may not be indicated.

Gemcitabine   Gemcitabine has shown activity as a single agent and in one study was as effective and less toxic than a cisplatin/vindesine combination.[61]

Gemcitabine/cisplatin is an active combination, showing superiority to cisplatin alone.[62] In a study comparing the combination to MIC (although with a higher dose of cisplatin than UK MIC, which uses 50 mg/m^2), the gemcitabine/cisplatin combination had a higher response rate (38% vs 26%, $p = 0.877$).[63] There was no improvement in survival, however, with gemcitabine/cisplatin, and there was more haematological toxicity and no difference in quality of life. A UK study comparing gemcitabine/carboplatin to either MVP or MIC has shown no difference in response rate or toxicity between the two treatments.[64] A further UK London Lung Group Study, however, suggests a significant improvement in survival with gemcitabine/carboplatin compared with MVP, $p = 0.04$.[65a] The combination of gemcitabine/cisplatin is used frequently in Europe.

Paclitaxel Paclitaxel has shown activity in NSCLC, and combinations of paclitaxel and cisplatin have shown response rates of around 30% and a 2-month improvement in median survival compared with an etoposide and cisplatin combination.[65b] This combination is favoured in the USA. A cisplatin/paclitaxel combination has been shown to be as effective as vinorelbine/paclitaxel.[66] The ECOG 1594 trial compared several of these newer doublets of chemotherapy and has shown similar activity.[67]

The newer doublets of chemotherapy – cisplatin/vinorelbine, cisplatin/gemcitabine and cisplatin/paclitaxel – show good activity, but there have been few comparison trials with MVP or MIC. The response rates of the newer combinations are a little higher, but in advanced disease they do have more toxicity. All three drugs – vinorelbine, gemcitabine and paclitaxel – have been approved by the National Institute for Clinical Excellence (NICE) for the use as first-line therapy, ideally in combination with cisplatin, for patients with stage III and IV NSCLC.[68]

Second-line chemotherapy

If a patient has had a good response to first-line therapy that is sustained for more than 6 months, and they still have a good performance status, then re-treating with chemotherapy when symptomatic may be beneficial. The response rate to second-line chemotherapy, however, drops substantially. In those patients who relapse within 6 months of chemotherapy, there is some evidence that docetaxel may have activity following a platinum-based combination. Compared with best supportive care, docetaxel chemotherapy has shown improved quality of life and a survival benefit at 1 year of 16%, $p = 0.003$.[69] On this basis it has been approved by NICE for consideration as second-line therapy following cisplatin combination therapy.[68]

NSCLC overexpresses epidermal growth factor receptor (EGFR), which is involved in cell growth. An orally active EGFR tyrosine kinase inhibitor ZD1839 (Iressa) has been developed and has shown efficacy in the treatment of NSCLC. An overall response rate of 18.7% (95% CI 13.7–24.7%), and symptom control rate of 38.7% (95% CI 30.5–47.4%) has been demonstrated in patients with NSCLC after one or two lines of chemotherapy, including a platinum-containing therapy.[70] Phase II studies with ZD1839 in combination with chemotherapy have shown no additional toxicity,[71] but results from phase III studies are disappointing.

Radiotherapy

Palliative radiotherapy can be very effective in the management of patients with advanced NSCLC. Treatment may be given to the primary site or to treat symptomatic problems, such as bone infiltration, skin deposits, or for superior vena cava (SVC) obstruction. Good palliation is often achieved. Endobronchial radiation may be a useful technique and whole brain radiotherapy may be required for brain metastases.

Other palliative treatments

Palliative care is an essential component of the management of patients with advanced lung cancer and must be involved early alongside any chemotherapy or radiotherapy treatments.

Some patients present or develop SVC obstruction and this can also be managed by a radiologically inserted SVC stent, which may give good palliation of symptoms in addition to radiotherapy. Endobronchial therapy – such as laser treatment, stent insertion or radiotherapy – can be useful for bronchial obstruction due to an endobronchial component to the tumour, and is particularly useful for haemoptysis. If recurrent pleural effusions are a problem, then rather than repeated aspiration, thoracoscopic drainage and pleurodesis can often provide excellent results.

Mesothelioma

No therapeutic intervention in mesothelioma has been shown to improve survival, although the natural history of the disease is variable and there are some long-term survivors.[72] Most patients present with advanced disease where treatment is aimed at palliation. A few patients may have more localised disease on presentation, or respond well to initial chemotherapy and be considered for more aggressive surgical approaches.

Surgery

Surgery for mesothelioma varies from a thoracoscopic biopsy and pleurodesis to an extrapleural pneumonectomy. Pleurectomy and decortication can produce a symptomatic benefit by removing painful tumour, and the procedure is associated with less morbidity and mortality than an extrapleural pneumonectomy.[73] Some centres have combined this approach with radiotherapy and chemotherapy in a phase II study.[74] Extrapleural pneumonectomy is occasionally performed in the UK, but there are several centres within the USA where this approach is combined with hemithorax radiotherapy and chemotherapy. These aggressive treatment programmes are only for those with good performance status and early-stage disease. The operative mortality from the surgery alone is 6–30%, although centres with experience in the techniques claim an operative mortality of <5%.[75] *There have been no randomised controlled trials of any of these treatment modalities and no evidence of a survival benefit.* Such a trial is planned to start in 2005 in the UK (the MARS trial). Surgery should be viewed as a palliative procedure and may be appropriate for some patients, but aggressive combined modality approaches are rarely undertaken in the UK.

Radiotherapy

Radiotherapy given within 6 weeks of thoracoscopy or pleural biopsy to the exit sites can reduce the frequency of disease seeding along the biopsy tract and causing chest wall nodules.[76] Palliative radiotherapy can be used for painful chest wall disease, especially when eroding bone, and also for brain metastases, although these are rare with mesothelioma.

Chemotherapy

There are several agents that have shown activity in malignant mesothelioma, although response rates are generally low, of the order of 15–20%. Drugs that have been used are doxorubicin, cisplatin, cyclophosphamide and premetrexed, alone or in combination. In our own institution, MVP has a response rate of 20% and good symptomatic response rate of 50%.[77] Similar response rates and symptomatic benefit have also been seen with single agent vinorelbine.[78] Gemcitabine, another newer chemotherapy agent, has shown very little activity in mesothelioma as a single agent,[79,80] but good activity in combination with cisplatin, although with more toxicity.[81] The first licensed chemotherapy drug for malignant mesothelioma is pemetrexed (Alimta). In combination with cisplatin, this drug was shown to be superior to cisplatin alone, including improved survival and is now the chemotherapy standard of care.[105]

It is important that patients with advanced mesothelioma who are considered for chemotherapy should be entered into clinical trials. In the UK we have the first national randomised clinical trial in mesothelioma underway comparing MVP, vinorelbine and supportive care. This and other studies will evaluate both clinical and symptomatic response rates.

Prognostic factors

Staging systems are often difficult to apply to many patients presenting with more advanced mesothelioma and are based on assessment for surgery rather than a guide to prognosis. What would be more useful is a prognostic score to stratify patients for entry and analysis of future trials. Two prognostic scoring systems have been proposed by the European Organisation for Research and Treatment of Cancer (EORTC) and the Cancer and Leukaemia Group B (CALGB). These have identified poor prognostic factors from large series of patients and proposed prognostic groupings; the EORTC have a high- and low-risk group and the CALGB six prognostic groups.[6,82] In the EORTC data, the low-risk group had a median survival of 10.8 months and high-risk group 5.5 months. One-year survival was 40% (95% CI 30–50) and 12% (95% CI 4–20), respectively. A recent study in the UK applied the prognostic factors to their population and found, on multivariate analysis, the following to be poor prognostic markers:

- sarcomatous histological subtype
- low plasma haemoglobin
- elevated blood white cell count
- poor performance status and
- male sex.[83]

NURSING CARE FOR PATIENTS RECEIVING CHEMOTHERAPY FOR LUNG CANCER

Suzanne Vizor

PALLIATIVE CARE

The majority of newly diagnosed patients have advanced disease for which no curative treatment is available.[86] Only 6% of patients are asymptomatic at diagnosis.[87]

Palliation should therefore be central to any management plan in this patient group.[88] Nurses are skilled at working with patients to help them clarify the symptoms they are experiencing[89] and facilitating self-help strategies. The skills of a clinical nurse specialist are invaluable, especially in supporting the family unit as a whole.

PSYCHOSOCIAL ISSUES

Generally, nurses have the most consistent and continuing relationship with cancer patients.[90] Therefore, they are ideally placed to help patients come to terms with the psychological trauma related to being diagnosed with lung cancer. The psychosocial impact of a lung cancer diagnosis can be more devastating than other cancers because of its rapid course and grave prognosis.[91] Patients may withdraw socially and isolate themselves as a way of coping with their symptoms.[92] Family disruptions may occur, with major shifts in family roles in a short period of time.[93] The nurse is often the facilitator who ensures appropriate communication and coordination of care.[94]

SMOKING

The majority of lung cancers can be attributed to smoking; these patients may feel guilty that they brought the cancer on themselves.[91] This can result in blame being voiced by family and friends and grieving shown as anger and bitterness. The desire to stop smoking should be supported and the benefits emphasised. Smoking cessation can increase quality of life even in advanced stages of the disease.[93] Sarna[95] supports this view by listing nine benefits, as shown in Box 37.3.

TREATMENT CHOICE

Lung cancer is primarily a disease of old age, with more than 70% of all new cases occurring in people

---

Box 37.3 Why smokers with lung cancer should quit

- Decrease shortness of breath and cough
- Decrease risk of recurrence
- Decrease risk of secondary tobacco-related malignancies
- Decrease risk/worsening of other tobacco-related diseases: heart disease, chronic obstructive pulmonary disease, stroke
- Decrease risk of treatment side effects
- Decrease risk of weight loss: improve food tastes and smells
- Increase feelings of well-being and being in control
- Decrease risk of lung cancer and heart disease from second-hand smoke for other members in the household
- Be a role model for family and friends[95]

---

aged 60 years or over, with a peak incidence at 75 years of age.[96] Generally, age on its own is a very weak predictor of the likelihood of toxicity or treatment failure.[97] However, the possibility of concurrent medical conditions increases with age, and can result in polypharmacy[98] and/or abnormal blood results. These two possible consequences can limit the chemotherapeutic agents used or dictate the dose level. This can also result in patients being ineligible to take part in certain clinical trials; few have age limits but most have biochemical eligibility criteria for study entry. Nurses have a key role in evaluating the balance of risk and benefits of chemotherapy.[99] Engelking's table of chemotherapy agents that are associated with increased toxicity in the elderly is a useful guide.[98]

Consent

In the treatment of lung cancer there are complex issues linked to consent. Due to the predominantly non-curative nature of this disease, patients need to be supported in discussions concerning treatment choices.[100] The chemotherapy toxicity predicted life expectancy and quality of life issues all impact on the patient's decision.

BREATHLESSNESS

Difficulty in breathing is reported by as many as 65% of lung cancer patients.[101] This symptom is often related to deep concerns about life, death and fears of suffocation.[91] The only research of the non-pharmaceutical management of breathlessness in lung cancer has been coordinated by Corner.[102] This research demonstrated that the holistic approach to patients' symptoms by specialist nurses could produce improvements in quality of life,[88] which are devoid of toxicity.[103]

Dyspnoea in this patient group can be further exacerbated by chemotherapy. Some cytotoxic drugs can cause chronic pulmonary fibrosis, particularly when the patient also receives radiotherapy or has had thoracic surgery.[104] Susan Holmes examines this issue in the 'Less common toxic effects' chapter of her book.[90] (See also Ch. 29.)

CONCLUSION

To improve treatment and care of patients with lung cancer in the future it is now acknowledged that a multidisciplinary approach is needed.[102] Nurses are in the ideal position to play a pivotal role in coordinating care and responding to the very complex needs of the individual with lung cancer and their family.

References

1. UK CR. Statistics – incidence. 2002. www. cancerresearchuk.org

2. Campaign CR. Lung cancer and smoking – UK. London: Cancer Research Campaign; 1992.

3. Campaign CR. Lung topples breast as biggest killer cancer of women. Cancer Research Campaign; 2000; 26.09.2000.

4. Peto J, Decarli A, La Vecchia C, et al. The European mesothelioma epidemic. Br J Cancer 1999; 79(3–4):666–672.

5. Suzuke Y. Pathology of human malignant mesothelioma. Semin Oncol 1980; 8:268.

6. Curran D, Sahmoud T, Therasse P, et al. Prognostic factors in patients with pleural mesothelioma: the European Organization for Research and Treatment of Cancer experience. J Clin Oncol 1998;16(1):145–152.

7. Lubin JH, Blot WJ, Berrino F, et al. Modifying risk of developing lung cancer by changing habits of cigarette smoking. Br Med J (Clin Res Ed) 1984; 288(6435):1953–1956.

8. Hansen HH, Goldstraw P, Gregor A, et al. Tumours of the trachea and lung. In: Peckham M, Pinedo H, Veronesi U, eds. Oxford textbook of oncology. 1st edn. Oxford: Oxford University Press; 1995:1553–1557.

9. Watson DCT. Mesothelioma. In: Peckham M, Pinedo H, Veronesi U, eds. Oxford textbook of oncology. 1st edn. Oxford: Oxford University Press; 1995:1557–1562.

10. Lee PN. Indoor Environment 1993; 2:129–142.

11. Sanders BM, Jay M, Draper GJ, et al. Non-ocular cancer in relatives of retinoblastoma patients. Br J Cancer 1989; 60(3):358–365.

12. Pieterman RM, van Putten JW, Meuzelaar JJ, et al. Preoperative staging of non-small-cell lung cancer with positron-emission tomography [comment]. N Engl J Med 2000; 343(4):254–261.

13. Rawson NS, Peto J. An overview of prognostic factors in small cell lung cancer. A report from the Subcommittee for the Management of Lung Cancer of the United Kingdom Coordinating Committee on Cancer Research [published erratum appears in Br J Cancer 1990; 62(3):550]. Br J Cancer 1990; 61(4):597–604.

14. Cerny T, Blair V, Anderson H, et al. Pretreatment prognostic factors and scoring system in 407 small-cell lung cancer patients. Int J Cancer 1987; 39(2):146–149.

15. Mountain CF. A new international staging system for lung cancer. Chest 1986; 89(4 Suppl):225S–233S.

16. Mountain CF. Revisions in the International System for Staging Lung Cancer [see comments]. Chest 1997; 111(6):1710–1717.

17. Rusch VW. A proposed new international TNM staging system for malignant pleural mesothelioma from the International Mesothelioma Interest Group. Lung Cancer 1996; 14(1):1–12.

18. Tockman MS. Survival and mortality from lung cancer in a screened population: the Johns Hopkins Study. Chest 1986; 89:324–325S.

19. Melamed MR, Flehinger BJ, Zaman MB, et al. Screening for early lung cancer. Results of the Memorial Sloan-Kettering study in New York. Chest 1984; 86(1):44–53.

20. Kubik A, Parkin DM, Khlat M, et al. Lack of benefit from semi-annual screening for cancer of the lung: follow-up report of a randomized controlled trial on a population of high-risk males in Czechoslovakia. Int J Cancer 1990; 45(1):26–33.

21. Fontana RS, Sanderson DR, Woolner LB, et al. Lung cancer screening: the Mayo program. J Occup Med 1986; 28(8):746–750.

22. Sone S, Takashima S, Li F, et al. Mass screening for lung cancer with mobile spiral computed tomography scanner [see comments]. Lancet 1998; 351(9111):1242–1245.

23. Henschke CI, McCauley DI, Yankelevitz DF, et al. Early Lung Cancer Action Project: overall design and findings from baseline screening [see comments]. Lancet 1999; 354(9173):99–105.

24. Prasad US, Naylor AR, Walker WS, et al. Long term survival after pulmonary resection for small cell carcinoma of the lung [see comments]. Thorax 1989; 44(10):784–787.

25. Pignon JP, Arriagada R, Ihde DC, et al. A meta-analysis of thoracic radiotherapy for small-cell lung cancer [see comments]. N Engl J Med 1992; 327(23):1618–1624.

26. Auperin A, Arriagada R, Pignon JP, et al. Prophylactic cranial irradiation for patients with small-cell lung cancer in complete remission. Prophylactic Cranial Irradiation Overview Collaborative Group [see comments]. N Engl J Med 1999; 341(7):476–484.

27. Arriagada R, Le Chevalier T, Borie F, et al. Prophylactic cranial irradiation for patients with small-cell lung cancer in complete remission [see comments]. J Natl Cancer Inst 1995; 87(3):183–190.

28. Murray N, Coy P, Pater JL, et al. Importance of timing for thoracic irradiation in the combined modality treatment of limited-stage small-cell lung cancer. The National Cancer Institute of Canada Clinical Trials Group. J Clin Oncol 1993; 11(2):336–344.

29. Thatcher N, Girling DJ, Hopwood P, et al. Improving survival without reducing quality of life in small-cell lung cancer patients by increasing the dose-intensity of chemotherapy with granulocyte colony-stimulating factor support: results of a British Medical Research Council Multicenter Randomized Trial. Medical Research Council Lung Cancer Working Party. J Clin Oncol 2000; 18(2):395–404.

30. Souhami RL, Spiro SG, Rudd RM, et al. Five-day oral etoposide treatment for advanced small-cell lung cancer: randomized comparison with intravenous chemotherapy [see comments]. J Natl Cancer Inst 1997; 89(8):577–580.

31. Girling DJ. Comparison of oral etoposide and standard intravenous multidrug chemotherapy for small-cell lung cancer: a stopped multicentre randomised trial.

Medical Research Council Lung Cancer Working Party [see comments]. Lancet 1996; 348(9027):563–566.

32. Saunders M, Dische S, Barrett A, et al. Continuous hyperfractionated accelerated radiotherapy (CHART) versus conventional radiotherapy in non-small-cell lung cancer: a randomised multicentre trial. CHART Steering Committee [see comments]. Lancet 1997; 350(9072):161–165.

33. Group NC. Chemotherapy in non-small cell lung cancer: a meta-analysis using updated data on individual patients from 52 randomised clinical trials. Non-small Cell Lung Cancer Collaborative Group [see comments]. BMJ 1995; 311(7010):899–909.

34. Stewart LA. Postoperative radiotherapy in non-small-cell lung cancer: systematic review and meta-analysis of individual patient data from nine randomised controlled trials. PORT Meta-analysis Trialists Group [see comments]. Lancet 1998; 352(9124):257–263.

35. Naruke T, Suemasu K, Ishikawa S. Lymph node mapping and curability at various levels of metastasis in resected lung cancer. J Thorac Cardiovasc Surg 1978; 76(6):832–839.

36. Pearson FG, DeLarue NC, Ilves R, et al. Significance of positive superior mediastinal nodes identified at mediastinoscopy in patients with resectable cancer of the lung. J Thorac Cardiovasc Surg 1982; 83(1):1–11.

37. Martini N, Flehinger BJ, Zaman MB, et al. Prospective study of 445 lung carcinomas with mediastinal lymph node metastases. J Thorac Cardiovasc Surg 1980; 80(3):390–399.

38. Vansteenkiste JF, De Leyn PR, Deneffe GJ, et al. Clinical prognostic factors in surgically treated stage IIIA-N2 non-small cell lung cancer: analysis of the literature [see comments]. Lung Cancer 1998; 19(1):3–13.

39. Vansteenkiste JF, Stroobants SG, De Leyn PR, et al. Lymph node staging in non-small-cell lung cancer with FDG-PET scan: a prospective study on 690 lymph node stations from 68 patients. J Clin Oncol 1998; 16(6):2142–2149.

40. Rosell R, Gomez-Codina J, Camps C, et al. A randomized trial comparing preoperative chemotherapy plus surgery with surgery alone in patients with non-small-cell lung cancer [see comments]. N Engl J Med 1994; 330(3):153–158.

41. Rosell R, Gomez-Codina J, Camps C, et al. Preresectional chemotherapy in stage IIIA non-small-cell lung cancer: a 7-year assessment of a randomized controlled trial. Lung Cancer 1999; 26(1):7–14.

42. Roth JA, Fossella F, Komaki R, et al. A randomized trial comparing perioperative chemotherapy and surgery with surgery alone in resectable stage IIIA non-small-cell lung cancer [see comments]. J Natl Cancer Inst 1994; 86(9):673–680.

43. Roth JA, Atkinson EN, Fossella F, et al. Long-term follow-up of patients enrolled in a randomized trial comparing perioperative chemotherapy and surgery with surgery alone in resectable stage IIIA non-small-cell lung cancer [see comments]. Lung Cancer 1998; 21(1):1–6.

44. Depierre A, Milleron B, Moro-Sibilot D, et al. Preoperative chemotherapy followed by surgery compared with primary surgery in resectable stage I (except T1N0), II, and IIIa non-small-cell lung cancer. J Clin Oncol 2002; 20(1):247–253.

45. Thongprasert S, Sanguanmitra P, Juthapan W, Clinch J. Relationship between quality of life and clinical outcomes in advanced non-small cell lung cancer: best supportive care (BSC) versus BSC plus chemotherapy. Lung Cancer 1999; 24(1):17–24.

46. Cullen MH, Billingham LJ, Woodroffe CM, et al. Mitomycin, ifosfamide, and cisplatin in unresectable non-small-cell lung cancer: effects on survival and quality of life [see comments]. J Clin Oncol 1999; 17(10):3188–3194.

47. Anderson H, Hopwood P, Stephens RJ, et al. Gemcitabine plus best supportive care (BSC) vs BSC in inoperable non-small cell lung cancer – a randomized trial with quality of life as the primary outcome. UK NSCLC Gemcitabine Group. Non-Small Cell Lung Cancer. Br J Cancer 2000; 83(4):447–453.

48. Ranson M, Davidson N, Nicolson M, et al. Randomized trial of paclitaxel plus supportive care versus supportive care for patients with advanced non-small-cell lung cancer. J Natl Cancer Inst 2000; 92(13):1074–1080.

49. Roszkowski K, Pluzanska A, Krzakowski M, et al. A multicenter, randomized, phase III study of docetaxel plus best supportive care versus best supportive care in chemotherapy-naive patients with metastatic or non-resectable localized non-small cell lung cancer (NSCLC). Lung Cancer 2000; 27(3):145–157.

50. Albain KS, Crowley JJ, LeBlanc M, et al. Survival determinants in extensive-stage non-small-cell lung cancer: the Southwest Oncology Group experience. J Clin Oncol 1991; 9(9):1618–1626.

51. Hickish TF, Smith IE, Ashley S, et al. Chemotherapy for elderly patients with lung cancer [letter]. Lancet 1995; 346(8974):580.

52. Dark GG, O'Brien ME. The evidence base for palliative chemotherapy. In: UK key advances in clinical practice series 2001. The effective management of lung cancer. Muers MF, Macbeth F, Wells FS et al (Eds) Aesculapims Medical Press, London 2001.

53. Hardy JR, Noble T, Smith IE. Symptom relief with moderate dose chemotherapy (mitomycin-C, vinblastine and cisplatin) in advanced non-small cell lung cancer. Br J Cancer 1989; 60(5):764–766.

54. Ellis PA, Smith IE, Hardy JR, et al. Symptom relief with MVP (mitomycin C, vinblastine and cisplatin) chemotherapy in advanced non-small-cell lung cancer. Br J Cancer 1995; 71(2):366–370.

55. Smith IE, O'Brien MER, Talbot DC, et al. Duration of chemotherapy in advanced non-small-cell lung cancer: a randomized trial of three versus six courses of mitomycin, vinblastine and cisplatin. J Clin Oncol 2001; 19:1336–1343.

56. Wozniak AJ, Crowley JJ, Balcerzak SP, et al. Randomized trial comparing cisplatin with cisplatin plus vinorelbine in the treatment of advanced

non-small-cell lung cancer: a Southwest Oncology Group study. J Clin Oncol 1998; 16(7):2459–2465.

57. Le Chevalier T, Brisgand D, Douillard JY, et al. Randomized study of vinorelbine and cisplatin versus vindesine and cisplatin versus vinorelbine alone in advanced non-small-cell lung cancer: results of a European multicenter trial including 612 patients. J Clin Oncol 1994; 12(2):360–367.

58. Le Chevalier T, Brisgand D, Soria JC, et al. Long term analysis of survival in the European randomized trial comparing vinorelbine/cisplatin to vindesine/cisplatin and vinorelbine alone in advanced non-small cell lung cancer. Oncologist 2001; 6(suppl 1):8–11.

59. Galetta D, Gebbia V, Riccardi F, et al. A randomised phase III trial of the Southern Italy Oncology Group (GOIM) of mitomycin C plus vindesine and cisplatin (MVP regimen) versus vinorelbine plus cisplatin (PV regimen) in stage III–IV non small cell lung cancer (abstract). Lung Cancer 2000; 29(suppl 1):21.

60. Costa A, Barradas P, Cristova M, et al. Preliminary results of a randomised phase III trial comparing four cisplatin (P) based regimens in the treatment of locally advanced and metastatic non-small cell lung cancer (NSCLC) (abstract). Lung Cancer 2000; 29(suppl 1):27.

61. Vansteenkiste J, Vandebroek J, Nackaerts K, et al. Symptom control in advanced non-small cell lung cancer (NSCLC): a multicenter prospective randomised phase III study of single agent gemcitabine (GEM) versus cisplatin-vindesine (PV). Proc Am Soc Clin Oncol 2000; 19:488a.

62. Sandler A, Nemunatis J, Dehnam C, et al. Phase III study of cisplatin with or without gemcitabine in patients with advanced nonsmall cell lung cancer. Proc Am J Clin Oncol 1998; 17(1747):454a.

63. Crino L, Scagliotti GV, Ricci S, et al. Gemcitabine and cisplatin versus mitomycin, ifosfamide, and cisplatin in advanced non-small-cell lung cancer: a randomized phase III study of the Italian Lung Cancer Project. J Clin Oncol 1999; 17(11):3522–3530.

64. Danson S, Clemons M, Middleton G, et al. A randomised study of gemcitabine with carboplatin (GC) versus mitomycin, vinblastine and cisplatin (MVP) or mitomycin, ifosphamide and cisplatin (MIC) as first line chemotherapy in advanced non-small cell lung cancer (NSCLC). Proc Am Soc Clin Oncol 2001; 20:1285.

65a. Rudd RM, Gower NH, James LE, et al. Phase III randomized comparison of gemcitabine and carboplatin with mitomycin, ifosfamide and cisplatin in advanced non-small cell lung cancer. Proc ASCO 2002, abstract 1164.

65b. Bonomi P, Kim K, Fairclough D, et al. Comparison of survival and quality of life in advanced non-small-cell lung cancer patients treated with two dose levels of paclitaxel combined with cisplatin versus etoposide with cisplatin: results of an Eastern Cooperative Oncology Group trial. J Clin Oncol 2000; 18(3):623–631.

66. Kelly K, Crowley J, Bunn PA Jr, et al. Randomized phase III trial of paclitaxel plus carboplatin versus vinorelbine plus cisplatin in the treatment of patients with advanced non-small-cell lung cancer: a Southwest Oncology Group trial. J Clin Oncol 2001;19(13):3210–3218.

67. Schiller JH, Harrington D, Sandler A, et al. A randomized phase III trial of four chemotherapy regimens in advanced non-small cell lung cancer (NSCLC). Proc Am Soc Clin Oncol 2000;19:abstract 2.

68. NICE. Guidance on the use of docetaxel, paclitaxel, gemcitabine and vinorelbine for the treatment of non-small cell lung cancer. London: National Health Service; June 2001.

69. Shepherd FA, Dancey J, Ramlau R, et al. Prospective randomized trial of docetaxel versus best supportive care in patients with non-small-cell lung cancer previously treated with platinum-based chemotherapy. J Clin Oncol 2000; 18(10):2095–2103.

70. Baselga J, Kris M, Yano S, et al. Phase II trials (IDEAL 1 and IDEAL 2) of ZD1839 in locally advanced or metastatic non-small-cell lung cancer (NSCLC) patients. Ann Oncol 2002; 13:481.

71. Miller VA, Johnson D, Heelan RT, et al. A pilot trial demonstrates the safety of ZD1839 ('Iressa'), an oral epidermal growth factor receptor tyrosine kinase inhibitor (EGFR-TKI), in combination with carboplatin (C) and paclitaxel (P) in previously untreated advanced non-small cell lung cancer (NSCLC). Proc Am Soc Clin Oncol 2001; 20:326a.

72. Murray PV, O'Brien MER, Smith IE, et al. The natural history of asymptomatic mesothelioma. Br J Cancer 2001; 85(suppl 1).

73. Soysal O, Karaoglanoglu N, Demiracan S, et al. Pleurectomy/decortication for palliation in malignant pleural mesothelioma: results of surgery. Eur J Cardiothorac Surg 1997; 11(2):210–213.

74. Rusch V, Saltz L, Venkatraman E, et al. A phase II trial of pleurectomy/decortication followed by intrapleural and systemic chemotherapy for malignant pleural mesothelioma. J Clin Oncol 1994; 12(6):1156–1163.

75. Grondin SC, Sugarbaker DJ. Pleuropneumonectomy in the treatment of malignant pleural mesothelioma. Chest 1999; 116(6 Suppl):450S–454S.

76. Boutin C, Rey F, Viallat JR. Prevention of malignant seeding after invasive diagnostic procedures in patients with pleural mesothelioma. A randomized trial of local radiotherapy. Chest 1995; 108(3):754–758.

77. Middleton GW, Smith IE, O'Brien ME, et al. Good symptom relief with palliative MVP (mitomycin-C, vinblastine and cisplatin) chemotherapy in malignant mesothelioma. Ann Oncol 1998; 9(3):269–273.

78. Steele JP, Sharmash J, Evans MT, et al. Phase II study of vinorelbine in patients with malignant mesothelioma. J Clin Oncol 2000; 18(23):3912–3917.

79. Kindler HL, Millard F, Herndon JE, et al. Gemcitabine for malignant mesothelioma: a phase II trial by the Cancer and Leukemia Group B. Lung Cancer 2001; 31(2–3):311–317.

80. van Meerbeeck JP, Baas P, Debruyne C, et al. A phase II study of gemcitabine in patients with malignant pleural mesothelioma. European Organization for Research

and Treatment of Cancer Lung Cancer Cooperative Group. Cancer 1999; 85(12):2577–2582.

81. Byrne MJ, Davidson JA, Musk AW, et al. Cisplatin and gemcitabine treatment for malignant mesothelioma: a phase II study [see comments]. J Clin Oncol 1999; 17(1):25–30.

82. Herndon JE, Green MR, Chahinian AP, et al. Factors predictive of survival among 337 patients with mesothelioma treated between 1984 and 1994 by the Cancer and Leukemia Group B. Chest 1998; 113(3):723–731.

83. Edwards JG, Abrams KR, Leverment JN, et al. Prognostic factors for malignant mesothelioma in 142 patients: validation of CALGB and EORTC prognostic scoring systems [see comments]. Thorax 2000; 55(9):731–735.

84. Le Chevalier T for the IALT investigators. Results of a randomized international adjuvant lung cancer trial (IALT): cisplatin-based chemotherapy (CT) vs no CT in 1867 patients with resected non-small cell lung cancer. Proc Am Soc Clin Oncol 2003; 6:2.

85. Curran WJ, Scott CB, Langer CJ, et al. Long-term benefit is observed in a phase III comparison of sequential vs concurrent chemo-radiation for patients with unresectable stage III nsclc. RTOG 9410. Proc Am Soc Clin Oncol 2003; 2499:621.

86. Office of National Statistics. Cancer survival trends: England and Wales 1971–1995. London: The Stationary Office; 1999.

87. Seale DD, Beaver BM. Pathophysiology of lung cancer. Nurs Clin N Am 1992; 27:603–613.

88. NHS Executive. Guidance on commissioning cancer services: improving outcomes in lung cancer: the manual. London: DOH; 1998.

89. Corner J, Bailey C. Cancer nursing in context. Oxford: Blackwell Science; 2001.

90. Holmes S. Cancer chemotherapy: a guide to practice. 2nd edn. Dorking: Asset Books; 1997.

91. Crowe M, Ultrino C. Psychosocial implications of lung cancer. J Pract Nurs 1990; March:36–38.

92. Iwamoto R. Lung cancer. In: Nevidjon BM, Sowers K, eds. A nurse's guide to cancer care. New York: Lippincott; 2000:44–61.

93. Knopp JM. Lung cancer. In: Dow KH, Bucholtz JD, Iwamoto R, et al. eds. Nursing care in radiation oncology. 2nd edn. Philadelphia: WB Saunders; 1997:293–315.

94. Ingle RJ. Lung cancers. In: Henke Yarbo C, Hansen Frogge M, Goodman M, et al., eds. Cancer nursing principles and practice. 5th edn. Sudbury: Jones and Bartlett; 2000:1298–1328.

95. Sarna L. Smoking cessation after the diagnosis of lung cancer. Dev Support Care 1998; 2:45–49.

96. Lee-Chiong TL, Matthay RA. Lung cancer in the elderly patient. Clin Chest Med 1993; 14:453–472.

97. Bailey C. The needs of older people. In: Corner J, Bailey C, eds Nursing care in context. Oxford: Blackwell; 2000:496–507.

98. Engelking C. Chemotherapy in the elderly: considerations for clinical practice. In: Barton-Burke M, Wilkes GM, Ingwersen KC, eds. Cancer chemotherapy: a nursing process approach. 3rd edn. Sudbury: Jones and Bartlett; 2001:519–534.

99. Estwing Ferrans C. Quality of life as an outcome of cancer care. In: Henke Yarbo C, Hansen Frogge M, Goodman M, et al, eds. Cancer nursing principles and practice. 5th edn. Sudbury: Jones and Bartlett; 2000:243–258.

100. Dean H. Multiple instruments for measuring quality of life. In: Frank-Stromborg M, Olsen SJ, eds. Instruments for clinical health-care research. 2nd edn. Sudbury: Jones and Bartlett; 1997:135–148.

101. Twycross RG, Lack SA. Therapeutics in terminal cancer. London: Churchill Livingstone; 1986.

102. Corner J. Management of breathlessness in advanced lung cancer: new scientific evidence for developing multidisciplinary care. In: Muers MF, Macbeth F, Wells FC, et al, eds. The effective management of lung cancer. London: Aesculapius Medical; 2001:129–140.

103. Muers MF, Macbeth F, Wells FC, et al, eds. The effective management of lung cancer. London: Aesculapius Medical; 2001.

104. Bisset M. Tumours of the lung. In: Tschudin V, ed. Nursing the patient with cancer. 2nd edn. London: Prentice Hall; 1996:202–218.

105. Vogelzang NJ, Rusthoven JJ, Symanowski J, et al. Phase III study of pemetrexed in combination with cisplatin versus cisplatin alone in patients with malignant pleural mesothelioma. J Clin Oncol 2003; 21(14):2629–2630.

Chapter **38**

Cancers of the upper gastrointestinal tract

Mark Hill

INTRODUCTION

The cancers that originate in the gastrointestinal (GI) tract form a heterogeneous group of malignant diseases. The epidemiology, pathology and clinical presentation vary quite considerably depending on the primary site, but stage is a common determinant of prognosis.[1] Together, these tumours account for 25–30% of cancer deaths in Europe, indicating the high incidence and relatively modest cure rate. Management strategies, while remaining focused around surgery when the tumour is localised, are becoming increasingly complex and multimodal, involving both chemotherapy and radiotherapy. These can be given together or sequentially, pre- or postoperatively. This chapter includes a section on each tumour site and describes current management options, highlighting the role of chemotherapy.

OESOPHAGEAL CANCER

Diagnosis and staging

The incidence of oesophageal cancer is rising. The disease is also changing in its predominant anatomical site, from proximal to distal, such that oesophago-gastric junction tumours are one of the most rapidly increasing of all cancers, especially in Western countries.[2,3] Smoking, alcohol consumption and chronic gastro-oesophageal reflux (associated with Barrett's oesophagus) are all risk factors for the subsequent development of oesophageal carcinoma.[4–8] Patients commonly present with dysphagia and weight loss. The diagnosis is usually made based on endoscopic appearances, with confirmation obtained by means of biopsy. Staging investigations include a computed tomography (CT) scan to exclude distant metastases, and in surgical candidates positron emission tomography (PET) scanning can provide additional information. Endoscopic ultrasound is required for accurate T-staging and local nodal status can also be assessed by this technique.[9]

Preoperative chemotherapy

The overall cure rate following surgical resection in apparently operable disease is in the order of 20%. Preoperative chemotherapy has been investigated extensively in recent years in an attempt to improve this dismal statistic. The results have been conflicting, although many clinicians have been confounded by the use of suboptimal chemotherapy, inadequate staging or lack of statistical power.[10–15] However, the latest evidence from a large well-conducted trial demonstrates a statistically significant and clinically relevant benefit with this approach.[16] This Medical Research Council initiated OE02 study randomised 802 patients with resectable oesophageal cancer to either immediate surgery or 2 cycles of a cisplatin/5-FU (5-fluorouracil) regimen prior to surgery. Overall survival was found to be higher at 2 years in the chemotherapy group (43% vs 34%, $p = 0.001$) and many centres have now adopted this strategy as standard. The next trial will compare this chemotherapy regimen to ECX (see below). Chemotherapy can also be used to shrink locally advanced tumours to permit consideration of subsequent surgical resection.

Chemoradiotherapy

Long-term survival and cure have been reported when chemotherapy is given in conjunction with radiotherapy for localised disease. Early trial evidence supporting this strategy came from an American Intergroup Study in which 121 patients with oesophageal cancer were randomised to receive either radiotherapy alone (64 Gy) or radiotherapy (50 Gy) plus 4 courses of cisplatin and 5-FU. In the combined modality arm, both median survival (14.1 months vs 9.3 months, $p = 0.001$) and the 5-year survival (27% vs 0%, $p <0.0001$) were significantly better than in the radiotherapy alone arm.[17] This approach is now considered standard for tumours that are inoperable because of their local extent or for patients medically unfit to undergo surgery. Chemoradiation has also been investigated preoperatively and 3 relatively small randomised trials have been published comparing this approach with surgery alone.[18–20] None has demonstrated convincing evidence of improved survival, although, again, poor trial design and statistical weaknesses may be obscuring a modest benefit.

Palliative chemotherapy

Once the tumour has metastasised, the main aims with currently available treatments are symptom control, improvement or maintenance of quality of life (QOL) and modest prolongations of survival. Combination chemotherapy has the potential to achieve all of these and a number of regimens have been investigated. The generally accepted 'gold standard', at least within the UK, is a combination of epirubicin, cisplatin and infused 5-FU (ECF). In a phase II trial in patients with squamous oesophageal cancer 57% responded objectively and 91% experienced a symptomatic improvement.[21] Phase III evidence in adenocarcinoma of the oesophagus comes from a trial comparing this regimen to the previous standard treatment, FAMTX (5-FU, doxorubicin and methotrexate).[22] Response rate, progression-free survival and survival were all superior with ECF.

GASTRIC CANCER

Diagnosis and staging

Stomach cancer is declining in incidence, although it remains a significant cause of cancer-related death worldwide. Infection with *Helicobacter pylori* is a recently recognised aetiological factor. It often presents late with locally advanced or metastatic disease that is not amenable to surgical resection. Common symptoms include weight loss, anorexia, early satiety, anaemia and epigastric pain. Diagnosis is usually made endoscopically and staging investigations include CT scan and laparoscopy.

Preoperative chemotherapy

Long-term cure rates following surgical resection for gastric cancer are unimpressive, except in the earliest stages of disease. This provides the rationale for studies investigating the role of chemotherapy prior to surgery. Two phase III trials have been initiated. The first was a Dutch study which closed early with only 56 patients entered, following an interim analysis showing no difference in resectability or evidence of down staging.[23] The trial employed suboptimal chemotherapy (FAMTX), however, and many patients were unable to complete the planned chemotherapy because of toxicity. The other study, which has recently been completed, compares 3 courses of ECF before and after surgery, with surgery alone (MRC MAGIC study). First results were reported in 2003 and showed an improvement in DFS with chemotherapy.

Adjuvant chemotherapy

The results from randomised trials of adjuvant chemotherapy vs observation have been conflicting. A meta-analysis and a systematic review have failed to demonstrate a major benefit, with at best very modest improvements in survival observed.[24,25] Adjuvant chemotherapy should therefore not be routinely offered outside of the context of a clinical trial. A single US study appears to show a survival benefit for postoperative chemoradiotherapy in high-risk patients, but this study has been criticised since the results in the surgery alone arm are poor, and the treatment has not been widely adopted outside of the United States.[26]

Palliative chemotherapy

Randomised studies of chemotherapy vs best supportive care have demonstrated statistically significant survival advantages for combination chemotherapy in patients with inoperable or metastatic disease. Median survival typically increases from 3–4 months to 8–10 months.[27] Improvements in QOL and symptom control are also associated with the use of chemotherapy in this setting. A cost-effectiveness analysis of palliative chemotherapy revealed equivalence to other established medical treatments such as antihypertensive therapy.[28]

A number of drugs have activity in gastric cancer, and a large number of combination regimens have been investigated. 5-FU is the most frequently employed agent, which, when given as an intravenous bolus, produces response rates of 7–20%, rising to 30% as a protracted venous infusion (PVI). Cisplatin can produce responses in tumours that have progressed on 5-FU-based chemotherapy regimens demonstrating a degree of non-cross-resistance. Consequently, modern regimens have these two drugs as a backbone. The anthracyclines or mitomycin C can be combined with them in tolerable but effective doses. Other active drugs include methotrexate, irinotecan and docetaxel.

Early studies focused on a combination of 5-FU, doxorubicin and mitomycin C (FAM). This regimen was superseded by FAMTX, in which mitomycin C was replaced by high-dose methotrexate.[29] The only regimen to have shown superiority to FAMTX in a randomised study is ECF (epirubicin, cisplatin and PVI 5-FU) developed at the Royal Marsden Hospital. Extended phase II studies showed objective response rates in the 60–70% range and very good symptom control.[30] A subsequent multicentre randomised trial showed improvements not only in response (45% vs 21%, $p = 0.002$) but also in failure-free survival

(7.4 months vs 3.4 months, $p = 0.0006$) and overall survival (8.9 months vs 5.7 months, $p = 0.009$).[22] QOL and economic analyses were also performed and demonstrated that global QOL was significantly better with ECF and that the cost in terms of life years gained was modest. This study confirms the efficacy of ECF and, given that it is the largest trial of its type, many now consider ECF as the treatment of choice in this disease. Moreover, the evidence from this study that the response rate was even more impressive in locally advanced disease (58% vs 28% with FAMTX) justifies the choice of this regimen as the perioperative therapy in the experimental arm of the MRC MAGIC study (see above). Substituting the new agents capecitabine (xeloda) and oxaliplatin for 5-FU and cisplatin are obvious next steps, and are being explored in the ongoing REAL II study.

PANCREATIC CANCER

Diagnosis and staging

The causes of pancreatic adenocarcinoma are ill-defined, but the risk does appear to be increased by tobacco consumption, diabetes and a history of pancreatitis. The symptomatology is often insidious, with vague epigastric discomfort and weight loss. When advanced, pancreatic cancer can present more acutely with additional symptoms such as jaundice, ascites and malabsorption. The diagnosis is made by a combination of radiological appearances (CT or ultrasound scan), tumour markers and tissue biopsy. The latter is important to exclude lymphoma and neuroendocrine tumours, although if biopsy is unsuccessful an elevated Ca19.9 tumour marker, associated with a typical history and radiology, is usually sufficient. Less than 10% of patients have operable disease but if surgery is to be considered,[31] magnetic resonance imaging (MRI) and, increasingly, endoscopic ultrasound (EUS) are required staging investigations.

Adjuvant therapy

Early small trials suggested a benefit from the use of postoperative adjuvant chemoradiotherapy. One such randomised study, performed by the Gastrointestinal Tumour Study Group (GITSG) in the mid 1980s, reported an improvement in median survival from 11 to 21 months ($p = 0.05$) for patients given adjuvant bolus 5-FU plus radiotherapy, compared with no adjuvant therapy.[32] A Norwegian study published a decade later demonstrated a doubling of median survival from 11 to 23 months ($p = 0.02$) when FAM was given postoperatively compared with patients receiving no adjuvant treatment, although 5-year survival was not improved.[33] More recently, the largest trial in this setting, conducted by the European Study Group for the Pancreatic Cancer (ESPAC-1), which compared 5-FU and folinic acid with or without radiotherapy to no adjuvant treatment, has been reported.[34] This showed no survival benefit for adjuvant chemoradiotherapy, but a significant benefit for adjuvant chemotherapy. The current trial (ESPAC-3) compares two chemotherapy regimens and chemoradiotherapy has now been largely abandoned in this setting.

Palliative treatment

As with other upper GI tract cancers, once the tumour has metastasised, therapy is aimed largely at symptom control. Chemotherapy can be modestly effective in achieving this. Randomised trials with 5-FU-based combination regimens vs best supportive care demonstrate advantages in terms of both QOL and survival for the chemotherapy-treated patients, increasing the median from approximately 3 to 9 with p values of <0.001.[35–38]

The Royal Marsden GI Unit has reported its experience with a combination of cisplatin and PVI 5-FU.[39] In the published series, 63 patients with locally advanced or metastatic disease were treated, 71% of whom experienced weight stabilisation or gain, 60% pain relief and 34% improved performance status. The overall objective response rate was 16% and the median survival 7.6 months. More recently, single agent gemcitabine has become the standard of care, based largely on a phase III comparison with short-infusion 5-FU.[39] A total of 126 patients were treated and the primary efficacy measure used was 'clinical benefit response' (CBR), an index measuring pain control, performance status and weight. CBR was significantly higher with gemcitabine compared to 5-FU (24% vs 5%, $p = 0.0022$). In terms of objective response, however, there was no significant difference detected in the patients with measurable disease: 3/56 (5%) gemcitabine, 0/57 5-FU. The median and 12-month survivals were significantly higher in the gemcitabine arm, 5½ months vs 4½ months and 18% vs 2%, respectively ($p = 0.0025$). Toxicity was minimal and the National Institute for Clinical Excellence (NICE) has ratified its use as first-line therapy in advanced disease. The Medical Research Council (MRC) has launched a study comparing gemcitabine with or without capecitabine.

NEUROENDOCRINE TUMOURS

Diagnosis and staging

Neuroendocrine tumours may arise in various organs of the GI tract, most commonly in the small bowel or appendix. Those with a non-carcinoid phenotype are often diagnosed serendipitously, following surgical resection. Carcinoid syndrome presents with diarrhoea, wheeze and flushing. Rare secretory tumours, e.g. insulinoma and glucagonoma, will present with the consequences of the elevated neuroendocrine product. In addition to CT scanning, measurement of the appropriate hormone is required, which for carcinoid tumours is urinary 5-HIAA (5-hydroxy-indoleacetic acid).

Systemic treatment

There are several systemic treatment options for both carcinoid and islet cell tumours. For patients with asymptomatic disease, if surgical resection is not possible, a watch and wait policy should be adopted, particularly for carcinoid tumours and well-differentiated islet cell tumours. The symptoms of carcinoid syndrome can often be improved and even abrogated by the use of parenteral synthetic somatostatin analogues, which suppress the production of peptides and hormones. Short-acting octreotide has now largely been superseded by a longer-acting analogue, lanreotide, which appears to offer similar efficacy but with the advantage of fortnightly dosing.[40] These drugs are also useful for the unpleasant rash (necrolytic migratory erythema) associated with glucagonomas. The duration of benefit is usually short in islet cell tumours (4–6 months), but can be considerably longer in carcinoid tumours (median 12 months). The serotonin ($5HT_3$) receptor antagonists are also helpful for the secretory diarrhoea syndromes. Targeted radiotherapy in the form of [131]I m-iodobenzylguanidine (MIBG) can also be effective.[41]

Interferon 5 MU subcutaneously three times weekly produces biochemical responses in 50% of patients and objective tumour responses in 10–15% of patients. The average duration of response is 20 months for islet cell tumours, but some patients may continue to respond for several years and for carcinoid tumours the average duration of response is 34 months.[42]

Carcinoid tumours are often resistant to chemotherapy. It is usually reserved for symptomatic patients unresponsive to other treatment. A number of regimens have been investigated incorporating one or more of the active agents: streptozocin, 5-FU, doxorubicin, interferon-α2b, mitomycin or cyclo-phosphamide. These induce short-lived regressions in 15–30% of patients.[43–45] Islet cell tumours are more sensitive to chemotherapy. A randomised Eastern Cooperative Oncology Group (ECOG) trial identified doxorubicin and streptozocin as superior to 5-FU and streptozocin in terms of both response rate (69% vs 45%) and survival (27 months vs 17 months).[46]

SMALL BOWEL TUMOURS

Diagnosis and staging

Small bowel tumours are uncommon and difficult to diagnose. They present with vague abdominal pain, weight loss, diarrhoea and sometimes bleeding. Investigation is with small bowel meal and CT scan, but the diagnosis is often not confirmed until laparotomy. Surgical resection is the treatment of choice, but this is often non-curative due to the frequent late presentation. There is insufficient data to recommend the routine administration of adjuvant chemotherapy, but it is sometimes used in fit patients at high risk of relapse.

Palliative chemotherapy

There is very little data to guide therapy, but the tumour does seem to be chemosensitive. One series investigating ECF in this setting reported a response rate of 38% and median survival of 13 months.[47]

HEPATOCELLULAR CARCINOMA

Diagnosis and staging

Historically uncommon in Western countries, the incidence of this tumour is now rising due to the increased prevalence of hepatitis C. It is already a major healthcare issue in Asia and the Third World. It is causally associated with viral hepatitis, alcohol abuse, autoimmune hepatitis, aflatoxins and haemochromatosis. Abdominal pain is by far the most common presenting symptom, followed by weight loss, abdominal swelling, lethargy and anorexia. A CT portogram is the staging investigation of choice, and is increasingly used in conjunction with MRI. Whole body CT detects distant metastases. Levels of α-fetoprotein are usually raised. Surgical resection and orthotopic transplantation are the only curative options when the tumour is small, but it is estimated that less than 10% of patients are suitable for this approach and long-term results are poor.[48] Other interventions such as cryosurgery and percutaneous intratumoural injections of alcohol are of limited value.

Palliative chemotherapy

Systemic chemotherapy is generally disappointing in hepatocellular carcinoma. Responses to treatment are infrequent (20% or less) and are of short duration. The anthracyclines remain the most widely used agents. Etoposide and cisplatin also have some activity and bolus 5-FU produces responses in 10% of patients. A small series (7 patients) treated with ECF revealed a response rate of 29%[49] and this combination deserves further investigation, although it should be emphasised that there is no established place for combination chemotherapy outside a clinical trial.

Regional chemotherapy via the hepatic artery has the advantage of delivering high concentrations of drug direct to the tumour. The most widely investigated drug is floxuridine but this has not shown substantial activity against hepatocellular carcinoma. An alternative approach has been chemoembolisation of the tumour followed by the administration of doxorubicin in a lipoidol suspension. This eventuates transient retention of the doxorubicin within the tumour microvasculature. Non-randomised studies suggest a survival benefit from such chemoembolization. However, two randomised studies have failed to show any benefit with this approach.[50,51] It would appear that any benefit (tumour regression) from chemoembolisation is offset by the hepatotoxicity of this treatment in a group of patients who usually have pre-existing liver impairment.

CHOLANGIOCARCINOMA

Diagnosis and staging

Cholangiocarcinoma is a rare tumour in Western countries, but is increasing in incidence. It usually presents with jaundice and the diagnostic investigation of choice is ERCP (endoscopic retrograde cholangiopancreatography), often with stent insertion at the same time. Curative surgical resection can be considered in the rare cases in which the tumour is localised.

Palliative chemotherapy

Chemotherapy may be offered for appropriate patients, usually in the form of one of the combination regimens active in gastric cancer. In phase II studies, objective response rates of 30–40% are usual. Survival and QOL benefits have been demonstrated for chemotherapy over best supportive care in a random assignment trial.[37] ECF is probably the most active tolerable regimen for this disease but further evaluation is required.[49]

References

1. Hamilton SR, Aaltonen LA, eds. WHO classification of tumours: pathology and genetics of tumours of the digestive system. Lyon: IARC Press; 2000.
2. Powell J, Robertson JE, McConkey CE. Increasing incidence of oesophageal cancer; in which sites and which histological types? Cancer 1987; 55:346–347.
3. Lund O, Hasenkam JM, Aagaard MT, et al. Time-related changes in characteristics of prognostic significance in carcinomas of the oesophagus. Br J Surg 1989; 76(12):1301–1307.
4. Day NE, Varghese C. Oesophageal cancer. Cancer Surv 1994; 19/20:43–54.
5. Lagergren J, Bergstrom, R, Lindgren A, et al. Symptomatic gastroesophageal reflux as a risk factor for esophageal adenocarcinoma. N Engl J Med 1999; 340:825–831.
6. Macfarlane GJ, Plesko I, Kramarova E, et al. Epidemiological features of gastric and oesophageal cancer in Slovakia. Br J Cancer 1994; 70:177–179.
7. Levine DS. Barrett's oesophagus and p53. Lancet 1994; 344:212–213.
8. Blount PL, Galipeu PC, Sanchez CA, et al. 17p allelic losses in diploid cells of patients with Barrett's esophagus who develop aneuploidy. Cancer Res 1994; 54:2292–2295.
9. Rösch T. Endoscopic ultrasonography. Endoscopy 1994; 26:148–168.
10. Roth JA, Pass HI, Flanagan MM, et al. Randomized clinical trial of preoperative and postoperative adjuvant chemotherapy with cisplatin, vindesine and bleomycin for carcinoma of the esophagus. J Thorac Cardiovasc Surg 1988; 96:242–248.
11. Ancona E, Ruol A, Castoro C, et al. First-line chemotherapy improves the resection rate and long-term survival of locally advanced (T4, any N, M0) squamous cell carcinoma of the thoracic esophagus: final report on 163 consecutive patients with 5-year follow-up. Ann Surg 1997; 226(6):714–723.
12. Hilgenberg AD, Carey RW, Wilkins EW, et al. Preoperative chemotherapy, surgical resection, and selective postoperative therapy for squamous cell carcinoma of the oesophagus. Ann Thorac Surg 1988; 45:357–363.
13. Law S, Fok M, Chow S, et al. Preoperative chemotherapy versus surgical therapy alone for squamous cell carcinoma of the esophagus: a prospective randomized trial. J Thorac Cardiovasc Surg 1997; 114:210–217.
14. Kelson D, Ginsburg R, Pajak TF, et al. Chemotherapy followed by surgery compared with surgery alone for localised esophageal cancer. N Engl J Med 1998; 339:1979–1984
15. Kok TC, Lanschot JV, Siersma PD, et al. Neoadjuvant chemotherapy in operable esophageal squamous cell cancer: final report of a phase III multicenter randomized controlled trial. Proc ASCO 1997; 16:984.
16. Medical Research Council Oesophageal Cancer Working Group. Surgical resection with or without preoperative chemotherapy in oesophageal cancer: a randomised controlled trial. Lancet 2002; 359:1727–1733.
17. Herskovic A, Martz K, Al-Sarraf SM, et al. Combined chemotherapy and radiotherapy compared with radiotherapy alone in patients with cancer of the oesophagus. N Engl J Med 1992; 326:1593–1598.
18. Walsh TN, Noonan N, Hollywood D, et al. A comparison of multimodal therapy versus surgery for esophageal adenocarcinoma. N Eng J Med 1996; 335:462–467.
19. Urba S, Orringer MB, Turrisi A, et al. Randomised trial of preoperative chemoradiation versus surgery alone in patients with locoregional esophageal carcinoma. J Clin Oncol 2001; 19:283–285.
20. Bosset J, Gignoux M, Triboulet J, et al. Chemoradiotherapy followed by surgery compared with surgery alone in squamous-cell cancer of the esophagus. N Engl J Med 1997; 337:161–167.
21. Andreyev HJ, Norman AR, Cunningham D, et al. Squamous oesophageal cancer can be downstaged using protracted venous infusion of 5-fluorouracil with epirubicin and cisplatin (ECF). Eur J Cancer 1995; 31A:1594–1598.
22. Webb A, Cunningham D, Scarffe JH, et al. A randomised trial comparing epirubicin, cisplatin and fluorouracil versus fluorouracil, doxorubicin and methotrexate in advanced oesophago-gastric cancer. J Clin Oncol 1997; 15:261–267.
23. Songun I, Keizer HJ, Hermans J, et al. Chemotherapy for operable gastric cancer: results of the Dutch randomised FAMTX trial. The Dutch Gastric Cancer Group. Eur J Cancer 1999; 35:558–562.
24. Hermans J, Bonenkamp JJ, Boon MC, et al. Adjuvant therapy after curative resection for gastric cancer: meta-analysis of randomized trials. J Clin Oncol 1993; 11:1441–1447.
25. Janugar KG, Hafstrom L, Nygren P, et al. A systematic overview of chemotherapy effects in gastric cancer. Acta Oncologica 2001; 40:309–325.
26. Macdonald JS, Smalley SR, Benedetti J, et al. Chemoradiotherapy after surgery compared with surgery alone for adenocarcinoma of the stomach or gastroesophageal junction. N Engl J Med. 2001; 345:725–730.
27. Murad AM, Santiago FF, Petroianu A, et al. Modified therapy with 5-fluorouracil, doxorubicin, and methotrexate in advanced gastric cancer. Cancer 1993; 72:37–41.
28. Glimelius B, Hoffman K, Graf W, et al. Cost-effectiveness of palliative chemotherapy in advanced gastrointestinal cancer. Ann Oncol 1995; 6:267–274.
29. Wils O, Klein H, Wagner D, et al. Sequential high dose methotrexate and fluorouracil combined with doxorubicin: a step forward in the treatment of gastric cancer. J Clin Oncol 1991; 9:827–831.
30. Findlay M, Cunningham D, Norman A, et al. A phase II study in advanced gastro-esophageal cancer using

epirubicin and cisplatin in combination with continuous infusion 5-fluorouracil (ECF). Ann Oncol 1994; 5:609–616.

31. Johnson C. Prognosis in pancreatic cancer. Lancet 1997; 349:1027–1028.

32. Gastrointestinal Tumour Study Group. Pancreatic cancer: adjuvant combined radiation and chemotherapy following curative resection. Arch Surg 1985; 120:899.

33. Bakkevold KE, Arnesjo B, Dahl O, et al. Adjuvant combination chemotherapy (DMF) following radical resection of carcinoma of the pancreas and papilla of Vater. Results of a controlled, prospective, randomised multicentre study. Eur J Cancer 1993; 29:698–703.

34. Neoptolemos JP, Dunn JA, Stocken DD, et al. Adjuvant chemoradiotherapy and chemotherapy in resectable pancreatic cancer: a randomised trial. Lancet 2001; 358:1576–1585.

35. Mallinson CN, Rake MO, Cocking JB. Chemotherapy in pancreatic cancer. Br Med J 1980; 281:1589–1591.

36. Palmer KR, Kerr M, Knowles G, et al. Chemotherapy prolongs survival in inoperable pancreatic carcinoma. Br J Surg 1994; 81:882–885.

37. Glimelius B, Hoffman K, Sjödé N P-O, et al. Chemotherapy improves survival and quality of life in advanced pancreatic and biliary cancer. Ann Oncol 1996; 7:593–600.

38. Nicolson M, Webb A, Cunningham D, et al. Cisplatin and protracted venous infusion 5-fluorouracil (CF) – good symptom relief with low toxicity in advanced pancreatic carcinoma. Ann Oncol 1995; 6:801–804.

39. Burris HA, Moore MJ, Anderson J, et al. Improvements in survival and clinical benefit with gemcitabine as first line therapy for patients with advanced pancreas cancer: a randomised trial. J Clin Oncol 1997; 15:403–413.

40. Ruszniewski P, Ducreux M, Chayvialle J-A, et al. Treatment of the carcinoid syndrome with the long acting somatostatin analogue lanreotide: a prospective study in 39 patients. Gut 1996; 39: 279–283.

41. Shapiro B. Summary, conclusions and future directions of [131I] metaidobenzylguanidine therapy in the treatment of neural crest tumours. J Nucl Biol Med 1991; 35:357–363

42. Eriksson M, Oberg K. Interferon therapy of malignant endocrine pancreatic tumours. Front Gastrointest Res 1995; 23:451–460.

43. Moertel CG. Treatment of the carcinoid tumour and the malignant carcinoid syndrome. J Clin Oncol 1983; 1:727–740.

44. Oberg K. The use of chemotherapy and the management of neuroendocrine tumours. End Met Clin N Am 1993; 22:9412–9452.

45. Andreyev HJN, Scott-Mackie P, Cunningham D, et al. A phase II study of continuous infusion fluorouracil and interferon alfa 2b in the palliation of malignant neuroendocrine tumours. J Clin Oncol 1995; 13(6):1486–1492.

46. Moertel CG, Lefkopoulo M, Lipsitz S, et al. Streptozocin-doxorubicin, streptozocin-fluorouracil or chlorozotocin in the treatment of advanced islet-cell carcinoma. N Engl J Med 1992; 326:519–523.

47. Crawley C, Ross P, Norman A, et al. The Royal Marsden experience of small bowel adenocarcinoma treated with protracted venous infusion 5-fluorouracil. Br J Cancer 1998; 78:508–510.

48. Mazzaferro V, Regalia E, Doci R, et al. Liver transplantation for the treatment of small hepatocellular carcinomas in patients with cirrhosis. N Engl J Med 1996; 334:693–729.

49. Ellis PA, Norman A, Hill A, et al. Epirubicin, cisplatin and infusional 5FU (ECF) in hepato-biliary tumours. Eur J Cancer 1995; 31A:1594–1598.

50. Pelletier G, Roche A, Ink O, et al. A randomized trial of hepatic arterial chemoembolization in patients with unresectable hepatocellular carcinoma. J Hepatol 1990; 11:181–184.

51. Groupe d'Etude et de Traitement du Carcinome Hepatocellulaire. A comparison of lipiodol chemo-embolization and conservative treatment for unresectable hepatocellular carcinoma. N Engl J Med 1995; 19:1256–1261.

Chapter **39**

Cancers of the lower gastrointestinal tract

Jillian Noble, Charlotte Rees, Paul J Ross
and David Cunningham

MEDICAL CARE FOR PATIENTS WITH LOWER GASTROINTESTINAL TRACT CANCER

COLORECTAL CANCER

Introduction

Colorectal cancer is the third most commonly diagnosed cancer in the UK and the second most common
cause of cancer death. In 2000, there were almost one
million cases diagnosed worldwide. Approximately
30 000 cases are diagnosed in the UK each year.[1] The
incidence of colorectal cancer is higher in men than
women. Wide global variation exists for colorectal
cancer. Ethnic and racial differences suggest environmental factors play a major role in aetiology; 80% of
tumours present over 60 years of age, whereas less
than 1% present under the age of 40. The commonest
histological subtype is adenocarcinoma.

Aetiology

Most colorectal cancers arise from benign adenomatous polyps. Development of colorectal cancer is a
multistep process involving genetic mutations, activation of oncogenes such as K-ras and c-myc and loss of
tumour suppressors such as APC, DCC, MCC and
p53. This process is known as the adenoma–carcinoma
sequence.[2] The majority of cases of colorectal cancers
are sporadic, but a minority occurs as a result of an
inherited genetic mutation.[3,4] Familial adenomatous
polyposis (FAP), the polyposis/hamartoma syndromes
(Peutz–Jeghers syndrome, juvenile polyposis) and
hereditary non-polyposis colorectal cancer (HNPCC)
account for 5% of all colorectal cancers. FAP is caused

by an inherited mutation in one of the alleles of the tumour suppressor gene adenomatous polyposis coli (APC) on chromosome 5,[5] whereas HNPCC is caused by mutations in any one of a number of mismatch repair genes.[6] Peutz–Jeghers syndrome results from a mutation in LKB1 and juvenile polyposis from a mutation in SMAD4. Inflammatory bowel disease, a positive family history or a history of adenomatous polyps also confers increased risk.[7]

Risk factors thought to be associated with the development of colorectal cancer include obesity, smoking and the consumption of meat and fat.[8,9] Physical activity, the consumption of fruit and vegetables and hormone replacement therapy are thought to be protective.[10–12]

Staging

Treatment and prognosis in colorectal cancer is highly dependent on stage of disease. Dukes' staging was originally described in 1929 and was subsequently modified to become the Astler–Coller staging system (Table 39.1). These systems have now been superseded by the TNM classification, which is based on primary tumour characteristics (T), lymph node involvement (N) and the presence of distant metastasis (M) (Table 39.2).

Investigations

The primary investigation is colonoscopy and biopsy of the tumour. This allows histological confirmation and is also necessary to exclude synchronous primaries in the colon. Computed tomography (CT) scanning of the thorax, abdomen and pelvis is used to look for distant disease. In patients with rectal cancers, a magnetic resonance imaging (MRI) scan of the pelvis is performed to give detailed loco-regional assessment of the primary tumour: in particular, information

Table 39.2   Union Internationale Control le Cancer (UICC) staging for colorectal cancer

UICC stage	Tumour	Regional lymph nodes	Distant metastasis
0	Tis	N0	M0
I	T1	N0	M0
	T2	N0	M0
IIA	T3	N0	M0
IIB	T4	N0	M0
IIIA	T1–T2	N1	M0
IIIB	T3–T4	N1	M0
IIIC	Any T	N2	M0
IV	Any T	Any N	M1

about the circumferential resection margin. Routine blood tests, including full blood count, urea and electrolytes, liver function tests and carcinoembryonic antigen (CEA), are also carried out.

Management of colorectal cancer

The management of primary colorectal cancer is determined according to the site of the tumour and is divided into colon cancers, which are above the peritoneal reflection, and rectal cancers, which are below the peritoneal reflection.

Colon cancer

Surgery remains the mainstay of treatment. Seventy-five to eighty per cent of patients present with localised disease. Five-year survival following curative surgery is shown in Table 39.3. The standard surgical treatment is resection of the tumour with primary anastomosis. The choice of operation/resection depends on the location of the tumour and its arterial supply. Postoperatively, patients should be considered for adjuvant chemotherapy based on final TNM stage. The aim of adjuvant treatment is to eliminate micrometastatic disease and therefore prevent recurrence. There is no role for adjuvant chemotherapy in stage I disease. The role of adjuvant chemotherapy

Table 39.1   Modified Astler–Coller classification

Type	Description
Dukes' A	Tumour confined to mucosa
Dukes' B1	Tumour extends into but not beyond muscularis
Dukes' B2	Tumour extends into/through serosa
Dukes' C1	Tumour found in local lymph nodes but muscularis propria not breached
Dukes' C2	Tumour found in local lymph nodes and the muscularis propria has been breached
Dukes' D	Distant metastases

Table 39.3   Five-year survival in colorectal cancer

Type	5-year survival
Dukes' A	80–90%
Dukes' B	60–70%
Dukes' C	20–30%

will be discussed separately in the following sections (Stage III colon cancer and Stage II colon cancer).

Stage III colon cancer   The role of adjuvant chemotherapy in stage III colon cancer is now well established. The first study to show a survival advantage reported in 1988 and was carried out by the National Surgical Adjuvant Breast and Bowel Project (NSABP) study group.[13] In this study, Wolmark et al assigned 1166 patients to observation, bacille Calmette-Guèrin (BCG) immunotherapy or chemotherapy with 5-fluorouracil (5-FU), semustine and vincristine. The chemotherapy arm had a 7% improvement in 5-year disease-free survival (DFS) (p = 0.02), and an 8% absolute improvement in 5-year overall survival (OS) (p = 0.05) compared with surgery alone. BCG conferred an overall survival benefit (67% vs 59% in controls; p = 0.03) but no gain in DFS.[14] This was thought to be due to decreasing death related to comorbid conditions.

In 1989, the North Central Cancer Treatment Group (NCCTG) reported a significant reduction in recurrence rate and a survival benefit with 5-FU and levamisole compared with levamisole alone or observation in stage II and stage III colon cancer.[15] Levamisole was reported to be an immunomodulator and synergistic with 5-FU, possibly through selective stabilization of mRNA. This prompted the pivotal Intergroup-0035 study that confirmed an advantage of 5-FU and levamisole for 1 year compared with observation alone.[16,17] Separate analyses were performed for stage II and stage III patients. A trend for a reduction in recurrence rate but no difference in OS was seen in the stage II patients in the 5-FU and levamisole arm. However, in the stage III patients, there was a 40% reduction in recurrence and a 33% reduction in death compared with observation at a median follow-up of 6.5 years. The absolute improvement in 5-year survival was 13% in the 5-FU and levamisole arm compared with observation alone. In 1990, 1 year of 5-FU and levamisole was recommended as adjuvant treatment for stage III colon cancer.[18]

In 1995, a trial carried out by the International Multicentre Pooled Analysis of Colon Cancer Trials (IMPACT) investigators, comparing observation with 5-FU and leucovorin, was reported.[19] The 3-year survival in the chemotherapy arm was 76% compared with 64% in the surgery alone arm in stage III patients. The Intergroup-0085 and the NSABP C-03 provided further evidence for this combination.[20,21] More recently, several European studies have compared leucovorin and levamisole in combination with 5-FU. The Netherlands Adjuvant Colorectal Cancer Project (NACCP) showed improved survival from 44% in the surgery alone arm to 56% in the 5-FU/levamisole arm.[22] The Arbeitgemeinshaft Gastrointestinale Onkologie compared 5-FU/leucovorin with 5-FU/levamisole and found a survival benefit in the leucovorin arm (63 months vs 55 months).[23] The Forschungsgruppe Onkologie Gastrointestinaler Tumoren-1 study confirms this data.[24] Finally, the Intergroup-0089 study randomised 3759 patients to 4 arms: 5-FU/levamisole for 12 months; 5-FU/low-dose leucovorin for 6 months; 5-FU/high-dose leucovorin for 8 months; or 5-FU with levamisole and low-dose leucovorin for 6 months.[25] This showed levamisole is not an essential component of adjuvant treatment, there is no difference between 6 months and 12 months of leucovorin and also no difference between low- and high-dose leucovorin. In addition to trials comparing levamisole and 5-FU, trials recently have compared infused vs bolus 5-FU. The Groupe d'Etude et de Recherche Clinique en Oncologie Radiotherapies show no difference in DFS or OS between infused and bolus 5-FU but found decreased toxicity with infused 5-FU.[26] Saini et al reported a similar study with protracted venous infusion (PVI) 5-FU vs bolus 5-FU and found similar survival but significantly less toxicity in the PVI arm.[27] Currently, the recommended regimen for stage III disease is 5-FU/leucovorin for 6 months, starting 6–12 weeks following surgery.

The latest data presented at the American Society of Clinical Oncology (ASCO) in 2003 shows promising results with 5-FU/leucovorin/oxaliplatin in the adjuvant setting.[28] The MOSAIC trial, a large phase III trial, randomised patients with stage II/III colon cancer to 5-FU/leucovorin or 5-FU/leucovorin/oxaliplatin. Preliminary results show 77.8% 3-year DFS in the 5-FU/leucovorin/oxaliplatin arm vs 72.9% in the 5-FU/leucovorin arm (p <0.01). This represents a 23% reduction in the risk of recurrence in the oxaliplatin-containing arm. Although these results are very encouraging, oxaliplatin-containing regimens are not yet considered the standard of care in the adjuvant setting. The NSABP C-07 trial is also currently investigating the role of oxaliplatin with bolus 5-FU/leucovorin as adjuvant therapy.

Trials are also examining the role of irinotecan in combination with 5-FU/leucovorin. The results of the PETACC-3 trial comparing 5-FU/leucovorin vs 5-FU/leucovorin/irinotecan in stage III patients are awaited.

The next step in adjuvant therapy will be the introduction of oral fluoropyrimidines, including capecitabine and uracil-tegafur (UFT). Capecitabine is an oral prodrug metabolised to 5-FU in the tumour site by thymidine phosphorylase. There are higher levels of this enzyme in tumour tissue than in normal tissue, which allows for targeted therapy.[29] The toxicity profile of capecitabine is superior to bolus 5-FU, apart from an increase in hand-foot syndrome.[30,31] Trials are ongoing to investigate the efficacy of oral fluoropyrimidines. The NSABP C-06 compares UFT/leucovorin vs 5-FU/leucovorin and the X-ACT trial is evaluating capecitabine vs 5-FU/leucovorin. Trials have also commenced combining capecitabine and oxaliplatin as adjuvant therapy. The use of oral fluoropyrimidines will simplify the administration of adjuvant chemotherapy in colorectal cancer.

Stage II colon cancer The benefits of adjuvant chemotherapy in stage II colon cancer are less clear cut. There are two contradictory pooled analyses. The IMPACT B2 study pooled 5 trials and found a benefit for adjuvant treatment that was not statistically significant.[32] In contrast, a pooled analysis carried out by NSABP showed a greater relative reduction in mortality than in stage III disease (30% vs 18%).[33] Possible reasons for these contradictory results include variations in regimens and lack of power. The most recent evidence comes from the Dutch NACCP trial where the survival rate was increased from 70% to 78%.[22] Further data may come from the ongoing Quick and Simple and Reliable Study (QUASAR) regarding the benefit of adjuvant treatment in stage II disease. Recruitment in the uncertain arm is due to be completed in late 2003.[34]

Adjuvant chemotherapy, therefore, remains controversial in stage II disease. The decision to recommend adjuvant chemotherapy is consequently often based on high-risk characteristics, including intestinal obstruction or perforation, T4 tumours, poorly differentiated tumours, extramural venous, lymphatic or perineural invasion.

Rectal cancer

Surgery remains the primary modality for localised rectal tumours but, unlike colon cancer, achieving a wide resection margin is limited by the bony pelvis and therefore local recurrence is more common. Attempts to reduce the local recurrence rates have concentrated on improving surgical techniques, radiotherapy and chemoradiation. Tumours can be divided into those that can proceed directly to surgery and those that may benefit from neoadjuvant treatment. Tumours with a low risk of a positive resection margin will undergo primary surgery. The remaining tumours can be divided into low tumours that require neoadjuvant treatment in order to try to preserve sphincter function or poor prognosis tumours with an at-risk circumferential resection margin as defined by high-resolution MRI of the rectum. These include tumours

within 1 mm of the mesorectal fascia, any T3 tumour below the levators, T3C/D and T4 tumours or any T stage with 4 or more lymph nodes.

Total mesorectal excision (TME) has become the standard surgical technique in rectal cancer in several European countries. This involves sharp dissection under clear vision, with the excision of the rectum and mesorectum within the mesorectal fascia. Recurrence rates of 6–10% have been reported using TME surgery compared with 25–40% using conventional surgery.[35–38]

Preoperative radiation Preoperative radiotherapy may be short-course radiotherapy (5 Gy daily for 5 days) or long-course radiotherapy (up to 45 Gy in 25 fractions). There have been two randomised trials comparing short course preoperative radiotherapy followed by surgery alone. The Swedish Rectal Cancer Trial compared short-course preoperative radiotherapy with conventional surgery alone.[39] It demonstrated an increased survival and reduced local recurrence rate in the radiotherapy arm. The rate of recurrence was 11% in the arm that received radiotherapy and 27% in the surgery alone arm (p <0.001). Overall survival was 58% in the radiotherapy arm vs 48% in the surgery alone arm (p = 0.004). In this trial patients underwent anterior resection or abdominoperineal resection but not total mesorectal excision, within 1 week of radiotherapy. The second trial was a multicentre, randomised trial comparing preoperative radiotherapy and TME with TME alone.[40] OS was similar in the two groups but the rate of local recurrence at 2 years was 2.4% in the radiotherapy + surgery group and 8.2% in the surgery-only group (p <0.001).

A trial by the Medical Research Council compared surgery alone vs surgery preceded by long-course radiotherapy (40 Gy in 20 fractions) in patients with clinically fixed rectal cancers.[41] The rate of local recurrence was significantly reduced (35.9% vs 46.4%, p = 0.04) in the radiotherapy arm but there was no difference in overall survival (31 months vs 24 months, p = 0.1). There have also been two meta-analyses looking at both short- and long-course radiotherapy. The first meta-analysis combined 19 trials comparing preoperative radiotherapy with surgery alone:[42] the majority used long-course radiotherapy. This meta-analysis showed a reduced risk of local recurrence, with preoperative radiotherapy (45.9% vs 52.9%, p <0.00001) and a trend towards improved OS. The second meta-analysis demonstrated a significant reduction in local recurrence and OS. Preoperative radiotherapy was superior to surgery alone in all but one trial, reaching statistical significance in six trials.[43]

Preoperative chemoradiation The benefits of preoperative chemoradiation (Table 39.4) include eliminating

Table 39.4   Preoperative chemoradiation

Stage	Description
Preoperative chemotherapy	5-FU (300 mg/m^2/day) continuous infusion for 12 weeks + mitomycin C (7 mg/m^2) bolus every 6 weeks
Chemoradiation	Pelvic radiotherapy (45 Gy in 25 fractions + boost 5.4–9 Gy) + 5-FU (200 mg/m^2/day) for 6 weeks
Surgery	Anterior resection or abdominoperineal resection
Postoperative chemotherapy	5-FU (300 mg/m^2/day) continuous infusion for 12 weeks + mitomycin C (7 mg/m^2) bolus every 6 weeks

micrometastatic disease and increased radiation sensitivity. The NSABP R-03 trial randomised 267 patients to pre- versus postoperative chemoradiation.[44] DFS at 1 year in the preoperative chemoradiation arm was 83% as compared to 78% in the postoperative arm ($p = 0.29$). The German CAO/ARO/AIO-94 study compared neoadjuvant chemoradiation with standard postoperative chemoradiation.[45] Preoperative chemotherapy was well tolerated and there was no increased risk of postoperative morbidity. Efficacy data are awaited.

A study by Chau et al evaluated the benefits of neoadjuvant chemotherapy prior to chemoradiation and surgery in patients with locally advanced rectal cancer. Patients received 12 weeks of chemotherapy with PVI 5-FU and mitomycin C prior to synchronous chemoradiation with PVI 5-FU followed by surgery and postoperative chemotherapy. Radiological response was seen in 27.8% after chemotherapy and 80.6% following chemoradiation.[46] Data was also presented at ASCO in 2003 from a trial evaluating neoadjuvant capecitabine and oxaliplatin prior to synchronous chemoradiation and TME in poor risk/locally advanced rectal cancer. Of 17 evaluable patients, all had partial responses following capecitabine and oxaliplatin. Following chemoradiation, response was sustained in all patients.[47]

Future trials include the NSABP R-04 trial, which will compare capecitabine and infusional 5-FU as part of a preoperative chemoradiation regimen.

Adjuvant treatment   Two trials have shown the benefit of adjuvant chemotherapy in stage II and stage III rectal cancer. The NSABP R-01 study showed an improvement in DFS with MOF (semustine, vincristine, 5-FU) chemotherapy compared to surgery alone. Radiation alone reduced local recurrence rate but did not affect DFS or OS.[48] NSABP R-02 confirmed these results and also found the addition of radiotherapy to chemotherapy conferred no advantage for DFS or OS but did reduce local recurrence rate.[49]

Two further trials examined chemotherapy combined with radiotherapy. The Gastrointestinal Tumor Study Group 7175 showed a survival advantage of chemoradiation over surgery alone.[50] NCCTG 79-47-51 found lower local recurrences and improved survival for chemoradiation compared with radiation alone.[51] Finally, two Intergroup trials have examined the scheduling of chemoradiation. Intergroup-0114 showed no difference between 5-FU, 5-FU/leucovorin, 5-FU/levamisole and 5-FU/levamisole/leucovorin.[52] The Gastrointestinal Intergroup compared infusional and bolus 5-FU and found DFS and OS advantages with infusional 5-FU.[53]

In summary, the treatment for patients with rectal cancer is based upon preoperative staging, including MRI of the rectum. Those at risk of a positive resection margin receive a preoperative schedule with neoadjuvant chemotherapy and chemoradiation. Patients suitable for primary surgery for rectal cancer will receive adjuvant chemotherapy according to their pathological staging, as for colon cancer. Patients with positive circumferential resection margins who did not receive preoperative irradiation receive postoperative synchronous chemoradiation.

Metastatic colorectal cancer

Colorectal cancer most commonly metastasises to the liver. Liver metastases develop in nearly 20% of stage II and 50% of stage III patients. Metastatic disease in the majority of patients is incurable, but increasingly patients with small volume liver and/or lung disease are considered for surgical resection.

Management of potentially resectable metastatic disease   In recent years surgical resection of liver metastases has become increasingly popular as it can result in long-term survival. Chemotherapy, portal vein embolisation and ablative techniques have also increased the number of patients thought to be resectable. In a large prospective study of 484 patients with untreated hepatic metastases, the median survival was 31% at 1 year, 7.9% at 2 years, 2.6% at 3 years and 0.9% at 4 years.[54] One trial that compared surgical resection in patients with potentially resectable disease with no treatment found 28% 5-year survival compared with 0%.[55] Operability depends on the patient's performance status, the extent of disease and liver function; 10–20% of patients have metastases that are amenable to surgery. Preoperative chemotherapy can be used to downstage liver metastases in order to increase the chance of operability. In one study chemotherapy with 5-FU/leucovorin and oxaliplatin permitted the resection of 16% of patients previously felt to be inoperable. The 3- and 5-year survival rates were comparable to those observed after resection of resectable lesions (54% and 40%, respectively).[56] 5-FU and folinic acid is effective in 20% of cases; when combined with irinotecan or oxaliplatin, this can rise to 50%. Douillard et al randomised 387 patients with metastatic colorectal cancer to irinotecan, 5-FU and leucovorin or 5-FU/leucovorin alone. The response rate was significantly higher in the irinotecan group (49% vs 31%, p <0.001). Overall survival was also higher (median 17.4 months vs 14.1 months, p = 0.031).[57] In March 2002, the National Institute for Clinical Excellence (NICE) approved the use of 5-FU, leucovorin and oxaliplatin for the downstaging of potentially resectable liver metastases.

The benefit of adjuvant chemotherapy following resection of hepatic metastases is controversial. Most studies have examined hepatic arterial infusion of the drugs. Lorenz and Rossian carried out a multicentre trial that failed to show any survival benefit of hepatic arterial infusion of 5-FU and folinic acid following liver resection over surgery alone.[58] A second study randomly assigned 156 patients to systemic chemotherapy +/− hepatic arterial infusion and found combined treatment reduced the hepatic recurrence rate and improved overall survival at 2 years (86% vs 72%, p = 0.03).[59] Finally, the Eastern Cooperative Oncology Group (ECOG) compared hepatic arterial infusion plus floxuridine and intravenous 5-FU with surgery alone.[60] The risk of recurrence was reduced in the combined group but there was no difference in OS. Only one trial has looked at the role of systemic chemotherapy with 5-FU and folinic acid over no treatment. There was a survival benefit in the 5-FU arm but it was not statistically significant.

The overall benefit of chemotherapy after surgical resection remains uncertain because many of the studies have been underpowered to detect a clinically important improvement in outcome. Despite the Kemeny data, hepatic arterial infusion of chemotherapy following hepatic resection has not been widely adopted, possibly because of logistical concerns. Neoadjuvant systemic chemotherapy can be used to downstage liver metastases prior to surgical resection. The European Organisation for Research and Treatment of Cancer (EORTC) has commenced a trial comparing surgery with or without neoadjuvant and adjuvant oxaliplatin, 5-FU and leucovorin in patients with resectable liver metastases. This will hopefully clarify the role of perioperative chemotherapy.

It is also possible to resect pulmonary metastases. Studies have shown 5-year survival in the order of 25–40% in appropriately selected patients.[61–63] Macroscopically, complete resection is the most important independent prognostic factor.[64]

Chemotherapy for metastatic disease   For over 40 years the treatment of colorectal cancer has been based on 5-fluorouracil. Recently, the introduction of two new classes of cytotoxic agent – irinotecan, a topoisomerase I inhibitor, and oxaliplatin, a third-generation platinum – have increased the treatment options available.

Fluoropyrimidines   5-FU alone produces a response rate of approximately 10%. The addition of leucovorin significantly improves response rates to 23%.[65] Trials have also shown that the administration of 5-FU as a continuous infusion results in a significant response advantage and improvement in progression-free survival over bolus 5-FU in advanced disease. A meta-analysis combining six trials showed a significant improvement in median overall survival in the infused group vs the bolus group (12.1 vs 11.3 months, p = 0.039). Toxicity profiles vary with increased haematological toxicity in the bolus group and more hand-foot syndrome in the infused group.[66]

Recently developed oral fluoropyrimidines represent an alternative to infused regimens. Capecitabine is an oral fluoropyrimidine converted to 5-FU by enzymes located in the liver and in tumours. Two studies have compared capecitabine with bolus 5-FU/leucovorin.[30,31] Data from these studies was pooled and showed improved overall response rate in the capecitabine arm (25.7% vs 16.7%, p <0.002).[67] Median time to disease progression, overall survival and duration of response showed no difference between the two treatment groups.

UFT, another oral fluoropyrimidine, combines uracil and tegafur. Tegafur is a prodrug of 5-FU and uracil inhibits dihydropyrimidine dehydrogenase, the main catabolic enzyme of 5-FU. Two trials have compared UFT/leucovorin with bolus 5-FU/leucovorin. The first trial randomised 816 patients and showed equivalent median overall survival in the two arms (12.4 vs 13.4 months) but significantly worse time to progression with UFT.[68] The second study randomised 380 patients, demonstrating similar survival in both arms (12.2 vs 10.3 months, p = 0.226). However, survival in the bolus 5-FU arm was lower than in other trials.[69]

Thymidylate synthase inhibitors   Raltitrexed inhibits thymidylate synthase. Phase III trials have compared raltitrexed with 5-FU/leucovorin and found similar median survival in both arms in three out of four studies. The remaining study showed 5-FU/leucovorin was superior. The only advantage of raltitrexed over 5-FU is in patients who develop 5-FU-induced chest pain, which does not occur with raltitrexed.

Topoisomerase I inhibitors   Irinotecan is a semisynthetic derivative of the natural alkaloid camptothecin, which interacts with topoisomerase I. Response rates in patients with advanced colorectal cancer who have previously received 5-FU-based chemotherapy vary from 11 to 17%.[70] There have been two studies in patients whose disease is resistant/refractory to 5-FU. One compared irinotecan with best supportive care in 279 patients, and demonstrated an improvement in 1-year survival from 13.8% in the best supportive care group to 36.2% in the irinotecan group ($p = 0.0001$). Pain-free survival and quality of life were also improved in the irinotecan group.[71] The other study compared irinotecan and infused 5-FU. One-year survival was 45% in the irinotecan arm, compared with 32% in the infused 5-FU arm. Median survival was 10.8 months in the irinotecan group vs 8.5 months in the fluorouracil group.[72] As a result of these trials, irinotecan became accepted as second-line treatment in advanced colorectal cancer.

Following on from the earlier studies, two phase III randomised trials of irinotecan in combination with 5-FU have been carried out. One trial compared irinotecan, leucovorin and bolus 5-FU (IFL) with bolus 5-FU and leucovorin and with irinotecan alone. The IFL regimen showed longer overall survival compared with 5-FU/leucovorin (17.4 months vs 14.1 months, $p = 0.031$).[57] In the second study, irinotecan, infused 5-FU and leucovorin was compared with infused 5-FU and leucovorin alone. Survival again was increased in the irinotecan arm (14.8 months vs 12.6 months, $p < 0.05$).[73] The first trial used bolus 5-FU, whereas the second trial used infusional 5-FU. This shows irinotecan is superior, regardless of the schedule of 5-FU.

Oxaliplatin   Oxaliplatin is a third-generation platinum compound. It has been evaluated as a single agent first-line treatment in metastatic colorectal cancer, with response rates of 12–24.3%.[74] Most studies, however, have examined oxaliplatin in combination with 5-FU/leucovorin, as synergy has been demonstrated. Giacchetti et al performed a phase III trial comparing oxaliplatin + chronomodulated 5-FU/leucovorin with 5-FU/leucovorin as first-line treatment.[75] This showed an improved response rate (53% vs 16%, $p < 0.0001$)

and median progression-free survival (8.7 months vs 6.1 months, $p = 0.048$), but no improvement in overall survival. A similar study by De Gramont et al using standard infused 5-FU/leucovorin showed the response rate (50.7% vs 22.3%, $p = 0.0001$) and progression-free survival (9.0 months vs 6.2 months, $p = 0.003$) were improved, but the improvement in OS was not significant (16.2 months vs 14.7 months, $p = 0.12$). In this trial there was significant crossover from the 5-FU/leucovorin alone arm to the oxaliplatin-containing arm on disease progression, possibly masking the survival advantage of oxaliplatin.[76] The US Intergroup study N9741 has recently reported an overall survival advantage with an oxaliplatin-containing regimen.[77] It began as a six-arm study, but three arms closed during the study due to poor tolerability or inferior efficacy. The three remaining arms were irinotecan/bolus 5-FU/leucovorin (IFL), oxaliplatin/infused 5-FU/leucovorin (FOLFOX4) and oxaliplatin/irinotecan (IROX). The FOLFOX4 regimen showed better OS (19.5 months vs 14.8 months, $p = 0.0001$), time to progression (8.7 months vs 6.9 months, $p = 0.0014$) and response rate (45% vs 31%, $p = 0.002$) compared with IFL. The difference in outcomes between the two arms could in part be due to bolus 5-FU in the IFL vs infused 5-FU in the FOLFOX4 regimen. In addition, 60% of the patients in the FOLFOX4 arm received irinotecan as second-line treatment, whereas 24% of patients in the IFL arm received oxaliplatin as second-line treatment, as it was not licensed at the time of study inception in the United States. The combination arm (IROX) also showed improved OS (17.4 months vs 14.8 months, $p = 0.04$) and response rate (34% vs 31%, $p = 0.03$) but not time to progression (6.5 months vs 6.9 months, $p > 0.5$) compared with the IFL arm. Oxaliplatin has also been evaluated as second-line treatment in combination with 5-FU/leucovorin (FOLFOX4) compared with 5-FU/leucovorin and oxaliplatin alone in patients who had progressed through irinotecan.[78] Response rates were 9.9% for FOLFOX4 vs 0% for 5-FU/leucovorin ($p < 0.0001$). Median time to progression was 4.6 months in the FOLFOX4 arm vs 2.7 months for 5-FU/leucovorin ($p < 0.0001$).

It has been established that both irinotecan and oxaliplatin combined with 5-FU/leucovorin improve response rate. Combination and sequential use has also been examined. A French study gave irinotecan/5-FU/leucovorin (FOLFIRI) followed by FOLFOX4 as second-line treatment or FOLFOX4 followed by FOLFIRI as second-line treatment.[79] Response rates were similar for first-line treatment (56% vs 53%), but FOLFIRI was inferior to FOLFOX4 for second-line treatment (4% vs 15%). There was no difference in time to progression after two lines (14.5 months vs 11.9 months). Combination regimens with oxaliplatin and irinotecan have been examined in phase II trials. One trial compared the combination with 5-FU/leucovorin and alternating irinotecan (FOLFIRI) and oxaliplatin (FOLFOX4):[80] 6% in the alternating arm had a partial response compared with 23% in the combination arm, and median OS was 9.8 months (95% confidence interval (CI) 6.4–13.2%) in the alternating arm and 12.3 months (95% CI 9.8–14.8%) in the combination arm. This may be due to the lower dose intensities in the alternating arm.

Molecularly targeted therapy   Two new monoclonal antibodies have recently been developed and are currently undergoing clinical trials. Both act by targeting growth factors.

Bevacizumab blocks angiogenesis by targeting vascular endothelial growth factor (VEGF). A trial was presented at ASCO in 2003. Patients were randomised to IFL + bevacizumab or + placebo.[81] Median survival was 20.3 months in the bevacizumab-containing arm compared with 15.6 months in the placebo-containing arm. Response rates were also improved in the bevacizumab arm (45% vs 35%). A second abstract was also presented comparing bevacizumab alone or in combination with oxaliplatin/5-FU/leucovorin (FOLFOX4) or oxaliplatin/5-FU/leucovorin alone. Survival data were not yet available.[82]

Cetuximab is a chimaeric monoclonal antibody that targets the epidermal growth factor receptor (EGFR). Phase I trials have confirmed activity in colorectal cancer. A phase II trial presented at ASCO in 2001 demonstrated major objective responses to cetuximab plus irinotecan in patients with EGFR-positive, irinotecan-refractory colorectal cancer.[83] Out of 21 patients 17% achieved a partial response (95% CI 11–25%) and an additional 31% had stable disease. A phase II trial presented at ASCO in 2003 compared irinotecan plus cetuximab with cetuximab alone in EGFR-positive patients who were irinotecan-refractory.[84] The response rate was 17.9% (95% CI 13.0–27.7%) in the combination arm vs 9.9% (95% CI 5.0–17.1%) in the cetuximab-alone arm. Time to progression in the cetuximab + irinotecan arm was 126 days compared with 45 days in the cetuximab-alone arm.

CARCINOMA OF THE ANUS

Anal cancer is uncommon and represents only 4% of lower gastrointestinal (GI) malignancies. Squamous cell carcinomas make up the majority of all primary cancers of the anus. Rarer histological subtypes include adenocarcinoma and basaloid carcinoma. Most anal cancers are curable by primary chemoradiation or local excision. Squamous cell carcinoma of the anus is associated with human papillomavirus and the human immunodeficiency virus (HIV).

Investigations and staging

Patients should be staged with a CT scan of the thorax, abdomen and pelvis and an MRI scan of the pelvis. Biopsy for histological confirmation is also required. Routine blood tests, including full blood count, urea and electrolytes and liver function tests, are also performed.

The anal canal extends from the rectum to the perianal skin. Staging of anal tumours has been described by the American Joint Committee on Cancer (AJCC) and is shown in Table 39.5.

Management

Surgery used to be the treatment of choice in anal cancer. This has now been superseded by chemoradiation, with surgery reserved as a salvage option. Treatment also depends on the extent of disease. In-situ carcinoma is removed surgically. For T1–T2 tumours, the options are surgery or radiotherapy. The standard treatment for T1–T2, N1–N3 or T3–T4 any N is chemoradiation.

Chemoradiation has been used since the mid-1970s, following a trial by Nigro et al where radiotherapy, 5-FU and mitomycin C were used in anal cancer and complete pathological responses were seen.[85,86] Two phase III trials have compared radiotherapy alone vs

Table 39.5   Union Internationale Control le Cancer (UICC) staging for anal cancers

Stage	T	N	M
Stage 0	Tis	N0	M0
Stage I	T1	N0	M0
Stage II	T2	N0	M0
	T3	N0	M0
Stage IIIA	T1	N1	M0
	T2	N1	M0
	T3	N1	M0
	T4	N0	M0
Stage IIIB	T4	N1	M0
	Any T	N2	M0
	Any T	N3	M0
Stage IV	Any T	Any N	M1

radiotherapy with 5-FU and mitomycin C and shown improved local control and disease-specific survival but no improvement in overall survival with the addition of chemotherapy.[87,88] Toxicity was similar in both groups. Flam et al examined the role of mitomycin C in combination with 5-FU and radiotherapy and found mitomycin C significantly improved results with 71% colostomy-free survival vs 59%, $p = 0.014$.[89]

Subsequent research has concentrated on finding the optimum schedule of chemoradiation. Cisplatin has been combined with 5-FU and radiation and response rates from 68 to 94% were seen. Colostomy-free survival up to 86% was reported.[90,91]

Finally, studies have examined the role of induction chemotherapy and higher doses of radiation. A French phase II study used two cycles of 5-FU and cisplatin followed by concomitant chemoradiation and a further two cycles of 5-FU/cisplatin.[92] Complete response rate was 67%. Three-year overall survival, colostomy-free and disease-free survival rates were 86%, 73% and 67%, respectively. The ACT II study is also currently investigating the role of cisplatin compared with mitomycin C and examining the role of adjuvant chemotherapy.

Our current standard management involves 5-FU and mitomycin C with radiotherapy. Radiotherapy is given in two phases with 45 Gy in 25 fractions followed by 15 Gy in 6 fractions after a 2–3 week break. 5-FU is given in week 1 and week 5 with mitomycin C on day 1. Surgery is used for residual disease.

Metastatic carcinoma of the anus

Distant metastases develop in 10–20% of patients. There are few studies on treatment, and therefore there is no recommended standard treatment. Responses have been seen with cisplatin alone and bleomycin and vinblastine in combination with cisplatin.[93,94] The combination of cisplatin and 5-FU has been studied in small numbers of patients and a 16% complete response rate and a 48% partial response rate have been found. Our current standard regimen is cisplatin or mitomycin C with 5-FU.

NURSING CARE FOR PATIENTS RECEIVING CHEMOTHERAPY FOR GASTROINTESTINAL CANCERS

Ramani Sitamvaram

INTRODUCTION

5-FU chemotherapy remains the mainstay of treatment for GI cancers. Chemotherapy is often delivered in the ambulatory or outpatient setting. More recently, new oral cytotoxic agents such as capecitabine are being used and increasing numbers of patients are receiving oral chemotherapy at home. Oncology nurses play a key role in the education and support of patients undergoing chemotherapy. (See also Ch. 12.)

COMPLEXITY OF TREATMENT

The majority of people diagnosed with GI cancers are over the age of 65. The physiological and social changes that occur with ageing are important considerations in making decisions on chemotherapy treatments. Patients may have other medical conditions that affect their ability to have the full dose of drugs. The ability of the immune system to cope with the risk of infection as well as decreased liver and renal functions need to be considered when choosing chemotherapy agents. In the older person, more than in any other, it is also important to consider the effect on the quality of life.[95] Many of these patients may be living alone or with an elderly relative. They may be the main carer for their husband or wife. When making treatment decisions, healthcare professionals need to be aware of what support services, if any, are available.

Treatments for GI cancers are often multimodal in nature. Patients may have had or go on to have surgery or radiotherapy prior to or after commencing chemotherapy. Patients' experience of chemotherapy plays a significant role in how they manage further treatment.

Patients often have beliefs and misconceptions of chemotherapy, which can cause them to be unduly worried or frightened. Nurses can help to alleviate these worries so that patients can cope better with the treatment and side effects.[96] Accurate information-giving and helping patients to understand the rationale for treatment, especially those having treatment for advanced cancers, may help reduce their anxiety and distress. Involving the patient and family in decision-making enables a good patient–professional relationship. Patients need to feel comfortable to be able to ask questions. Family and friends are often the main support system for the patients as they try to cope with treatment and its effect. (See also Ch. 5.)

PATIENT EDUCATION AND SUPPORT

Chemotherapy for this group of patients is mainly in the ambulatory or outpatient setting. Effective education is important for the successful completion of ambulatory chemotherapy. The safe use of protracted infusions of chemotherapy by patients while at home requires structured, well-planned teaching by the nurses prior to a patient's discharge.[97] Nurses need to take into account patients' individual needs and abilities. Practical demonstrations and clearly written and concise handouts will enable the patient and family to acquire skills and knowledge about the drugs and their side effects as well as the equipment being used.[98] Ensuring that there is community support available for patients alleviates their anxieties and will help with compliance and early reporting of side effects.

Oral chemotherapy

In recent years, increasing numbers of patients are receiving self-administering oral chemotherapy at home. The support of oncology nurses will be central to the effective management of these patients. Patients often think of chemotherapy in terms of needles, and sometimes think that oral tablets may not have as severe side effects, or that it may be like taking a vitamin pill.[99] Nurses have a primary role in ensuring that patients understand the administration of chemotherapy tablets and potential side effects and the early reporting of them. Patient compliance is critical to successful administration of oral chemotherapy. Nurses working with this group of patients have a role in identifying and supporting patients who are able to cope with home chemotherapy and those who need close supervision and additional support. There may be limitations to a patient's ability to cope with oral chemotherapy. There may be issues with gut absorption and function due to their illness, making oral chemotherapy inappropriate. Elderly patients can have problems with sight or have limited manual dexterity in managing tablets.[99] These patients may also be taking other medication, and adding oral chemotherapy may not be feasible. Nurses need to foster a good relationship with the patient and carer so that the patient can feel comfortable in asking questions and reporting side effects.

NUTRITION

Cancer treatments can affect the nutritional status of a patient. Their digestive system is often disturbed due to diarrhoea and constipation, leading to weight loss (more of an issue with upper GI cancer). (See also Ch. 19.)

Eating is a basic body function and often a social activity. Difficulty in eating or the inability to eat can have a profound physical and psychological impact on the patient and family. The families' own beliefs or their desire to encourage the patient to eat as a way of helping may cause additional stress. Family members feel that preparing food and feeding their loved one is something they can actively do and often there is frustration, despair and anger when the patient is unable to eat.

Tube feeding

Some patients may require tube feeding. Understanding the psychological and social needs of patients requiring tube feeding is an important nursing issue.

Patients requiring long-term feeding lose control over food selection and consumption. As eating is a social, cultural and religious activity, adaptation may be difficult. In helping patients to adapt, nurses need to understand the patient's lifestyle and perception of the importance of food and eating.[95] They can then identify areas of concern. Patients can feel self-conscious surrounded by their feeding equipment, and their mobility may also be reduced, as they have to be attached to a pump.

BODY IMAGE

GI cancer and chemotherapy can further impact on a patient's already altered body image. Symptoms of weight loss, dysphagia, diarrhoea, hair loss and lethargy can worsen as a result of treatment. Diarrhoea and stomatitis are common side effects of GI chemotherapy. Patients who already have altered bowel habits due to their disease may get an increase in their diarrhoea. This can lead to increased flatus and incontinence. Furthermore, some patients may have to cope with a stoma following surgery. The effect of chemotherapy may increase their worries on issues such as changes in stoma appearance, increased diarrhoea, unpleasant smells and bags leaking, causing concerns about social and public situations and leading to feelings of body function failure.[100] Patients may be embarrassed to go out, further increasing their sense of isolation. This, in turn, can cause barriers in socialisation with family and friends. Isolation can also bring about feelings of despair and further impact on family relationships. Patients often feel a sense of loss of control, leading to low self-esteem. Therefore, nursing care needs to encompass both physical and psychological aspects.

CONCLUSION

Oncology nurses need to have a good understanding of the issues that affect cancer patients as they undergo treatment as nurses play a major role in facilitating patient education, support, communication and acting as liaison between the patient, family and other disciplines.

References

1. Ferlay J, Bray F, Pisani P, et al. GLOBOCAN 2000: Cancer incidence, mortality and prevalence worldwide, Version 1.0. IARC CancerBase No 5. Lyon: IARC; 2001. www.dep.iarc.fr/globocan/globocan.htm. 2003.

2. Vogelstein B, Fearon ER, Hamilton SR, et al. Genetic alterations during colorectal-tumor development. N Engl J Med 1988; 319:525–532.

3. Arvanitis ML, Jagelman DG, Fazio VW, et al. Mortality in patients with familial adenomatous polyposis. Dis Colon Rectum 1990; 33:639–642.

4. Voskuil DW, Vasen HF, Kampman E, et al. Colorectal cancer risk in HNPCC families: development during lifetime and in successive generations. National Collaborative Group on HNPCC. Int J Cancer 1997; 72:205–209.

5. Cottrell S, Bicknell D, Kaklamanis L, et al. Molecular analysis of APC mutations in familial adenomatous polyposis and sporadic colon carcinomas. Lancet 1992; 340:626–630.

6. Peltomaki P, Vasen HF. Mutations predisposing to hereditary nonpolyposis colorectal cancer: database and results of a collaborative study. The International Collaborative Group on Hereditary Nonpolyposis Colorectal Cancer. Gastroenterology 1997; 113:1146–1158.

7. Levin B. Inflammatory bowel disease and colon cancer. Cancer 1992; 70:1313–1316.

8. Willett WC, Stampfer MJ, Colditz GA, et al. Relation of meat, fat, and fiber intake to the risk of colon cancer in a prospective study among women. N Engl J Med 1990; 323:1664–1672.

9. Giovannucci E. An updated review of the epidemiological evidence that cigarette smoking increases risk of colorectal cancer. Cancer Epidemiol Biomarkers Prev 2001; 10:725–731.

10. Thune I, Lund E. Physical activity and risk of colorectal cancer in men and women. Br J Cancer 1996; 73:1134–1140.

11. Steinmetz KA, Potter JD. Vegetables, fruit, and cancer prevention: a review. J Am Diet Assoc 1996; 96:1027–1039.

12. MacLennan SC, MacLennan AH, Ryan P. Colorectal cancer and oestrogen replacement therapy. A meta-analysis of epidemiological studies. Med J Aust 1995;162: 491–493.

13. Wolmark N, Fisher B, Rockette H, et al. Postoperative adjuvant chemotherapy or BCG for colon cancer: results from NSABP protocol C-01. J Natl Cancer Inst 1988; 80:30–36.

14. Wieand HS, Smith R, Colangelo L. Adjuvant chemotherapy in carcinoma of the colon: 10 year results of NSABP protocol C-01. Proc Am Soc Clin Oncol 2003; 20:138a.

15. Laurie JA, Moertel CG, Fleming TR, et al. Surgical adjuvant therapy of large-bowel carcinoma: an evaluation of levamisole and the combination of levamisole and fluorouracil. The North Central Cancer Treatment Group and the Mayo Clinic. J Clin Oncol 1989; 7:1447–1456.

16. Moertel CG, Fleming TR, Macdonald JS, et al. Levamisole and fluorouracil for adjuvant therapy of resected colon carcinoma. N Engl J Med 1990; 322:352–358.

17. Moertel CG, Fleming TR, Macdonald JS, et al. Fluorouracil plus levamisole as effective adjuvant therapy after resection of stage III colon carcinoma: a final report. Ann Intern Med 1995; 122:321–326.

18. NIH Consensus Conference. Adjuvant therapy for patients with colon and rectal cancer. JAMA 1990; 264:1444–1450.

19. Efficacy of adjuvant fluorouracil and folinic acid in colon cancer. International Multicentre Pooled Analysis of Colon Cancer Trials (IMPACT) investigators. Lancet 1995; 345:939–944.

20. Wolmark N, Rockette H, Fisher B, et al. The benefit of leucovorin-modulated fluorouracil as postoperative adjuvant therapy for primary colon cancer: results from National Surgical Adjuvant Breast and Bowel Project protocol C-03. J Clin Oncol 1993; 11:1879–1887.

21. O'Connell MJ, Mailliard JA, Kahn MJ, et al. Controlled trial of fluorouracil and low-dose leucovorin given for 6 months as postoperative adjuvant therapy for colon cancer. J Clin Oncol 1997; 15:246–250.

22. Taal BG, Van Tinteren H, Zoetmulder FA. Adjuvant 5FU plus levamisole in colonic or rectal cancer: improved survival in stage II and III. Br J Cancer 2001; 85:1437–1443.

23. Porschen R, Bermann A, Loffler T, et al. Fluorouracil plus leucovorin as effective adjuvant chemotherapy in curatively resected stage III colon cancer: results of the trial adjCCA-01. J Clin Oncol 2001; 19:1787–1794.

24. Staib L, Link KH, Beger HG. Toxicity and effects of adjuvant therapy in colon cancer: results of the German prospective, controlled randomized multicenter trial FOGT-1. J Gastrointest Surg 2001; 5:275–281.

25. Haller DG, Catalano PJ, Macdonald JS. Fluorouracil, leucovorin and levamisole adjuvant therapy for colon cancer: five year final report of Int-0089. Proc Am Soc Clin Oncol 2003; 17:256a.

26. Andre T, Colin P, Louvet C, et al. Semimonthly versus monthly regimen of fluorouracil and leucovorin administered for 24 or 36 weeks as adjuvant therapy in

stage II and III colon cancer: results of a randomized trial. J Clin Oncol 2003; 21:2896–2903.

27. Saini A, Norman AR, Cunningham D, et al. Twelve weeks of protracted venous infusion of fluorouracil (5-FU) is as effective as 6 months of bolus 5-FU and folinic acid as adjuvant treatment in colorectal cancer. Br J Cancer 2003; 88:1859–1865.

28. de Gramont A, Banzi M, Navarro J, et al. Oxaliplatin/ 5-FU/LV in adjuvant colon cancer: results of the international randomized mosaic trial. Proc Am Soc Clin Oncol 2003; 21:253.

29. Miwa M, Ura M, Nishida M, et al. Design of a novel oral fluoropyrimidine carbamate, capecitabine, which generates 5-fluorouracil selectively in tumours by enzymes concentrated in human liver and cancer tissue. Eur J Cancer 1998; 34:1274–1281.

30. Hoff PM, Ansari R, Batist G, et al. Comparison of oral capecitabine versus intravenous fluorouracil plus leucovorin as first-line treatment in 605 patients with metastatic colorectal cancer: results of a randomized phase III study. J Clin Oncol 2001; 19:2282–2292.

31. Van Cutsem E, Twelves C, Cassidy J, et al. Oral capecitabine compared with intravenous fluorouracil plus leucovorin in patients with metastatic colorectal cancer: results of a large phase III study. J Clin Oncol 2001; 19:4097–4106.

32. Efficacy of adjuvant fluorouracil and folinic acid in B2 colon cancer. International Multicentre Pooled Analysis of B2 Colon Cancer Trials (IMPACT B2) Investigators. J Clin Oncol 1999; 17:1356–1363.

33. Mamounas E, Wieand S, Wolmark N, et al. Comparative efficacy of adjuvant chemotherapy in patients with Dukes' B versus Dukes' C colon cancer: results from four National Surgical Adjuvant Breast and Bowel Project adjuvant studies (C-01, C-02, C-03, and C-04). J Clin Oncol 1999; 17:1349–1355.

34. Comparison of fluorouracil with additional levamisole, higher-dose folinic acid, or both, as adjuvant chemotherapy for colorectal cancer: a randomised trial. QUASAR Collaborative Group. Lancet 2000; 355:1588–1596.

35. Havenga K, Enker WE, Norstein J, et al. Improved survival and local control after total mesorectal excision or D3 lymphadenectomy in the treatment of primary rectal cancer: an international analysis of 1411 patients. Eur J Surg Oncol 1999; 25:368–374.

36. Heald RJ, Moran BJ, Ryall RD, et al. Rectal cancer: the Basingstoke experience of total mesorectal excision, 1978–1997. Arch Surg 1998; 133:894–899.

37. Wibe A, Rendedal PR, Svensson E, et al. Prognostic significance of the circumferential resection margin following total mesorectal excision for rectal cancer. Br J Surg 2002; 89:327–334.

38. Nagtegaal ID, Marijnen CA, Kranenbarg EK, et al. Circumferential margin involvement is still an important predictor of local recurrence in rectal carcinoma: not one millimeter but two millimeters is the limit. Am J Surg Pathol 2002; 26:350–357.

39. Improved survival with preoperative radiotherapy in resectable rectal cancer. Swedish Rectal Cancer Trial. N Engl J Med 1997; 336:980–987.

40. Kapiteijn E, Marijnen CA, Nagtegaal ID, et al. Preoperative radiotherapy combined with total mesorectal excision for resectable rectal cancer. N Engl J Med 2001; 345:638–646.

41. Randomised trial of surgery alone versus surgery followed by radiotherapy for mobile cancer of the rectum. Medical Research Council Rectal Cancer Working Party. Lancet 1996; 348:1610–1614.

42. Adjuvant radiotherapy for rectal cancer: a systematic overview of 8,507 patients from 22 randomised trials. Lancet 2001; 358:1291–1304.

43. Camma C, Giunta M, Fiorica F, et al. Preoperative radiotherapy for resectable rectal cancer: a meta-analysis. JAMA 2000; 284:1008–1015.

44. Roh MS, Petrelli NJ, Wieand HS. Phase III randomized trial of pre-operative versus post-operative multimodality therapy in patients with carcinoma of the rectum. Proc Am Soc Clin Oncol 2001; 20:123a.

45. Sauer R, Fietkau R, Wittekind C, et al. Adjuvant vs. neoadjuvant radiochemotherapy for locally advanced rectal cancer: the German trial CAO/ARO/AIO-94. Colorectal Dis 2003; 5:406–415.

46. Chau I, Allen M, Cunningham D, et al. Neoadjuvant systemic fluorouracil and mitomycin C prior to synchronous chemoradiation is an effective strategy in locally advanced rectal cancer. Br J Cancer 2003; 88:1017–1024.

47. Chau I, Cunningham D, Tait D, et al. Twelve weeks of neoadjuvant capecitabine (cap) and oxaliplatin (ox) followed by synchronous chemoradiation (CRT) and total mesorectal excision (TME) in MRI defined poor risk locally advanced rectal cancer resulted in promising tumour regression and symptomatic relief. Proc Am Soc Clin Oncol 2003; 21.

48. Fisher B, Wolmark N, Rockette H, et al. Postoperative adjuvant chemotherapy or radiation therapy for rectal cancer: results from NSABP protocol R-01. J Natl Cancer Inst 1988; 80:21–29.

49. Wolmark N, Wieand HS, Hyams DM, Colangelo L, Dimitrov NV, Romond EH et al. Randomized trial of postoperative adjuvant chemotherapy with or without radiotherapy for carcinoma of the rectum: National Surgical Adjuvant Breast and Bowel Project Protocol R-02. J Natl Cancer Inst 2000;92:388-96.

50. Prolongation of the disease-free interval in surgically treated rectal carcinoma. Gastrointestinal Tumor Study Group. N Engl J Med 1985; 312:1465–1472.

51. Krook JE, Moertel CG, Gunderson LL, et al. Effective surgical adjuvant therapy for high-risk rectal carcinoma. N Engl J Med 1991; 324:709–715.

52. Tepper JE, O'Connell M, Niedzwiecki D, et al. Adjuvant therapy in rectal cancer: analysis of stage, sex, and local control – final report of intergroup 0114. J Clin Oncol 2002; 20:1744–1750.

53. O'Connell MJ, Martenson JA, Wieand HS, et al. Improving adjuvant therapy for rectal cancer by combining protracted-infusion fluorouracil with radiation therapy after curative surgery. N Engl J Med 1994; 331:502–507.

54. Stangl R, Altendorf-Hofmann A, Charnley RM, et al. Factors influencing the natural history of colorectal liver metastases. Lancet 1994; 343:1405–1410.

55. Wilson SM, Adson MA. Surgical treatment of hepatic metastases from colorectal cancers. Arch Surg 1976; 111:330–334.

56. Bismuth H, Adam R, Levi F, et al. Resection of non-resectable liver metastases from colorectal cancer after neoadjuvant chemotherapy. Arch Surg 1996; 224:509–520.

57. Douillard JY, Cunningham D, Roth AD, et al. Irinotecan combined with fluorouracil compared with fluorouracil alone as first-line treatment for metastatic colorectal cancer: a multicentre randomised trial. Lancet 2000; 355:1041–1047.

58. Lorenz M, Rossion I. [Adjuvant and palliative regional therapy of liver metastases in colorectal tumors]. Dtsch Med Wochenschr 1995; 120:690–697.

59. Kemeny N, Huang Y, Cohen AM, et al. Hepatic arterial infusion of chemotherapy after resection of hepatic metastases from colorectal cancer. N Engl J Med 1999; 341:2039–2048.

60. Kemeny MM, Adak S, Gray B, et al. Combined-modality treatment for resectable metastatic colorectal carcinoma to the liver: surgical resection of hepatic metastases in combination with continuous infusion of chemotherapy – an intergroup study. J Clin Oncol 2002; 20:1499–1505.

61. Pastorino U. Lung metastasectomy for colorectal cancer. Tumori 1997; 83:S28–S30.

62. Mountain CF, McMurtrey MJ, Hermes KE. Surgery for pulmonary metastasis: a 20-year experience. Ann Thorac Surg 1984; 38:323–330.

63. Goya T, Miyazawa N, Kondo H, et al. Surgical resection of pulmonary metastases from colorectal cancer. 10-year follow-up. Cancer 1989; 64:1418–1421.

64. Long-term results of lung metastasectomy: prognostic analyses based on 5206 cases. The International Registry of Lung Metastases. J Thorac Cardiovasc Surg 1997; 113:37–49.

65. Modulation of fluorouracil by leucovorin in patients with advanced colorectal cancer: evidence in terms of response rate. Advanced Colorectal Cancer Meta-Analysis Project. J Clin Oncol 1992; 10:896–903.

66. Efficacy of intravenous continuous infusion of fluorouracil compared with bolus administration in advanced colorectal cancer. Meta-analysis Group In Cancer. J Clin Oncol 1998; 16:301–308.

67. Twelves C. Capecitabine as first-line treatment in colorectal cancer. Pooled data from two large, phase III trials. Eur J Cancer 2002; 38(Suppl 2):15–20.

68. Douillard JY, Hoff PM, Skillings JR, et al. Multicenter phase III study of uracil/tegafur and oral leucovorin versus fluorouracil and leucovorin in patients with previously untreated metastatic colorectal cancer. J Clin Oncol 2002; 20:3605–3616.

69. Carmichael J, Popiela T, Radstone D, et al. Randomized comparative study of tegafur/uracil and oral leucovorin versus parenteral fluorouracil and leucovorin in patients with previously untreated metastatic colorectal cancer. J Clin Oncol 2002; 20:3617–3627.

70. Vanhoefer U, Harstrick A, Achterrath W, et al. Irinotecan in the treatment of colorectal cancer: clinical overview. J Clin Oncol 2001; 19:1501–1518.

71. Cunningham D, Pyrhonen S, James RD, et al. Randomised trial of irinotecan plus supportive care versus supportive care alone after fluorouracil failure for patients with metastatic colorectal cancer. Lancet 1998; 352:1413–1418.

72. Rougier P, Van Cutsem E, Bajetta E, et al. Randomised trial of irinotecan versus fluorouracil by continuous infusion after fluorouracil failure in patients with metastatic colorectal cancer. Lancet 1998; 352:1407–1412.

73. Saltz LB, Cox JV, Blanke C, et al. Irinotecan plus fluorouracil and leucovorin for metastatic colorectal cancer. Irinotecan Study Group. N Engl J Med 2000; 343:905–914.

74. Cvitkovic E, Bekradda M. Oxaliplatin: a new therapeutic option in colorectal cancer. Semin Oncol 1999; 26:647–662.

75. Giacchetti S, Perpoint B, Zidani R, et al. Phase III multicenter randomized trial of oxaliplatin added to chronomodulated fluorouracil-leucovorin as first-line treatment of metastatic colorectal cancer. J Clin Oncol 2000; 18:136–147.

76. de Gramont A, Figer A, Seymour M, et al. Leucovorin and fluorouracil with or without oxaliplatin as first-line treatment in advanced colorectal cancer. J Clin Oncol. 2000; 18:2938–2947.

77. Goldberg RM, Morton RF, Sargent DG. N9741: oxaliplatin (oxal) or CPT-11 + 5-fluorouracil(5-FU)/leucovorin (LV) or oxal + CPT-11 in advanced colorectal cancer. Updated efficacy and quality of life (QOL) data from an intergroup study. Proc Am Soc Clin Oncol 2003; 21.

78. Rothenberg ML, Oza AM, Bigelow RH, et al. Superiority of oxaliplatin and fluorouracil-leucovorin compared with either therapy alone in patients with progressive colorectal cancer after irinotecan and fluorouracil-leucovorin: interim results of a phase III trial. J Clin Oncol 2003; 21:2059–2069.

79. Achille E, Tournigand C, Andre T. FOLFIRI then FOLFOX or FOLFOX then FOLFIRI in metastatic colorectal cancer: results of a phase III trail. Eur J Cancer 2001; 37(Suppl 6):S289.

80. Becouarn Y, Gamelin E, Coudert B, et al. Randomized multicenter phase II study comparing a combination of fluorouracil and folinic acid and alternating irinotecan and oxaliplatin with oxaliplatin and irinotecan in fluorouracil-pretreated metastatic colorectal cancer patients. J Clin Oncol 2001; 19:4195–4201.

81. Hurwitz H, Fehrenbacher L, Cartwright T, et al. Bevacizumab (a monoclonal antibody to vascular endothelial growth factor) prolongs survival in first-line colorectal cancer (CRC): results of a phase III trial of bevacizumab in combination with bolus IFL (irinotecan/5-fluorouracil/leucovorin) as a first-line therapy in subjects with metastatic CRC. Proc Am Soc Clin Oncol 2003; 21.

82. Benson AB, Catalano PJ, Meropol NJ, et al. Bevacizumab (anti-VEGF) plus FOLFOX4 in previously treated advanced colorectal cancer (advCRC): an interim toxicity analysis of th Eastern Cooperative Group (ECOG) study E3200. Proc Am Soc Clin Oncol 2003; 21.

83. Saltz LB, Rubin M, Hochster H, et al. Cetuximab (IMC-C225) plus irinotecan (CPT-11) is active in CPT-11-refractory colorectal cancer (CRC) that expresses epidermal growth factor receptor (EGFR). Proc Am Soc Clin Oncol 2003; 21.

84. Cunningham D, Humblet S, Siena S, et al. Cetuximab (C225) alone or in combination with irinotecan (CPT-11) in patients with epidermal growth factor receptor (EGFR)-positive, irinotecan refractory metastatic colorectal cancer (MCRC). Proc Am Soc Clin Oncol 2003; 21.

85. Nigro ND, Seydel HG, Considine B, et al. Combined preoperative radiation and chemotherapy for squamous cell carcinoma of the anal canal. Cancer 1983; 51:1826–1829.

86. Nigro ND, Vaitkevicius VK, Considine B Jr. Combined therapy for cancer of the anal canal: a preliminary report. Dis Colon Rectum 1974; 17:354–356.

87. Bartelink H, Roelofsen F, Eschwege F, et al. Concomitant radiotherapy and chemotherapy is superior to radiotherapy alone in the treatment of locally advanced anal cancer: results of a phase III randomized trial of the European Organization for Research and Treatment of Cancer Radiotherapy and Gastrointestinal Cooperative Groups. J Clin Oncol.1997; 15:2040–2049.

88. Epidermoid anal cancer: results from the UKCCCR randomised trial of radiotherapy alone versus radiotherapy, 5-fluorouracil, and mitomycin. UKCCCR Anal Cancer Trial Working Party. UK Co-ordinating Committee on Cancer Research. Lancet 1996; 348:1049–1054.

89. Flam M, John M, Pajak TF, et al. Role of mitomycin in combination with fluorouracil and radiotherapy, and of salvage chemoradiation in the definitive nonsurgical treatment of epidermoid carcinoma of the anal canal: results of a phase III randomized intergroup study. J Clin Oncol 1996; 14:2527–2539.

90. Doci R, Zucali R, La Monica G, et al. Primary chemoradiation therapy with fluorouracil and cisplatin for cancer of the anus: results in 35 consecutive patients. J Clin Oncol 1996; 14:3121–3125.

91. Martenson JA, Lipsitz SR, Wagner H Jr, et al. Initial results of a phase II trial of high dose radiation therapy, 5-fluorouracil, and cisplatin for patients with anal cancer (E4292): an Eastern Cooperative Oncology Group study. Int J Radiat Oncol Biol Phys 1996; 35:745–749.

92. Peiffert D, Giovannini M, Ducreux M, et al. High-dose radiation therapy and neoadjuvant plus concomitant chemotherapy with 5-fluorouracil and cisplatin in patients with locally advanced squamous-cell anal canal cancer: final results of a phase II study. Ann Oncol 2001; 12:397–404.

93. Salem PA, Habboubi N, Anaissie E, et al. Effectiveness of cisplatin in the treatment of anal squamous cell carcinoma. Cancer Treat Rep 1985; 69:891–893.

94. Ajani JA, Carrasco CH, Jackson DE, et al. Combination of cisplatin plus fluoropyrimidine chemotherapy effective against liver metastases from carcinoma of the anal canal. Am J Med 1989; 87:221–224.

95. Otto SE (ed.). Oncology nursing: chemotherapy. 4th edn. St Louis: Mosby; 2000:659–662.

96. Holmes S. Cancer chemotherapy. A guide for practice. Dorking: Asset Books; 1997.

97. Groenwald SL, Hansen Frogge M, Goodman M, et al, eds. Cancer nursing, principles and practice. 4th edn. Boston: Jones and Bartlett; 1997.

98. Dougherty L, Viner C, Young J. Establishing ambulatory chemotherapy at home. Prof Nurse 1998; 13(6):356–358.

99. Hollywood E, Semple D. Nursing strategies for patients on oral chemotherapy. Oncology (Huntingt) 2001; 15(1 suppl 2):37–39.

100. White CE. Living with a stoma. London: Sheldon; 1997.

Chapter **40**

Gynaecological cancers

CHAPTER CONTENTS

MEDICAL CARE FOR PATIENTS WITH GYNAECOLOGICAL CANCERS

Justin Stebbing, Stanley Kaye and Martin Gore

INTRODUCTION

Cancers of the female reproductive organs are heterogeneous with regard to histology, natural history, clinical behaviour and methods of treatment. Appropriate therapy requires careful diagnostic evaluation to distinguish from other malignancies of the pelvis (e.g. rectal and bladder cancers) as well as from metastatic lesions. Accurate staging is critical, as treatment is virtually always guided by the extent of disease spread. Optimal conditions for diagnosis, staging and therapy require excellent communication between oncologists, surgeons, radiologists and histopathologists. It is becoming increasingly evident that patients do better when managed within the context of multidisciplinary teams whose personnel have expertise in a particular type of cancer. For example, surgery should be performed by gynaecological oncologists and nurses should have both oncology and gynaecological expertise.[1]

Tumours in this section include epithelial and non-epithelial ovarian cancers, cervix and endometrial tumours.

EPITHELIAL OVARIAN CANCER

Introduction

Epithelial ovarian cancer (EOC) is the commonest form of gynaecological cancer in the Western world and the leading cause of death in this category: it affects approximately 6500 women each year in the United Kingdom, with an annual death rate of 4500, making it the fourth most common cause of death from malignancy in women.[2] Aetiology and risk factors include advanced age, nulliparity, European or North American descent and any history of the familial cancer syndromes. Screening with CA125 and/or transvaginal ultrasound has not thus far been shown to be cost-effective. However, patients at increased risk, including those with a strong family history or those with known BRCA-1 or -2 mutations, may benefit from transvaginal ultrasound, CA125 measurement and salpingo-oophorectomy.[3]

Diagnosis and staging

The diagnosis and staging of EOC requires a laparotomy and the recommended surgical intervention is a total abdominal hysterectomy, bilateral salpingo-oophorectomy, omentectomy and 'debulking' of tumour. The two most important and consistently defined prognostic factors in EOC are FIGO (International Federation of Gynaecology and Obstetrics) stage at diagnosis (Table 40.1) and the size of residual disease after initial surgery.[4]

Table 40.1   FIGO staging for ovarian cancer[5]

Stage	Description
Stage I	IA – one ovary, capsule intact, no ascites
Disease confined to the ovaries	IB – both ovaries, capsule intact, no ascites
	IC – IA or IB with tumour on surface of one or both ovaries, or capsule rupture or positive ascites or peritoneal fluid
Stage II	Disease confined to the pelvis
Stage III	
Extrapelvic tumour present	IIIA – negative nodes and microscopic seedlings on peritoneum
	IIIB – negative nodes, peritoneal tumour " 2 cm
	IIIC – positive nodes and/or peritoneal tumour >2 cm
Stage IV	Spread to extra-abdominal site (including positive cytology from a pleural effusion)

Prognosis

Residual disease after surgery is described in virtually every multivariate analysis for prognostic factors that appears in the literature. This is a continuous variable but investigators use a cut-off dimension of 1 cm to define whether patients have been optimally or sub-optimally debulked and thus have a good or bad prognosis. The 3-year survival is approximately 75%, 50% and 25% for those with no macroscopic residuum, residuum of ≤1 cm, 1–5 cm and >5 cm respectively.[6] Other factors that have been shown in some multivariate analyses to be of prognostic significance include age of the patient, histology, performance status and tumour grade.[4] The chemosensitivity of EOC can often provide the basis for good palliation and prolongation of life.

Patients with early-stage ovarian cancer (stage I) have a good prognosis, with 5-year survival exceeding 80%. The 5-year survival of patients where the tumour has spread within the abdominal cavity is only 20%. The reason why overall survival in EOC is so poor (5-year survival 30%) is that the majority of patients (70–80%) present with advanced disease.[4]

First-line chemotherapy

It is widely accepted that all patients with stage II–IV disease should receive chemotherapy, as the relapse rate following surgery without further treatment approaches 100%. The role of chemotherapy for early-stage disease has recently been addressed in a large randomised trial (ICON1/ACTION).[7] These data suggest that there is a survival benefit (7%) absolute for the use of adjuvant platinum-based chemotherapy. However, a subset analysis suggests that this may only apply to patients who have been inadequately staged. Thus, for such patients and for those with poor prognosis early-stage ovarian cancer (e.g. stage IC, clear cell histology, grade III differentiation who have a 30–40% relapse rate), adjuvant chemotherapy should be considered. There remains debate as to whether those with stage IA grade I or II disease require more than surgery.[8,9]

Platinum-based chemotherapy

Trials of cytotoxic agents in ovarian cancer have been based on the identification of the high level of activity of platinum compounds, and these remain the cornerstone of therapy.[10,11] Once the use of platinum-based therapy was established in the 1980s, the next issue concerned the use of platinum-based combination therapy. These combinations were undoubtedly more toxic (especially with regards to myelosuppression) and, although response rates were generally higher than with single agent platinum, most trials failed to show a survival benefit. However, a number of trials showed an improvement in progression-free survival.[12]

Taxanes

In the early 1990s phase II trials in patients with relapsed and refractory EOC suggested that a new class of compounds, the taxanes, was active. These studies demonstrated an improved response rate associated with higher doses[13] and there was also a suggestion that efficacy was related to infusion time. For example, a European–Canadian study randomised patients with platinum pretreated relapsed ovarian cancer to receive either 175 mg/m^2 or 135 mg/m^2 of paclitaxel over either 24 or 3 hours[14] (bifactorial design). There were no statistically significant differences in response rate between these groups, although neutropenia was more pronounced with 24-hour infusions. However, progression-free survival was significantly longer in the higher-dose group (19 weeks vs 14 weeks, $p = 0.02$). A further GOG (Gynecologic Oncology Group) study randomised patients with recurrent disease to either paclitaxel 175 mg/m^2 or 250 mg/m^2 given by a 24-hour infusion[15] and this showed no statistically significant differences in time to disease progression or survival. The activity of paclitaxel in relapsed/refractory disease led to the initiation of trials where paclitaxel was given as part of first-line therapy.[16]

Platinum/paclitaxel chemotherapy

There are four large studies comparing the combination of platinum and paclitaxel with non-paclitaxel-containing platinum-based chemotherapy (Table 40.2). Two of these four trials demonstrated a benefit of combining cisplatin with paclitaxel and two failed to demonstrate an advantage for platinum–paclitaxel.

Randomised trials have shown that carboplatin–paclitaxel is equivalent in efficacy to cisplatin–paclitaxel and is less toxic (reviewed in Refs 21–24). The combination of carboplatin (dosed to an area under the curve of 5.0–7.5 – see Dosing of platinum compounds section below) + paclitaxel (175 mg/m^2 in a 3-hour infusion) for 6 cycles at 3-weekly intervals with paclitaxel has therefore become the standard first-line treatment for patients with epithelial ovarian cancer. There is no evidence of an impact on survival by any type of additional therapy, dose escalation strategies or prolonged infusion times.[25]

Dosing of platinum compounds

Carboplatin is an analogue of cisplatin which was introduced in 1981 because of its favourable toxicity profile, with reduced nephrotoxicity, ototoxicity and peripheral neuropathy.[26,27] Its dose-limiting toxicity was found to be myelosuppression, particularly thrombocytopenia, the severity of which was found to be related to pretreatment renal function.[28] Increased myelosuppression observed with combination chemotherapy containing carboplatin[29] necessitated a method by which its pharmacokinetic profile could be kept constant with repeated administrations.

The renal clearance of carboplatin is closely correlated with the glomerular filtration rate (GFR).[30] This suggests that the area under the concentration versus time curve (AUC) for carboplatin and, consequently, the toxicity and therapeutic efficacy of the drug, is directly related to the pretreatment GFR. Calvert and colleagues showed that the GFR, as measured by the ^{51}Cr-EDTA, can predict the carboplatin AUC, independent of BSA.[31] They derived a dosing formula from a retrospective analysis of carboplatin pharmacokinetics in 18 patients who had pretreatment GFRs in the range of 33–136 ml/min. They redefined the formula following its prospective use in 44 patients as follows:

$$\text{Dose of carboplatin (mg)} = \text{target AUC} \times (\text{GFR} + 25)$$

This formula provides a simple and consistent method of determining carboplatin dose in adults, although inaccuracies occur with low GFRs (<40 ml/min).

Estimation of glomerular filtration rate

The Calvert formula was developed using ^{51}Cr-EDTA clearance as a highly accurate measure of GFR. This technique is expensive and time-consuming (measurement is advised prior to cycles 1, 3 and 5) and some centres have replaced it with creatinine clearance as an estimate of GFR. Creatinine clearance may be measured by a 24-hour urine collection or estimated using one of a number of equations (including the Cockcroft–Gault or Jellife equations below) or nomograms.

The Cockroft and Gault equation

$$\text{GFR (ml/min)} = \frac{F \times (140 - \text{age}) \times \text{IBW (kg)}}{\text{Serum creatinine (}\mu\text{mol/l)}}$$

where $F = 1.04$ (females) and 1.23 (males) and ideal body weight (IBW in kg) = Y + (0.906 to each cm over 152.4 cm). Y = 45.5 (females) and 50 (males).

The Jeliffe equation

$$\text{GFR (ml/min)} = \frac{[98 - (0.8\,(\text{Age} - 20))] \times 0.9}{\text{Serum creatinine (}\mu\text{mol/l)} \times 88.4}$$

Table 40.2   Randomised trials of platinum and paclitaxel chemotherapy

Trial	Treatment arms	Response rate (%)	Median survival (months)
GOG protocol 111[17]	1. cyclophosphamide 750 mg/m² and cisplatin 75 mg/m²	60	24
	2. paclitaxel 135 mg/m² over 24 hours and cisplatin 75 mg/m²	73	38
European–Canadian	1. cyclophosphamide 750 mg/m² and cisplatin 75 mg/m²	66	25
OV protocol 10[18]	2. paclitaxel 175 mg/m² over 3 hours and cisplatin 75 mg/m²	77	35
GOG protocol 132[19]	1. cisplatin 100 mg/m²	67	30.2
	2. paclitaxel 200 mg/m² over 24 hours	43	26
	3. paclitaxel 135 mg/m² over 24 hours and cisplatin 75 mg/m²	67	26.6
ICON3 Study[20]	1. paclitaxel 175 mg/m² over 3 hours and carboplatin (AUC 6)	NE	38.7
	2. cyclophosphamide 500 mg/m², doxorubicin 50 mg/m² and cisplatin 50 mg/m²	NE	36
	3. carboplatin (AUC 6)	NE	36

NE = not evaluated.

More recently, Chatelut and colleagues[32] developed a formula for estimating carboplatin clearance, derived from a non-linear Bayesian estimation of information in a large pharmacokinetic database.

The Chatelut equation

$$GFR = \{[0.134 \times wt] + 218 \times wt \times [1 - (0.00457 \times age)] \times$$
$$[1 - (0.314 \times gender)]\}/\text{Serum creatinine (µmol/l)}$$

where GFR is in ml/min, weight (wt) is in kilograms, age is in years and gender is 0 for males and 1 for females.

It is worthwhile noting that older trials involving carboplatin administered the drug according to body surface area.[33] The optimal dose of platinum compounds has been evaluated in a number of randomised trials.[34] Data from these trials have failed to show any significant difference between double doses of cisplatin and double doses of carboplatin.[35] One study randomised patients to receive six cycles of cyclophosphamide (750 mg/m²) with cisplatin at doses of either 50 mg/m² or 100 mg/m².[36] The survival benefit with the higher dose of cisplatin seen at 2 years[37] was partially lost with time. Furthermore, long-term neurotoxicity and ototoxicity was more frequent in those patients receiving higher doses. A further trial by

Gore and colleagues[38] at the Royal Marsden Hospital randomised patients to treatment with carboplatin at an AUC of 6 or 12 and a Danish trial[39] randomised patients to an AUC of 4 or 8 (plus cyclophosphamide), with neither demonstrating a statistically significant difference in overall survival. (See also Ch. 2.)

Further surgery

Second-look laparotomy is not recommended, as evidence has shown that secondary debulking, following completion of platinum-based chemotherapy, failed to impact on survival.[40] The option of interval debulking surgery (during chemotherapy usually between cycles 3 and 4) in patients with suboptimally debulked disease (>1–2 cm) is increasingly pursued. This has followed the demonstration of a survival advantage in one randomised trial at 2 years in those patients who underwent interval debulking. These results, however, remain the subject of controversy (e.g. intent-to-treat analysis was not performed; only 37 out of 130 patients randomised to surgery were optimally cytoreduced) and further data are required.

Palliative surgery (or radiotherapy), which is designed to alleviate symptoms, has a role, and observational studies support its use in some circumstances such as removal of painful pelvic side wall disease (see Palliation of symptoms section below).

Neoadjuvant chemotherapy

The presence of residual disease after initial surgery is one of the most important adverse prognostic factors for survival.[4] This has led to the evaluation of neoadjuvant (or preoperative) chemotherapy, which has been proposed as an alternative approach to conventional initial surgery. The goal of this is to improve subsequent surgical quality, and patients with stage IV disease and those with a poor performance status are probably the best candidates for this approach. A prospective randomised study of neoadjuvant chemotherapy vs primary cytoreductive surgery is being conducted by the European Organisation for Research and Treatment of Cancer (EORTC).

Chemotherapy for relapsed disease

Patients with relapsed EOC are incurable, and chemotherapy for these women must be viewed as palliative. The toxicity of treatment is therefore a very important consideration. The likelihood of response to second-line treatment is based on a number of factors that have been identified in non-randomised studies and include:

- the length of time between initial treatment to the start of second-line therapy
- previous response
- the bulk of disease
- the number of sites of disease and
- histology.[41]

Three studies have shown that patients who relapse with a disease-free interval of greater than 1 year have a good chance of responding again to platinum-based chemotherapy, whereas patients who relapse soon (6 months to 1 year) after first-line therapy are unlikely to benefit from further platinum.[42–44] Failing one platinum compound usually means resistance to another.[45] (See also Ch. 14.)

Thus, patients who relapse within 1 year are frequently entered into phase II trials. The new compounds that have been studied in this patient population (e.g. topotecan,[46,47] liposomal doxorubicin preparations[48,49] and gemcitabine[50,51]) have all given similar response rates of approximately 20% with durations of response of 6–8 months.[8] Future trials will address the role of these agents with first-line chemotherapy in addition to platinum–paclitaxel regimens. Oral chemotherapy with etoposide (50 or 100 mg twice daily for 7 days of a 28-day cycle) has shown activity in paclitaxel- and platinum-resistant disease,[52] and administration of this drug can occur entirely in the outpatient environment.

Combination chemotherapy for relapsed disease

There are no randomised studies comparing chemotherapy with best supportive care, although the randomised trials performed that compare one treatment vs another provide useful data (Table 40.3).[53,54] For example, a trial comparing topotecan with paclitaxel in relapsed disease demonstrated similar response rates, which were lower than in previous single arm phase II trials.[55]

Some of the highest response rates in relapsed disease can be seen with the combination of epirubicin (50 mg/m^2), cisplatin (75 mg/m^2) and infusional 5-fluorouracil ($200 \text{ mg/m}^2/\text{day}$) administered through a central venous access device (CVAD).[56] One rationale here is that 5-fluorouracil is S-phase specific with a short serum half-life, a continuous infusion therefore allowing maintained plasma levels with prolonged exposure to cancer cells in the sensitive part of their cycle.[57] Two recent large randomised trials have confirmed the benefit of combination platinum-based therapy over single agent carboplatin in patients with potentially chemo-sensitive relapse.[100,101]

Schedule of chemotherapy

There have been four studies that have shown that paclitaxel can be safely given weekly by 1-hour infusion at a dose of $90–100 \text{ mg/m}^2$,[58–61] leading to a recent trial which randomised platinum pretreated patients

Reference	Number of patients	Regimen	Response rate	Overall survival
Cantu et al[54]	97	CAP vs	55%	35 months
		paclitaxel	45%	26 months
Bolis et al[53]	190	Carbo-Epi vs	62%	20 months
		Carbo	56%	16 months

Table 40.3 Combination vs single agent chemotherapy in advanced disease

CAP, cyclophosphamide, doxorubicin and cisplatin; Carbo, carboplatin; Carbo-Epi, carboplatin and epirubicin.

to receive either weekly paclitaxel (67 mg/m² over 3 hours) or 3-weekly paclitaxel (200 mg/m² over 3 hours).[62] There were no significant differences in response rate (35 vs 37%, $p = 0.89$), time to progression (6.1 vs 8.4 months, $p = 0.85$) or overall survival (13.6 months vs 14.7 months, $p = 0.98$). The frequencies of World Health Organisation grade III or IV neutropenia, neuropathy, alopecia and arthralgia/myalgia were, however, decreased in those patients randomised to receive weekly paclitaxel. In addition, there was no difference in the number of hypersensitivity reactions in patients randomised to receive either oral or intravenous steroids intended to prevent hypersensitivity.

Other methods of chemotherapy administration

Intraperitoneal chemotherapy provides an opportunity to increase the concentration of cytotoxic agents in close proximity to scattered tumour deposits throughout the peritoneum. It has the potential to cause a number of problems, including peritonitis, adhesion formation, loculation of fluid and obstruction, and these factors may render this route of administration impractical. Benefits seen in several randomised studies[63–65] suggest that it is reasonable to investigate its use within the context of clinical trials, and future studies are required that compare this route of administration with standard intravenous regimens.

The use of high doses of chemotherapy requiring haematological support in the form of peripheral blood stem cell transplantation or autologous bone marrow transplantation does not have an established role in the treatment of any subset of patients with ovarian cancer. Phase II trials have failed to demonstrate any efficacy for such an approach in patients with bulky or drug-resistant disease.[66]

New therapies

At the present time, patients with relapsed disease should be offered palliative chemotherapy and, where possible, entered into clinical trials, including studies of new platinum analogues designed to overcome known mechanisms of platinum resistance.

For example, BBR3464 is a charged (4+) triplatinum complex that is administered daily for 5 days. It is 40- to 80-fold more potent than cisplatin on a molar dose basis and achieves a high proportion of interstrand and intrastrand DNA adducts (cisplatin produces the latter effect only) that are not recognised by DNA repair proteins (unlike cisplatin-induced adducts). This observation may explain resistance to cisplatin and lack of resistance to BBR3464 in tumours expressing mutations of the p53 oncosuppressor gene.[67] (See also Ch 1.)

Patients who relapse with a disease-free interval of more than 1 year should at some stage receive further platinum-based treatment, either as a single agent or a combination (e.g. epirubicin, cisplatin and 5-fluorouracil). Patients with truly refractory disease should probably not receive more than two lines of chemotherapy, as they are unlikely to benefit from repeated treatments with different drugs.

A difficult management problem is the optimal timing of second- or third-line treatment and whether this should commence at the first sign of relapse (e.g. a rising CA125 with no macroscopic evidence of disease on computed tomography (CT scan)) or whether one should wait for measurable progression without symptoms. Current trials will address this question, although in view of previous data, one should probably treat patients before disease becomes very bulky (3–5 cm).[40] Hormonal therapy, either with tamoxifen (40 mg daily) or medroxyprogesterone acetate (300 mg daily) is often used in this setting and, although objective responses are rare, their appetite-stimulating properties are beneficial to patients with a poor prognosis.

NON-EPITHELIAL OVARIAN TUMOURS

Introduction

Ovarian tumours of non-epithelial origin comprise approximately 25% of malignant ovarian cancers and must be distinguished from those of epithelial origin, as their natural history and management differ. These tumours are rare, and histological review by an expert is essential. The FIGO staging system, as described for EOC, applies for non-epithelial ovarian cancer. Surgery in stage Ia and Ib disease is often curable, although late relapses may occur. Use of combination chemotherapy after initial surgery has improved the prognosis for many of these tumours.[68]

Non-epithelial ovarian tumours may also include lymphomas and metastatic tumours (e.g. breast cancer) and these should be treated the same as when found in other sites. Theca cell, Sertoli–Leydig cell tumours and gynandroblastomas are benign and these will not be discussed further.

Granulosa cell tumours

Granulosa cell tumours are derived from the sex cords of the developing gonad; the mean age at diagnosis is 53 years old, although 5% of cases are diagnosed before puberty. Presentation is commonly as stage I disease and unilateral and, unlike EOC, symptoms due to oestrogen or occasionally androgen secretion lead to early diagnosis. Inhibin, which is secreted by granulosa cells and inhibits follicle-stimulating hormone

(FSH) secretion, is elevated in most patients with active granulosa cell tumour although testing is not widely available. Levels of this hormone can be used to monitor response to treatment and indicate relapsed disease, but it may also be elevated during menstruation, pregnancy and with other tumours[69] (as for the CA125 level in EOC).

The natural history of granulosa cell tumours is of very slow growth, and late recurrence contributes to a steady decline in survival except for those patients who are truly stage IA. Stage II–IV tumours have a 10-year survival of approximately 50% and it is often possible to resect local recurrences and hold chemotherapy in reserve for unresectable disease. A common 3-weekly regimen used is BEP chemotherapy: bleomycin (days 2, 8 and 15: 30 000 IU/m^2; omitted courses 4, 5 and 6); etoposide (100 mg/m^2 days 1–5) and cisplatin (20 mg/m^2 days 1–5). One prospective study has attained a response rate of 83% with this combination; myelotoxicity was tolerable.[70] Granulosa cell tumours tend to be radiosensitive and others may be amenable to hormonal treatment or surgery.

Mixed mesodermal tumours

There is debate as to the sarcomatous or carcinomatous histiogenesis of these tumours and, consequently, whether platinum- or anthracycline-based chemotherapy would be more effective. Mixed mesodermal tumours usually present at a late stage and a reasonable strategy has been to combine platinum (cisplatin 75 mg/m^2 or carboplatin AUC6), paclitaxel (175 mg/m^2 over 3 hours) and doxorubicin (50 mg/m^2) or epirubicin (60 mg/m^2) every 3 weeks with granulocyte colony-stimulating factor (G-CSF; dosed at 5 µg/kg) at the neutrophil nadir, a regimen known as G-CAT.[71] Sequential doublets may be a less toxic way of delivering the three drugs (i.e. cisplatin–doxorubicin followed by cisplatin–paclitaxel) and remains unproven.[102]

Germ cell tumours

These uncommon but aggressive tumours seen often in young women are frequently unilateral. Fertility-sparing surgery should be the first treatment choice, as cures can be attained even in the presence of metastatic disease. Elevated levels of α-fetoprotein (indicates yolk sac elements) and human chorionic gonadotrophin (associated with trophoblastic elements) can help in diagnosis. These markers may also be used to monitor response to surgery or chemotherapy as well as disease recurrence during follow-up (as for CA125 levels in EOC, inhibin in granulosa cell tumours).

Salvage VIP (vincristine, ifosfamide and cisplatin) and paclitaxel-containing regimens can be used in relapsed disease (as they have shown activity against testicular teratomas).[72] Another regimen used is 3-weekly ACE chemotherapy (doxorubicin 40 mg/m^2, cyclophosphamide 600 mg/m^2 and etoposide 100 mg/m^2; all intravenous). This is also used in the treatment of rare primary small cell cancers of the ovary.[73]

CANCER OF THE UTERINE CERVIX

Introduction

Cancer of the uterine cervix affects approximately 3100 women in the United Kingdom each year[2] and is more common in:

- lower socioeconomic groups
- women who have had early first intercourse and
- multiple partners and
- multiple pregnancies
- individuals who smoke
- those who are immunosuppressed (with HIV).

There is a close association between infection with specific subtypes of human papillomavirus (specifically types 16, 18, 31, 33 and 35) and the development of carcinoma in-situ and subsequent cancer. Diagnosis is usually straightforward (as opposed to the diagnosis of EOC), because the cervix can be visually inspected and easily biopsied. Thus, 75% of cervix cancers are diagnosed at early stages when they are potentially curable. International studies have demonstrated a significant reduction in the death rate from cervix cancer since the introduction of the Pap smear (cytological evaluation of cervix cells), which is a sensitive, specific and cost-effective method of screening.[74] Long-term survival rates are 76% for stage I (confined to the cervix), 55% for stage II (local spread to adnexae or upper vagina), 31% for stage III (spread to pelvic side walls or lower vagina) and 7% for stage IV (distant spread). As for ovarian cancer, a chest radiograph should be obtained to exclude pulmonary involvement.

Treatment of cancer of the cervix

Early-stage cervical cancer (stage I or II) can be treated with radical hysterectomy, yielding equivalent results to pelvic radiation, which has been the standard, definitive therapy. The radiotherapy dose given is 45–50 Gy to the pelvis + an additional intracavitary boost. Phase I and II studies have established that platinum-based chemotherapy can be safely combined with pelvic irradiation. This combination of treatment modalities has a number of theoretical advantages, including platinum-induced sensitisation of tumour cells to the effects of radiotherapy. The complete response rate expected with use of radiotherapy alone is generally high, depending on stage of disease, and therefore any incremental benefit from added chemotherapy has required assessment in phase III trials. The results of five randomised trials evaluating this strategy in over 1500 women have demonstrated that the risk of death is decreased by 30–50% by concurrent cisplatin-based therapy (usually 40 mg/m^2 weekly) given concurrently with radiation therapy (Table 40.4).

The success of this strategy has been seen with squamous cell cancers of the head and neck. Available data do not allow conclusions to be drawn as to which drugs or regimens are optimal in the treatment of cervical cancer and it is unclear whether surgery should precede chemoradiation, follow it, or whether it is necessary at all. (See Ch. 42 for discussion of chemoradiation.)

No trials of neoadjuvant or adjuvant chemotherapy have been large enough to detect a 10% difference in overall survival. Current data suggest that the effect of neoadjuvant or adjuvant chemotherapy may range from a small benefit, to a small decrement in survival. The trials performed illustrate the importance of using chemotherapy regimens with manageable toxicity.[80] The treatment of women with recurrent disease remains difficult and, despite the reasonable response rates observed, the role of chemotherapy still needs to be defined. Phase II studies of 3-weekly cisplatin and infusional 5-fluorouracil (metastatic squamous cervical cancer) and epirubicin, cisplatin and infusional 5-fluorouracil (metastatic adenocarcinoma of the cervix) are currently accruing patients with disseminated disease.

ENDOMETRIAL CANCER

Introduction

Cancer of the endometrium affects approximately 4500 women in the United Kingdom per year[2] and is highly curable as it tends to present with bleeding at an early stage. Aetiological factors include prolonged, uninterrupted stimulation of the endometrium with oestrogen (and its analogues) or familial cancer syndromes, notably hereditary non-polyposis colorectal cancer (HNPCC). Associations include obesity and diabetes and the majority of endometrial tumours are adenocarcinomas. (See also Ch. 39.)

Treatment for endometrial cancer

For patients with low-risk disease (stage I or II confined to the endometrium), treatment consists of a total abdominal hysterectomy + surgical staging. Those with intermediate-risk disease (stage I grade 3; stage II – cervix involvement; stage IIIA – serosal invasion or positive peritoneal cytology) are treated with surgical resection of all gross disease followed by pelvic and/or vaginal irradiation. High-risk disease (stage IIIB – vaginal metastases; IIIC – positive nodes; IVA – bladder or rectal involvement) are treated with surgery and radiotherapy. The radiotherapy dose is usually 45 Gy to the pelvis post-surgery (an intracavitary boost is added when surgery has not been performed). The role of chemotherapy for high-risk disease is currently being investigated in randomised trials. Patients with advanced, recurrent or disseminated disease should receive systemic therapy. In patients with disease no longer amenable to surgery and radiotherapy, hormonal therapy with progestins (medroxyprogesterone acetate 300–400 mg daily) yields response rates of 40%, progression-free survivals of 9 months and overall survivals of 14 months in patients whose tumours are oestrogen- and progesterone-receptor positive.[81] Higher dose schedules have not yielded better results, although tamoxifen (20 mg daily) gives a response rate of 20% in those who do not respond to standard progesterone therapy. Response rates in patients with hormone-receptor negative tumours are significantly lower and chemotherapy is often considered as initial therapy.

As for EOC, active cytotoxic agents identified in phase II studies include platinum compounds, taxanes,

Table 40.4 Randomised trials of concurrent chemotherapy and radiotherapy (RT)

Study	FIGO stage	Control group	Comparison group	Relative risk of death in comparison group
Keys et al[75]	IB	RT	RT + weekly cisplatin	0.54
Rose et al[76]	IIB–IVA	RT plus hydroxyurea	RT + cisplatin *or*	0.61
			RT + cisplatin + 5-fluorouracil + hydroxyurea	0.58
Morris et al[77]	IB–IVA	Extended field RT	RT + cisplatin + 5-fluorouracil	0.52
Whitney et al[78]	IIB–IVA	RT + hydroxyurea	RT + cisplatin + 5-fluorouracil	0.72
Peters et al[79]	IB or IIA	RT	RT + cisplatin + 5-fluorouracil	0.5

etoposide, topotecan and doxorubicin or epirubicin, and response rates of approximately 20% are observed. One study has shown no advantage for doxorubicin–paclitaxel as compared with doxorubicin–cisplatin,[82] and randomised trials are underway. The most commonly used off-trial regimen is cisplatin–doxorubicin (both 50 mg/m²), which is given 3-weekly, and patients with a poor performance status are considered for single agent carboplatin (AUC 6; 4-weekly).

PALLIATION OF SYMPTOMS

The main symptoms suffered by patients with gynaecological cancers are recurrent ascites and abdominal pain, often associated with intestinal obstruction. Other common problems include fistula formation, malodorous discharge, thromboembolic events and deterioration in renal function. Patients who respond to chemotherapy or radiotherapy are likely to have these symptoms palliated, and therefore the decision to use these treatments to palliate these symptoms is based on the likelihood of a response. In general, chemotherapy does not palliate patients with intestinal obstruction and is used infrequently, except when there is intestinal obstruction at presentation of EOC and patients are chemonaive. An extensive systematic review of the literature on the palliation of intestinal obstruction in patients with advanced gynaecological and intestinal malignancy examined the use of corticosteroids, antiemetics, analgesics, somatostatin, surgery, gastrostomy tubes, chemotherapy, radiotherapy and total parenteral nutrition.[83] The evidence base for these interventions was poor in terms of prospective randomised clinical trials, although many uncontrolled retrospective series have examined the use of all these modalities in the management of intestinal obstruction. There are two randomised trials of the use of corticosteroids in bowel obstruction due to gynaecological and gastro-intestinal malignancy and although there is a suggestion that patients treated with steroids benefited, the number of patients involved is too small to make any firm conclusions.[84,85] In patients being actively considered for surgical intervention as part of multimodality care, steroids should not be given. (See also Chs 7 and 14.)

CONCLUSIONS

Future and currently accruing randomised studies will help address many unanswered questions, including the role of new chemotherapeutic agents. Strategies involving the eradication of minimal residual disease following first-line therapy for epithelial ovarian cancer or for the consolidation and maintenance of complete remission need to be pursued. Communication between laboratory scientists and clinicians will help ensure that advances in molecular understanding (e.g. mechanisms of drug resistance) are translated into useful therapies. A further challenge is to ensure that all patients are treated under the auspices of multidisciplinary care teams.

NURSING CARE FOR PATIENTS RECEIVING CHEMOTHERAPY FOR GYNAECOLOGICAL CANCERS

Karen Handscomb

INTRODUCTION

The complexity of multimodality treatment for gynaecological cancers brings about increasing challenges for the multiprofessional team. The nurses' expertise is pivotal in ensuring women and their carer's perspective is central to all discussion and in addressing the complex implications of treatment.

ASSESSING WOMEN

When a woman first presents with gynaecological cancer, the determinant of her nursing management may not be the diagnostic evaluation but whether she has had, or has hopes to have, a family.

For those women who have not yet thought about having a family, there is a limited amount of time to consider techniques that may preserve fertility,[86] if appropriate. This needs careful discussion and consideration and, whatever the outcome, there is an associated sense of loss and anger that needs to be carefully addressed over time. (See Ch. 32.)

THE IMPACT OF CHEMOTHERAPY

For many women, treatment on the female reproductive organs is viewed as an assault on their sense of self. This is reinforced by a sometimes premature menopause,[87] an often diminished sexual function[88] and the change in ability of the woman to continue in her roles both inside and outside the family unit.[89] This may be for a variety of reasons, such as:

- daily hospital visits, especially for women having chemoradiotherapy (where often there is overwhelming side effects of treatment).

- the fact that she may have just had major surgery or be undergoing interval debulking as part of her treatment plan:

- Interval, or intervention, debulking surgery is the term used for a planned procedure performed in advanced ovarian cancer, where primary surgery is incomplete and has been followed by several courses of chemotherapy. Following surgery, chemotherapy is continued.[90]

- the disease itself.

THE ROLE OF THE NURSE

Practical help

In helping the women and her carer's plan for treatment and the changes it brings, the nurse may enable her to carry on with 'normal life' as far as possible. This may mean looking at practical help, financial support and a careful explanation of what they may be able to expect. Themed counselling based on information and education about cancer and providing positive health strategies has been found to be more beneficial by women than supportive care alone.[91]

Male partners

Often for male partners it will be the first time they have had to take on the caring role in what men themselves have called a 'crisis situation,'[92] and this should be addressed by acknowledging their particular needs.

Patient advocacy

The role of the nurse as patient advocate in the decision-making process is vital. A sound knowledge of the side effects of treatment and the potential benefits of treatment are paramount to effectively support women and their carers and to facilitate collaboration, participation and empowerment.[93] This is important in both the initial decision to have treatment, and in decisions that may have to be made along the way such as equating potential long-term benefits with seemingly insurmountable side effects, particularly for those women who know there can be no cure.

Information–giving

A study by Elit et al[94] in women with gynaecological cancer showed that providing information and encouraging participation improved mood and patient satisfaction. It should be remembered that many women are unaware of their reproductive anatomy (Fig. 40.1).

Sometimes the nurse is able to reassure women that the treatment they will be having will be able to take away the symptoms of a tumour in the pelvis that may have been plaguing their lives for months, and sometimes years. These debilitating symptoms will vary according to the site of gynaecological cancer, but can include those given in Box. 40.1.

Relief, potentially, happens very quickly once treatment has started, but skilled management of these symptoms is vital until this time.

PLANNING FOR DISCHARGE

The safe administration of chemotherapy within a controlled hospital environment is often the least difficult part of having chemotherapy for the woman. It is when women get home that the side effects begin and the uncertainty sets in. The method, and complexity of administration of chemotherapy, can often complicate this, as well as being administered by conventional intravenous and oral methods:

- occasionally, intraperitoneal chemotherapy is given for ovarian cancer
- topical chemotherapy may be given for cancer of the vulva
- alongside radiotherapy and surgery.

It is important that women and their carers are able to maintain contact with the team. Wherever possible, a flexibility of roles, such as that of the Gynaecological Oncology Clinical Nurse Specialist, allows for proactive supportive care across operational boundaries and the flagging up of potentially life-threatening side effects such as neutropenia. This will go hand in hand with ensuring, whenever appropriate, that a relationship is established early on with the local community teams and contact made with support organisations such as Ovacome (ovarian cancer) and Jo's Trust (cervical cancer).

COPING WITH THE LONG–TERM CONSEQUENCES OF TREATMENT

Women are left with changes due to the chemotherapy long after treatment. Stacey[97] eloquently talks about the bodily impression that chemotherapy has left her with and how 'music listened to during chemotherapy became unbearable and favourite food from that time inedible'.

Clearly, nursing care should not finish when treatment has finished – often, it is then that problems come to the fore.[98] These problems may include relationship difficulties, a change in sexual activity and

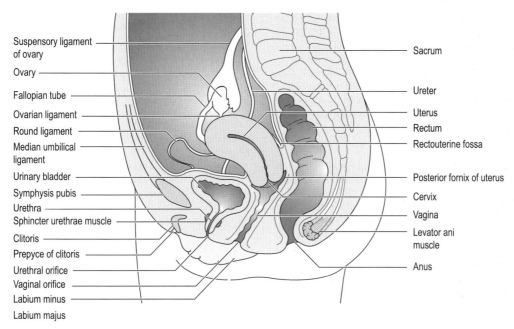

Suspensory ligament of ovary

Ovary

Fallopian tube

Ovarian ligament

Round ligament

Median umbilical ligament

Urinary bladder

Symphysis pubis

Urethra

Sphincter urethrae muscle

Clitoris

Prepyce of clitoris

Urethral orifice

Vaginal orifice

Labium minus

Labium majus

Sacrum

Ureter

Uterus

Rectum

Rectouterine fossa

Posterior fornix of uterus

Cervix

Vagina

Levator ani muscle

Anus

Figure 40.1   The female reproductive system.[95]

Box 40.1   Presenting symptoms of gynaecological cancers

Cancer of the cervix
  Abnormal vaginal bleeding
  Offensive vaginal discharge
  Lower back pain

Cancers of the ovary and fallopian tubes
  Malignant ascites[96] and 'tight band' just under their breasts
  Early saiety and indigestion
  Vague abdominal symptoms

Cancer of the vulva and vagina
  History of vulval irritation and soreness
  Vaginal discharge

Cancer of the uterus
  Abnormal vaginal bleeding

coping with infertility. Women feel reassured by long-term follow-up, as many view remission merely as another stage of illness.[99] The Gynaecological Oncology Clinical Nurse Specialist can play a vital role at this time by providing expertise, continuity and a contact point for the multiprofessional team.

References

1. Junor EJ, Hole DJ, Gillis CR. Management of ovarian cancer: referral to a multidisciplinary team matters. Br J Cancer 1994; 70:363–370.

2. CRC. Cancer Research Campaign. Cancer stats: 2001 http://www. crc. org. uk

3. Jacobs I. Overview – progress in screening for ovarian cancer. In: Sharp F, Blackett T, Berek J, et al, eds. Ovarian cancer 5. Oxford: Isis Medical Media; 1998:199–216.

4. Friedlander M. Prognostic factors. In: Sharp F, Blackett T, Berek J, et al, eds. Ovarian cancer 5. Oxford: Isis Medical Media; 1998:199–216.

5. Pettersson F. Annual report of the results of treatment in gynaecologic cancer. International Federation of Gynaecology and Obstetrics (FIGO), Vol. 20, 1988.

6. Neijt JP, ten Bokkel Huinink W, van der Burg ME, et al. Long-term survival in ovarian cancer. Mature data from the Netherlands Joint Study Group for Ovarian Cancer. Eur J Cancer 1991; 27:1367–1372.

7. Vergote IB, Trimbos BJ, Guthrie D, et al. Results of a randomized trial in 923 patients with high-risk early ovarian cancer, comparing adjuvant chemotherapy with no further treatment following surgery. Proc Am Soc Clin Oncol 2001; 20:201a.

8. Ahmed FY, Wiltshaw E, A'Hern RP, et al. Natural history and prognosis of untreated stage I epithelial ovarian cancer. J Clin Oncol 1996; 14:2968–2975.

9. Gore M. The evidence base for medical intervention in ovarian cancer. In: MacLean AB, Gore M, Miles A, eds. The effective management of ovarian cancer. London: Aesculapius Medical Press; 1999:76–89.

10. Harries M, Gore M. Part I: chemotherapy for epithelial ovarian cancer – treatment at first diagnosis. Lancet Oncol 2002; 3(9):529–536.

11. Taylor AE, Wiltshaw E, Gore ME, et al. Long-term follow-up of the first randomized study of cisplatin versus carboplatin for advanced epithelial ovarian cancer. J Clin Oncol 1994; 12(10):2066–2070.

12. Advanced Ovarian Cancer Trialists Group. Chemotherapy in advanced ovarian cancer: an overview of randomised clinical trials. BMJ 1991; 303:884–893.

13. Kohn EC, Sarosy G, Bicher A, et al. Dose-intense Taxol: high response rates in patients with platinum resistant recurrent ovarian cancer. J Natl Cancer Inst 1994; 86:18–24.

14. Eisenhauer EA, ten Bokkel Huinink WW, Swenerton KD, et al. European–Canadian randomised trial of paclitaxel in relapsed ovarian cancer: high-dose versus low-dose and long versus short infusion. J Clin Oncol 1994; 12:2654–2666.

15. Omura GA, Brady MF, Delmore JE, et al. A randomised trial of paclitaxel (T) at two dose levels and filgastrim (G) at 2 doses in platinum pre-treated epithelial ovarian cancer (OVCA). Proc Am Soc Clin Oncol 1996;(15):280A.

16. Du Bois A, Neijt JP, Thigpen JT. First line chemotherapy with carboplatin plus paclitaxel in advanced ovarian cancer – a new standard of care. Ann Oncol 1999; 10(suppl 1):35–41.

17. McGuire WP, Hoskins WJ, Brady MF, et al. Cyclophosphamide and cisplatin compared with paclitaxel and cisplatin in patients with stage III and IV ovarian cancer. N Engl J Med 1996; 334:1–6.

18. Stuart G, Bertelsen K, Mangioni C, et al. Updated analysis shows a highly significant improved overall survival (OS) for cisplatin-paclitaxel as first line treatment of advanced ovarian cancer: mature results of the EORTC-GCCG, NOCOVA, NCIC CTG and Scottish Intergroup Trial. Proc Am Soc Clin Oncol 1998; 17:361a.

19. Muggia FM, Braly PS, Brady MR, et al. Phase III trial of cisplatin or paclitaxel, versus paclitaxel versus cisplatin and paclitaxel in patients with suboptimal stage III or IV ovarian cancer. J Clin Oncol 2000; 18:106–115.

20. Columbo N. Randomised trial of paclitaxel and carboplatin versus a control arm of carboplatin or CAP (cyclophosphamide, doxorubicin & cisplatin): the Third International Collaborative Ovarian Neoplasm Study. Proc Am Soc Clin Oncol 2000; 19:379a.

21. Stebbing J, Gore M. The dosing and schedule of cytotoxics in ovarian cancer. CME J Gynecol 2000; 3:362–364.

22. Aabo K, Adams M, Adnitt P, et al. Chemotherapy in advanced ovarian cancer: four systematic meta-analyses of individual patient data from 37 randomised trials. Br J Cancer 1998; 78:1479–1487.

23. Go RS, Adjei AA. Review of the comparative pharmacology and clinical activity of cisplatin and carboplatin. J Clin Oncol 1999; 17:409–422.

24. Neijt JP, Engelholm SA, Malgorzata E, et al. Exploratory phase III study of paclitaxel and cisplatin versus paclitaxel and carboplatin in advanced ovarian cancer. J Clin Oncol 2000; 18:3084–3092.

25. Mainwaring PN, Gore ME. The importance of dose and schedule in cancer chemotherapy: epithelial ovarian cancer. Anticancer Drugs 1995; 6(suppl 5):29–41.

26. Harrap KR. Preclinical studies identifying carboplatin as a viable cisplatin alternative. Cancer Treat Rev 1985; 12:21–33.

27. Canetta R, Rozencweig M, Carter SK. Carboplatin: the clinical spectrum to date. Cancer Treat Rev 1985; 12:125–136.

28. Calvert AH, Harland SJ, Newell DR, et al. Early clinical studies with cis-diammine-1,1-cyclobutane dicarboxylate platinum II. Cancer Chemother Pharmacol 1982;9:140–147.

29. Shibata K, Nakatsumi Y, Kasahara K, et al. Analysis of thrombocytopenia due to carboplatin combined etoposide in elderly patients with lung cancer. J Cancer Res Clin Oncol 1996; 122:437–442.

30. Harland SJ, Newell DR, Sidduck ZH, et al. Pharmacokinetics of cis-diammine-1,1-cyclobutane dicarboxylate platinum II in patients with normal and impaired renal function. Cancer Res 1984; 44:1693–1697.

31. Calvert AH, Newell DR, Gumbrell LA, et al. Carboplatin dosage: prospective evaluation of a simple formula based on renal function. J Clin Oncol 1989; 7:1748–1756.

32. Chatelut E, Canal P, Brunner V, et al. Prediction of carboplatin clearance from standard morphological and biological patient characteristics. J Natl Cancer Inst 1995; 87(8):573–580.

33. Vaughan M, Sapunar F, Gore M. Clinical experience – platinum and taxanes. In: Kelland LR and Farrell N, eds. Platinum-based drugs in cancer therapy. Totowa, New Jersey: Humana Press; 2000:195–231.

34. McGuire WP, Ozols RF. Chemotherapy of advanced ovarian cancer. Semin Oncol 1998; 25:340–348.

35. Thigpen JT. Dose intensity in ovarian carcinoma: hold, enough? J Clin Oncol 1997; 15:1291–1293.

36. Kaye SB, Paul J, Cassidy J, et al. Mature results of a randomised trial of two doses of cisplatin for the treatment of ovarian cancer. J Clin Oncol 1996; 14:2113–2119.

37. Kaye SB, Lewis CR, Paul J, et al. Randomised study of two doses of cisplatin with cyclophosphamide in epithelial ovarian cancer. Lancet 1992; 340:329–333.

38. Gore M, Mainwaring P, A'Hern R, et al. Randomised trial of dose intensity with single agent carboplatin in patients with epithelial ovarian cancer. J Clin Oncol 1998; 16:2426–2434.

39. Jakobsen A, Bertelsen K, Andersen JE, et al. Dose–effect study of carboplatin in ovarian cancer: a Danish Ovarian Cancer Group Study. J Clin Oncol 1997; 15:193–198.

40. Poole CH, Raghunadharao D. Monitoring and follow-up of patients treated with chemotherapy for epithelial ovarian cancer. In: MacLean AB, Gore M, Miles A, eds. The effective management of ovarian cancer. London: Aesculapius Medical Press; 1999:30–47.

41. Eisenhauer EA, Vermorken JB, van Glabbeke M. Predictors of response to subsequent chemotherapy in platinum-pretreated ovarian cancer. Ann Oncol 1997; 8:963–968.

42. Blackledge G, Lawton F, Redman C, et al. Response of patients in phase II studies of chemotherapy in ovarian cancer: implications for patient treatment and design of phase II trials. Br J Cancer 1989; 59:650–653.

43. Gore ME, Fryatt I, Wiltshaw E, et al. Treatment of relapsed ovarian cancer with cisplatin or carboplatin following treatment with these compounds. Gynecol Oncol 1990; 36:207–211.

44. Markham M, Rothman R, Hawkes T, et al. Second-line platinum therapy in patients with ovarian cancer previously treated with cisplatin. J Clin Oncol 1991; 9:389–393.

45. Taylor AE, Wiltshaw E, Gore ME, et al. Long-term follow up of the first randomised study of cisplatin versus carboplatin for advanced epithelial ovarian cancer. J Clin Oncol 1994; 12:2066–2070.

46. Hoskins P, Eisenhauer E, Fisher B, et al. Sequential couplets of cisplatin/topotecan and cisplatin/paclitaxel as first-line therapy for advanced epithelial ovarian cancer. An NCIC Clinical Trials Group Phase II Study. Proc Am Soc Clin Oncol 1999; 18:357a.

47. Blessing JA, Bookman MA, Lentz SS, et al. Topotecan has substantial antitumor activity as first-line salvage therapy in platinum-sensitive epithelial ovarian carcinoma: a gynecologic oncology group study. J Clin Oncol 2000; 18:1062–1068.

48. Gibbs D, Pyle L, Allen M, et al. A phase I dose finding study of carboplatin (C), paclitaxel (P) and liposomal doxorubicin (LD) in advanced epithelial ovarian carcinoma (EOC). Proc Am Soc Clin Oncol 2000; 19:389a.

49. Israel VP, Garcia AA, Roman L, et al. Phase II study of liposomal doxorubicin in advanced gynecologic cancers. Gynecol Oncol 2000; 78:143–147.

50. Hansen SW, Anderson H, Boman K, et al. Gemcitabine, carboplatin, and paclitaxel as first-line treatment of ovarian cancer FIGO stages IIB-IV. Proc Am Soc Clin Oncol 1999; 18:357a.

51. Silver DF, Piver MS. Gemcitabine salvage chemotherapy for patients with gynecologic malignancies of the ovary, fallopian tube, and peritoneum. Am J Clin Oncol 1999; 22:450–452.

52. Rose PG, Blessing JA, Mayer AR. Prolonged oral etoposide as second-line therapy for platinum-resistant and platinum-sensitive ovarian carcinoma: a Gynecologic Oncology Group study. J Clin Oncol. 1998; 16:405–410.

53. Bolis G, Scarfone G, Villa A, et al. A randomised study in recurrent ovarian cancer comparing the efficacy of single agent versus combination chemotherapy, according to time to relapse. Proc Am Soc Clin Oncol 1996; 15:750.

54. Cantu MG, Buda A, Parma G, et al. Randomized controlled trial of single-agent paclitaxel versus cyclophosphamide, doxorubicin, and cisplatin in patients with recurrent ovarian cancer who responded to first-line platinum-based regimens. J Clin Oncol 2002; 20:1232–1237.

55. ten Bokkel Huinink W, Gore M, Carmichael J, et al. Topotecan versus paclitaxel for the treatment of recurrent epithelial ovarian cancer. J Clin Oncol 1997; 15:2183–2193.

56. Webb A, A'Hern R, Everard M, et al. High activity of epirubicin, cisplatin, protracted venous infusional (PVI) 5-fluorouracil (ECF) after platinum and taxanes in relapsed epithelial ovarian cancer (EOC). Proc Am Soc Clin Oncol 2000; 19:1566.

57. Lokich J. Phase I study of peripheral venous infusional 5-fluorouracil. Cancer 1981; 48:2565–2568.

58. Loeffler TM, Freund W, Lipke J, et al. Schedule and dose intensified paclitaxel as weekly one hour infusion. Evidence for improved toxicity profile and response activity in pretreated solid tumours. Proc Am Soc Clin Oncol 1995; 14:470.

59. Alvarez A, Mickiewicz E, Piris N, et al. Weekly taxol high dose intensity treatment phase II study, Proc Am Soc Clin Oncol 1996; 15:183.

60. Fennely D, Aghajanian C, Shapiro F, et al. Phase I and pharmacologic study of paclitaxel administered weekly in patients with relapsed ovarian cancer. J Clin Oncol 1997; 15:187–192.

61. Klaasen U, Wilke H, Strumberg D, et al. Phase I study with a weekly 1 hour infusion of paclitaxel in heavily pretreated patients with metastatic breast and ovarian cancer. Eur J Cancer 1996; 32A:547–549.

62. Andersson H, Boman K, Ridederheim M, et al. An updated analysis of a randomised study of single agent paclitaxel (p) given weekly vs 3 weekly to patients with ovarian cancer treated with prior platinum therapy. Proc Am Soc Clin Oncol 2000; 19:380a.

63. Alberts DS, Liu PY, Hannigan EV, et al. Intraperitoneal cisplatin plus intravenous cyclophosphamide versus intravenous cisplatin plus intravenous cyclophosphamide for stage III ovarian cancer. N Engl J Med 1996; 335:1950–1955.

64. Markman M, Bundy BN, Alberts DS, et al. Phase III trial of standard-dose intravenous cisplatin plus paclitaxel versus moderately high-dose carboplatin followed by intravenous paclitaxel and intraperitoneal cisplatin in small-volume stage III ovarian carcinoma: an intergroup study of the Gynecologic Oncology Group, Southwestern Oncology Group, and Eastern Cooperative Oncology Group. J Clin Oncol 2001; 19:1001–1007.

65. Armstrong DK, Bundy BN, Beargen R, et al. Randomized phase III study of intravenous (IV) paclitaxel and cisplatin versus IV paclitaxel, intraperitoneal (IP) cisplatin and IP paclitaxel in optimal stage III epithelial ovarian cancer (OC): a Gynaecologic Oncology Group trial (GOG 172). Pro Am Soc Clin Oncol 2002; 21:201a.

66. Stiff PJ, Bayer R, Kerger C, et al. High dose chemotherapy with autologous transplantation for persistent/relapsed ovarian cancer. A multivariate analysis of survival for 100 consecutively treated patients. J Clin Oncol 1997; 15:1309–1317.

67. Sessa C, Capri G, Gianni L, et al. Clinical and pharmacological phase I study with accelerated titration design of a daily times five schedule of BBR 3464, a novel cationic triplatinum complex. Ann Oncol 2000; 11:977–985.

68. Gershenson DM. Update on malignant ovarian germ cell tumours. Cancer 1993; 71(suppl 4):1581–1590.

69. Bridgewater JA, Rustin GJS. Management of non-epithelial ovarian tumours. Oncology 1999; 57:89–98.

70. Columbo N, Parma G, Franchi D. An active chemotherapy regimen for advanced ovarian sex cord-stromal tumours. Gynecol Oncol 1999; 72:129–130.

71. Gregory RK, Hill ME, Moore J, et al. Combining platinum, paclitaxel and anthracycline in patients with advanced gynaecological malignancy. Eur J Cancer 2000; 36:502–507.

72. Bower M, Fife K, Holden L, et al. Cisplatin-based chemotherapy for ovarian germ cell tumours. Eur J Cancer 1996; 32A:593–597.

73. Tewari K, Brewer C, Cappuccini F, et al. Advanced-stage small cell carcinoma of the ovary in pregnancy: long-term survival after surgical debulking and multi-agent chemotherapy. Gynecol Oncol 1997; 66:531–534.

74. National Cancer Institute Workshop. The 1988 Bethesda system for reporting cervical/vaginal cytological diagnoses. JAMA 1989; 262:931–934.

75. Keys HM, Bundy BN, Stehman FB, et al. Cisplatin, radiation, and adjuvant hysterectomy compared with radiation and adjuvant hysterectomy for bulky stage IB cervical carcinoma. N Engl J Med 1999; 340:1154–1161.

76. Rose PG, Bundy BN, Watkins EB, et al. Concurrent cisplatin-based radiotherapy and chemotherapy for locally advanced cervical cancer. N Engl J Med 1999; 340:1144–1153.

77. Morris M, Eifel PJ, Lu J, et al. Pelvic radiation with concurrent chemotherapy compared with pelvic and para-aortic radiation for high-risk cervical cancer. N Engl J Med 1999; 340:1137–1143.

78. Whitney CW, Sause W, Bundy BN, et al. A randomised comparison of fluorouracil plus cisplatin versus hydroxyurea as an adjunct to radiation therapy in stages IIB–IVA carcinoma of the cervix with negative para-aortic nodes. J Clin Oncol 1999; 17:1339–1348.

79. Peters WA, Liu PY, Barrett R, et al. Cisplatin, 5-fluorouracil plus radiation are superior to radiation therapy as adjunctive high-risk early-stage carcinoma of the cervix after radical hysterectomy and lymphadenectomy. Presented at 30th meeting of Society for Gynecologic Oncologists, San Francisco; 1999.

80. Gibbs DD, Blake PR, Gore ME. Cytotoxic chemotherapy in the treatment of carcinoma of the uterine cervix. Curr Obst Gynecol 1999; 9:130–136.

81. Lentz SS. Advanced and recurrent endometrial carcinoma: hormonal therapy. Sem Oncol 1994; 21:100–106.

82. Di Paola GR, Sardi J. Treatment of endometrial cancer. In: International Gynecologic Oncology Society Book. Bologna: International Proceedings Division; 2000:8–9.

83. Feuer DJ, Broadley KE, Tate AT. Systematic review of the management of intestinal obstruction due to advanced gynaecologic and intestinal cancer. NHS executive research and development project NCP 2/1211, 1998.

84. Hardy JR. Leading article: medical management of bowel. Br J Surg 2000; 87:1281–1283.

85. Laval G, Girardier J, Lassauniere JM, et al. The use of steroids in the management of inoperable intestinal obstruction in terminal cancer patients: do they remove the obstruction? Palliat Med 2000; 14:3–10.

86. Schilsku RL, Lewis BJ, Sherings RJ, et al. Gonadal dysfunction in patients receiving chemotherapy for cancer. Ann Intern Med 1980; 93(1):109–114.

87. Wren BG. Hormonal therapy following female genital tract cancer. Int J Gynaecol Cancer 1994; 4:217–224.

88. Crowther ME, Corney RH, Shepherd JH. Psychosexual implications of gynaecological cancer. British Medical Journal 1994; 308:869–870.

89. Auchincloss SS. Psychosocial issues in gynecologic cancer survivorship. Cancer 1995; 76(10):2117–2124.

90. Blake P, Lambert H, Crawford R. Gynaecological oncology: a guide to clinical management. Oxford: Oxford Medical Publications; 1998.

91. Cain EN, Kohorn EI, Quinlan DM, et al. Psychological benefits of a cancer support group. Cancer 1986; 57:183–189.

92. Carlsson ME, Strang PM. Educational group support for patients with gynaecological cancer and their families. Supp Care Cancer 1996; 4:102–109.

93. Corner J. Inaugural lecture: nursing and the counter culture for cancer. Eur J Cancer Care 1997; 6(3):174–181.

94. Elit LM, Levine MN, Gafni A. A patient's preferences for therapy in advanced epithelial ovarian cancer: development, testing and application of a bedside decision instrument. Gynecol Oncol 1996; 62:329–335.

95. www.gynaesurgeon.co.uk

96. Preston N. New strategies for the management of malignant ascites. Eur J Cancer Care 1995; 4:178–183.

97. Stacey J. Teratologies: a cultural study of cancer. London: Routledge; 1997.

98. Anderson BL, van der Does J. Surviving gynecological cancer and coping with sexual morbidity: an international problem. Int J Gynecol Cancer 1994; 4:225–240.

99. Bradley EJ, Potts MK, Redman CWE, et al. The experience of long-term hospital follow-up for women who have suffered early stage gynecological cancer: a qualitative interview study. Int J Gynecol Cancer 1999; 9:491–496.

100. Parmar MK, Ledermann JA, Colombo N, et al. Paclitaxel plus platinum-based chemotherapy versus conventional platinum-based chemotherapy in women with relapsed ovarian cancer. Lancet 2003; 361(9375): 2099–2106.

101. Pfisterer J, Plante M, Vergote I, et al. Gemcitabine/carboplatin (GC) vs carboplatin (C) in platinum sensitive recurrent ovarian cancer (OVCA). Results of a Gynecologic Cancer Intergroup randomised phase III trial of the AGO OVAR, the NCIC CTG and the EORTC GCG. Proc Am Soc Clin Oncol 2004; 23: Abs 5005.

102. Hess V, A'Hern R, Nasiri N, et al. Mucinous epithelial ovarian cancer: a separate entity requiring specific treatment. J Clin Oncol 2004; 22(6):1040–1044.

Chapter **41**

Urological cancers

CHAPTER CONTENTS

MEDICAL CARE FOR PATIENTS WITH BLADDER CANCER

Robert Huddart and Rahul Mukherjee

GENERAL INFORMATION

Bladder cancer represents 7.9% of all new cancer cases in men and 3.2% in women. It accounts for 4.4% of cancer deaths in men and 2.4% in women. Incidence varies from country to country, with rates being higher in Western Europe and North America.

The main aetiological factors in bladder cancer are chemical carcinogens. Increased mortality rates are seen in workers in the dye and rubber industries (10–50-fold risk increase).[1] The two chemicals felt most likely to be responsible are 2-naphthylamine and benzidine.[2] Cigarette smoking is associated with a 2–3-fold increase in the risk of bladder cancer.[3] Drugs such as phenacitin[4] and cyclophosphamide[5] and its metabolites are also bladder carcinogens. Exposure to ionising radiation increases the risk of bladder cancer, with a latent period of around 20 years.[6] Chronic irritation of the bladder increases the risk of cancer, and is associated with chronic or recurrent infection, bladder calculi, indwelling catheters and anatomical variations and abnormalities.[7] Chronic infection by *Schistosoma haematobium*, endemic in some developing countries is responsible for increased rates of squamous cell cancer (SCC) of the bladder.[8] There may be a small increased risk in relatives of patients with a family history of bladder cancer.[9]

The most common pathology of bladder cancer is transitional cell carcinoma (90%), followed by squamous cell carcinoma (5%). Other histological types include adenocarcinoma, small cell carcinoma, sarcoma, lymphoma and melanoma.

STAGING INFORMATION

The clinical staging of carcinoma of the bladder is determined by the depth of invasion of the bladder wall by the tumor. This determination requires a cystoscopic examination that includes a biopsy, and examination under anesthesia to assess the size and mobility of palpable masses, the degree of induration of the bladder wall and the presence of extravesical extension or invasion of adjacent organs. Clinical staging, even when computed tomographic (CT) and/or magnetic resonance imaging (MRI) scans and other imaging modalities are used, often underestimates the extent of tumour, particularly in cancers that are less differentiated and more deeply invasive.

The American Joint Committee on Cancer (AJCC) has designated staging by TNM classification to define bladder cancer.

TNM definitions

Primary tumour (T)
The suffix 'm' should be added to the appropriate T category to indicate multiple lesions. The suffix 'is' may be added to any T to indicate the presence of associated carcinoma in situ.

TX	primary tumour cannot be assessed
T0	no evidence of primary tumour
Ta	noninvasive papillary carcinoma
Tis	carcinoma in situ: 'flat tumour'
T1	tumour invades subepithelial connective tissue
T2	tumour invades muscle
T2a	tumour invades superficial muscle (inner half)
T2b	tumour invades deep muscle (outer half)
T3	tumour invades perivesical tissue

T3a	microscopically
T3b	macroscopically (extravesical mass)
T4	tumour invades any of the following: prostate, uterus, vagina, pelvic wall, or abdominal wall
T4a	tumour invades the prostate, uterus, vagina
T4b	tumour invades the pelvic wall, abdominal wall

Regional lymph nodes (N)
Regional lymph nodes are those within the true pelvis; all others are distant lymph nodes.

NX	regional lymph nodes cannot be assessed
N0	no regional lymph node metastasis
N1	metastasis in a single lymph node, 2 cm or less in greatest dimension
N2	metastasis in a single lymph node, more than 2 cm but not more than 5 cm in greatest dimension; or multiple lymph nodes, none more than 5 cm in greatest dimension
N3	metastasis in a lymph node more than 5 cm in greatest dimension

Distant metastasis (M)

MX	distant metastasis cannot be assessed
M0	no distant metastasis
M1	distant metastasis

AJCC stage groupings

Stage 0a
Ta, N0, M0

Stage 0is
Tis, N0, M0

Stage I
T1, N0, M0

Stage II
T2a, N0, M0 T2b, N0, M0

Stage III
T3a, N0, M0 T3b, N0, M0 T4a, N0, M0

Stage IV
T4b, N0, M0 Any T, N1, M0 Any T, N2, M0 Any T, N3, M0 Any T, Any N, M1

UNTREATED BLADDER CANCER

The natural history of untreated bladder cancer is determined by the grade of the tumour and the depth of invasion. Because of the progressive nature of the disease, even early disease will generally progress on to multiple lesions and worsening symptoms. Patients with metastatic disease, if untreated, have a median survival of 3–6 months.[10] Because of these characteristics, it is usually only patients with extremely poor performance status who are not treated.

TREATMENT OPTION OVERVIEW

Superficial bladder tumours

The commonest presentation of bladder cancer is with a tumour restricted to the bladder surface or subepithelial connective tissue. For all these patients, initial treatment is by surgical, usually transurethral, resection (TUR) of all visible tumour. Following resection, there is a substantial risk of recurrence in a proportion of patients. The most important risk factor for recurrence, progression and survival is grade. Progression occurs without additional treatment in over 50% of high-grade (G3) patients compared with 10% of low-grade (G1) tumours. Other risks factors for recurrence and progression are stage (T1>Ta), presence of multiple tumours, tumour size (>2 cm) and early recurrence after initial resection.[11] The overall survival at 5 years for Ta tumours is 90%, falling to 75% for T1 disease.

Low-grade superficial tumours

The primary treatment of superficial bladder cancer is surgical resection of all visible tumour. Postoperative intravesical chemotherapy has been shown to decrease recurrence rates and prolong disease-free survival.[13] Agents that have been evaluated as intravesical treatment in superficial bladder cancer include thiotepa, doxorubicin, mitomycin c and epirubicin. All of these agents can cause chemical cystitis.

Early postoperative instillation of a single dose of mitomycin C has been shown to reduce the risk of recurrence by 40–50%.[14] The decision to use initial intravesical treatment depends on the patient's risk of recurrence and is advised for patients with multiple lesions (who have a higher risk of recurrence than solitary lesions (56% vs 26%)) and for lesions greater than 2 cm in size.

In recurrent disease, the role of intravesical treatment is more clearly defined. Single-dose postoperative treatment may still be recommended for solitary recurrences. There is evidence that a course of weekly instillations are more effective than single-shot treatment but the optimal duration and dosage is yet to be defined.[15] It is, however, more toxic and is therefore most suitable for higher-risk patients with multiple or frequent relapses. A commonly used schedule is mitomycin C 40 mg/40 ml instilled into the bladder for 1 hour given weekly for 6 weeks.

High-grade superficial tumours

High-grade superficial tumours have an increased risk of progressing to invasive disease. Once again, the initial management is local surgical resection. Early repeated resection is increasingly advised, as understaging has been frequently reported.

Some authors advise that because of the high rate of progression to invasive disease, patients should be treated by immediate cystectomy. However, overall results for initial cystectomy are similar to those for salvage cystectomy following conservative intravesical treatment,[16] allowing the option of organ preservation.

The use of intravesical chemotherapy in high-grade Tis and T1 tumours has shown good initial response rates, but the progression-free survival rates have been poor and there is little evidence that it affects the risk of progression to invasive disease.

Immunotherapy using bacille Calmette-Guérin (BCG), used intravesically, produces higher response rates. Compared to TUR alone, TUR + BCG shows reductions in tumour recurrence and progression to invasive disease. Trials comparing BCG with chemotherapy have demonstrated the superiority of BCG and it is therefore considered treatment of choice.[17,18] BCG has greater local toxicity than chemotherapy, causing a profound inflammatory reaction on bladder mucosa. Twenty five per cent of patients develop an influenza-like syndrome lasting 12–24 hours after instillation. A small number of patients can develop tuberculosis, which usually responds to antituberculous therapy, although deaths have been reported, especially in association with bladder trauma. There is no consensus of the preferred strain, dose or details of schedules. Common UK practice would be 50 mg of TICE strain or 120 mg of Connaught given weekly for 6 weeks. The role of subsequent maintenance is controversial, although booster courses of 3 weeks at 3 months, 6 months for 3 years has been shown to be superior to no maintenance in one randomised trial.[19] But this significantly increases toxicity and repeated treatments at relapse could be as good.

Of patients with carcinoma in situ (CIS) treated with intravesical BCG, 30% fail to respond to initial treatment and normally will undergo cystectomy. Of those achieving a complete response (CR), 30% will fail at 5 years; the management of such failures is controversial, with most advocating immediate cystectomy, although further remissions may be induced by repeated intravesical treatment. Overall, at 10 years, 31% of patients treated with BCG will remain disease-free.

Invasive bladder cancer

Local treatment
Patients presenting with invasive bladder cancer require local radical treatment. The choice usually lies between radical cystectomy and radical radiotherapy. Surgical treatment offers the most secure way of obtaining local control but at the risk of surgical morbidity/mortality and in most patients the need for a urinary diversion. Radiotherapy allows the possibility of organ conservation but suffers from a limited long-term control which requires salvage cystectomy. Overall there is little difference in results, with approximately a 30–50% 5-year survival from invasive disease.

Neoadjuvant chemotherapy
Neoadjuvant chemotherapy has been studied in patients with invasive bladder cancer to try and improve bladder preservation rates and improve survival. Phase II studies have shown response rates of 60–70% and complete response rates of 30%. Several randomised trials have been reported and although individually the results have been equivocal a recent meta-analysis has shown a clear survival advantage for chemotherapy. In this study the use of chemotherapy in combination with surgery or radiotherapy reduced the risk of death by 13%, with an absolute 5% improvement in survival.[20]

Neoadjuvant chemotherapy can be combined with complete TUR to select patients for bladder preservation. Patients in CR after chemotherapy are treated with radiotherapy; those with residual disease go on to salvage cystectomy. A Radiation Therapy Oncology Group (RTOG) study of this technique achieved bladder preservation rates of 60%, with no demonstrable survival detriment.

Concurrent chemoradiation
The use of chemotherapy, particularly cisplatin and 5-fluorouracil (5-FU) as a radiation sensitiser, has been examined in a number of phase II studies. Bladder preservation rates of over 60% have been reported.[21] A randomised trial performed by the National Cancer Institute of Canada of concurrent cisplatin/radiotherapy vs radiotherapy alone showed improved recurrence-free survival in the chemotherapy arm and a trend to improved overall survival.[22]

Advanced/metastatic disease
Systemic chemotherapy is the mainstay of active treatment in patients with metastatic disease. The most active single agents reported are cisplatin, doxorubicin, mitomycin C and methotrexate and, more recently, gemcitabine and the taxanes. These single agents give response rates in the order of 15–20%, with CR rates of <5%. Higher response rates and improved survival have been obtained with the use of combination chemotherapy. For many years the two most effective regimens have been combinations of methotrexate, cisplatin and vinblastine with (MVAC[23]) or without doxorubicin (CMV[24]). MVAC is generally seen as the gold standard against which other schedules are judged, and achieves response rates of 40–50%, and CR rates of 10%. However, this is at the cost of high toxicity. The initial MVAC series showed mucositis rates of 40%, renal toxicity in 31%, neutropenic sepsis in 20% and a toxic death rate of 4%. Therefore, the treatment is only suitable for patients with good performance status and limited comorbidity. Accelerated MVAC with G-CSF (granulocyte colony-stimulating factor) support has achieved equivalent or better results with lower toxicity in an EORTC (European Organisation for Research and Treatment of Cancer) trial.[25]

Such multi-agent cisplatin-based chemotherapy improves median survival from 3–6 months to approximately 9–12 months and has been shown to be better than single-agent[26] or non-platinum-based chemotherapy[27] in randomised trials.

New regimens using taxanes and gemcitabine have been investigated, because of their reduced toxicity. A phase III trial comparing MVAC to gemcitabine/cisplatin showed equivalent response rates and survival, with significantly reduced toxicity for the gemcitabine/cisplatin arm.[28]

Patients not suitable for such treatment represent a difficult problem. Schedules based around carboplatin or MV are often tried, but data on their success are limited.[27,29] Recently, the MRC have tested infusional 5-FU in this setting, but a 17% response rate and 6 months median survival only were achieved.[30] The EORTC are currently testing carboplatin and gemcitabine vs carboplatin, methotrexate and vinblastine in this patient group.

REGIMENS

MVAC

N saline	1 litre + 20 mmol KCl IV 6 hours × 2	day 1
Methotrexate	30 mg/m²	days 2, 15 and 22
Vinblastine	3 mg/m²	days 2, 15 and 22
Adriamycin	30 mg/m²	day 2
Mannitol 10%	200 ml over 30 min	day 2
Cisplatin	70 mg/m²	day 2

Escalated MVAC

Methotrexate	30 mg/m^2	day 1
Vinblastine	3 mg/m^2	day 1
Adriamycin	30 mg/m^2	day 1
Cisplatin	70 mg/m^2	day 1
with GCSF		days 4–11

Cycle repeated every 14 days

CMV

Methotrexate	40 mg/m^2	days 1 and 8
Vinblastine	5 mg/m^2	days 1 and 8
Cisplatin	100 mg/m^2	day 2

Cycle repeated every 21 days

Gemcitabine/cisplatin*

Gemcitabine	1000 mg/m^2	days 1, 8 and 15
Cisplatin	70 mg/m^2	day 2

Cycle repeated every 28 days
or

Gemcitabine	1000 mg/m^2	days 1 and 8
Cisplatin	70 mg/m^2	day 1

Cycle repeated every 21 days

*The 28-day schedule is the schedule used in the randomised trial of gemcitabine and cisplatin vs methotrexate, vinblastine, doxorubicin and cisplatin in advanced or metastatic bladder cancer.[28] The day 15 gemcitabine is frequently omitted due to thrombocytopenia. Hence, the 21-day cycle is increasingly used by many investigators.

'Low-toxicity' schedules

Gemcitabine	1250 mg/m^2	days 1 and 8 every 21 days

MV

Methotrexate	30 mg/m^2	days 1 and 8
Vinblastine	4 mg/m^2	days 1 and 8 every 21 days

CM

Carboplatin	AUC5	day 1
Methotrexate	60 mg/m^2	day 1 every 21 days

MEDICAL CARE FOR PATIENTS WITH PROSTATE CANCER

Robert Huddart and Rahul Mukherjee

GENERAL INFORMATION

Prostate cancer is predominantly a disease of older men, with median age at diagnosis of 72 years old. Consequently, many patients will die of unrelated comorbid conditions; thus, immediate treatment is not always required.

With the earlier detection of prostate cancer by virtue of the increasing prostate-specific antigen (PSA) testing of asymptomatic men, defining the patient population requiring treatment is becoming increasingly important.

There are racial variations in prostate cancer mortality. African-Americans have the highest mortality rate in the world, followed by Scandinavians. Mortality rates are lowest in people of oriental descent. Men who have a first-degree relative with prostate cancer are at a two–three times higher risk of developing prostate cancer.[31] This risk increases with multiple-affected family members or with relatives diagnosed at an early age.

Linkage analysis in families with multiple cases of prostate cancer has found suggestive evidence for prostate cancer susceptibility loci on several chromosomes.[32]

There is some epidemiological data which suggest that increased dietary fat intake, particularly saturated fat, may increase the risk of prostate cancer. Cohort studies have been less conclusive.[33]

Ninety five per cent of prostate cancers are adenocarcinoma.

TNM classification of prostate cancer

Primary tumour (T)

TX	primary tumour cannot be assessed
T0	no evidence of primary tumour
T1	clinically inapparent tumour not palpable nor visible by imaging
T1a	tumour incidental histologic finding in 5% or less of tissue resected
T1b	tumour incidental histologic finding in more than 5% of tissue resected
T1c	tumour identified by needle biopsy (e.g. because of elevated PSA)
T2	tumour confined within prostate*
T2a	tumour involves one lobe
T2b	tumour involves both lobes

T3 tumour extends through the prostatic capsule**
T3a extracapsular extension (unilateral or bilateral)
T3b tumour invades seminal vesicle(s)
T4 tumour is fixed or invades adjacent
    structures other than seminal vesicles:
    bladder neck, external sphincter, rectum,
    levator muscles, and/or pelvic wall

*Note: tumour found in 1 or both lobes by needle biopsy, but not palpable or reliably visible by imaging, is classified as T1c.

**Note: invasion into the prostatic apex or into (but not beyond) the prostatic capsule is not classified as T3, but as T2.

Regional lymph nodes (N)

Regional lymph nodes are the nodes of the true pelvis, which essentially are the pelvic nodes below the bifurcation of the common iliac arteries. They include the following groups (laterality does not affect the N classification): pelvic (NOS), hypogastric, obturator, iliac (internal, external, NOS), periprostatic and sacral (lateral, presacral, promontory (Gerota's) or NOS). Distant lymph nodes are outside the confines of the true pelvis and their involvement constitutes distant metastasis. They can be imaged using ultrasound, CT, MRI or lymphangiography, and include: aortic (para-aortic, periaortic, lumbar), common iliac, inguinal, superficial inguinal (femoral), supraclavicular, cervical, scalene and retroperitoneal (NOS) nodes.

NX regional lymph nodes cannot be assessed
N0 no regional lymph node metastasis
N1 metastasis in regional lymph node or nodes
NOS not otherwise specified.

Distant metastasis*** (M)

MX distant metastasis cannot be assessed
M0 no distant metastasis
M1 distant metastasis
M1a nonregional lymph node(s)
M1b bone(s)
M1c other site(s)

***Note: when more than one site of metastasis is present, the most advanced category (pM1c) is used.

Several grading systems have been proposed, of which the Gleason system is the most commonly used. This grading system recognises the fact that prostate cancer is a multifocal disease with heterogeneous glandular patterns. Thus, two individual scores, each ranging from 1 to 5, are given to the two most predominant histologic patterns of prostate cancer. The two scores are added together to give the Gleason sum. Sums of 2–4 represent well-differentiated disease; 5–7, moderately differentiated disease; and 8–10, poorly differentiated disease.[34,35]

UNTREATED PROSTATE CANCER

The prognosis of untreated prostate cancer is related to the Gleason score, clinical stage and presenting PSA. Patients with localised prostate cancer and a Gleason score ≤4 who were untreated or had hormones for disease progression have 4–7% chance of dying of prostate in the 15 years following diagnosis. In contrast, those having a Gleason score of 8 or more have a 60–87% chance of dying of prostate cancer in the same period (and less than 5% chance of being alive[36]).

In patients with grade 1 or 2 cancers and a life expectancy of less than 10 years, watchful waiting is a reasonable approach.

TREATMENT OPTION OVERVIEW

Localised disease: T1–T2,N0,M0; Gleason sum ≤ 7, PSA <20 ng/ml of blood

Watchful waiting and active surveillance

Active surveillance closely monitors patients with early cancers who are otherwise suitable for radical treatment. Data suggest that 70% will not show signs of progression within 5 years. Thus surveillance aims to radically treat patients with significant cancers but avoids treatment and its attendant morbidity in patients with indolent cancers. Watchful waiting is a more palliative approach generally considered in asymptomatic patients with life expectancy less than 10 years (due to age or comorbid medical conditions). If patients do get PSA progression, hormone therapy is usually instituted.[37]

Radical prostatectomy

Patients must be medically fit for major surgery and thus radical prostatectomy is most commonly considered for younger patients (age <65 years old). The treatment is potentially curative and has the potential side effects of impotence and incontinence.[38]

Radical radiotherapy ± neoadjuvant hormones

Radical radiotherapy ± neoadjuvant hormones is also a curative option. Overall cure rates are similar to that achieved by surgery.[39] Neoadjuvant hormone treatment with an LHRH (luteinising hormone releasing hormone) agonist for 3 months prior to radiotherapy has been shown to improve local control and disease-free survival but not overall survival.[40] The major risks of radiotherapy are impotence and bowel toxicity in the long term.[41]

Brachytherapy implant

Long-term follow-up data for brachytherapy implants using iodine-125 or palladium seeds is less mature than for surgery or external beam radiotherapy. In patients with Gleason grade ≤6 disease, PSA <10 ng/ml blood results are similar to surgery and external beam radiotherapy.[39] Current data suggest reduced long-term toxicity with respect to impotence, bowel toxicity and incontinence. Major toxicity is dysuria for up to 6 months after treatment. Glands larger than 50 cm³ or smaller than 20 cm³ or patients who have had a transurethral prostate resection are generally not suitable for brachytherapy.[42]

Hormones alone

Treatment with hormone therapy alone does not eradicate the prostate cancer but may provide disease control for a period of years. It is therefore an option in symptomatic patients with a shorter life expectancy.

T3,N0,M0 and/or Gleason ≥8 and/or PSA >20 ng/ml of blood

Radiotherapy + adjuvant hormones

These patients with locally advanced tumours are most frequently treated by radical radiotherapy. Addition of pelvic radiotherapy to local treatment improved survival in a recent RTOG study.[43] These patients have a high risk of biochemical failure and have been shown to benefit from adjuvant hormones (LHRH agonists for 3 years) in two large phase III trials examining the use of adjuvant hormones.[44–46]

Hormone therapy

Patients with locally advanced disease are commonly treated by hormone therapy alone. The relative merits of this strategy compared to use of radiotherapy and hormone therapy in this patient population is unknown and is being tested in an international trial (MRC PR07).

T4 or N1 or M1

These patients are not thought to be curable using local treatment. They are generally treated with hormone therapy.

Failure after radical treatment

Patients who develop biochemical failure (a detectable and rising PSA on three occasions) after radical prostatectomy may be treated with radical radiotherapy to the prostate bed if there is no evidence of distant disease on restaging. There is evidence that salvage radiotherapy is more effective if the patient has a PSA less than 1 ng/ml.[47]

Patients with biochemical failure after radical radiotherapy are generally treated with hormone therapy (see below). The optimal timing of this intervention has not been defined, but patient factors include symptoms or anxiety. In asymptomatic patients the presenting PSA and the PSA doubling time as well as the absolute PSA value should be taken into account.

Hormonal therapy

For patients requiring systemic management, the first standard manipulation in patients with prostate cancer is hormonal therapy. Response rates of over 80% are anticipated. The duration of response depends on disease extent and differentiation of tumours. A median response duration of 12–18 months is anticipated for patients with metastatic disease compared to median response duration in the order of 5 years for those with localised disease.[48]

Indications for hormonal therapy include:

- metastatic disease
- treatment of locally advanced disease
- adjuvant or neoadjuvant therapy in combination with radiotherapy
- treatment of patients failing radical therapy

The timing of therapy for patients not receiving radical treatment or relapsing following radical treatment remains controversial. This is in part due to the sensitivity of the PSA assay, which can detect relapse/progression months/years before clinical symptoms develop. Data from the adjuvant trials (see above) suggest that treating small volume disease may be advantageous. An MRC trial suggested that immediate treatment prolonged survival, particularly in non-metastatic patients, and reduced the risk of major complications.[49,50] We therefore advise immediate hormonal therapy for patients with demonstrable metastatic disease and for non-metastatic patients with rapidly rising PSA (doubling <6 months). For non-metastatic patients with slowly rising PSA, we individualise treatment, balancing the benefits of early treatment vs the problems of prolonged therapy.

Hormonal effect is largely directed at abrogating the stimulatory effect of testosterone on prostate cancer cells. First-line treatment is usually with an LHRH agonist (e.g goserelin 3.6 mg 4 weekly depot injection or leuprorelin 3.75 mg 4-weekly depot). LHRH agonists reduce LH levels by down-regulating LHRH receptors and produce castrate levels of testosterone within 2–3 weeks. The efficacy of this treatment is equivalent to surgical castration (subcapsular orchidectomy) and is preferred to surgery by the majority of men. The mode of action of these drugs leads to an initial LH/testosterone surge, which is usually blocked by administration of cyproterone acetate 100 mg three times a day for 1 week prior and

2 weeks post the first LHRH injection. The major toxicities of this treatment are loss of libido, hot flushes and fatigue. Long-term treatment is associated with reduced muscle bulk, accelerated osteoporosis and, possibly, an increased risk of cardiovascular disease.

A recent alternative is to block the androgen receptor with a non-steroidal antiandrogen, bicalutamide (150 mg daily). This drug leads to raised testosterone levels. A proportion of patients remain potent on this therapy, and it is thus particularly applicable to sexually active patients. Gynaecomastia (50%) and breast discomfort (30%) can be problematic and may require preventative treatment with radiotherapy or tamoxifen (20 mg orally weekly).[51,52] Trials suggest overall better quality of life and equivalent efficacy to LHRH therapy for patients with locally advanced disease but inferior results for patients with metastatic disease.

Following castration, low levels of adrenal androgens are still produced and there has been debate as to whether there is an advantage for combined LHRH therapy with an antiandrogen (CAB) (e.g. flutamide 250 mg three times daily or bicalutamide 50 mg once daily) to block adrenal androgen production. A meta-analysis of trials suggests a possible 2% advantage (range 0–5%) for this approach.[53] The extra cost and toxicity of this approach has not led to routine usage of this treatment in the UK.

PSA failure after first–line hormone treatment

For patients requiring treatment after failing first-line hormone therapy, the options include:

- antiandrogen withdrawal
- second-line hormonal therapy
- chemotherapy
- isotope therapy
- bisphosphonate treatment
- palliative radiotherapy.

These are discussed below.

Antiandrogen withdrawal
When CABs have been used, there is a documented withdrawal response to hormonal agents. PSA response rates of 21% have been reported after cessation of flutamide. The median response duration was 5 months. Similar effects have been reported with bicalutamide, megestrol acetate and diethylstilbestrol.[54]

Second-line hormonal therapy
Blocking adrenal androgens is a common second step after first-line failure. This can be achieved by an antiandrogen, either non-steroidal or steroidal (see above). Alternatively, a steroid such as prednisolone 7.5 mg once daily or dexamethasone 1.5–2 mg once daily can be used. Steroids decrease ACTH (adrenocorticotrophic hormone) production via negative feedback, thus reducing adrenal androgens production, which are produced as part of the steroid metabolism of the adrenals. Used in low doses, hormonal therapy can also have symptomatic benefits in addition to causing PSA responses.[55] In an EORTC trial, it achieved better results than anti-androgen treatment.[56]

Oestrogens such as diethylstilbestrol have complex action. In doses ≥3 mg they produce castrate testosterone levels due to negative feedback on LH at the pituitary level. In addition, they may have a direct cytotoxic effect on prostate cancer, as evidenced by responses in patients failing combined androgen blockade.[57,58] In a Royal Marsden phase II study, 29% of men had a PSA fall >50% for 4 weeks and over 50% had improvement in pain scores when used as third-line therapy.[59] This treatment is more toxic than other therapies with >50% of patients developing gynaecomastia, 10% risk of thromboembolic complications and risk of gastrointestinal disturbance. Prophylactic breast bud irradiation prior to commencing treatment and concurrent low-dose aspirin (75 mg once daily) is recommended for all patients.[52]

Chemotherapy for advanced hormone refractory disease
Mitoxantrone (mitozantrone) There have been two phase III studies comparing mitoxantrone (mitozantrone) plus a corticosteroid to corticosteroid alone. Tannock et al reported statistically significant improvement in palliation of bone pain as well as increased duration of symptom improvement but not survival for the addition of mitoxantrone (mitozantrone).[60] The Cancer and Leukaemia Group B (CALGB) study included asymptomatic patients; no survival difference was detected but patients receiving mitoxantrone (mitozantrone) had better quality of life indices, particularly for pain control.

Typically, mitoxantrone (mitozantrone) is used at a dosage of 12 mg/m^2, repeated 3 weekly. Dose reductions (25–50%) should be undertaken in patients with extensive bone metastases and evidence of bone marrow suppression.

Estramustine Estramustine is a combination of an oestrogen with a non-nitrogen mustard. A recent trial of 201 patients using estramustine plus vinblastine vs vinblastine alone showed increased time to progression with the addition of estramustine.[61] Survival difference was not statistically significant, although there was a trend favouring the estramustine arm (11.9 vs 9.2 months). Estramustine is more toxic than mitoxantrone (mitozantrone), with toxicities that include lethargy, nausea/vomiting, thromboembolism, myelosuppression and fluid retention. Evidence of greater efficacy than oestrogen alone (diethylstilbesterol) is lacking.

Taxanes   Taxanes have been shown to have activity in a number of small phase II trials, either alone or in combination with other cytotoxics. Most work has focused on docetaxel, given either 75 mg/m^2 3 weekly or 30–36 mg/m^2 weekly (for 3–6 weeks). Sustained PSA of >50% in PSA and palliative benefit has been reported in 45–55% of patients.[62–64] It has been suggested the combination of a taxane and estramustine may be synergistic and more active than either alone.[65] US and European trials have been undertaken comparing docetaxel (± estramustine) with mitoxantrone (mitozantrone) and prednisone showing improved palliation and survival for docetaxel.

Bisphosphonates   Metastatic bone pain is a major problem for prostate cancer patients. Treatment with bisphosphonates, such as pamidronate 90 mg or sodium clodronate 1500 mg, can lead to reduction in bone pain in patients with bony metastases.[66] A new more potent bisphosphonate (zoledronate 4 mg) has recently been licensed for treatment of symptomatic bony disease in prostate cancer and in a recently reported trial (in abstract) has been shown to reduce the incidence of new skeletal-related events.[67] A recent MRC study has suggested bony progression may be delayed by early administration of an oral bisphosphonate.[68]

Unsealed radioisotopes   Strontium, samarium and rhenium have been shown to improve bone pain from prostate cancer. Strontium (150 MBq) seems to have equal efficacy for relief of bone pain to either local or extended field radiotherapy, with the added advantage of reducing the onset of new sites of bone pain and with lower toxicity than extended field radiotherapy.[69] There is randomised evidence to show improvement in survival with the use of strontium in combination with doxorubicin,[70] although data in this small study need confirmation.

MEDICAL CARE FOR PATIENTS WITH TESTICULAR CANCER

Robert Huddart and Rahul Mukherjee

EPIDEMIOLOGY

Testicular cancers account for 1% of all male cancer, with 1400 new cases diagnosed in the United Kingdom each year. They are the commonest malignancy in men aged 20–40 years old. The peak incidence is at 25–35 years old. The incidence of testicular tumours has been steadily rising through the last 100 years, with an increase of 15–20% being seen over successive 5-year periods.

Risk factors for testicular tumours include a family history (relative risk 6–10) and testicular maldescent (relative risk 3.8), as well as low birth weight and infantile hernias.

PATHOLOGICAL CLASSIFICATION

The pathology of testicular germ cell tumours is broadly divided into seminoma or non-seminoma (or teratomas).

The World Health Organisation histological classification of testicular germ cell tumours is shown below. The British Testicular Tumour Board nomenclature is given in parentheses.

A. Tumour showing single cell type
1. Seminoma
2. Embryonal carcinoma (malignant teratoma undifferentiated; MTU)
3. Teratoma (malignant teratoma differentiated; MTD)
4. Choriocarcinoma (malignant teratoma trophoblastic; MTT)
5. Yolk sac tumour.

The majority of non-seminomas have more than one cell type, and the relative proportions of each cell type should be specified. The cell type of these tumours is important for estimating the risk of metastases and response to chemotherapy.

B. Tumour showing more than one histological pattern
1. Embryonal carcinoma and teratoma with or without seminoma (malignant teratoma intermediate; MTI)
2. Embryonal carcinoma and yolk sac tumour with or without seminoma
3. Embryonal carcinoma and seminoma
4. Yolk sac tumour and teratoma with or without seminoma
5. Choriocarcinoma and any other element.

Approximately 40% of patients have pure seminoma, and a further 14% have mixed seminoma and non-seminoma. Of non-seminomas, most are embryonal carcinomas (MTU) (37%) or mixed embryonal carcinoma/teratoma (50%). The other subtypes, teratoma (5%), yolk sac and choriocarcinoma (7%), are less common.

Box 41.1   Royal Marsden Hospital Staging

I   Testicular involvement alone. No evidence
    of metastases

Is   Stage I on surveillance

Im   Stage I on CT but marker (AFP or hCG) above
    normal range

II   Infradiaphragmatic lymph node involvement
    Stage II A / B/ C: maximum diameter
    <2/ 2–5/ >5 cm

III   Supradiaphragmatic nodes involved
    Stages A / B / C as for stage II.

IV   Visceral metastases
    Lung substaging: L1, <3 metastases;
       L2: >3 metastases; L3, >3 metastases + one
       or more metastases >2 cm
    Organ involved: H+, liver metastases;
       Br+, brain metastases; M+, mediastinum;
       N+, neck lymph nodes

PATIENT ASSESSMENT

Decisions regarding patient management are made according to patient stage and prognostics category. Stage/prognostic category are assigned by the nature of primary site and extent of disease determined by tumour marker levels – alpha fetoprotein (AFP), β human chorionic gonadotrophin (hCG) and lactate dehydrogenase (LDH) – and CT scanning of chest abdomen and pelvis (± brain if multiple lung metastases or high tumour markers). The Royal Marsden Staging system (Box 41.1) remains the most widely used for documenting disease extent. For decision-making in patients with metastatic disease, it has been superseded by the International Germ Cell Cancer Consensus Group (IGCCCG) prognostic classification (Table 41.1).

TREATMENT OVERVIEW

Stage I

Seminoma

The primary is removed by radical inguinal orchidectomy. Of those men with clinical stage I disease, approximately 15–20% will have occult metastatic disease. Risk factors for relapse are tumour size >4 cm and rete testis invasion. In the presence of both factors, there is a 33% risk of relapse compared with a 12–15% risk with 0 or 1 of these factors.[71] This can be reduced by adjuvant para-aortic irradiation to a dose of 20–30 Gy. This treatment reduces the risk of relapse to under 3%. The MRC TE 18 trial has compared doses of 20 vs 30 Gy. Early results suggest that 20 Gy achieves equivalent results to 30 Gy, with lower toxicity, and is thus

Table 41.1   IGCCCG prognostic classification

Nonseminoma	Seminoma
GOOD PROGNOSIS	
Testis or retroperitoneal primary and no nonpulmonary visceral metastases and	Any primary site and no non-pulmonary visceral metastases and normal AFP, any hCG, any LDH
Good markers (all of the following): AFP <1000 ng/ml	
hCG <5000 IU/L (1000 ng/ml)	
LDH <1.5 upper limit of normal	
56% of nonseminomas	90% of seminomas
5-year, PFS, 89%	5-year PFS, 82%
5-year survival, 92%	5-year survival, 86%
INTERMEDIATE PROGNOSIS	
Testis or retroperitoneal primary and no non-pulmonary visceral metastases and Intermediate markers (any of the following)	Any primary site and no non-pulmonary visceral metastases and normal AFP, any hCG, any LDH
AFP >1000 and <10 000 ng/ml	
or	
hCG >5000 IU/L and <50 000 IU/L	
or	
LDH >1.5 x N and <10 × N	
28% of non-seminomas	10% of seminomas
5-year PFS, 75%	5-year PFS, 67%
5-year survival, 80%	5-year survival, 72%

Table 41.1   IGCCCG prognostic classification—cont'd

Nonseminoma	Seminoma
POOR PROGNOSIS	
Mediastinal primary	No patients classified as poor prognosis
or	
Non-pulmonary visceral metastases	
or	
Poor markers (any of the following):	
AFP >10 000 ng/ml	
or	
hCG >50 000 IU/L	
or	
LDH >10 x upper limit of normal	
16% of non-seminomas	
5-year PFS, 41%	
5-year survival, 48%	

AFP, alpha fetoprotein; hCG, human chorionic gonadotrophin; LDH, lactate dehydrogenase; PFS, progression-free survival.

the current preferred dose.[72] An MRC trial (TE 19) has compared single agent carboplatin[73] with para-aortic radiation (results due 2003/4).

Alternatively, patients may be managed by a surveillance policy after orchidectomy. Similar cure rates can be achieved (approaching 100%), with relapses salvaged using radiotherapy or chemotherapy.[73] However, relapses are more difficult to detect and less predictable in time to development, making this approach more difficult than for non-seminoma (see below). This approach is gaining popularity in low-risk patients in view of data on the risk of late second malignancy in these patients. Patients need regular cross-sectional imaging for 5 years and should be followed up for at least 10 years as late relapses do occur.

Non-seminoma

The primary is treated by radical inguinal orchidectomy. Approximately 30% of men with clinical stage I disease will go on to develop overt metastases.[74] Those patients whose primary tumour histology showed vascular invasion have a 50% risk of recurrence; those without vascular invasion have a 15% risk. Low-risk patients are generally managed with surveillance. High-risk patients may also undergo surveillance but may be offered two courses of adjuvant cisplatin-based chemotherapy, e.g. BEP[75] or BOP,[76] which reduces relapse risk to <1%.

Metastatic disease

Seminoma

Stage II   The primary is removed by radical inguinal orchidectomy. Stage II seminomas are treated based on the size of the nodal mass. With patients with masses <5 cm in diameter, the standard treatment is radiotherapy to the mass, para-aortic and ipsilateral pelvic lymph nodes. The large volume is treated to a dose of 30 Gy with a 5 Gy boost to the enlarged nodes. If radiotherapy is contraindicated, then chemotherapy is used. A single cycle of carboplatin (AUC 7) reduces the risk of subsequent out-of-field relapse.[77]

For patients with nodal masses greater than 5 cm, standard therapy after orchidectomy is 3 cycles of BEP chemotherapy.[78]

Stage III/IV   The primary is removed by radical inguinal orchidectomy. The metastatic disease is treated by 3 cycles of BEP chemotherapy in low-risk patients, 4 cycles in intermediate-risk patients. Bleomycin is often omitted with no obvious loss of efficacy in patients at high risk of lung toxicity (poor renal function, age >40 years old),[79,80] but 4 cycles of therapy should be used in these cases. Single agent carboplatin can cure many patients, but is associated with more relapses and is an alternative for patients unable to tolerate BEP.[81]

Non-seminoma

BEP chemotherapy remains the standard treatment for metastatic non-seminoma germ cell tumours (NSGCT). Recent trials have shown that 3 cycles of BEP are as effective as 4 cycles for patients with good prognosis disease. A total of 500 mg/m^2 of etoposide is used and the treatment can be scheduled over 3 days.[82] Bleomycin lung toxicity is a major toxicity of this treatment and, although uncommon at cumulative dose of less than 300 000 units, it affects about

1% of patients in most series. Omitting bleomycin reduces the effectiveness of the treatment.[83–85] Other regimens have been shown to be more toxic (ifosfamide)[86] or less effective (carboplatin).[87]

Approximately one-third of patients with stage II–IV NSGCT will have residual masses after treatment. These may contain active undifferentiated tumour, differentiated teratoma or fibrotic/necrotic tissue. Differentiated teratoma may grow and transform into undifferentiated tumour or develop into other tumours, so surgical resection of residual masses is recommended.[88]

Recurrent disease

Patients who fail standard chemotherapy are treated with regimens including ifosfamide, cisplatin and vinblastine or etoposide in combination with surgery or radiotherapy wherever possible. Taxol- and gemcitabine-containing regimens are currently in phase II trials. High-dose chemotherapy and autologous stem cell rescue is frequently utilised and may improve cure rates, although this remains to be proved.

REGIMENS

BEP (3 day) $B_{30}E_3P_2$

Prehydration

1 L N saline + 20 mmol KCl (hydration) 4 hourly × 2	Day 0

Etoposide

165 mg/m^2 in 500 ml N saline over 1 hour	Repeated days 1, 2, 3

Bleomycin

30 000 units IV stat	Days 2, 8* and 15*

Hydrocortisone

100 mg IV given before bleomycin

Cisplatin

Mannitol 10%, 200 ml over 30 min pre-chemo	
Cisplatin 50 mg/m^2 in 1 L N saline + 20 mmol KCl over 6 hours	
1 L N saline + 20 mmol KCl + 10 mmol Mg^{2+} 6 hourly × 3	Repeated days 1,2

Aim to administer 3 cycles for good prognosis patients or 4 cycles for intermediate and 4–6 cycles for poor prognosis patients.
*Bleomycin to be given if total white count >0.8 × 10^9/L; platelet count > 80 000 × 10^9/L.

Carboplatin

Carboplatin dose to be based on accurate (3-point) EDTA clearance (not corrected for BSA). Dose of first course to be based on clearance and subsequent courses adjusted for previous myelosuppression. Dosage based on Calvert formula:

$$\text{Single agent dosage} = 7 \times (\text{EDTA clearance in ml/min} + 25)$$
$$(\text{e.g. clearance} = 80; \text{dose} = 105 \times 7 = 735\text{mg})$$

Given in 500 ml, 5% dextrose over 1 hour	Day 1

Ifosfamide/cisplatin/etoposide (IPE) 21-day cycles

Prehydration

1 litre N saline + 20 mmol KCl 6 hours × 2

Etoposide

100 mg/m^2 in 500 ml N saline over 1 hour	Days 1, 3 and 5

Cisplatin

Mannitol 10%, 200 ml over 30 min pre cisplatin	
Cisplatin 20 mg/m^2 in 1 L N saline + 20 mmol KCl over 6 hours	
1 L N saline + 20 mmol KCl + 10 mmol Mg^{++} 4 hours × 2	Repeated days 1, 2, 3, 4 and 5

Ifosfamide*

1g/m^2 + mesna (0.5 g/m^2) in 500 ml N saline over 1 hour then mesna 0.5 g/m^2 over 7 hours in 1 litre N saline + 20 mmol KCl	Days 1, 2, 3, 4 and 5

TIP

As used MRC trial
Cisplatin 20 mg/m^2 daily IV for 5 days
Ifosfamide 1g/m^2 IV daily for 5 days
Mesna 1g IV daily over 5 days
Paclitaxel 175 mg/m^2 IV over 3 hours

HIGH-DOSE CHEMOTHERAPY SCHEDULES

2 DRUG: CARBO/ETOPOSIDE (RMH Standard)

Carboplatin

AUC 6 in 500 ml 5% dextrose over 1 hour	Days −6, −5, −4, −3

Etoposide

360 mg/m^2, given in   Days –6, –5, –4, –3
  two divided doses of
  180 mg/m^2, each given
  over 2 hours in
  1 litre N saline
followed by 1 L N saline +   Days –6, –5, –4, –3
  20 mmol KCl +
  10 mmol MgCl
  over 4 hours

Return of stem cells   Day 0

3 DRUG: CARBOPEC
As used in IT94 study
  randomised trial.

Carboplatin

550 mg/m^2 in 1 L 5%   Days –7, –6, –5, –4
  dextrose over 2 hours
  (see trial protocol for dose
  modification if normalised

EDTA <100 ml/min)
(maximum AUC 30)

Etoposide

450 mg/m^2 (in divided doses   Days –7, –6, –5, –4
  of 225 mg/m^2 over 2 hours)
  in 1 L N saline

Cyclophosphamide

1600 mg/m^2 in 250 ml 5%
  dextrose over 1 hour

Mesna

(pre-cyclo) 400 mg/m^2 in   Days –7, –6, –5, –4
  250 ml of 5% dextrose
  over 1 hour (post-cyclo)
  400 mg/m^2 in 250 ml of
  5% dextrose over 30 min
  4 hourly × 5

Return of stem cells   Day 0

MEDICAL CARE FOR PATIENTS WITH RENAL CANCER

Riyaz NH Shah and Timothy G Eisen

GENERAL INFORMATION

Renal tumours account for 2% of all cancers (150 000 new cases per year worldwide).[89] This section discusses the management of renal cell carcinomas (RCC), which constitute 75% of adult renal tumours.

There are twice as many male cases as female, with a mean age at diagnosis of 50–70 years old. The incidence is increasing in the West.[90,91] Associations have been described with cigarette smoking,[92] obesity, high fat diet, renal stone formation, chronic dialysis and exposure to carcinogens (e.g. cadmium, derivatives of aromatic amines, tryptophan and phenacetin abuse), as reviewed by Moyad et al.[93]

The risk of developing RCC is greatly increased in first-degree relatives of patients, suggesting genetic factors. There is a known relationship between RCC and germline mutations in the von Hippel–Lindau (VHL) gene[94] and this is occasionally part of the VHL syndrome characterized by haemangioblastomas (in the cerebellum, spinal cord and retina), phaeochromocytoma, pancreatic and renal cysts and RCC.[95] Tuberous sclerosis is also associated with an increased incidence of RCC.

Pathologically, RCCs are thought to arise from a mitotic process involving the renal tubular epithelium.

Morphological classification using the Heidelberg system is commonly used.[96,97] The main groups are clear cell, chromophillic and chromophobic, which account for 60–80%, 7–14% and 4–10% of RCCs, respectively. Clear cell morphology is associated with an increased incidence of distant metastases and vena caval involvement, with a resultant poorer prognosis.[98] Sarcomatoid features are also associated with an adverse prognosis.[99] Each of these subtypes has associations with a variety of cytogenetic abnormalities, and newer molecular classification systems will undoubtedly come into routine practice.[100]

Tumours are usually graded using the Fuhrman grading system,[101] from 1 to 4, which classifies the morphology from most to least differentiated and has important prognostic implications (Table 41.2).

STAGING INFORMATION

Patients are staged using the TNM classification system (see Table 41.3). Stage I is defined as T1 N0 M0 and stage II as T2 N0 M0. Stage III as T1-2 N1 M0 or T3 N0/1 M0. Stage IV is defined as any M1 or T4. Survival of differing stages is given in Table 41.4.

Apart from grade and stage, other features have been defined as indicating a poorer prognosis. There include a low Karnofsy performance score (<80%),

Table 41.2 Grading of RCC and survival

Fuhrman grade	Incidence of all RCC (%)	Probability of distant metastases after nephrectomy (%)	Five–year survival (%)
I	10	2	76
II	35	72	72
III	35	51	51
IV	20	35	35

Source: based on Bretheau et al[102] and Delahunt et al.[103]

LDH >1.5 × upper limit of normal (ULN), haemoglobin <lower limit of normal, high serum Ca, the absence of a nephrectomy, time from diagnosis, number of metastatic sites, weight loss, high erythrocyte sedimentation rate (ESR) and high neutrophil count.[105]

Patients can present with a variety of symptoms from the primary, metastases, systemic effects or paraneoplastic phenomena. The commonest symptoms include haematuria, pain, abdominal mass, weight loss and anaemia[106] Other common systemic features include pyrexia, sweats, hypercalcaemia and fatigue. Metastases can cause a variety of problems, including pain, pathological fractures, neurological deficits or pulmonary symptoms. Paraneoplastic production of hormones is well described (especially erythropoietin and renin).

Investigations of a new patient with suspected RCC should include full blood count, urea, electrolytes, liver function, calcium and lactate dehydrogenase (LDH) and urine cytology. Imaging of the renal system should include CT/ultrasonography scanning. A chest X-ray is usually sufficient in excluding significant pulmonary disease. Plain X-rays of painful regions are effective methods of excluding bony involvement, especially in combination with bone scans. Post-surgical follow-up should include regular blood tests, as detailed above, as well as imaging to detect relapse. In our institution we recommend 3-monthly chest X-ray and 6-monthly CT scanning of the chest and abdomen for 2 years in resected RCC.

MANAGEMENT OF RENAL CELL CARCINOMAS

The management of RCC involves the three classical modalities of cancer treatment: namely surgery, radiotherapy and systemic therapy.

In the case of stage I and II disease, a radical nephrectomy is a potentially curative procedure and the treatment of choice. In some patients this may not be appropriate, due to factors such as comorbidity. In such cases, embolisation or radical radiotherapy may be considered. The role of nephron sparing surgery in

Table 41.3 The TNM staging system

T	N	M
x = not assessable	x = not assessable	x = not assessable
0 = No primary	0 = no regional nodal mets	0 = no distant mets
1= primary ≤7 cm	1 = met in a single regional node	1 = distant mets
2= primary >7 cm but confined to kidney	2 = in more than one regional node	
3 = invasion to adrenal, perinephric tissue, vessels, etc., but not beyond Gerota's fascia		
4 = beyond Gerota's fascia		

mets = metastases.

Table 41.4 Survival and stage

Stage	Per cent of patients (suspected to have RCC)	Per cent of patients (incidentally discovered)	Survival (%)
I	4	14	65–85
II	49	64	45–80
III	26	19	15–35
IV	22	3	0–10

Source: based on Siow et al.[104]

patients with bilateral synchronous disease or a solitary kidney is under active review.

The indications for nephrectomy in patients with metastatic disease include, first, palliation of the renal bed. Progressive renal bed involvement can be difficult to manage and the early use of nephrectomy, just as the patient is developing local symptoms, can prevent this problem arising. Most relapses after radical nephrectomy are distant, with only 5–10% of patients developing a local recurrence.[107] In addition, nephrectomy can palliate symptoms such as weight loss, sweats, pain and haematuria and may improve hypertension and hypercalcaemia. Secondly, spontaneous regression of metastases is described as occurring in about 1% of cases post nephrectomy. It occurs more commonly with pulmonary metastases but can occur in the presence of spread to other distant organs.[108,109] Thirdly, nephrectomy is also indicated in patients with advanced disease if they are to be candidates for systemic cytokine therapy, as the data to date suggest a 10% increase in response rate and survival in this subgroup.[110,111] In addition, surgical resection of solitary metastases in lung, brain or bone is also indicated, as these patients seem to have a longer than expected survival.[112]

RCC is a relatively radio-resistant disease. Currently, there is no role for adjuvant radiotherapy post nephrectomy. Radiotherapy is given radically in some patients with inoperable local disease; however, this does not prolong survival but palliates local symptoms for a while.[113] Radiotherapy can be used to palliate painful bony metastases.

Various 'mainstream' chemotherapy drugs have been used to treat RCC, including vinblastine, CCNU (lomustine), anthracyclines and cyclophosphamide. These agents all seem to have low levels of activity against RCC, either singly or in combination and are not routinely used.[114] In trial settings newer chemotherapeutic agents such as capecitabine and gemcitabine are being investigated. Combination therapy with gemcitabine and infusional 5-FU has shown promise.[115] Thalidomide is an agent showing promise in RCC. Its mechanism of action is unknown but phase II data are encouraging (reviewed by Eisen[116]).

Hormonal agents such as medroxyprogesterone acetate (MPA) have been used in RCC treatment. Although there are anecdotal reports of complete responders and prolonged survival, these are rare. Most patients do, however, get some palliation in terms of appetite improvement, reduction in weight loss and increased performance status. In patients not fit for entry into a clinical trial or cytokine therapy, MPA is a standard treatment within the UK at a dose of 300 mg/day.

The cytokines interferon-2α (IFN-α) and interleukin-2 (IL-2) have activity in RCC. IFNα at a dose of 10 MU given 3 times per week has been shown to improve survival when compared to MPA with acceptable toxicity.[117] This result has been reinforced by a meta-analysis, including other randomised trials.[118] At this dose, IFNα is well tolerated, with flu-like symptoms being the major toxicity. This can be ameliorated with night-time administration and paracetamol. Other toxicities include anorexia, vomiting, altered taste, myelosuppression, liver dysfunction and mood changes. IFNα is immunomodulatory to NK cells, T cells and macrophages. In addition, it is thought to have cytostatic and anti-angiogenic effects.

IL-2 has been shown to have similar activity to IFN-α in terms of overall survival;[119] however, toxicity can be more problematic as it is commonly associated with a capillary leak syndrome, which can lead to multiorgan failure.

Treatment with IL-2 and IFN-α in combination with chemotherapy (initially fluoropyrimidines) has also been investigated.[120] Combination regimens have been shown to be superior to tamoxifen[121] and pooling phase II data of biochemotherapy suggests higher response rates. Many different regimens of IL-2 + IFN-α + 5-FU exist, and consensus has not been reached; however, the highest response rate described has been with infusional 5-FU.[122] An EORTC study is underway comparing a single cycle of the Atzpodien regimen to observation in the high-risk adjuvant setting.

NURSING CARE FOR PATIENTS WITH UROLOGICAL CANCER

Maria Caulfield and Amanda Baxter

INTRODUCTION

For the majority of urology patients, chemotherapy is not the primary treatment for their disease. Therefore, many come into the chemotherapy setting with pre-existing problems caused not only by their disease but also as a result of other treatments such as surgery. Healthcare professionals also need to be aware that, for many, the reason they need chemotherapy is because of recurring and/or advanced disease. Consequently, they may not only need support in dealing with the side effects of chemotherapy but also with the emotional issues of coming to terms with recurring disease or the possibility of death.

Urological cancers on the whole affect people aged 60 years old and over. Patients may have other health problems, which may impact on their ability to tolerate and/or cope with chemotherapy regimens. The effects of the ageing process and their social circumstances must all be taken into account when considering chemotherapy.

Testicular cancer patients are the exception to these points. They are young, generally between the ages of 15 and 35 years old[123] and therefore tolerate chemotherapy well. Testicular tumours are extremely chemosensitive and, even with metastatic disease, a cure rate of over 80% can be achieved with chemotherapy.[124] However these patients then have to live with the long-term side effects from their chemotherapy, some of which will be discussed further.

FERTILITY

Although chemotherapy can have an adverse effect on fertility, the effects vary according to the patient's age, the drugs used and the dose.[125] Alkylating agents, such as cisplatin, which is used commonly in urology regimens, have the most recognised side effects on fertility.[126]

Testicular patient fertility

Although infertility can be a potentially important issue for all patients, it is those with testicular cancer for whom the implications may be more significant as they tend to be diagnosed at an age when many young men have not even started to think about having children. However, as the use of neoadjuvant and adjuvant chemotherapy expands, other groups of patients, such as those with bladder cancers aiming to undergo bladder-conserving treatment, will also need to consider the implications of chemotherapy-induced infertility.

However, for many with bladder and prostate cancer, their fertility may have been already affected by previous surgery, radiotherapy and hormone manipulation.

Chemotherapy causes damage to rapidly dividing sperm cells and the higher the total dose the slower the recovery of sperm cell production and the more likely it is to stop completely.[126] The sort of abnormalities caused to sperm as a result of chemotherapy include reduced sperm counts, reduced semen volume, altered sperm motility, structure and maturation.

Contraception

It cannot be assumed that chemotherapy automatically induces infertility. Patients and their partners should always be informed that they need to use contraception to avoid pregnancy. Barrier methods are preferred so as to avoid chemotherapy metabolites being excreted in semen, which can be a potential hazard for partners.[127] Advice should also be given to avoid attempting conception for at least 2 years post chemotherapy, not only to decrease the mutational risks but also to assess treatment response. The risk of disease recurrence has been shown to be highest within the first 2 years post treatment.[128]

Sperm banking

For men, the option of sperm banking is an increasingly successful method of preserving fertility. Even for men who present with poor quality sperm, the introduction of intracytoplasmic sperm injection (ICSI), where a single sperm is injected directly into an egg, means fertility can be retained. The Human Fertilisation and Embryology Authority require all patients having semen cryopreservation to be tested for hepatitis C and HIV before sperm can be stored long term. These men need counselling and support about these tests and their possible implications. For those presenting with advanced and life-threatening testicular cancer, where there is an urgent need to commence chemotherapy, there may not be time to undertake sperm banking or patients may not be able to produce a sample to be stored. Therefore, it is these patients who may need additional ongoing emotional support, as unfortunately they are also the patients who will need more intensive chemotherapy regimens, thus increasing the risk of long-term infertility. (See also Chs 32 and 48.)

Female fertility management

In contrast to men, the age of a woman when she commences chemotherapy is a key issue to her future fertility. The older a women is, the less likely she is to preserve her fertility and after the age of 35 it is highly likely that chemotherapy will push her in to the menopause.[126] Therefore, not only do women need emotional support in coming to terms with such issues but also they may need practical support in dealing with menopausal symptoms such as hot flushes. (See also Ch. 33.)

The ability to offer fertility treatment is more difficult for women. There are a number of options:

- Embryo freezing (IVF) – where fertilised eggs are frozen. Women either need to be in an established relationship or use donated sperm. This is well-established treatment which has been used for more than 20 years.
- Oocyte freezing – where unfertilised eggs are frozen. This is a relatively new and experimental treatment; eggs can be damaged during the freezing and thawing process.
- Ovarian tissue freezing – where ovarian tissue, which has been removed by laparoscopic biopsy or oophrectomy, is frozen. The aim is to reimplant the tissue or collect the eggs, which are then fertilised before being reimplanted. This is an experimental treatment that is in its early stages.

Harvesting eggs for the treatment outlined above means there would be a delay of at least 3 weeks before chemotherapy could start and may be life-threatening. Support and information will be needed by these women in order to help them make decisions. (See also Chs 32 and 48.)

SEXUAL FUNCTION

The majority of people with cancer experience some degree of sexual difficulty.[128] For those with cancers of the prostate and bladder, the physical effects of surgery, radiotherapy and hormone treatment may have already caused long-term sexual problems, whereas for patients with testicular and renal cancers the experience of having chemotherapy may be the first time they encounter sexual problems.

Chemotherapy-induced side effects such as fatigue, nausea and hair loss can produce both physical and emotional responses that can cause sexual function problems such as altered sexual desire, which can in turn lead to erectile dysfunction and decreased vaginal secretions. Although these effects tend to be short term, they may take many months to resolve after treatment finishes. Patients who have radiotherapy and/or surgery as well as chemotherapy have an increased risk of developing difficulties with sexual function. Decreased sexual enjoyment and desire have been reported as a long-term outcome of treatment of testicular cancer.[129] Altered ejaculatory function, erectile dysfunction, vaginal dryness, loss of sensation in the vagina and dyspareunia are all consequences of treatment for urological cancers.[130]

Although the effects of chemotherapy on sexual function are thought to be short term, there are few studies which have examined this. Those that do, such as that of Ozen et al,[131] have only looked at small numbers of patients over short periods of time. Therefore, healthcare professionals should not assume that patients who achieve long-term remission no longer have sexual problems, as there may be unresolved issues and these patients may still need information and support. The majority of patients do not need psychotherapy or medical intervention to recover satisfying sex lives but they do need accurate information and support about what to expect.[126]

ALTERED BODY IMAGE

Considering the side effects from the various treatments on fertility and sexual function for urology cancers, there is very little research exploring the psychological impact on this group of patients. This may be because the majority of patients are men, who, unlike women, cope differently and do not readily talk about their experiences.[132] Indeed, very little is known about testicular cancer patients' support and survivorship issues, despite the increase in survival rates for testicular cancer.[133]

It has been clearly demonstrated that surgical treatments can have negative effects on body image;[134,135] therefore, it can be assumed that the added side effects of hair loss and fatigue can only enhance negative images. A negative body image has been proposed to be the most common cause of sexual problems in cancer patients.[136] Consequently, a vicious circle begins where sexual problems caused by treatment negatively alter body image, which in turn enhances any sexual problems.

Altered body image not only affects the individual's sexuality but also his self-esteem and self-concept.[137] Facing a life-threatening illness, treatment regimens and the outcomes of those treatments may lead patients to question their role in their family and society in general. Support, information-giving and active listening can all assist the patient in dealing with these issues.

It is not clear at present what information and support urology patients actually want. Healthcare professionals should not assume that the information and support they give is actually what the patient wants or needs to know. There is a great need for further research in this area.[132] (See also Ch. 5.)

References

1. Case RAM, Hosker ME, McDonald DB, et al. Tumours of the urinary bladder in workmen engaged in the manufacture and use of certain dyestuff intermediates in the British chemical industry. Br J Ind Med 1954; 11:75–104.

2. Decarli A, Peto J, Piolatto G, La Vecchia C. Bladder cancer mortality of workers exposed to aromatic amines: analysis of models of carcinogenesis. Br J Cancer 1985; 51(5):707–712.

3. McLaughlin JK, Hrubec Z, Blot WJ, et al. Smoking and cancer mortality among U.S. veterans: a 26-year follow-up. Int J Cancer 1995; 60(2):190–193.

4. Piper JM, Tonascia J, Matanoski GM. Heavy phenacetin use and bladder cancer in women aged 20 to 49 years. N Engl J Med 1985; 313(5):292–295.

5. Travis LB, Curtis RE, Glimelius B, et al. Bladder and kidney cancer following cyclophosphamide therapy for non-Hodgkin's lymphoma. J Natl Cancer Inst 1995; 87(7):524–530.

6. Boice JD Jr, Engholm G, Kleinerman RA, et al. Radiation dose and second cancer risk in patients treated for cancer of the cervix. Radiat Res 1988; 116(1):3–55.

7. Dolin PJ, Cook-Mozaffari P. Occupation and bladder cancer: a death-certificate study. Br J Cancer 1992; 66(3):568–578.

8. Badawi AF, Mostafa MH, Probert A, et al. Role of schistosomiasis in human bladder cancer: evidence of association, aetiological factors, and basic mechanisms of carcinogenesis. Eur J Cancer Prev 1995; 4(1):45–59.

9. Kiemeney LA, Schoenberg, M. Familial transitional cell carcinoma. J Urol 1996; 156(3):867–872.

10. Raghavan D, Shipley WU, Garnick MB, et al. Biology and management of bladder cancer. N Engl J Med 1990; 322(16):1129–1138.

11. Parmar MK. Re: Recurrence of superficial bladder carcinoma after intravesical instillation of Mitomycin-C. Br J Urol 1989; 64(6):659.

12. Kurth KH, Denis L, Bouffioux C, et al. Factors affecting recurrence and progression in superficial bladder tumours. Eur J Cancer 1995; 31a(11):1840–1846.

13. Pawinski A, Sylvester R, Bouffioux C, et al. A combined analysis of EORTC/MRC randomized clinical trials for the prophylactic treatment of TaT1 bladder cancer. Eortc Genito-Urinary Tract Cancer Cooperative Group and the Medical Research Council Working Party on Superficial Bladder Cancer. Acta Urol Belg 1996; 64(2):27.

14. Tolley DA, Parmar MK, Grigor KM, et al. The effect of intravesical mitomycin C on recurrence of newly diagnosed superficial bladder cancer: a further report with 7 years of follow up. J Urol 1996; 155(4):1233–1238.

15. Bouffioux CH, Kurth KH, Bono A, et al. Intravesical adjuvant chemotherapy for superficial transitional cell bladder carcinoma: results of 2 European Organization for Research and Treatment of Cancer randomised trials with mitomycin C and doxorubicin comparing early versus delayed instillations and short-term versus long-term treatment. J Urol 1995; 153(3):934–941.

16. Lamm DL, Griffith JG. The place of intravesical chemotherapy as defined by results of prospective randomized studies (substances and treatment schemes). Prog Clin Biol Res 1992; 378:43–53.

17. Lamm DL. Comparison of BCG with other intravesical agents. Urology 1991; 37(5 Suppl):30–32.

18. Pagano F, Olvia G, Maio G, et al. Surgical treatment of stage I-II testicular cancer. Oncology, München, Sympomed 1992; 2:121–123.

19. Lamm ML, Long DD, Goodwin SM, et al. Transforming growth factor-beta1 inhibits membrane association of protein kinase C alpha in a human prostate cancer cell line, PC3. Endocrinology 1997; 138(11):4657–4564.

20. Abol-Enein H, Bassi P, Boyer M, et al. Neoadjuvant chemotherapy in invasive bladder cancer: a systematic review and meta-analysis. Lancet 2003; 361(9373):1927–1934.

21. Hussain M, Vaishampayan U, Du W, et al. Combination paclitaxel, carboplatin, and gemcitabine is an active treatment for advanced urothelial cancer. J Clin Oncol 2001; 19(9):2527–2533.

22. Coppin CM, Gospodarowicz MK, James K, et al. Improved local control of invasive bladder cancer by concurrent cisplatin and preoperative or definitive radiation. The National Cancer Institute of Canada Clinical Trials Group. J Clin Oncol 1996; 14(11):2901–2907.

23. Sternberg CN, Yagoda A, Scher HI, et al. M-VAC (methotrexate, vinblastine, doxorubicin and cisplatin) for advanced transitional cell carcinoma of the urothelium. J Urol 1988; 139(3):461–469.

24. Harker WG, Meyers FJ, Freiha FS, et al. Cisplatin, methotrexate, and vinblastine (CMV): an effective chemotherapy regimen for metastatic transitional cell carcinoma of the urinary tract. A Northern California Oncology Group Study. J Clin Oncol 1985; 3(11):1463–1470.

25. Sternberg C, de Mulder P, Schornagel J, et al. Randomized phase III trial in advanced urothelial tract tumors of high dose intensity M-VAC chemotherapy and G-CSF versus classic M-VAC. Program/Proc Am Soc Clin Oncol 2000; 19:329a.

26. Loehrer PJ Sr, Einhorn LH, Elson PJ, et al. A randomized comparison of cisplatin alone or in combination with methotrexate, vinblastine, and doxorubicin in patients with metastatic urothelial carcinoma: a cooperative group study [published erratum appears in J Clin Oncol 1993;11(2):384]. J Clin Oncol 1992; 10(7):1066–1073.

27. Mead G, Russell M, Clark P, et al. A randomized trial comparing methotrexate and vinblastine (MV) with cisplatin, methotrexate and vinblastine (CMV) in advanced transitional cell carcinoma: results and

a report on prognostic factors in a Medical Research Council study. Br J Cancer 1998; 78(8):1067–1075.

28. von der Maase H, Hansen SW, Roberts JT, et al. Gemcitabine and cisplatin versus methotrexate, vinblastine, doxorubicin, and cisplatin in advanced or metastatic bladder cancer: results of a large, randomized, multinational, multicenter, phase III study. J Clin Oncol 2000; 17(17):3068–3077.

29. Huddart R, Lau F, Guerrero-Urbano T, et al. Accelerated chemotherapy in the treatment of urothelial cancer. Clin Oncol 2001; 13(4):279–283.

30. Highley M, Griffiths G, Uscinska B, et al. A phase II trial of continuous 5-fluorouracil (5-FU) in recurrent locally advanced or metastatic transitional cell carcinoma of the urinary tract. In: British Cancer Research Meeting (BCRM) 1–4 July 2001, Leeds, UK. BJC; 2001:52.

31. Kalish LA, McDougal WS, McKinlay JB. Family history and the risk of prostate cancer. Urology 2000; 56(5):803–806.

32. Jarvik GP, Stanford JL, Goode EL, et al. Confirmation of prostate cancer susceptibility genes using high-risk families. J Natl Cancer Inst Monogr 1999 26:81–87.

33. Ramon JM, Bou R, Romea S, et al. Dietary fat intake and prostate cancer risk: a case-control study in Spain. Cancer Causes Contr 2000; 11(8):679–685.

34. Gleason DF, Mellinger GT. The Veterans Administration Cooperative. Prediction of prognosis for prostatic adenocarcinoma by combined histological grading and clinical staging. J Urol 1974; 111(1):58–64.

35. Gleason DF. Histologic grading of prostate cancer: a perspective. Hum Pathol 1992; 23(3):273–279.

36. Albertsen P, Gleason D, Barry M. Competing risk analysis of men aged 55 to 74 years at diagnosis managed conservatively for clinically localized prostate cancer. JAMA 1998; 280:975–980.

37. Chodak GW, Thisted RA, Gerber GS, et al. Results of conservative management of clinically localised prostate cancer. N Engl J Med 1994; 330(4):242–248.

38. Zincke H, Bergstralh EJ, Blute ML, et al. Radical prostatectomy for clinically localized prostate cancer: long-term results of 1,143 patients from a single institution. J Clin Oncol 1994; 12(11):2254–2263.

39. D'Amico AV, Whittington R, Malkowicz SB. Biochemical outcome after radical prostatectomy, external beam radiation therapy or interstitial radiation therapy for clinically localised prostate cancer. JAMA 1998; 280:969–974.

40. Pilepich MV, Krall JM, al Sarraf M, et al. Androgen deprivation with radiation therapy compared with radiation therapy alone for locally advanced prostatic carcinoma: a randomized comparative trial of the Radiation Therapy Oncology Group. Urology 1995; 45(4):616–623.

41. Pilepich MV, Bagshaw MA, Asbell SO, et al. Definitive radiotherapy in resectable (stage A2 and B) carcinoma of the prostate – results of a nationwide overview. Int J Radiat Oncol Biol Phys 1987; 13(5):659–663.

42. Wallner KE, Roy J, Harrison L. Tumour control and morbidity following transperineal Iodine[125] implantation for stage T1/T2 prostate carcinoma. Int J Radiat Oncol Biol Phys 1996; 14(2):449–453.

43. Roach M 3rd, DeSilvio M, Lawton C, et al. Phase III trial comparing whole-pelvic versus prostate-only radiotherapy and neoadjuvant versus adjuvant combined androgen suppression: Radiation Therapy Oncology Group 9413. J Clin Oncol 2003; 21(10):1904–1911.

44. Bolla M, Gonzalez D, Warde P, et al. Improved survival in patients with locally advanced prostate cancer treated with radiotherapy and goserelin (see comments). N Engl J Med 1997; 337(5):295–300.

45. Pilepich MV, Caplan R, Byhardt RW, et al. Phase III trial of androgen suppression using goserelin in unfavorable-prognosis carcinoma of the prostate treated with definitive radiotherapy: report of Radiation Therapy Oncology Group protocol 85-31. J Clin Oncol 1997; 15(3):1013–1021.

46. Pilepich MV, Winter K, Lawton C, et al. Phase III trial of androgen suppression adjuvant to definitive radiotherapy. Long term results of RTOG study 85-31. In: ASCO 2003 Proc Thirty-Ninth Annual Meeting, May 31–June 3, 2003, Chicago, Illinois: JCO:381.

47. Do T, Parker RG, Do C, et al. Salvage radiotherapy for biochemical and clinical failures following radical prostatectomy. Cancer J Sci Am 1998; 4(5):324–330.

48. Traynor A. Recent advances in hormonal therapy for cancer. Curr Opin Oncol 1995; 7(6):572–581.

49. Kirk D. CTSU. Immediate versus deferred treatment for advanced prostatic cancer: initial results of the Medical Research Council Trial. The Medical Research Council Prostate Cancer Working Party Investigators Group. Br J Urol 1997; 79(2):235–246.

50. Kirk D. Re: A structured debate: immediate versus deferred androgen suppression in prostate cancer – evidence for deferred treatment. J Urol 2002; 167(2 Pt 1):652; author reply 653.

51. Boccardo F, Rubagotti A, Garofalo L, et al. Tamoxifen (T) is more effective than anastrozole (A) in preventing gynecomastia induced by bicalutamide (B) monotherapy in prostate cancer (pca) patients (pts). In: American Society of Clinical Oncology (ASCO), Thirty-Ninth Annual Meeting, May 31–June 3, 2003; Chicago, Illinois. JCO; 2003:400.

52. Waterfall NB, Glaser MG. A study of the effects of radiation on prevention of gynaecomastia due to oestrogen therapy. Clin Oncol 1979; 5(3):257–260.

53. Prostate Cancer Trialists Collaborative Group (Dearnaley DP member). Maximum androgen blockade in advanced prostate cancer: an overview of the randomised trials. Lancet 2000; 355(9214): 1491–1498.

54. Schellhammer PF, Venner P, Haas GP, et al. Prostate specific antigen decreases after withdrawal of anti-androgen therapy with bicalutamide or flutamide in patients receiving combined androgen blockade. J Urol 1997; 157(5):1731–1735.

55. Sartor O, Weinberger M, Moore A, et al. Effect of prednisone on prostate-specific antigen in patients with hormone-refractory prostate cancer. Urology 1998; 52(2):252–256.

56. Fossa SD, Slee PH, Brausi M, et al. Flutamide versus prednisone in patients with prostate cancer symptomatically progressing after androgen-ablative therapy: a phase III study of the European organization for research and treatment of cancer genitourinary group. J Clin Oncol 2001; 19(1):62–71.

57. Farrugia D, Ansell W, Singh M, et al. Stilboestrol plus adrenal suppression as salvage treatment for patients failing treatment with luteinizing hormone-releasing hormone analogues and orchidectomy. BJU Int 2000; 85(9):1069–1073.

58. Smith DC, Redman BG, Flaherty LE, et al. A phase II trial of oral diethylstilbesterol as a second-line hormonal agent in advanced prostate cancer. Urology 1998;52(2):257–260.

59. Shahidi M, Norman A, Gadd J, et al. Prospective review of diethylstilbestrol in advanced prostate cancer no longer responding to androgen suppression. In: ASCO Thirty-Seventh Annual Meeting, May 12–15, 2001. San Francisco, CA; 2001:176b.

60. Tannock IF, Osoba D, Stockler MR, et al. Chemotherapy with mitroxantrone plus prednisone or prednisone alone for symptomatic hormone-resistant prostate cancer: a Canadian randomised trial with palliative end points. J Clin Oncol 1996; 14(6):1756–1764.

61. Hudes G, Einhorn L, Ross E, et al. Vinblastine versus vinblastine plus oral estramustine phosphate for patients with hormone-refractory prostate cancer: A Hoosier Oncology Group and Fox Chase Network phase III trial. J Clin Oncol 1999; 17(10):3160–3166.

62. Beer TM, Pierce WC, Lowe BA, et al. Phase II study of weekly docetaxel in symptomatic androgen-independent prostate cancer. Ann Oncol 2001; 12(9):1273–1279.

63. Berry W, Dakhil S, Gregurich MA, et al. Phase II trial of single-agent weekly docetaxel in hormone-refractory, symptomatic, metastatic carcinoma of the prostate. Semin Oncol 2001; 28(4 Suppl 15):8–15.

64. Picus J, Schultz M. Docetaxel (Taxotere) as monotherapy in the treatment of hormone-refractory prostate cancer: preliminary results. Semin Oncol 1999; 26(5 Suppl 17):14–18.

65. Petrylak DP, Macarthur R, O'Connor J, et al. Phase I/II studies of docetaxel (Taxotere) combined with estramustine in men with hormone-refractory prostate cancer. Semin Oncol 1999; 26(5 Suppl 17):28–33.

66. Heidenreich A, Hofmann R, Engelmann UH. The use of bisphosphonate for the palliative treatment of painful bone metastasis due to hormone refractory prostate cancer. J Urol 2001; 165(1):136–140.

67. Garfield D. New bisphosphonate shows promise in bone metastases. Lancet Oncol 2001; 2(9):525.

68. Dearnaley D, Sydes M, on behalf of the MRC PR05 collaborators; The Institute of Cancer Research, Sutton, UK; MRC Clinical Trials Unit, London, UK.

Preliminary evidence that oral clodronate delays symptomatic progression of bone metastases from prostate cancer: first results of the MRC Pr05 Trial. In: ASCO Thirty-Seventh Annual Meeting; May 12–15, 2001, San Francisco, CA. Program/Proceedings of ASCO, Part 1 of 2; 2001:174a.

69. Quilty PM, Kirk D, Bolger JJ, et al. A comparison of the palliative effects of strontium-89 and external beam radiotherapy in metastatic prostate cancer. Rad Oncol 1994; 31:33–40.

70. Tu SM, Millikan RE, Mengistu B, et al. Bone-targeted therapy for advanced androgen-independent carcinoma of the prostate: a randomised phase II trial. Lancet 2001; 357(9253):336–341.

71. Warde P, Specht L, Horwich A, et al. Prognostic factors for relapse in stage I seminoma managed by surveillance: a pooled analysis. J Clin Oncol 2002; 20(22):4448–4452.

72. Jones W, Fossa S, Meas G, et al. A randomised trial of two radiotherapy schedules in the adjuvant of stage I seminoma (MRC TE18) – preliminary report. In: Germ cell tumours V. London: Springer; 2002:235–236.

73. Oliver RTD, Edmonds PM, Ong JYH, et al. Pilot studies of 2 and 1 course carboplatin as adjuvant for stage I seminoma: should it be tested in a randomized trial against radiotherapy? Int J Radiat Oncol Biol Phys 1994; 29(1):3–8.

74. Read G, Stenning SP, Cullen MH, et al. Medical Research Council prospective study of surveillance for stage I testicular teratoma. Medical Research Council Testicular Tumors Working Party. J Clin Oncol 1992; 10(11):1762–1768.

75. Cullen MH, Stenning SP, Parkinson MC, et al. Short-course adjuvant chemotherapy in high-risk stage I nonseminomatous germ cell tumors of the testis: A Medical Research Council report. J Clin Oncol 1996; 14(4):1106–1113.

76. Dearnaley D, Fossa S, Kaye S, et al. Adjuvant bleomycin, vincristine and cisplatin (BOP) for high risk clinical stage I (HRCS1) non-seminomatous germ cell tumours (NSGCT) – A Medical Research Council (MRC) pilot study. In: ASCO Thirty-Fourth Annual Meeting, May 16–19, 1998, Los Angeles, CA: ASCO Program/Proceedings; 1998:309a.

77. Patterson H, Norman A, Mitra S, et al. Combination carboplatin and radiotherapy in the management of Stage II testicular seminoma: comparison with radiotherapy treatment alone. Radiother Oncol 2001; 59(1):5–11.

78. Gregory C, Peckham MJ. Results of radiotherapy for stage II testicular seminoma. Radiother Oncol 1986; 6(4):285–292.

79. Simpson A, Paul J, Graham J, et al. Fatal bleomycin pulmonary toxicity in the west of Scotland 1991–1995: a review of patients with germ cell tumours. BJC 1998; 78(8):1061–1066.

80. O'Sullivan JM, Huddart RA, Norman AR, et al. Predicting the risk of bleomycin lung toxicity in patients with germ-cell tumours. Ann Oncol 2003; 14(1):91–96.

81. Horwich A, Oliver R, Wilkinson P, et al. A Medical Research Council randomized trial of single agent carboplatin versus etoposide and cisplatin for advanced metastatic seminoma. B J Cancer 2000; 83(12):1623–1629.

82. de Wit R, Roberts J, Wilkinson P, et al. Equivalence of three or four cycles of bleomycin, etoposide, and cisplatin chemotherapy and of a 3- or 5-day schedule in good-prognosis germ cell cancer: a randomized study of the European Organization for Research and Treatment of Cancer Genitourinary Tract Cancer Cooperative Group and the Medical Research Council. J Clin Oncol 2001; 19(6):1629–1640.

83. Toner GC, Stockler MR, Boyer MJ, et al. Comparison of two standard chemotherapy regimens for good-prognosis germ-cell tumours: a randomised trial. Australian and New Zealand Germ Cell Trial Group. Lancet 2001; 357(9258):739–745.

84. Loehrer PJ, Johnson D, Elson P, et al. Importance of bleomycin in favourable-prognosis disseminated germ cell tumors: an Eastern Cooperative Oncology Group Trial. J Clin Oncol 1995; 13(2):470–476.

85. Levi J, Raghaven D, Harvey V, et al. The importance of bleomycin in combination chemotherapy for good prognosis germ cell carcinoma. J Clin Oncol 1993; 11(7):1300–1305.

86. Nichols CR, Catalano PJ, Crawford ED, et al. Randomized comparison of cisplatin and etoposide and either bleomycin or ifosfamide in treatment of advanced disseminated germ cell tumors: an Eastern Cooperative Oncology Group, Southwest Oncology Group, and Cancer and Leukemia Group B Study. J Clin Oncol 1998; 16(4):1287–1293.

87. Horwich A, Sleijfer DT, Fossa SD, et al. Randomized trial of bleomycin, etoposide, and cisplatin compared with bleomycin, etoposide, and carboplatin in good-prognosis metastatic nonseminomatous germ cell cancer: a Multiinstitutional Medical Research Council/European Organization for Research and Treatment of Cancer Trial. J Clin Oncol 1997; 15(5):1844–1852.

88. Hendry W, Norman A, Dearnaley D, et al. Metastatic nonseminomatous germ cell tumours of the testis – results of elective and salvage surgery for patients with residual retroperitoneal masses. Cancer 2002; 94(6):1668–1676.

89. Parkin DM, Pisani P, Ferlay J. Estimates of the worldwide incidence of 25 major cancers in 1990. Int J Cancer JID – 0042124, 1999; 80:827–841.

90. Katz DL, Zheng T, Holford TR, et al. Time trends in the incidence of renal carcinoma: analysis of Connecticut Tumor Registry data, 1935–1989. Int J Cancer 1994; 58:57-63.

91. Chow WH, Devesa SS, Warren JL, et al. Rising incidence of renal cell cancer in the United States. JAMA JID – 7501160, 1999; 281:1628–1631.

92. Doll R, Peto R. The causes of cancer: quantitative estimates of avoidable risks of cancer in the United States today. J Natl Cancer Inst 1981; 66:1191–1308.

93. Moyad MA. Review of potential risk factors for kidney (renal cell) cancer. Semin Urolog Oncol 2001; 19:280–293.

94. Latif F, Tory K, Gnarra J, et al. Identification of the von Hippel–Lindau disease tumor suppressor gene. Science 1993; 260:1317–1320.

95. Melmon KL, Rosen SW. Lindau's disease. Am J Med 1964; 36:595–617.

96. Kovacs G, Akhtar M, Beckwith BJ, et al. The Heidelberg classification of renal cell tumours. J Pathol 1997; 183:131–133.

97. Storkel S, Eble JN, Adlakha K, et al. Classification of renal cell carcinoma: Workgroup No. 1. Union Internationale Contre le Cancer (UICC) and the American Joint Committee on Cancer (AJCC). Cancer 1997; 80:987–989.

98. Ljungberg B, Alamdari FI, Stenling R, et al. Prognostic significance of the Heidelberg classification of renal cell carcinoma. Eur Urol 1999; 36:565–569.

99. de Peralta-Venturina M, Moch H, Amin M, et al. Sarcomatoid differentiation in renal cell carcinoma: a study of 101 cases. Am J Surg Pathol 2001; 25:275–284.

100. Zambrano NR, Lubensky IA, Merino MJ, et al. Histopathology and molecular genetics of renal tumors toward unification of a classification system. J Urol 1999; 162:1246–1258.

101. Fuhrman SA, Lasky LC, Limas C. Prognostic significance of morphologic parameters in renal cell carcinoma. Am J Surg Pathol 1982; 6:655–663.

102. Bretheau D, Lechevallier E, de Fromont M, et al. Prognostic value of nuclear grade of renal cell carcinoma. Cancer 1995; 76:2543–2549.

103. Delahunt B, Nacey JN. Renal cell carcinoma. II. Histological indicators of prognosis. Pathology 1987; 19:258–263.

104. Siow WY, Yip SK, Ng LG, et al. Renal cell carcinoma: incidental detection and pathological staging. J R Coll Surg Edinb 2000; 45:291–295.

105. Motzer RJ, Mazumdar M, Bacik J, et al. Survival and prognostic stratification of 670 patients with advanced renal cell carcinoma. J Clin Oncol 1999; 17:2530–2540.

106. Skinner DG, Colvin RB, Vermillion CD, et al. Diagnosis and management of renal cell carcinoma. A clinical and pathologic study of 309 cases. Cancer 1971; 28:1165–1177.

107. Rabinovitch RA, Zelefsky MJ, Gaynor JJ, et al. Patterns of failure following surgical resection of renal cell carcinoma: implications for adjuvant local and systemic therapy. J Clin Oncol 1994; 12:206–212.

108. Lokich J. Spontaneous regression of metastatic renal cancer. Case report and literature review. Am J Clin Oncol 1997; 20:416–418.

109. Mims MM, Christenson B, Schlumberger FC, et al. A 10-year evaluation of nephrectomy for extensive renal-cell carcinoma. J Urol 1966; 95:10–15.

110. Motzer RJ, Mazumdar M, Bacik J, et al. (2000) Effect of cytokine therapy on survival for patients with advanced renal cell carcinoma. J Clin Oncol 2000; 18:1928–1935.

111. Flanigan RC, Salmon SE, Blumenstein BA, et al. Nephrectomy followed by interferon alfa-2b compared with interferon alfa-2b alone for metastatic renal-cell cancer. N Engl J Med 2001; 345:1655–1659.

112. O'Dea, MJ, Zincke H, Utz DC, et al. The treatment of renal cell carcinoma with solitary metastasis. J Urol 1978; 120:540–542.

113. Halperin EC, Harisiadis L. The role of radiation therapy in the management of metastatic renal cell carcinoma. Cancer 1983; 51:614–617.

114. Yagoda A, Abi-Rached B, Petrylak D. Chemotherapy for advanced renal-cell carcinoma: 1983–1993. Semin Oncol 1995; 22:42–60.

115. Rini BI, Vogelzang NJ, Dumas MC, et al. Phase II trial of weekly intravenous gemcitabine with continuous infusion fluorouracil in patients with metastatic renal cell cancer. J Clin Oncol 2000; 18:2419–2426.

116. Eisen T. Thalidomide in solid malignancies. J Clin Oncol 2002; 20:2607–2609.

117. MRC Collaborators. Interferon-alpha and survival in metastatic renal carcinoma: early results of a randomised controlled trial. Medical Research Council Renal Cancer Collaborators. Lancet 1999; 353:14–17.

118. Hernberg M, Pyrhonen S, Muhonen T. Regimens with or without interferon-alpha as treatment for metastatic melanoma and renal cell carcinoma: an overview of randomized trials. J Immunother 1999; 22:145–154.

119. Negrier S, Escudier B, Lasset C, et al. Recombinant human interleukin-2, recombinant human interferon alfa-2a, or both in metastatic renal-cell carcinoma. Groupe Francais d'Immunotherapie. N Engl J Med 1998; 338:1272–1278.

120. Atzpodien J, Kirchner H, Hanninen EL, et al. Interleukin-2 in combination with interferon-alpha and 5-fluorouracil for metastatic renal cell cancer. Eur J Cancer 1993; 29A(Suppl 5): S6–S8.

121. Atzpodien J, Kirchner H, Fuhrman SA. Results of a randomised clinical trial comparing sc Interleukin-2, sc Interferon-alpha and bolus iv 5-flourouracil against oral tamoxifen in progressive metastatic renal cell carcinoma. Proc Am Soc Clin Oncol 1997; 16:1164.

122. Allen MJ, Vaughan M, Webb A, et al. Protracted venous infusion 5-fluorouracil in combination with subcutaneous interleukin-2 and alpha-interferon in patients with metastatic renal cell cancer: a phase II study. Br J Cancer 2000; 83:980–985.

123. O'Rourke M. Genitourinary cancers. In: Otto SE, ed. Oncology nursing. 4th edn. St Louis: Mosby; 2001.

124. Chaudhary U, Haldas J. Long term complications of chemotherapy for germ cell tumours. Drugs 2003; 63(15):1565–1577.

125. Lamb M. Effects of cancer on the sexuality and fertility of women. Semin Oncol Nurs 1995; 11(2):120–127.

126. Foster R. Fertility issues in patients with cancer. Cancer Nurs Pract 2002; 1(1):26–30.

127. Davies C. The impact of cancer treatment on male fertility. Cancer Nurs Pract 2003; 2(4):25–31.

128. Shrover L. Sexuality and fertility after cancer. New York: John Wiley and Sons; 1997.

129. Joly F, Heron JF, Kalusinski L, et al. Quality of life in long-term survivors of testicular cancer: a population-based case-control study. J Clin Oncol 2002; 20(1):73–80.

130. Jenkins M, Ashley J. Sex and the oncology patient. Discussing sexual dysfunction helps the patient optimize quality of life. Am J Nurs 2002; 102(Suppl 4):13–15.

131. Ozen H, Sahin A, Toklu C, et al. Psychosocial adjustment after testicular cancer treatment. J Urol 1998; 159(6):1947–1950.

132. Clark A, Jones P, Newbold S. Practice development in cancer care: self help for men with testicular cancer. Nurs Stand 2002; 14(50):41–46.

133. Moynihan C. Strength in silence. The Guardian 20th October 1998.

134. Boy D, Carl P. Acceptance of silicone testicular prostheses in long term follow up. Urologe 2002; 41(5):462–469 [in German].

135. Herr H. Quality of life of incontinent men after radical prostatectomy. J Urol 1994; 151(3):652–654.

136. Fann A. Psychological and psychosocial effects of prostate cancer. Nurs Stand 2002; 17 (13):33–37.

137. Salter M. Altered body image. The nurse's role. London: Baillière Tindall; 1997.

Chapter **42**

Chemotherapy for cancers of the head and neck

CHAPTER CONTENTS

MEDICAL CARE FOR PATIENTS WITH HEAD AND NECK CANCERS

Paul J Ross, Kevin J Harrington and Martin Gore

INTRODUCTION

Cancers of the head and neck are a varied group, being the sixth commonest type of malignancy worldwide.[1] Squamous cell carcinoma is the most common histological subtype of tumour, occurring in the head and neck region, with approximately 400 000 cases per annum worldwide.[2] The principal sites of involvement with squamous carcinoma are the oral cavity and larynx.[3] Other histological subtypes considered in this chapter are undifferentiated carcinomas of nasopharyngeal type (UCNT) and adenoid cystic carcinomas of salivary glands.

Cancers of the head and neck region account for approximately 3% of all new cases of malignant disease in the USA,[1] and 4% in the United Kingdom. However, there is significant global variation in the incidence of head and neck cancers. High rates are observed in India (30% of cancer in males; 13% in females) and Southeast Asia.[1] In Korea cancers of the head and neck account for 14% of cancers in men and 10% of cancers in women.[1] In addition, incidence rates can vary between different regions of one country. In Austria, cancers of the oral cavity and oropharynx are higher in rural than in urban areas. In Italy head and neck cancer is more common in the northern than central and southern parts of the country.

Aetiology of squamous head and neck cancer

The most important aetiological factor for squamous head and neck cancer is smoking or chewing tobacco.

Alcohol, particularly spirit ingestion, is also an important aetiological factor and these two factors are synergistic. Betel nut and paan chewing is an important aetiological factor in India. Other less important aetiological factors include dental and mechanical trauma, and the Plummer–Vinson (Paterson–Kelly) syndrome. Premalignant lesions, including leukoplakia and erythroplakia, carry an increased risk of the development of head and neck cancer. Many head and neck cancers are associated with somatic mutations, including mutations of the *p53* tumour suppressor gene. Growth factor overexpression is frequently involved in carcinogenesis with amplification and/or gene rearrangement of the epidermal growth factor receptor (*EGFR*, *c-erb B-2*). Other oncogenes observed to be mutated or overexpressed in squamous head and neck cancer include *EMS1*, *erb B-3*, *Prad-1* (cyclin D1), *Hst-1*, *Int-2*, *c-myc*, and the *ras* gene family. In addition, patients with a number of inheritable syndromes are at increased risk of head and neck cancer (Box 42.1). Viral infection may also have a role in squamous head and neck cancer. Human papillomaviruses (HPV) are identified in both benign and malignant lesions of the upper aerodigestive tract. Certain HPV subtypes, such as 6, 11, 16, 18, 30, 31 and 33, are associated with head and neck cancer. Furthermore, patients with human immunodeficiency virus (HIV) infection are at increased risk for the development of squamous cell carcinomas. (See also Ch. 1.)

Aetiology of undifferentiated nasopharyngeal cancers

There are also significant differences in the global incidence of UCNT; it is particularly common in Hong Kong and South China, whereas in Taiwan it is the most common cause of death in males. It is also common in the Philippines, Malaysia, Greenland, Malta, North Africa and Saudi Arabia.[4] In the remainder of the world, UCNT is rare, with an incidence rate of less than 1/100 000 per annum. Furthermore, there appears to be a bimodal age distribution, with 20% of all cases (in high-prevalence areas) occurring in patients under 30 years old. A number of possible dietary causes have been identified, including consumption of salted fish, particularly in childhood. Other possible dietary factors include deficient intake of fresh fruit and vegetables, consumption of salted and preserved plums, fermented fish sauce and preserved shrimp paste. Apart from the possible dietary causes, it is known that patients have evidence of Epstein–Barr virus (EBV) in the epithelial tumour cells.[5] This is associated with elevated EBV titres of immunoglobulin A (IgA) viral capsid antigen and IgA early antigen. In addition, recent studies have demonstrated that tumour-derived EBV DNA can be detected in the plasma and serum of patients with UCNT and that this can be used as a tumour marker.

STAGING

The AJCC/UICC (American Joint Committee on Cancer/Union Internationale Contre le Cancer) staging system is based on primary tumour characteristics (T), lymph node involvement (N) and the presence of distant metastasis (M).[6] This system has been facilitated by the adoption of the same staging notation for lymph node spread regardless of the primary head and neck site (except for nasopharyngeal tumours where a different system is used) (Box 42.2). Unfortunately, this uniformity has not been possible for staging of the primary tumour and the reader is referred to the AJCC Cancer Staging Manual for details.

INVESTIGATION

Staging should include inspection of the primary site, with measurement of its dimensions and examination for direct extension into adjacent tissues and local lymph node areas. Most patients require both outpatient nasendoscopy and an examination under anaesthetic, with direct endoscopic, evaluation. Biopsies should be taken from any obvious primary lesion, areas of field change and, in the case of an occult primary tumour, the most likely sites (nasopharynx, tongue base, tonsil and pyriform fossa).

Computed tomography (CT) is the predominant imaging tool for patients with head and neck cancer.[7] Magnetic resonance imaging (MRI) may provide supplemental information and is particularly useful for evaluating perineural tumour spread and for the determination of the submucosal extent of a pharyngeal tumour when its margins are not entirely clear on CT scan. MRI is used preferentially for imaging nasopharyngeal cancers, and when intracranial structures are at risk. Haematogenous spread is uncommon at presentation, but most frequently involves the lungs. Consequently, the chest should be imaged with a plain

---

Box 42.1	**Inheritable syndromes associated with an increased risk of head and neck cancer**[1]

Lynch type II syndrome
Bloom's syndrome
Fanconi's anaemia
Xeroderma pigmentosum
Ataxia telangiectasia
Li–Fraumeni syndrome

Box 42.2 Staging of nodes and metastases in head and neck cancer

N_x Regional lymph node cannot be assessed
N_0 No regional lymph node metastasis
N_1 Metastasis in a single ipsilateral lymph node, 3 cm or less in greatest dimension
N_2 Metastasis in a single ipsilateral lymph node, more than 3 cm but not more than 6 cm in greatest dimension, or multiple ipsilateral lymph nodes, none more than 6 cm in greatest dimension, or in bilateral or contralateral lymph nodes, none more than 6 cm in greatest dimension
N_{2a} Metastasis in a single ipsilateral lymph node, more than 3 cm but not more than 6 cm in greatest dimension
N_{2b} Metastasis in multiple ipsilateral lymph nodes, not more than 6 cm in greatest dimension
N_{2c} Metastasis in bilateral or contralateral lymph nodes, none more than 6 cm in greatest dimension
N_3 Metastasis in a lymph node more than 6 cm in greatest dimension
M_x Presence of distant metastasis cannot be assessed
M_0 No distant metastasis
M_1 Distant metastasis

chest radiograph, or preferably CT scan. A full blood count, urea and electrolytes and liver function tests should also be performed. In patients with a diagnosis of UCNT, liver ultrasound and bone scan are mandatory.

CHEMOTHERAPY FOR SQUAMOUS CELL CANCER OF THE HEAD AND NECK

Chemotherapy in the management of locoregional head and neck cancer

Surgery and/or radiotherapy are the mainstay of locoregional treatment, with attitudes to cytotoxic chemotherapy ranging from enthusiasm[8] to disdain.[9,10] Despite more than 70 randomised trials involving over 12 000 patients, the benefits of adding chemotherapy to locoregional treatment of head and neck cancer are unresolved. However, most of the randomised trials evaluating this subject were too small to detect even a moderate effect on survival.[11] In an effort to determine the role of chemotherapy in locoregional head and neck cancer, three separate meta-analyses have been published during the 1990s.[11-13]

Meta-analyses of chemotherapy trials

Meta-analyses assessing the role of chemotherapy in locoregional head and neck cancer were published in 1995 and 1996.[12,13] These largely included the same patients from the same trials. Both meta-analyses concluded that there was a small but significant reduction in the risk of death with chemotherapy (Table 42.1). There was significant heterogeneity between the

Table 42.1 Meta-analyses of chemotherapy trials [11-13]

Reference		Number of trials	Number of patients	Hazard ratio	95% CI	p	Absolute benefit	
							At 2 years	At 5 years
12	Overall	54	7,443	0.73	0.86–0.81	NR	NR	NR
	Concomitant	16	2,506	0.56	0.48–0.66	NR	NR	NR
	Neoadjuvant	28	4,141	0.83	0.74–0.96	NR	NR	NR
13	Overall	42	5,079					
	Available for survival	25	3,708	0.99	0.81–0.99	<0.05	NR	NR
	Concomitant	11		0.78	0.67–0.92	<0.005	NR	NR
	Neoadjuvant			0.95	0.83–1.10	NS	NR	NR
11	Overall	63	10,741	0.9	0.8–0.94	<0.0001	4%	4%
	Concomitant	26	3,727	0.81	0.76	<0.0001	7%	8%
	Neoadjuvant			0.95	0.88–1.01	0.10	2%	2%
	Adjuvant			0.98	0.85–1.19	0.74	1%	1%

NR, not reported; NS, not significant.

studies included in both analyses. However, both observed that chemotherapy given concomitantly with radiotherapy improves survival compared to locoregional treatment alone, whereas neoadjuvant treatment was less effective (see Table 42.1).

The analysis by El-Sayed and Nelson also demonstrated that there was an increase in toxicity with the addition of chemotherapy (Table 42.2).[13] Subsequent to these two meta-analyses, Henk[14] reviewed the acute and late radiation morbidity of the 19 publications of trials of concurrent chemoradiotherapy reviewed by Munro.[12] These 19 trials included 3 using multi-agent chemotherapy and 16 using single agent chemotherapy. In 17 trials the same dose of radiotherapy was given with or without chemotherapy; in 2 an effectively lower radiation dose was given in the chemotherapy group. Chemotherapy resulted in increased acute toxicity (odds ratio 2.86; $p <0.001$) in all but 2 trials, and this was significant in 6 trials (Table 42.3). In addition, late toxicity was increased (odds ratio 1.82; $p <0.05$).

The most comprehensive study conducted by the Meta-Analysis of Chemotherapy on Head and Neck Cancer (MACH-NC) collaborative group reported in 2000.[11] This meta-analysis addressed three questions:

1. What was the effect of the addition of chemotherapy to locoregional treatment on survival?
2. What was the effect of the timing of the chemotherapy?
3. Did neoadjuvant chemotherapy permit laryngeal preservation?

Trials were eligible if recruitment began after 1 January 1965 and completed before 31 December 1993. The first meta-analysis included 63 trials involving 10 741 patients. Survival was significantly improved with the addition of chemotherapy (see Table 42.1). As with the previous meta-analyses, adjuvant and neoadjuvant chemotherapy were not observed to have

Table 42.3   Acute and late toxicity from concurrent chemoradiation[14]

Drug	Acute toxicity	Late toxicity
5-Fluorouracil	2.63 (1.58–4.37)	2.14 (0.39–11.67)
Bleomycin	6.92 (4.01–11.94)	4.88 (0.63–37.8)
Methotrexate	2.38 (1.19–4.75)	1.48 (0.64–3.44)
Cisplatin	2.58 (0.73–9.15)	No data
Mitomycin C	0.42 (0.16–1.15)	1.15 (0.43–3.03)
Overall	2.86 (2.15–3.81)	1.82 (1.02–3.26)
p value	<0.001	<0.05

a significant effect on survival (see Table 42.1). In contrast, concomitant therapy resulted in a significant improvement in survival (see Table 42.1). However, considerable heterogeneity was found between the trials of concomitant chemoradiotherapy. One relatively homogeneous group was identified of 12 trials (2516 patients) with conventional radiotherapy as locoregional treatment and the same dose in the two arms. In this group the hazard ratio for death was 0.89 (95% CI 0.81–0.97). A second heterogeneous group of 14 trials (1211 patients) used various study designs: surgery plus preoperative radiotherapy or postoperative radiotherapy with or without concomitant chemotherapy (5 trials); a lower effective dose of radiotherapy in the chemotherapy arm (7 trials, 2 confounded); chemotherapy alternated with radiotherapy (4 trials, 2 confounded). This group had a hazard ratio of 0.67 (95% CI 0.59–0.77). Thus, the survival benefit from chemotherapy resulted from this small group of concomitant trials evaluating a variety of treatments. Nonetheless, the findings are consistent with previous meta-analyses. In addition, a further 18 trials including approximately 5000 patients are either in progress or have closed since 1994 and will further define the benefits of concomitant chemoradiotherapy.

The concomitant trials were also grouped by the MACH–NC collaborative group into single agent chemotherapy (17 trials, 2634 patients) vs polychemotherapy (9 trials, 1093 patients). The effect of concomitant chemoradiotherapy was significantly greater with polychemotherapy than with single agent chemotherapy (hazard ratio 0.69 vs 0.87). However, there was a non-significant increase in the risk of death with platinum-containing polychemotherapy, but not with polychemotherapy without platinum. Furthermore, no such increase in risk of death was observed with 5-fluorouracil (5-FU) and platinum combinations. Thus, this trial does not clearly identify the optimal choice of concomitant chemotherapy regimen.

Table 42.2   Relative risks of toxicity with addition of chemotherapy to locoregional treatment of head and neck cancer[13]

Toxicity	Relative risk of occurrence	p
Nausea	77	<0.001
Mucositis	3.0	<0.001
Skin reaction	1.4	0.010
Delayed radiotherapy	2.9	<0.001
Treatment-related death	2.4	<0.001
Bone marrow toxicity	16	<0.001
Overall toxicity	2.2	<0.001

The second meta-analysis conducted by the MACH-NC collaborative group examined the timing of chemotherapy. Six trials, involving 861 patients, that compared neoadjuvant with or without adjuvant chemotherapy plus radiotherapy to concomitant or alternating chemoradiotherapy were included in this analysis. This analysis also showed a trend towards improved survival, with alternating or concomitant chemoradiation (hazard ratio 0.91, 95% CI 0.79–1.06) but this did not reach statistical significance ($p = 0.23$).

Finally, the MACH-NC collaborative group examined the role of chemotherapy in larynx preservation. Three trials, including 602 patients, compared radical surgery plus radiotherapy to neoadjuvant chemotherapy with cisplatin and 5-FU followed by radiotherapy in responders or radical surgery plus radiotherapy in non-responders. In contrast to other results, a non-significant trend in favour of radical surgery was observed (hazard ratio 1.19, 95% CI 0.97–1.46; $p = 0.1$).

New directions in chemoradiotherapy for head and neck cancer

The data reviewed above make a compelling case for the use of concomitant chemoradiation in the primary management of locally advanced squamous cell head and neck cancer. Indeed, in many centres this approach is now accepted as the standard of care. Nonetheless, there remain significant uncertainties about the optimal means of integrating concomitant chemoradiotherapy into current practice. The issues can be summarised as follows:

Chemoradiotherapy in the context of altered radiotherapy fractionation regimens   Most of the published trials of concomitant chemoradiotherapy have been conducted using conventional radiation fractionation schedules (2 Gy per day, 5 days a week to a total dose of 64–72 Gy). However, a recent phase III study from the Radiation Therapy Oncology Group (RTOG) has reported the results of a comparison between conventional fractionation and three altered fractionation regimens in patients with head and neck cancer. The conventional regimen was shown to be inferior to two of the altered fractionation regimens (hyperfractionation to 81.6 Gy in 68 fractions of 1.2 Gy twice daily; concomitant boost radiotherapy to 72 Gy in 42 fractions of 1.8 Gy per fraction plus a second daily fraction of 1.5 Gy in the last 12 treatment days).[15] As a consequence, a new series of trials will need to be conducted looking at the integration of chemotherapy into these altered fractionation regimens. An early report of the use of concomitant cisplatin (6 mg/m²/day) in patients receiving hyperfractionated radiotherapy

(77 Gy in 70 fractions over 7 weeks) has demonstrated a progression-free survival advantage at 5 years.[16]

Neoadjuvant chemotherapy followed by chemoradiotherapy   Despite the findings detailed above relating to the use of neoadjuvant chemotherapy before radical radiotherapy, there is increasing interest in the use of chemotherapy before embarking on a full course of radical chemoradiotherapy. At present, at the Royal Marsden Hospital, patients with locally advanced stage III and IV disease receive two cycles of induction chemotherapy (cisplatin 75 mg/m² on day 1, 5-FU 1 g/m² on days 1–4) followed by radical radiotherapy using concomitant chemotherapy (cisplatin 100 mg/m²) on days 1 and 29. It is likely that this approach will receive increasing attention in future study design.

Introduction of new cytotoxic agents into chemoradiotherapy practice   As presented above, the studies of concomitant chemoradiotherapy have employed a limited number of drugs. In recent years there has been a general acceptance that cisplatin (or carboplatin) should be included in these regimens. However, a number of newer cytotoxic agents may yield an improved degree of activity with radiation and are currently the subject of active study. Taxanes (paclitaxel, docetaxel), irinotecan and gemcitabine have all been shown to be active against head and neck cancer and to enhance the radiation response.[17] The integration of these agents into existing and altered fractionation radiotherapy schedules and definition of the associated toxicity and efficacy end points will be a major challenge for the future.

Introduction of novel agents into chemoradiotherapy practice   Elucidation of the underlying molecular biology of head and neck cancer is opening the way for novel targeted therapy approaches to this disease. For example, dysregulation of normal epidermal growth factor receptor-mediated signalling has been implicated in head and neck cancer progression. This pathway can be blocked by monoclonal antibodies (IMC-C225, cetuximab) or small molecules (ZD1839, gefitinib). Each of these agents may have the ability to enhance the tumour response to radiotherapy and trials are currently under way (reviewed in Harrington and Nutting[18]).

Chemotherapy of recurrent and metastatic head and neck cancer

Squamous cell carcinoma of the head and neck is a chemosensitive disease with single agent activity observed with many cytotoxic agents (Table 42.4).

Table 42.4 Cytotoxic agents with single agent activity in squamous cell carcinoma of the head and neck

Chemotherapy	Response rate (%)	Reference
Cisplatin	28	19
Carboplatin	26	19
5-Fluorouracil	17	19
Methotrexate	30	19
Bleomycin	10–30	19
Ifosfamide	26	19
Docetaxel	30–45	30–32
Paclitaxel	20–40	27–29
Topotecan	12	46
Gemcitabine	13	44

Chemotherapy is generally reserved for the management of locoregional disease recurrence not amenable to further surgery and/or radiotherapy, or metastatic disease. Until the mid 1990s methotrexate was the standard cytotoxic agent used by virtue of its documented activity, acceptable toxicity, convenience of administration, and low cost.[19,20] Methotrexate was administered at a dose of 40–50 mg/m^2/week. Mucositis and myelosuppression were the main dose-limiting toxicities. Reported response rates varied between 8 and 50% and averaged approximately 30%. However, in a multi-institutional randomised study involving 277 patients a response rate of only 10% was observed with methotrexate, with a median duration of response of just 4 months.[21]

Cisplatin is probably the most active single agent in head and neck cancer, with response rates of 14–41%

in phase II studies.[19] Cisplatin is also the only agent demonstrated to improve survival compared to supportive care alone. One study randomised 116 patients between single agent cisplatin, single agent bleomycin, cisplatin + bleomycin, or supportive care alone.[22] Single agent cisplatin resulted in a significant improvement in survival compared with supportive care alone (p <0.05). Furthermore, single agent cisplatin and cisplatin + bleomycin improved survival compared with supportive care alone and single agent bleomycin (p <0.01). In addition, another trial has indicated that cisplatin results in improved survival compared with methotrexate (p <0.025).[23]

The most widely used combination chemotherapy regimen is cisplatin in combination with 4–5 days of infusional 5-FU (CF). Three large randomised trials have compared CF with single agent cisplatin (Table 42.5).[23–25] Two of these studies demonstrated a significant improvement in response rates with CF compared to single agent cisplatin. Both studies that reported time to progression demonstrated that this was increased with CF compared to single agent cisplatin. However, none demonstrated a significant improvement in survival with CF, with a median survival for all patients of between 5 and 6 months. The study by Jacobs and colleagues observed a survival trend in favour of CF with 40% surviving more than 9 months compared to 24% treated with cisplatin and 27% with 5-FU. One further large randomised study evaluated CF chemotherapy. This study included 277 patients in a comparison with carboplatin/5-FU and methotrexate.[21] There was a significantly higher

Table 42.5 Randomised trials of cisplatin and 5-fluorouracil (5-FU)

Reference	Regimen	No. of patients	Response rate (%)	TTP (months)
23	Cisplatin	50	28	NR
	Methotrexate	50	12	NR
	CF	50	24	NR
	Cisplatin and methotrexate	50	22	NR
24	Cisplatin	83	17	2.0
	5-FU	83	13	1.7
	CF	79	32*	2.4**
25	CABO	127	37†	4.4
	CF	116	33.5††	4.0
	Cisplatin	122	16	2.8

CABO = methotrexate, bleomycin, vincristine and cisplatin.
NR = not reported.
*CF vs cisplatin p = 0.035; CF vs 5-FU p = 0.005.
**p = 0.023.
†p = 0.003.
††p <0.001.

response rate with CF (32%) compared to methotrexate (10%; p <0.001) but, as with the comparisons with single agent cisplatin, this improvement in response rate did not achieve a survival advantage (6.6 months and 5.6 months, respectively).

A major limitation of these studies is that none assessed the effects of treatment on symptoms or on quality of life. A study from the Royal Marsden Hospital has evaluated the role of chemotherapy in symptom control.[26] This study identified 57 patients treated with palliative chemotherapy between 1989 and 1995. Forty-three patients were treated with CF, 6 CF + interferon and 8 either methotrexate or bleomycin/epirubicin/cisplatin. There were 52 evaluable patients with a response rate of 35%. Symptoms assessed included pain, swelling, dysphagia, stomatitis, speech, trismus, breathing difficulties and appetite. A total of 103 symptoms were reported, with 44 (43%) improving and 52 (50%) stabilising with treatment. Symptoms most frequently reported to improve were pain (39%), swelling (52%) and dysphagia (33%). Symptomatic response was most frequent in patients with an objective response, although symptomatic improvement was observed in 33% of patients whose tumours failed to respond or progressed through chemotherapy. (See Ch. 7 and Sec 2.)

New cytotoxic agents

New cytotoxic agents are currently being evaluated, both as single agent therapy and also in polychemotherapy schedules. Taxanes (paclitaxel and docetaxel) have both been observed to have single agent activity.

Paclitaxel functions by promoting stabilisation of microtubules during cell division, resulting in arrest of the cell cycle at G2/M and subsequent apoptosis. Response rates of 20–40% have been reported with single agent paclitaxel (Table 42.6).[27–29] Docetaxel has also demonstrated response rates of 30–40% as a single agent in phase II studies (see Table 42.6).[30–32] The major toxicities with both these drugs are neutropenia and peripheral neuropathy.

Both taxanes have been evaluated in polychemotherapy regimens, most frequently involving the combination of taxane with either cisplatin or carboplatin with or without 5-FU (Table 42.7).[33–41] In phase II studies response rates increased to 77% from the combination of paclitaxel with cisplatin.[33] However, in the only reported randomised study involving 210 patients response rates were around 35%.[36] Furthermore, no response or survival advantage from dose intensification with growth factor support was observed. Two studies have evaluated the combination of paclitaxel, ifosfamide and cisplatin (TIP).[42,43] The phase II study involved 52 assessable patients with a response rate of 58% and median survival of 8.8 months.[43] It is not yet known whether taxane-containing regimens have a response, quality of life or survival advantage compared to CF and this question needs to be addressed in phase III trials. In addition, trials need to evaluate quality of life and survival benefits from treatment with a taxane-containing regimen after failure of CF.

Other new cytotoxic drugs evaluated in head and neck cancer include gemcitabine and topotecan.

Table 42.6   Phase II trials of taxanes

Ref	Regimen	Disease stage	Evaluable patients (No.)	Response rate (%)	Overall survival; median (months)	Grade 3/4 toxicity
27	Paclitaxel 175 mg/m^2 over 3 h q21	Recurrent and/or metastatic	20	20	NR	Leucopenia & thrombocytopenia
29	Paclitaxel 250 mg/m^2 over 24 h q21	Locally advanced, recurrent or metastatic	30	40	9.2	Neutropenic fever; neuropathy
28	Paclitaxel 250 mg/m^2 over 24 h q21	Locally advanced, recurrent or metastatic	17	36	NR	Neutropenic sepsis; neuropathy
30	Docetaxel 100 mg/m^2 over 1 h q21	Recurrent or metastatic	37	32	NR	Neutropenia
31	Docetaxel 100 mg/m^2 over 1 h q21	Locally advanced or recurrent	31	42	NR	Febrile leucopenia, fatigue, diarrhoea
32	Docetaxel 60 mg/m^2 over 1 h q21	Locally advanced or metastatic	23	30	NR	Neutropenia, thrombocytopenia

^{a}q21 = every 3 weeks (21 days).

Table 42.7 Studies of taxanes containing polychemotherapy regimens in advanced squamous head and neck carcinoma

Ref	Phase	Regimen	Disease stage	Evaluable patients (No.)	Response rate (%)	Overall survival	Grade 3/4 toxicities*
33	I/II	Paclitaxel 175–300 mg/m^2 day 1 + cisplatin 75 mg/m^2 day 2 q21	Locally advanced, recurrent or metastatic	27	77	–	Myalgia
35	II	Paclitaxel 200 mg/m^2 + carboplatin AUC = 7 q28	Recurrent or metastatic	14 NPC 35 non-NPC	57 23	Not reached 7.3 months	None
36	III	Paclitaxel 200 mg/m^2 + cisplatin 75 mg/m^2 + G-CSF q21 vs Paclitaxel 135 mg/m^2 + cisplatin 75 mg/m^2 q21	Locally advanced, recurrent or metastatic	105 105	35 36	7.3 months 7.3 months	Neutropenia and febrile neutropenia in both arms
38	I/II	Paclitaxel 135 mg/m^2 day 1 + cisplatin 75 mg/m^2 day 2 + 5-FU 1000–800 mg/m^2/day days 2–5 (2–6) q21	Locally advanced, recurrent or metastatic	25	60 (58)†	11 months (6 months)†	Neutropenia Mucositis
39	II	Docetaxel 100 mg/m^2 + cisplatin 75 mg/m^2 q21	Locally advanced, recurrent or metastatic	41	54	–	Febrile neutropenia Leucopenia
40	II	Docetaxel 80 mg/m^2 day 1 + cisplatin 40 mg/m^2 days 2 and 3, + CI 5-FU 1g/m^2 days 1–3 q21	Locally advanced or recurrent	19	44	11	Febrile neutropenia Leucopenia
41	I/II	Docetaxel 75 mg/m^2 day 1 + cisplatin 75–100 mg/m^2 day 1 + CI 5-FU 1g/m^2 days 1–4 q21	Locally advanced	43	40		Hypomagnesaemia Hypocalcaemia Neutropenia Febrile neutropenia

*≥10%.
†Patients with recurrent and metastatic disease.
G-CSF = granulocyte colony-stimulating factor; AUC = area under the curve; CI 5-FU = continuous infusion 5-fluorouracil; NPC = nasopharyngeal carcinoma; q21 = every 3 weeks; q28 = every 4 weeks.

Gemcitabine is a water-soluble analogue of deoxycytidine, a pyrimidine antimetabolite. The only published phase II study included 62 patients.[44] Gemcitabine 1 g/m² weekly for 3 weeks followed by 1 week of rest achieved a response rate of 13% in 54 evaluable patients. Treatment was generally well tolerated, with 15% grade 3/4 neutropenia, and the most frequent non-haematological toxicities were nausea/vomiting, fatigue and fever. One group have shown that the combination of gemcitabine and cisplatin has a favourable toxicity profile.[45] The topoisomerase I inhibitor topotecan has also shown activity in advanced squamous cell cancer of the head and neck.[46]

Chemotherapy of recurrent and metastatic disease – conclusions

There is reasonable justification for the use of CF chemotherapy in patients with recurrent or metastatic squamous cell carcinoma of the head and neck. Cisplatin has been demonstrated to improve survival compared with supportive care alone. Objective tumour responses are observed more frequently with CF than with single agent cisplatin, and consequently are predicted to result in higher rates of symptomatic response. Consequently, at the Royal Marsden Hospital, as at many other centres, standard therapy is cisplatin (100 mg/m² day 1) plus 5-FU (1 g/m² days 1–4) every 21 days. Furthermore, CF should be considered a reference treatment against which new therapies for the treatment of advanced head and neck cancer are compared.

To date, new cytotoxic drugs have not demonstrated any obvious improvement in outcomes for patients, although a randomised trial comparing a taxane + cisplatin to CF would be justified. Consequent to these poor results, investigators are evaluating novel strategies, including immunotherapy and gene therapy. Such strategies have recently been reviewed by Ganly and Kaye.[47]

CHEMOTHERAPY IN THE MANAGEMENT OF NASOPHARYNGEAL CANCERS

The primary treatment for patients with nasopharyngeal cancer is traditionally radiotherapy.[48] The 5-year survival rate reported for patients with stage III nasopharyngeal cancer treated by radiotherapy is 46% and for stage IV approximately 30%.[49] In 1998 an intergroup study reported improved outcomes for patients with stage III and IV nasopharyngeal cancers treated with a combination of chemotherapy and radiotherapy.[50] One hundred and ninety-three (147 eligible) patients were randomised to either 70 Gy of radiotherapy alone or combined with cisplatin 100 mg/m² on days 1, 22 and 43 during radiotherapy, followed by 3 cycles of

adjuvant chemotherapy. The adjuvant chemotherapy was cisplatin 80 mg/m² on day 1 and 5-FU 1000 mg/m²/day on days 1–4 every 4 weeks. Median survival was 34 months for radiotherapy alone and had not been reached for chemoradiation at the time of reporting. Three-year survival had improved from 47% with radiotherapy alone to 78% with chemoradiation ($p = 0.005$). Similar improvements in 3-year progression-free survival were observed (24% vs 69%; $p < 0.001$). Consequently, chemoradiation has become the standard of care for patients with stage III and IV undifferentiated nasopharyngeal carcinoma. Currently, patients are treated in accordance with the protocol described by Al-Sarraf et al.[50] However, grade 3/4 toxicity is increased with combined modality therapy, particularly leucopenia, neutropenia, nausea and vomiting, and stomatitis. Therefore, consideration should be given to the cisplatin dose in individual cases and it may be appropriate to reduce the dose of cisplatin to 80 mg/m².

The use of neoadjuvant chemotherapy followed by radiotherapy represents an alternative strategy to chemoradiation for the management of locally advanced nasopharyngeal cancers. Sixty-nine patients with locally advanced nasopharyngeal cancer were included in a phase II trial evaluating the combination of bleomycin, epirubicin and cisplatin (BEC) chemotherapy.[51] Patients were treated with three cycles of BEC chemotherapy followed by conventional radiotherapy (70 Gy). The overall response rate to initial chemotherapy was 98%, with 62% achieving complete response. Three months after radiotherapy 94% of patients achieved local control. Median disease-free survival had not been reached with 90 months follow-up; 4-year disease-free survival is 60% and 4-year overall survival 66%. Similar results were observed in a subsequent study evaluating a four drug combination (5-FU, bleomycin, epirubicin, cisplatin; FBEC) in 23 patients with locally advanced disease.[52] The overall response rate was 91.5%, with 22% achieving complete response to initial chemotherapy. Twenty-two patients (87%) achieved a complete response following radiotherapy. With a median follow-up of 51 months, 65% of patients are still in first remission and 4-year survival is 58%. This group have subsequently undertaken a randomised trial to establish the benefit of neoadjuvant chemotherapy in patients with locally advanced nasopharyngeal cancer. Three hundred and thirty-nine patients were randomised to three cycles of BEC followed by radiotherapy or radiotherapy alone.[53] Preliminary results with a median follow-up of 49 months demonstrated a significant improvement in progression-free survival with neoadjuvant chemotherapy (55% vs 33%; $p < 0.01$).

Patients with recurrent or metastatic undifferentiated nasopharyngeal carcinoma may be effectively treated with chemotherapy. Single agent activity has been noted with a number of cytotoxic agents, including bleomycin, etoposide, epirubicin, cisplatin, 5-FU, mitoxantrone (mitozantrone) and paclitaxel.[51,54,55] A French group have reported a series of four studies that have established the standards of care for patients with recurrent or metastatic nasopharyngeal cancer (Table 42.8).[51,52,56,57] These studies observed response rates of between 45% and 78%, with around 20% of patients demonstrating complete responses following treatment with three or four drug cisplatin-based combination regimens. Median overall survival is around 15 months, with a range from 7 months to more than 78 months.

Two other groups have reported similar response rates with cisplatin-based combination regimens in recurrent or metastatic undifferentiated nasopharyngeal carcinoma. A Canadian group evaluated a combination of cyclophosphamide, doxorubicin, cisplatin, methotrexate and bleomycin.[58] A response rate of 82% was observed, with median survival durations of 16 months and 14 months for recurrent locoregional and metastatic disease, respectively. The toxicity of this regimen was unacceptable, with 7 treatment-related deaths. A study from Taiwan evaluated cisplatin, 5-FU and leucovorin.[59] The response rate was 68% and the median survival was between 14 and 16 months.

There have been fewer studies of new drugs in nasopharyngeal cancer compared to the work being undertaken in squamous head and neck cancer. Paclitaxel has been found to have a 22% response rate in previously untreated metastatic disease.[55] Paclitaxel combined with carboplatin has been evaluated in patients with previously untreated metastatic nasopharyngeal carcinoma.[60] The response rate was 75%, with 1 patient demonstrating a complete response. The median time to progression was 7 months and median survival was 12 months. On the basis of this small study, a combination of paclitaxel and carboplatin has similar efficacy to other platinum-based regimens in nasopharyngeal cancer. Further larger studies will be required for verification.

In conclusion, patients presenting with locally advanced nasopharyngeal carcinoma should be treated with either chemoradiation or neoadjuvant chemotherapy followed by conventional radiotherapy. At the Royal Marsden Hospital patients are currently offered treatment with chemoradiation, according to the regimen described by Al-Sarraf et al.[50] In patients with recurrent and/or metastatic disease, a platinum-based chemotherapy, either cisplatin + 5-FU or BEC, remains the standard chemotherapy. At the Royal Marsden Hospital, BEC is currently used as the standard chemotherapy. Long-term survival is documented after chemotherapy for metastatic undifferentiated nasopharyngeal carcinoma and it is suggested that the dose–response effect of aggressive cisplatin-based combinations has played a major role in obtaining long-term complete responses.[61] Thus, further exploration with alternative regimens is warranted. One approach could examine the incorporation of paclitaxel into a platinum-based polychemotherapy regimen. An alternative strategy that may be of benefit in selected young patients achieving complete response is high-dose chemotherapy with peripheral blood progenitor cell rescue.

THE ROLE OF CHEMOTHERAPY IN THE MANAGEMENT OF ADVANCED ADENOID CYSTIC CARCINOMA

Adenoid cystic carcinomas are relatively rare slow-growing tumours that arise in the submandibular gland and minor salivary glands. Management of a primary adenoid cystic carcinoma is with surgery, often followed by radiotherapy. However, local relapse occurs in approximately 50% of patients and distant metastases are detected in up to 40%. The disease frequently runs an indolent course, with chemotherapy held in reserve for symptomatic tumours that cannot be controlled by other means. Numerous single agents have been used, including cyclophosphamide, vincristine, methotrexate, bleomycin, cisplatin, 5-FU and doxorubicin. In addition, various combinations of these drugs have been evaluated with little evidence of improved response rates compared to single agent chemotherapy. The objective and symptomatic response rates achieved with a number of single agent or polychemotherapy regimens are presented in Table 42.9. The majority of studies have a very small number of patients due to the rarity of the tumour. Despite this, it can be concluded that some drugs have activity as a single agent, in particular cisplatin and 5-FU. In addition, there is the suggestion that combination chemotherapy is more effective than single agent therapy. In the four studies that examined symptomatic benefits of treatment, symptomatic improvement was seen most frequently in patients with stable or responding disease. The highest recorded symptom response rate was observed with cisplatin and 4-day infusional 5-FU,[62] but higher objective response rates have been observed with other combinations. Therefore, in an effort to improve response rates and optimise symptom control, patients are currently offered treatment with the ECF regimen (epirubicin 50 mg/m^2 day 1, cisplatin 60 mg/m^2 day 1 and protracted venous infusion 5-FU 300 mg/m^2/day every 21 days).

Table 42.8 Results for chemotherapy for metastatic nasopharyngeal cancer

Regimen	No. of patients	Response rate	Complete response	Mean duration of survival in complete responders	Overall survival median (range)	Ref	Notes
PBF Cisplatin 100 mg/m² day 1, bleomycin 15 mg day 1 and 16 mg/m²/day continuous infusion days 1–5, 5-FU 650 mg/m²/day for three monthly cycles	49	78%	19% (9)	25 months	(7–58 + months)	56	
BEC Bleomycin 15 mg/m² day 1 and 16 mg/m²/day continuous infusion days 1–5; epirubicin 80 mg/m² day 1 and cisplatin 100 mg/m² day 1	44	45%	20% (9)	30 months	(12–72+ months)	51	Grade 3/4 neutropenia 57% with 2 toxic deaths from neutropenic sepsis Grade 3/4 mucositis in 27%
FMEP 5-FU 800 mg/m²/day days 1–4, epirubicin 70 mg/m² day 1, mitomycin C 10 mg/m² day 1, and cisplatin 100mg/m² day 1 every 4 weeks for 6 cycles	44	52%			14 months	57	Grade 3/4 neutropenia in 89%, febrile neutropenia in 36%. Grade 3/4 thrombocytopenia in 61%
FBEC 5-FU 700 mg/m²/day continuous infusion days 1–4 plus a modified BEC regimen	26	78%	35% (9)		15 months	52	Grade 3/4 neutropenia in 85%, febrile neutropenia in 35%. Three toxic deaths (2 from sepsis). Severe mucositis in 42%
Cyclophosphamide, methotrexate, bleomycin	69	82%			16 months for locoregional disease, 14 months for metastatic disease	58	Seven treatment-related deaths doxorubicin, cisplatin, recurrent
Cisplatin, 5-FU and leucovorin	22	68%	23%		14–16 months	59	
Paclitaxel		22%				55	
Paclitaxel 175 mg/m² Carboplatin AUC = 6	32	75%	3% (1)		12 months	60	

AUC, area under the curve; 5-FU, 5-fluorouracil.

Table 42.9   Objective and symptomatic responses to chemotherapy in advanced adenoid cystic carcinoma

Regimen	Number treated	Objective response (%)	Symptomatic response (%)	Reference
5-FU	12	33	33[a]	63
Cisplatin	10	50	70	64
Cisplatin, doxorubicin	5	40	NR	65
Cisplatin, doxorubicin, 5-FU	9	22	NR	66
Cyclophosphamide, doxorubicin, cisplatin	9	33	NR	67
Cyclophosphamide, vincristine, 5-FU	8	25	25[a]	68
Cyclophosphamide, doxorubicin, cisplatin	11	18	NR	69
Cyclophosphamide, doxorubicin, cisplatin	4	25	NR	70
5-FU, doxorubicin, cyclophosphamide, cisplatin	7	43	NR	71
Cisplatin	10	0	NR	72
Cisplatin, doxorubicin, bleomycin	9	33	NR	72
Cyclophosphamide, doxorubicin, cisplatin	6	33	NR	73
Epirubicin	20	10	29	74
Cyclophosphamide, doxorubicin, cisplatin	12	25	NR	75
Mitoxantrone (mitozantrone)	32	12	NR	76
Cisplatin, 5-FU	11	0	64	62

Source: Reproduced with permission from Hill et al.[62]
[a]Pain only.
NR = not reported; 5-FU = 5-fluorouracil.

NURSING CARE FOR PATIENTS RECEIVING CHEMOTHERAPY FOR HEAD AND NECK CANCERS

Caroline Soady

THE ROLE OF CHEMOTHERAPY IN HEAD AND NECK CANCER

The role of chemotherapy in the management of head and neck cancer will depend primarily on the histology of the head and neck tumour. The majority are squamous cell carcinoma in origin, which accounts for 90% of all head and neck tumours.[77] Curative treatment for squamous cell carcinoma will predominantly focus on the use of surgery and/or radiotherapy.[78] In this context concomitant chemotherapy is used to enhance the efficacy of curative radiotherapy. Concomitant chemotherapy and radiotherapy has resulted in statistically significant improved disease-free and overall survival for patients with head and neck cancer.[79–81] Chemotherapy is also used neoadjuvantly to debulk larger or advanced tumours prior to surgical resection and/or radiotherapy, or palliatively to provide relief from symptoms such as pain and to achieve some control over local recurrent disease or distant metastases, with the emphasis on quality of life.[82]

Chemotherapy drugs commonly used include cisplatin or carboplatin and 5-FU, which are administered intravenously in a regimen over a period of between 4 and 5 days. Although cisplatin-based chemotherapy has been found to have a major response in 90% of these tumours, randomised studies have repeatedly failed to demonstrate any associated survival advantage.[83]

THE IMPACT OF HEAD AND NECK CANCER ON THE INDIVIDUAL

Head and neck cancer and its treatment can have a considerable and devastating impact on both function and aesthetics. Due to the nature of the disease, the individual's fight against cancer often becomes an immensely public battle, potentially resulting in alterations to the airway, to communication, to nutrition and to anatomy. Emphasis should be placed on rehabilitation, assisting the patient to adjust to the changes in body image and to reintegrate into society. In order to address these and other complex needs, a multiprofessional team approach is required[84–86] at all stages of the patient's disease trajectory. (See also Chs 5 and 19.)

DECISION-MAKING IN CURATIVE HEAD AND NECK CANCER CHEMOTHERAPY

Following diagnosis, many patients suffer overwhelming feelings of loss of control, which may in turn lead to feelings of both helplessness and hopelessness and a belief that they have no influence over what is happening to them.[87]

The multiprofessional team will need to spend time with the patient and family, providing verbal and written information as appropriate and contact telephone numbers. Nursing staff should discuss the options of support available in the community, such as Macmillan and district nurses who can advise on chemotherapy side effects and other important issues. (See also Chs 5 and 19.)

DECISION-MAKING IN PALLIATIVE HEAD AND NECK CANCER CHEMOTHERAPY

The decision on palliative chemotherapy can be complex and should take into consideration the following factors:

- patient preference
- an assessment of current and likely future symptoms
- likelihood of symptom relief from specific treatments
- physical and psychosocial effects of treatment
- inconvenience of treatment
- the age of the patient
- comorbidity.[85]

Some patient groups may require a skin-tunnelled catheter in order to administer specific regimens of palliative chemotherapy, e.g. recurrent adenocarcinoma of the trachea with lung metastases, which can be treated with ECF. The patient who already has a tracheostomy tube and a gastrostomy tube in situ may decide to refuse further treatment to avoid the encumbrance of another indwelling appliance that potentially can encroach further on his remaining quality of life. The patient and his family will need time to discuss the options available. The World Medical Assembly, cited in McGrath,[88] states that there are five points which are important in obtaining consent from a patient for medical intervention:

- explanation of the proposed treatment must be given, using appropriate language that is understood by the patient

- risks and benefits of the treatment should be clearly stated
- any alternatives to treatment should be included
- adequate time for the patient's questions must be given
- the patient should be aware of the option to withdraw at any time from treatment, with that decision respected and with the implied expectation of the continuation of support from the multiprofessional team involved.

(For further information see Ch. 5.)

Other influences in palliative treatment

Many patients who present with recurrence will already have undergone a combination of treatment modalities involving surgery (with or without reconstruction), chemotherapy and/or radiotherapy. As recurrence can sometimes closely follow a difficult radical phase, acknowledging the incurable nature of the disease may be very difficult.[85] The patient and family will require immense support at this time and nursing staff should, through effective communication, ensure that links are established in the community with Macmillan or Marie Curie nurses and the general practitioner. This will enable the patient and family to discuss various issues and receive guidance on the management of symptoms. (For further information see Ch. 14.)

ASSESSMENT PRIOR TO CHEMOTHERAPY

A thorough clinical assessment is required to identify the patient's performance status. This will include a detailed examination and history by the medical oncology team. Early and prompt referral to members of the multiprofessional team is essential.

Dental assessment

A dental assessment should be performed to identify if any treatment is required prior to commencing chemotherapy. All too often, oral/dental care is overlooked until an actual problem develops.[89] Once treatment has started, any essential dental work can only be performed once pancytopenia resolves, to prevent complications from bleeding and infection. Some patients will undergo a combination of chemotherapy followed by radiotherapy and may require dental extractions prior to commencing treatment to prevent the development of complications, e.g. osteoradionecrosis. Osteoradionecrosis appears as decreased marrow cellularity and vascularity, fibrosis and fatty degeneration, as a result of radiation damage to the maxilla or mandible.[90]

Functional assessment

All staff should be aware of the impact of the disease process on the individual's function and look out for signs and symptoms that indicate that further decisions must be made before starting chemotherapy. Staff working within the speciality of head and neck oncology should be experienced at asking appropriate questions to elicit specific information, on such topics as dysphagia, stridor and aspiration of diet and fluids on swallowing. Nursing staff (due to the nature of their role) are ideally placed to pick up on any changes in condition or new symptoms.

Dysphagia

Swallowing may be impaired due to the presence of a malignant tumour, which ultimately can result in deterioration in nutritional status. By referring the patient promptly to the dietitian and to the speech and language therapist, assessments can be performed and an action plan established accordingly. The dietitian may suggest that enteral tube feeding is required to maintain nutrition during this time. A nasogastric tube is used for the short term (3–4 weeks), while a gastrostomy or jejunostomy tube is used for a longer-term period. The individual needs of the patient should be carefully considered by all members of the multiprofessional team. A gastrostomy or jejunostomy tube is visually less obtrusive than a nasogastric tube.

As some chemotherapy protocols have the potential for high emetogenicity, patients may avoid the distress and discomfort of repeated nasogastric tube insertions (due to risk of vomiting the tube out) by having an enteral tube inserted. The decision should be made prior to commencing chemotherapy, enabling the patient and/or family to familiarise themselves with the different aspects of essential care. (See also Ch. 19.)

Aspiration

Aspiration of diet and/or fluids may occur due to the presence of mechanical obstruction such as an oral or oropharyngeal tumour. Staff will need to use appropriate questions to ascertain whether the patient is coughing after taking diet and/or fluids, in conjunction with assessing for signs of a chest infection. The speech and language therapist will be able to assess the swallowing and devise an action plan to enable the patient to learn specific techniques to protect the airway on swallowing different consistencies or may advise temporary nil by mouth until treatment has begun and a reassessment can take place. Assessment prior to commencing chemotherapy is essential, as the development of a chest infection while undergoing chemotherapy will result in complications that can jeopardise not only the continuation of treatment but also patient survival.[91]

Stridor

Stridor (difficulty breathing) can occur due to the presence of a tumour occluding part of the airway. An elective tracheostomy may be performed to maintain the airway and bypass the tumour. The patient and family will require immense support in order to adjust to this aspect of care, in addition to coping with the side effects of the chemotherapy.

Ongoing assessment during chemotherapy

In order to provide ongoing assessment of chemotherapy side effects at home, the patient should be referred to appropriate members of the community team, e.g. district nurses. Through collaboration, this enables community and hospital teams to identify key issues that require intervention and to establish action plans to manage this accordingly, e.g. district nurse may be aware that the patient's hearing has deteriorated since commencing cisplatin chemotherapy and a hearing test will be arranged to assess the changes.

IMPACT OF PREVIOUS HEAD AND NECK SURGERY AND RADIOTHERAPY ON PATIENT UNDERGOING CHEMOTHERAPY

Management of the patient with head and neck cancer undergoing chemotherapy must focus on the patient's past treatment as well as the side effects of current chemotherapy protocols, as past treatment will impact on current treatment.

Radiotherapy for nasopharyngeal, maxillary sinus and palatal tumours often causes muscle and ligament trismus to the muscles of mastication.[92] Trismus is defined as difficulty in opening the mouth caused by scarring and fibrosis of the masticatory muscles (the temporalis, masseter, medial pterygoid and lateral pterygoid), causing restricted mobility of the temporomandibular joint.[93] This will affect the patient's ability to perform effective mouth care as part of the chemotherapy protocol, and will require adaptation of existing mouth care protocols for this specialist patient group. Educating the patient on the use of regular jaw exercises and using wooden spatulas to gradually increase mouth opening may help in the management of this difficult problem.

Surgery involving reconstruction using flaps and skin grafts can result in anatomical changes that can impact on finding a suitable vein for peripheral intravenous access, e.g. free radial forearm flap repair. (See also Ch. 10.)

Xerostomia (dryness of the mouth) is one of the major side effects of radical radiotherapy to the head and neck and occurs as a result of the salivary glands being involved in the radiation field. Salivary secretions are decreased in volume, with a lower buffering capacity and pH and an increase in viscosity.[94] Mouth care will therefore need to address this existing problem in addition to oral mucositis, one of the side effects of 5-FU. (See also Ch. 18.)

References

1. Kelly D, Shah J. Global incidence and etiology. In: Close L, Larson D, Shah J, eds. Essentials of head and neck oncology. New York: Thieme; 1998:3–10.

2. Parkin D, Muir C, Whelan S, et al. Cancer incidence in five continents. Vol 6. Lyon: IARC; 1992.

3. Campaign CR. Oral cancer. CRC Factsheet 1993; 14:1.

4. Souhami R, Tobias J. Cancer and its management. 3rd edn. Oxford: Blackwell Science; 1998.

5. Lyn T, Hsieh R, Chuang C, et al. Epstein-Barr virus associated antibodies and serum biochemistry in nasopharyngeal carcinoma. Laryngoscope 1984; 94:485–488.

6. Fleming I, Cooper J, Henson D, et al (eds). Head and neck sites. In: AJCC cancer staging manual. 5th edn. Philadelphia: Lippincott-Raven; 1997:21–64.

7. Schmalfuss I, Mancuso A. Global incidence and etiology. In: Close L, Larson D, Shah J, eds. Essentials of head and neck oncology. New York: Thieme; 1998:59–76.

8. Dimery I, Hong W. Overview of combined modality therapies for head and neck cancer. J Natl Cancer Inst 1993; 85:95–111.

9. Tannock I, Browman G. Lack of evidence for a role of chemotherapy in the routine management of locally advanced head and neck cancer. J Clin Oncol 1986; 4:1121–1126.

10. Taylor S. Why has so much chemotherapy done so little in head and neck cancer? J Clin Oncol 1987; 5:1–3.

11. Pignon J, Bourhis J, Domenge C, et al. Chemotherapy added to locoregional treatment for head and neck squamous-cell carcinoma: three meta-analyses of updated individual data. Lancet 2000; 355:949–955.

12. Munro A. An overview of randomised controlled trials of adjuvant chemotherapy in head and neck cancer. Br J Cancer 1995; 71:83–91.

13. El-Sayed S, Nelson N. Adjuvant and adjunctive chemotherapy in the management of squamous cell carcinoma of the head and neck region: a meta-analysis of prospective and randomised trials. J Clin Oncol 1996; 14:838–847.

14. Henk J. Controlled trials of synchronous chemotherapy with radiotherapy in head and neck cancer: overview of radiation morbidity. Clin Oncol 1997; 9:308–312.

15. Fu K, Pajak T, Trotti A, et al. A Radiation Therapy Oncology Group (RTOG) phase III randomized study to compare hyperfractionation and two variants of accelerated fractionation to standard fractionation radiotherapy for head and neck squamous carcinomas: first report of RTOG 9003. Int J Radiat Oncol Biol Phys 2000; 48:7–16.

16. Jeremic B, Shibamoto Y, Milicic B, et al. Hyperfractionated radiation therapy with or without concurrent low-dose daily cisplatin in locally advanced squamous cell carcinoma of the head and neck: a prospective randomized trial. J Clin Oncol 2000; 18:1458–1464.

17. Hennequin C, Favaudon V. Biological basis for chemo-radiotherapy interactions. Eur J Cancer 2002; 38:223–230.

18. Harrington K, Nutting C. Interactions between ionizing radiation and drugs in head and neck cancer: how can we maximize the therapeutic index? Curr Opin Investig Drugs 2002; 3:807–811.

19. Vokes E, Athanaisiadis I. Chemotherapy for squamous cell carcinoma of head and neck: the future is now. Ann Oncol 1996; 7:15–29.

20. Browman G, Cronin L. Standard chemotherapy in squamous cell head and neck cancer: what we have learned from randomized trials. Semin Oncol 1994; 21:311–319.

21. Forastiere A, Metch B, Schuller D, et al. Randomized comparison of cisplatin plus fluorouracil and carboplatin plus fluorouracil versus methotrexate in advanced squamous-cell carcinoma of the head and neck: a Southwest Oncology Group Study. J Clin Oncol 1992; 10:1245–1251.

22. Morton R, Rugman F, Dorman E, et al. Cisplatinum and bleomycin for advanced or recurrent squamous cell carcinoma of the head and neck: a randomised factorial phase III controlled trial. Cancer Chemother Pharmacol 1985; 15:283–289.

23. Liverpool Head and Neck Oncology Group. A phase III randomised trial of cisplatinum, methotrexate, cisplatinum + methotrexate and cisplatinum + 5-FU in end stage squamous carcinoma of the head and neck. Br J Cancer 1990; 61:311–315.

24. Jacobs C, Lyman G, Velez-Garcia E, et al. A phase III randomized study comparing cisplatin and fluorouracil as single agents and in combination for advanced squamous cell carcinoma of the head and neck. J Clin Oncol 1992; 10:257–263.

25. Clavel M, Vermoken J, Cognetti F, et al. Randomized comparison of cisplatin, methotrexate, bleomycin and vincristine (CABO) versus cisplatin and 5-fluorouracil

(CF) versus cisplatin (C) in recurrent or metastatic squamous cell carcinoma of the head and neck. A phase III study of the EORTC Head and Neck Cancer Cooperative Group. Ann Oncol 1994; 5:521–526.

26. Constenla D, Hill M, A'Hern R, et al. Chemotherapy for symptom control in recurrent squamous cell carcinoma of the head and neck. Ann Oncol 1997; 8:445–449.

27. Gebbia V, Testa A, Cannata G, et al. Single agent paclitaxel in advanced squamous cell head and neck carcinoma. Eur J Cancer 1996; 32A:901–902.

28. Smith R, Thornton D, Allen J. A Phase II trial of paclitaxel in squamous cell carcinoma of the head and neck with correlative laboratory studies. Semin Oncol 1995; 22:41–46.

29. Forastiere A, Shank D, Neuberg D, et al. Final report of a phase II evaluation of paclitaxel in patients with advanced squamous cell carcinoma of the head and neck. An Eastern Cooperative Group Oncology Trial (PA390). Cancer 1998; 82:2270–2274.

30. Catimel G, Verweij J, Mattijssen V, et al. Docetaxel (Taxotere): an active drug for the treatment of patients with advanced squamous cell carcinoma of the head and neck. Ann Oncol 1994; 5:533–537.

31. Dreyfuss A, Clark J, Norris C, et al. Docetaxel: an active drug for squamous cell carcinoma of the head and neck. J Clin Oncol 1996; 14:1672–1678.

32. Ebihara S, Fujii H, Sasaki Y. A late phase II study of docetaxel (Taxotere) in patients with head and neck cancer (HNC). Proc Am Soc Clin Oncol 1997; 16:399a.

33. Hitt R, Hornedo J, Colomer R, et al. Study of escalating doses of paclitaxel plus cisplatin in patients with inoperable head and neck cancer. Semin Oncol 1997; 24:58–64.

34. Schilling T, Heinrich B, Kau R, et al. Paclitaxel administration over 3 h followed by cisplatin in patients with advanced head and neck squamous cell carcinoma: a clinical phase I study. Oncology 1997; 54:89–95.

35. Fountzilas G, Skarlos D, Athanassiades A, et al. Paclitaxel by three-hour infusion and carboplatin in advanced carcinoma of the nasopharynx and other sites of the head and neck. A phase II study conducted by the Hellenic Cooperative Oncology Group. Ann Oncol 1997; 8:451–455.

36. Forastiere A, Leong T, Rowinsky E, et al. Phase III comparison of high-dose paclitaxel + cisplatin + granulocyte colony-stimulating factor versus low-dose paclitaxel + cisplatin in advanced head and neck cancer: Eastern Cooperative Oncology Group study E1393. J Clin Oncol 2001; 19:1088–1095.

37. Benasso M, Numico G, Rosso R, et al. Chemotherapy for relapsed head and neck cancer: paclitaxel, cisplatin, and 5-fluorouracil in chemotherapy-naive patients. A dose-finding study. Semin Oncol 1997; 24:46–50.

38. Hussain M, Gadgeel S, Kucuk O, et al. Paclitaxel, cisplatin, and 5-fluorouracil for patients with advanced or recurrent squamous cell carcinoma of the head and neck. Cancer 1999; 86:2364–2369.

39. Schoffski P, Catimel G, Planting A, et al. Docetaxel and cisplatin: an active regimen in patients with locally advanced, recurrent or metastatic squamous cell carcinoma of the head and neck. Results of a phase II study of the EORTC Early Clinical Studies Group. Ann Oncol 1999; 10:119–122.

40. Janinis J, Papadakou M, Xidakis E, et al. Combination chemotherapy with docetaxel, cisplatin and 5-fluorouracil in previously treated patients with advanced/recurrent head and neck cancer: a phase II feasability study. Am J Clin Oncol 2000; 23:128–131.

41. Posner M, Glisson B, Frenette G, et al. Multicenter phase I-II trial of docetaxel, cisplatin, and fluorouracil induction chemotherapy for patients with locally advanced squamous cell cancer of the head and neck. J Clin Oncol 2001; 19:1096–1104.

42. Benner S, Lippman S, Huber M, et al. Phase I trial of paclitaxel, cisplatin and ifosfamide in patients with recurrent or metastatic squamous cell cancer of the head and neck. Semin Oncol 1995; 22:22–25.

43. Shin D, Glisson B, Khuri F, et al. Phase II trial of paclitaxel, ifosfamide and cisplatin in patients with recurrent head and neck squamous cell carcinoma. J Clin Oncol 1998; 16:1325–1330.

44. Catimel G, Vermoken J, Clavel M, et al. A phase II study of gemcitabine (LY 188011) in patients with advanced squanous cell carcinoma of the head and neck. Ann Oncol 1994; 5:543–547.

45. Hitt R, Castellano D, Hidalgo M, et al. Phase II trial of cisplatin and gemcitabine in advanced squamous cell carcinoma of the head and neck. Ann Oncol 1998; 9:1347–1349.

46. Robert F, Soong S-j, Wheeler R. A phase II study of topotecan in patients with recurrent head and neck cancer. Identification of an active new agent. Am J Clin Oncol 1997; 20:298–302.

47. Ganly I, Kaye S. Recurrent squamous-cell carcinoma of the head and neck: overview of current therapy and future prospects. Ann Oncol 2000; 11:11–16.

48. Fee W Jr. Nasopharynx. In: Close L, Larson D, Shah J, eds. Essentials of head and neck oncology. New York: Thieme; 1998:205–210.

49. Qin D, Hu Y, Yan J, et al. Analysis of 1379 patients with nasopharyngeal carcinoma treated by radiation. Cancer 1988; 61:1117–1124.

50. Al-Sarraf M, LeBlanc M, Shanker Giri P, et al. Chemoradiotherapy versus radiotherapy in patients with advanced nasopharyngeal cancer: phase III randomized Intergroup study 0099. J Clin Oncol 1998; 16:1310–1317.

51. Azli N, Fandi A, Bachouchi M, et al. Final report of a phase II study of chemotherapy with bleomycin, epirubicin, and cisplatin for locally advanced and metastatic/recurrent undifferentiated carcinoma of the nasopharyngeal type. Cancer J Sci Am 1995; 1:222–229.

52. Taamma A, Fandi A, Azli N, et al. Phase II trial of chemotherapy with 5-fluorouracil, bleomycin, epirubicin, and cisplatin for patients with locally advanced, metastatic, or recurrent undifferentiated carcinoma

of the nasopharyngeal type. Cancer 1999; 86:1101–1108.

53. Trial INCSGVI. Preliminary results of a randomized trial comparing neoadjuvant chemotherapy (cisplatin, epirubicin, bleomycin) plus radiotherapy vs. radiotherapy alone in stage IV (≥N2, M0) undifferentiated nasopharyngeal carcinoma: a positive effect on progression-free survival. Int J Radiat Oncol Biol Phys 1996; 35:463–469.

54. Dugan M, Choy D, Ngai A, et al: Multicenter phase II trial of mitoxantrone in patients with advanced nasopharyngeal carcinoma in Southeast Asia: an Asian-Oceanian Clinical Oncology Association Group study. J Clin Oncol 1993; 11:70–76.

55. Au E, Tan E, Ang P. Activity of paclitaxel by three-hour infusion in Asian patients with metastatic undifferentiated nasopharyngeal cancer. Ann Oncol 1998; 9:327–329.

56. Boussen H, Cvitkovic E, Wendling J, et al. Chemotherapy of metastatic and/or recurrent undifferentiated nasopharyngeal carcinoma with cisplatin, bleomycin, and fluorouracil. J Clin Oncol 1991; 9:1675–1681.

57. Hasbini A, Mahjoubi R, Fandi A, et al. Phase II trial combining mitomycin with 5-fluorouracil, epirubicin, and cisplatin in recurrent and metastatic undifferentiated carcinoma of nasopharyngeal type. Ann Oncol 1999; 10:421–425.

58. Siu L, Czaykowski P, Tannock I. Phase I/II of the CA-PABLE regimen for patients with poorly differentiated carcinoma of the nasopharynx. J Clin Oncol 1998; 16:2514–2521.

59. Chi K, Chan W, Shu C, et al. Elimination of dose limiting toxicities of cisplatin, 5-fluorouracil, and leucovorin using a weekly 24-hour infusion schedule for the treatment of patients with nasopharyngeal carcinoma. Cancer 1995; 76:2186–2192.

60. Tan E, Khoo K, Wee J, et al. Phase II trial of a paclitaxel and carboplatin combination in Asian patients with metastatic nasopharyngeal carcinoma. Ann Oncol 1999; 10:235–237.

61. Fandi A, Bachouchi M, Azli N, et al. Long-term disease-free survivors in metastatic undifferentiated carcinoma of nasopharyngeal type. J Clin Oncol 2000; 18:1324–1330.

62. Hill M, Constenla D, A'Hern R, et al. Cisplatin and 5-fluorouracil for symptom control in advanced salivary adenoid cystic carcinoma. Eur J Cancer 1997; 33:275–278.

63. Tannock I, Sutherland D. Chemotherapy for adenoid cystic carcinoma. Cancer 1980; 46:452–454.

64. Schramm V, Srodes C, Myers E. Cisplatin therapy for adenoid cystic carcinoma. Arch Otolaryngol 1981; 107(12):739–741.

65. Posner M, Ervin T, Weichselbaum R, et al. Chemotherapy of advanced salivary gland neoplasms. Cancer 1982; 50:2261–2264.

66. Venook A, Tseng AJ, Myers F, et al. Cisplatin, doxorubicin, and 5-fluorouracil chemotherapy for salivary gland malignancies: a pilot study of the Northern

California Oncology Group. J Clin Oncol 1987; 5:951–955.

67. Dreyfuss A, Clark J, Fallon B, et al. Cyclophosphamide, doxorubicin, and cisplatin combination chemotherapy for advanced carcinomas of salivary gland origin. Cancer 1987; 60:2869–2872.

68. Triozzi P, Brantley A, Fisher S, et al. 5-Fluorouracil, cyclophosphamide and vincristine for adenoid cystic carcinoma of the head and neck. Cancer 1987; 59:887–890.

69. Creagan E, Woods J, Rubin J, et al. Cisplatin-based chemotherapy for neoplasms arising from salivary glands and contiguous structures in the head and neck. Cancer 1988; 62:2313–2319.

70. Belani C, Eisenberger M, Gray W. Preliminary experience with chemotherapy in advanced salivary gland neoplasms. Med Pediatr Oncol 1988; 16:197–202.

71. Dimery I, Legha S, Shirinian M, et al. Fluorouracil, doxorubicin, cyclophosphamide and cisplatin combination chemotherapy in advanced or recurrent salivary gland carcinoma. J Clin Oncol 1990; 8:1056–1062.

72. Haan Ld, Mulder Pd, Vermoken J, et al. Cisplatin based chemotherapy in advanced adenoid cystic carcinomas of the head and neck. Head Neck 1992; 14:273–277.

73. Tsukada M, Kokatsu T, Ito K, et al. Chemotherapy for recurrent adeno- and adenoid cystic carcinomas in the head and neck. J Cancer Res Clin Oncol 1993; 119:756–758.

74. Vermoken J, Verweij J, Mulder Pd, et al. Epirubicin in patients with advanced or recurrent adenoid cystic carcinoma of the head and neck. Ann Oncol 1993; 4:785–788.

75. Licitra L, Cavina R, Grandi C, et al. Cisplatin, doxorubicin and cyclophosphamide in advanced salivary gland carcinomas. Ann Oncol 1996; 7:640–642.

76. Verweij J, Mulder Pd, Graeff Ad, et al. Phase II study of mitoxantrone in adenoid cystic carcinomas of the head and neck. Ann Oncol 1996; 7:867–869.

77. Carew JF, Shah JP. Advances in multimodality therapy for laryngeal cancer. CA Cancer J Clin 1998; 48(4):211–228.

78. Weissler MC, Melin S, Sailer S, et al. Simultaneous chemoradiation in the treatment of advanced head and neck cancer. Arch Otolaryngol Head Neck Surg 1992; 118:806–810.

79. Vokes EE, Awan AM, Weichselbaum RR. Radiotherapy with concomitant chemotherapy for head and neck cancer. Haematol Oncol Clin North Am 1991; 5:753–767.

80. Forastiere AA. Chemotherapy of head and neck cancer. Ann Oncol 1992; 3:11–14.

81. al-Sarraf M. Cisplatin combinations in the treatment of head and neck cancer. Semin Oncol 1994; 21:28–34.

82. Bildstein CY, Blendowski C. Head and neck malignancies. In: Groenwald SL, Hansen Frogge M, Goodman M, et al, eds. Cancer nursing. Principles and practice. 4th edn. Boston: Jones and Bartlett; 1998:1199–1234.

83. Robbins KT. Targeted chemoradiation for advanced head and neck cancer. In: Robbins KT, Murry T, eds.

Head and neck cancer. London: Singular Publishing Group; 1998:51–53.

84. Whale Z. Head and neck cancer: an overview of literature. Eur J Oncol Nurs 1998; 2(2):99–105.

85. Scholes C, Frankum L, Maher J. Management of advanced head and neck cancer. Prog Palliat Care 1997; 5(2):54–59.

86. Cremonese G, Bryden G, Bottcher C. A multidisciplinary team approach to preservation of quality of life for patients following oral cancer surgery. ORL Head Neck Nurs 2000; 18(2):6–11.

87. Holmes S. Cancer chemotherapy. A guide for practice. Surrey: Asset Books; 1997.

88. McGrath P. It's OK to say no! Cancer Nurs 1985; 18(2):97–103.

89. Toth BB, Frame RT. Dental oncology: the management of disease and treatment – related oral/dental complications associated with chemotherapy. Curr Probl Cancer 1983; 10:7–35.

90. Iwamoto RR. Cancers of the head and neck. In: Hassey Dow K, Dunn Bucholtz J, Iwamoto R, et al. Nursing care in radiation oncology. Philadelphia: WB Saunders; 1997:239–260.

91. Stevens Fisher P. Nursing management of dysphagia. In: Sullivan PA, Guilford AM, eds. Swallowing intervention in oncology. London: Singular Publishing Group; 1999:181–194.

92. Davis RHL, Roberts D. Nursing care of the patient with head and neck cancer. Oncol Nurs Today 1999; 4(1):9–15.

93. Feber T (ed.). Head and neck oncology nursing. London: Whurr; 2000.

94. Marunick MT. The oral effects of radiation therapy. In: Robbins KT, Murry T, eds. Head and neck cancer. London: Singular Publishing Group; 1998:85–91.

Chapter **43**

Malignant melanoma

CHAPTER CONTENTS

MEDICAL MANAGEMENT OF MALIGNANT MELANOMA

Paul J Ross, Timothy G Eisen and Martin Gore

INTRODUCTION

Melanoma is an increasingly common disease. The incidence of melanoma has increased more rapidly over the last 50 years than all other forms of cancer, except lung cancer in female smokers. The lifetime risk of developing melanoma is 1 in 75 in the United States, rising to 1 in 25 in Australia.[1] In the United Kingdom there were 4980 new cases in 1998, with a male-to-female ratio of 0.67[2] and 1640 deaths distributed equally between men and women.[3] The reasons for this rapid increase in melanoma incidence are unclear, but probably result from a combination of increased exposure to sunlight,[4,5] increased amounts of ultraviolet B (UVB) irradiation reaching the Earth's surface and earlier detection of melanoma.[6]

Most patients present with early-stage disease and surgical excision results in cure rates of at least 90%. However, its behaviour is unpredictable and the Breslow thickness (Fig. 43.1), an indicator of vertical invasion, is the most useful prognostic factor.[7] Very thin melanomas (<1 mm) are rarely associated with relapse. However, patients with a thick primary melanoma (>4 mm) are at high risk of relapse and have a mortality rate of 50–90%. For patients with clinical evidence of regional lymph node involvement, 5-year survival declines to 25%.[8]

Melanoma may present or relapse with either locoregional disease, including intransit metastases or regional lymph node metastases, or distant disease, including

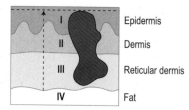

I		Epidermis
II		Dermis
III		Reticular dermis
IV		Fat

Stage 0 Also called melanoma *in situ*. The tumour is on the top layer of the epidermis.

Stage IA The tumour is less than 0.75 mm in thickness and/or has not penetrated to the papillary dermis (directly under the epidermis).

Stage IB The tumour is between 0.75 mm and 1.5mm thick and/or has penetrated to the reticular dermis, the layer of skin under the epidermis.

Stage IIA The tumour is between 1.5 mm and 4 mm thick and/or has penetrated the lower reticular dermis or deep dermis.

Stage IIB The tumour is more that 4 mm in thickness and/or invades subcutaneous fat. Additional tumours called satellites may be found within 2 cm of the primary melanoma.

Stage III The melanoma has spread to regional lymph nodes draining the involved area of skin.

Stage IV Distant metastases.

Figure 43.1 Breslow thickness.

non-regional nodal metastases and visceral metastases. There are two large overviews of survival for patients with metastatic melanoma. An analysis comprising 1521 patients reported a median survival of 7.5 months,[9] while a more recent meta-analysis comprising 5392 patients in 74 studies demonstrated a median survival of 7.9 months.[10] Survival with metastatic melanoma has been observed to correlate with:

- number of organ sites involved
- visceral involvement (except lung)
- elevated serum lactate dehydrogenase (LDH)
- reduced albumin
- male gender.[11]

However, treatment has no effect on survival of patients with metastatic melanoma. This emphasises the need to identify more effective therapies in patients with metastatic melanoma.

INVESTIGATION

Patients with melanoma are usually staged with full blood count, urea and electrolytes, liver function tests and serum LDH. Radiological studies should generally be limited to chest X-ray and liver ultrasound. Further investigation is only required if clinically indicated. For instance, if palliative surgery is to be considered, the greater accuracy of a computed tomography (CT) scan of thorax, abdomen and pelvis may help to determine if such surgery is appropriate.

There is considerable interest in the use of serum S100-beta levels and positron emission tomography (PET) for staging patients with melanoma. S100-beta is a calcium-binding protein found in melanoma cells. The proportion of patients with elevated serum levels of S100-beta increases with advancing stage of melanoma. Two studies have shown that elevated serum levels of S100-beta correlated with disease progression and shorter survival but did not give relevant additional information to that provided by serum LDH.[12,13] PET is a highly sensitive technique in melanoma,[14–16] being more sensitive than conventional radiology for the detection of lymph node and bone metastases. However, it is less sensitive for lung and brain metastases, and studies give conflicting data on the relative sensitivity of PET compared to conventional radiology for the detection of liver metastases. The precise role of PET in the management of patients with melanoma has yet to be defined and its use should be limited to trials evaluating its role.

Sentinel node biopsy following complete excision of a primary melanoma is increasingly used but remains controversial. This is based on the concept that regions of the skin have specific patterns of lymphatic drainage and drain preferentially to selected (sentinel) nodes. It should not be offered to patients with melanomas of less than 0.8 mm thickness, as this was the thickness used in studies evaluating sentinel node biopsy. Before undergoing sentinel node biopsy, patients should be staged with chest radiograph and liver ultrasound to exclude metastatic disease. No survival benefit has been demonstrated from sentinel node biopsy;[17] however, it does provide prognostic information. Thus, the controversy surrounding sentinel node biopsy is an ethical debate as to whether it is appropriate to seek prognostic information in a disease in which there is no established adjuvant therapy.

ADJUVANT THERAPY

Adjuvant chemotherapy

There is no established role for adjuvant chemotherapy in melanoma following the resection of either a primary melanoma or regional lymph node metastases. Four randomised trials with observation-only control arms have demonstrated no benefit for adjuvant dacarbazine (DTIC) chemotherapy in patients at high risk of relapse following surgery for primary melanoma and/or nodal metastases.[18–21] In the largest of these trials, 395 patients were randomised to DTIC (200 mg/m^2 days 1–5 every 4 weeks for 6 cycles) or observation. After a median follow-up of 41 months, disease-free and overall survival rates were not significantly different in the two arms.

Adjuvant immunotherapy

In 1996, the United States Food and Drug Administration (FDA) approved high-dose interferon α-2b (HDI) as adjuvant therapy for patients at high risk of relapse after resection of melanoma (American Joint Committee on Cancer (AJCC) stage IIB–III). This decision was based on the results of an Eastern Cooperative Oncology Group trial (ECOG 1684) in which 287 patients with T4 N0 or Tany N1 melanoma were randomised to HDI (induction phase: intravenous (IV) 20 MU/m^2 daily for 5 out of 7 days for 4 weeks; maintenance subcutaneous (sc) 10 MU/m^2 three times weekly for 48 weeks) or no treatment.[22] After a median follow-up of 6.9 years, the median survival (3.8 vs 2.8 years; $p = 0.002$) and 5-year survival (46% vs 37%; $p = 0.02$) were significantly improved with HDI. In addition, relapse-free survival was significantly improved with HDI ($p = 0.002$). The greatest impact of HDI was observed early in the trial, suggesting that the 4 weeks of IV therapy were necessary and may be sufficient for the clinical benefit. A North Central Cancer Treatment Group trial randomised 262 patients to 12 weeks of intramuscular (IM) HDI (20 MU/m^2) or observation. This study did not confirm the survival benefit but an intention-to-treat analysis demonstrated a trend towards improved disease-free survival with HDI ($p = 0.09$). Although moderate-to-severe toxicity, including fever, chills and flu-like symptoms, myelosuppression, hepatic and neurological, was observed in the majority of patients, a survival analysis adjusted for quality of life suggested the clinical benefit of treatment outweighed the toxic effects.[23]

A subsequent randomised trial ECOG 1690 randomised 642 patients to receive either HDI, low-dose interferon (3 MU three times per week sc for 2 years) or observation.[24] In this study no survival benefit was observed with either HDI or low-dose interferon. As with the ECOG 1684 study, a significant improvement in relapse-free survival was observed with HDI ($p = 0.054$) with a median follow-up of 52 months. The major difference between the ECOG 1690 and ECOG 1684 trials was a significantly better survival of patients in the observation arm of ECOG 1690

($p = 0.001$). One possible explanation for this is that patients in the observation arm of the ECOG 1690 trial who relapsed were rescued with interferon. In ECOG 1690, 36 (31%) of the 121 observation patients who relapsed were treated with interferon. Interferon salvage resulted in a significant improvement in median survival (2.22 years vs 0.82 years; $p = 0.002$).

The ECOG have now presented preliminary data from a third trial, ECOG 1694, including 880 patients randomised to HDI or the G_{M2} vaccine sc, weekly for 1 month, and then 3-monthly for 2 years. G_{M2} is a neuraminic acid containing glycosphingolipid G_{M2} ganglioside, and was one of the most active vaccines in phase II trials. In April 2000, the data monitoring committee, having reviewed data on 774 eligible patients with a median follow-up of 16.1 months, closed the trial. HDI resulted in a significant improvement in relapse-free ($p = 0.0015$) and overall ($p = 0.009$) survival. Due to the early closure of this trial, many investigators and clinicians treating melanoma do not accept this trial confirms the survival benefit from adjuvant treatment with HDI.

Two European studies provide further evidence in support of adjuvant interferon. These trials, in patients with intermediate-risk disease (AJCC stage II; T3 or T4 N0), randomised patients to low-dose interferon-α or observation. One study, with a median follow-up of 41 months, demonstrated an improvement in disease-free survival ($p = 0.02$) but no overall survival advantage.[25] The second study, with a median follow-up of 5 years, observed significant improvement in disease-free survival ($p = 0.02$) and overall survival ($p = 0.06$).[26]

Results from two further large studies are currently awaited. The European Organisation for Research and Treatment of Cancer (EORTC) 18592 study included more than 1200 patients with stage II–III melanoma. Patients were randomised to observation or IFN-α2b (10 MU/m^2 sc days 1–5 for 4 weeks followed by 10 MU/m^2 three times per week sc for 1 year or 5 MU/m^2 three times per week sc for 2 years) and results are anticipated later this year. The United Kingdom Coordinating Committee on Cancer Research (UKCCCR) AIM HIGH (adjuvant interferon in melanoma – high risk) study randomised patients with stage IIB–III melanoma to observation or low-dose interferon for 2 years. The EORTC has recently opened a trial assessing the role of pegylated interferon.

In conclusion, adjuvant therapy with HDI has a consistent effect on disease-free survival in patients at high risk of relapse after resection of melanoma (stage IIB–III). Only one trial with sufficient follow-up (E1684) has demonstrated a significant improvement. Furthermore, no survival benefit from HDI has been detected by separate meta-analyses from the ECOG.[27,103] Consequent to the lack of a clear beneficial impact of HDI on long-term survival and because of its high toxicity profile, HDI has not been adopted as standard adjuvant therapy in Europe. It is too early for definitive analysis of further trials and thus the mature results of these trials are awaited. In addition, the impact of dose and duration of treatment awaits further evaluation.

TREATMENT OF METASTATIC MELANOMA

Single agent chemotherapy

Four classes of chemotherapy have demonstrated activity in melanoma: DTIC, nitrosoureas, tubular agents and platinum compounds. In addition, newer agents found to have activity in melanoma include temozolomide, fotemustine and taxanes.

DTIC

DTIC, synthesised in 1959, is the most active single agent, with response rates of approximately 20%.[28,29] In contrast, response rates of approximately 15% are observed with nitrosoureas,[28] platinum compounds and tubular toxins.[29] The highest response rates (25–35%) with DTIC are observed with skin, subcutaneous and lymph node metastases; 15% with lung metastases; declining to 5–10% with liver, bone and brain metastases.[30] The median duration of response is 5–6 months. Complete responses are observed in 5% of patients, mostly in subcutaneous and lymph node metastases.[29] Overall, only 2% of patients treated with DTIC achieved durable complete responses and were disease-free for more than 6 years.

DTIC has been administered using a variety of doses and schedules. However, none has demonstrated a survival advantage relative to other schedules; consequently, most centres now use a dose of 1 g/m^2 as a 1 hour infusion three-weekly, administered together with a 5HT3 (5-hydroxytryptamine or serotonin) antagonist.

Fotemustine

Fotemustine is a chloroethyl nitrosourea that effectively crosses the blood–brain barrier and induces responses in brain metastases. Two studies administering fotemustine demonstrated a response rate of around 24%, including patients with cerebral metastases.[31,32]

Temozolomide

Temozolomide, a novel alkylating agent, is the prodrug of methyltriazeno-imidazole-carboxamide (MTIC), the active metabolite of DTIC. Unlike DTIC, which requires hepatic activation, temozolomide converts spontaneously to MTIC under physiological conditions. In a randomised trial of 305 patients, response rates of 12.1% with oral (po) temozolomide (200 mg/m^2/day for 5 days every 28 days) and 13.5% with DTIC (250 mg/m^2/day for 5 days every 21 days) were reported.[33] Median survival was similar: 7.7 months with temozolomide and 6.4 months with DTIC ($p = 0.2$). Temozolomide was well tolerated, with no statistically significant differences in toxicity compared to DTIC. Quality of life studies reported significantly better physical functioning and less insomnia for patients treated with temozolomide after 12 weeks. However, temozolomide is not currently licensed for use in the treatment of melanoma, as the FDA do not recognise DTIC as the standard of care in melanoma and have indicated a randomised trial against best supportive care alone would be required.

Taxanes

The taxanes paclitaxel and docetaxel have been evaluated in the treatment of metastatic melanoma. Two small studies evaluating paclitaxel observed response rates of 12% and 14%, respectively.[34,35] Single agent docetaxel has been evaluated in three small phase II trials.[36–38] Response rates were 17%, 12.5% and 6%, respectively. The activity of taxanes in melanoma has not been compared with DTIC in a randomised trial, and taxanes have no established role in the treatment of melanoma.

Combination chemotherapy

Many investigators examined combination chemotherapy in an effort to improve efficacy. Frequently, single institution phase II studies indicated higher response rates with combination chemotherapy. However, multicentre studies did not confirm such improvement. This was illustrated with the combination of vinblastine, bleomycin and cisplatin (VBD). Early phase II data suggested a response rate of 71%,[39] which fell to 43% with increased patient numbers.[40] Subsequently, a randomised comparison with DTIC observed a response rate of only 10% with VBD.[41] Furthermore, there was a trend towards longer progression-free and overall survival with DTIC.

A combination of DTIC (220 mg/m^2 days 1–3), cisplatin (25 mg/m^2 days 1–3), carmustine (150 mg/m^2 day 1 alternate cycles) and tamoxifen (10 mg orally twice daily) (the Dartmouth regimen) was initially reported to have a response rate of 55%.[42] A total of 384 patients were included in eight confirmatory unrandomised trials, with an overall response rate of 44% (95% CI 41.7–56.5%), with a complete response rate of

Table 43.1 Randomised trials including the Dartmouth regimen

Reference	No. patients	Response rate (%)	Median survival (months)
82	106	30	7
65	30	27	5.5
83	39	22	8
84	8	22	6.5
67	52	27	15.8
44	119	17	7.7

14%.[43] However, the hope generated by unrandomised observations was not confirmed in subsequent randomised trials. Six randomised trials included the Dartmouth regimen as one of the arms (Table 43.1); the response rates did not appear to be superior to single agent DTIC. The most recently reported trial included 240 patients in a randomised comparison to DTIC (1 g/m² 3-weekly).[44] Response rates (10% vs 18.5%; $p = 0.09$) and survival (6.3 months vs 7.7 months; $p = 0.38$) were similar with DTIC and the Dartmouth regimen. However, the Dartmouth regimen resulted in significantly increased toxicity. Consequently, there is no advantage to treatment with the Dartmouth regimen and single agent DTIC (1 g/m² 3-weekly) remains the gold standard for patients with metastatic melanoma.

Immunotherapy

The natural history of malignant melanoma is thought to be significantly influenced by the host immune response, and there have been attempts to treat melanoma by immunotherapy since the 1960s. The identification and availability of interferon-α (IFN-α) and interleukin-2 (IL-2) has resulted in considerable interest in the treatment of melanoma with these agents.

Interferon-α

IFN-α may act via antiproliferative activity, stimulating natural killer (NK) cell and cytotoxic T lymphocytes (CTL) and the up-regulation of cell surface antigens on tumour in vitro, in particular major histocompatibility complexes (MHC) I and II. IFN-α was observed to have antitumour activity in melanoma in phase II studies. An overview of 11 trials, including 315 patients treated with doses ranging from 10–50 MIU/m² sc three times weekly, to 20 MIU/m² IV daily, demonstrated an overall response rate of 15% (48/315) and one-third of responses were complete.[45] Prognostic factors were similar to those predicting response to cytotoxic chemotherapy: performance status and sites of disease (soft tissue, skin and nodal being good prognostic factors). The median duration of response was 8 months (range 1 to >60 months).

Toxicities Flu-like symptoms, the major toxicity of IFN-α, are dose-dependent and were previously discussed in the Adjuvant Immunotherapy section. Constitutional symptoms may resolve over time; the management of these symptoms is discussed in the Nursing Management of Malignant Melanoma section. Rare side effects include pancytopenia, abnormal liver function and neuropsychiatric symptoms. (The management of immunotherapy toxicity is also discussed in the Nursing Management of Melanoma section.)

In conclusion, IFN-α appears to have similar response rates to single agent DTIC, but no randomised comparisons have been undertaken. Therefore, its role in the treatment of advanced melanoma remains undefined and should be limited to clinical trials.

Interleukin-2

IL-2 is an immunostimulatory cytokine with antitumour effects mediated via activation of NK and specific cytotoxic T cells, lymphokine-activated killer (LAK) cells. An overview of 15 trials – comprising 540 patients, treated with bolus doses ranging from 12 MIU/m² three times per week to 50 MIU/m² three times per day, and continuous infusion schedules from 3 to 7 MIU/m²/day – reported a response rate of 15% (range 3–50%), with 2% achieving complete response. The largest study in this overview involved 134 patients treated with high-dose bolus IL-2 three times daily until grade 3 or 4 toxicity was reached for 2 cycles.[46] The overall response rate was 17%, and 9% demonstrated complete response. Complete responses were maintained for 9–91 months, with partial responses maintained for 2–34 months. A retrospective analysis of 266 patients treated with high-dose bolus IL-2 three times daily demonstrated a response rate of 17%.[47] Six per cent (16/266) achieved a complete response, with the median duration not reached at the time of analysis. Ten complete responders were progression-free at a median follow-up of 5 years.

Response to IL-2 does not appear to depend upon site of disease, with similar response rates at visceral and non-visceral metastases. High-dose IV bolus IL-2 appears to be more effective than low-dose continuous infusion. As with IFN-α, the toxicity of IL-2 depends upon dose and route of delivery, and the most frequent side effect is flu-like symptoms. Hypotension, vascular leak syndrome, renal, gastrointestinal and haematological toxicities are frequently dose-limiting.

IL-2 has similar response rates to DTIC and to IFN-α, but no randomised comparisons have been undertaken. Furthermore, no factors predictive of response to IL-2 have been identified. Consequently, the role of single agent IL-2 is yet to be established and its use should be restricted to clinical trials.

Interferon-α and interleukin-2

Murine (mouse) models suggested that the different mechanisms of action of IFN-α and IL-2 resulted in synergistic activity. Moreover, phase I and II trials suggested response rates of 20–40%. However, in a meta-analysis, including 911 patients treated with IFN-α and IL-2, a response rate of 17% was reported with combination treatment, which was not significantly better than IL-2 alone (15%) and was inferior to chemotherapy (29%).[48] The median survival was 11 months with combination therapy, which was not significantly better than treatment with IL-2 alone (8 months) or chemotherapy (8.6 months). One study randomised 85 patients between IL-2 alone and IL-2 combined with IFN-α.[49] Response rates were 5% with IL-2 alone compared to 10% with IL-2 + IFN-α ($p = 0.3$), with no complete responses in either arm. Furthermore, there was no significant difference in overall survival (9.7 months vs 10.2 months). In conclusion, no clear advantage for combination IL-2/IFN-α therapy has been demonstrated, and it remains experimental.

Combined chemotherapy and immunotherapy

Chemotherapy and immunotherapy drugs have different mechanisms of action and a number of preclinical studies indicated additive or synergistic effects for such combinations. In addition, chemotherapy and immunotherapy have different toxicity profiles. Consequently, this has become one of the most active areas of clinical research in metastatic melanoma.

Interferon-α and chemotherapy

Five randomised trials compared DTIC alone to the combination of IFN-α and DTIC (Table 43.2). One single institution trial, involving 64 patients, reported response, time to treatment failure (2.5 months vs 9.0 months) and overall survival (9.6 months vs 17.6 months) advantages with combination therapy.[50] Furthermore, the numbers of patients achieving complete response increased from 2 (7%) to 12 (40%) with combination therapy. However, these response and survival advantages were not confirmed in subsequent larger randomised studies.[51–53] Consequently, it is unlikely that the addition of IFN-α to DTIC results in significant therapeutic benefit.

Others have examined the addition of IFN-α to the BOLD (bleomycin, vincristine, lomustine (CCNU) and DTIC), Dartmouth or CVD (cisplatin, vinblastine, and DTIC) regimens. Response rates ranged from 26 to 68%.[54–58] However, these regimens did not improve

Table 43.2 Randomised trials comparing dacarbazine (DTIC) alone with DTIC + interferon-α (IFN-α)

Regimen	No. patients	Response rate (%)	Median survival (months)	Reference
DTIC	24	21	–	85
IFN-α	23	4	–	
DTIC + IFN-α	21	19	–	
DTIC	31	20	10	50
DTIC + IFN-α	30	53*	18	
DTIC	83	17	8	51
DTIC + IFN-α	87	21	9	
DTIC	82	20		52
DTIC + IFN-α 9 MIU/day	76	28		
DTIC + IFN-α 3 MIU three times per week	84	23		
DTIC	67	12	9	53
DTIC + IFN-α	65	21	9	

*$p = 0.007$.

survival and many resulted in unacceptable levels of myelosuppression.

Interleukin-2 and chemotherapy

Data from a meta-analysis of 19 studies, including 523 patients treated with combinations of IL-2 and chemotherapy, demonstrated a response rate of 22% and a median survival of 9.4 months. However, neither response nor survival was significantly improved compared to single agent chemotherapy or immunotherapy.

Biochemotherapy

Biochemotherapy refers to treatment with a combination of IFN-α, IL-2 and chemotherapy. Several studies reported the combinations of IL-2 and IFN-α with DTIC and/or cisplatin. These trials included patients with progressive and metastatic melanoma, good performance status, no brain metastasis and no prior exposure to any treatment component. Patients entering trials of biochemotherapy will often be required to have a CT brain scan, to prevent patients with cerebral metastases being treated in such trials. This is because there is a risk of exacerbating the space-occupying effect of cerebral metastases with both interferon and interleukin-2.

Khayat et al treated 39 patients with cisplatin, IL-2 and IFN-α. A response rate of 54% was observed, with 5 patients (13%) achieving complete response.[59] Other groups examined the addition of biological therapy to polychemotherapy. Phase II studies demonstrated these regimens to have response rates greater than 50% (Table 43.3). The combination of biological therapy with the Dartmouth regimen was first reported in 1992, and updated results were presented in 1999.[60,61] A response rate of 55% was observed among 83 assessable patients, with 12 complete responses (CR). The median survival was 12.2 months, with a plateau at 10.7%, 52 months from initial treatment. The MD

Anderson Cancer Center evaluated the combination of CVD with biological therapy. Three schedules have been studied (alternating, sequential and concurrent). In the alternating schedule, patients receive either two 5-day courses of CVD followed by one 5-day course of biological therapy, or three 5-day courses of biological therapy followed 3 weeks later by a 5-day course of CVD. Sequential scheduling involved CVD followed immediately by IL-2 and IFN-α, or the reverse sequence. Response rates of 33% (5% CR), 60% (23% CR) and 64% (21% CR) were observed with the alternating, sequential and concurrent schedules respectively.[62,63] Patients achieving complete remission with each of the three schedules demonstrated durable remissions lasting for 40+ to 75 months.

Thus, the most notable observation from phase II studies was that of durable CRs. A total of 278 patients have been treated with biochemotherapy, with CRs in 16%. CR was durable in at least 24 patients (8%) and 13 were maintained for at least 2 years. Toxicity varied, depending on dose and schedule. Frequently observed toxicities include myelosuppression, gastrointestinal toxicity, capillary leak syndrome, cardiac toxicity and autoimmune phenomena. It has been suggested that autoimmune phenomena, including vitiligo, are associated with responses and improved survival.

There are four randomised trials in which biochemotherapy has been evaluated (Table 43.4). A study from the EORTC has demonstrated the benefits of the addition of cisplatin to biological therapy.[64] One hundred and thirty-eight patients were treated with IL-2 + IFN-α alone or in combination with cisplatin. Response (33% vs 18%; $p = 0.04$) and progression-free survival (92 days vs 53 days; $p = 0.02$) were significantly better with cisplatin. However, there was no difference in overall survival, with a 9-month median duration of survival for all patients. A Royal Marsden Hospital study randomised 65 patients to the

Table 43.3   Phase II studies of biochemotherapy

Chemotherapy	No.	Complete response (%)	Overall response (%)	Duration complete response	Median survival (months)	Ref
Cisplatin	39	13	54	89+, 75+, 73+, 14, 13 weeks	11	59
CVD (alternating)	40	5	33	72+, 75+ months	Not stated	62
CVD (sequential)	62	23	60	40+, 40+, 41+, 42+, 48+, 48+, 52+, 52+ months	13	62
CVD (concurrent)	53	21	64	10, 12, 17, 23, 35, 50+, 50+, 52+, 54+, 56+, 61+ months	11.8	63
Dartmouth regimen	84	14	55	Not stated	12.2	61

CVD = cisplatin, vinblastine and dacarbazine (DTIC).

Table 43.4   Randomised studies of biochemotherapy

Regimen	Number	Response rate (%)	Survival (months)	Reference
BCDT +/– IL-2 + IFN-α	65	27 vs 22	5 vs 5.5	65
CDT +/– IL-2 + IFN-α	102	44 vs 27	10.7 vs 15.8	67
DT + IL-2 + IFN	92	13		66
CVDT + IFN		35		
CVDT + IFN + IL-2		37		
CD + IFN-α +/– IL-2	118	28 vs 22	Not stated	86

BCDT = carmustine (BCNU), cisplatin, dacarbazine (DTIC) and tamoxifen; IL-2 = interleukin-2; IFN-α = interferon-α; CVDT = cisplatin, vindesine, DTIC and tamoxifen.

Dartmouth regimen alone or combined with IL-2 and IFN-α.[65] This study did not detect any difference in response rate, progression-free survival or overall survival following the addition of biological therapy. Furthermore, the response rates were lower than for previous biochemotherapy studies and only 1 patient demonstrated a complete response. However, the doses of IL-2 and IFN-α were deliberately low to reduce toxicity. In a randomised phase II trial comprising 92 patients, no significant difference in response rates was observed from the addition of IL-2 to cisplatin, vindesine, DTIC, tamoxifen and IFN-α (37% v 35%).[66] The fourth study randomised 102 patients to cisplatin, DTIC and tamoxifen alone or combined with biological therapy.[67] A non-significant improvement in response was observed (44% vs 27%; $p = 0.07$), but there was no difference in survival. A fifth study performed by the EORTC, comprising 350 patients randomised to DTIC, cisplatin and IFN-α with or without IL-2, recently completed accrual. Preliminary data suggest no difference in objective response rates (28% vs 22%; $p = 0.12$), but the number of patients without relapse was higher in the IL-2-containing arm (10 vs 2 patients; $p = 0.028$).

In conclusion, randomised trials have failed to demonstrate response or survival benefits with biochemotherapy. Indeed, durable complete responses were not observed in randomised studies. Nonetheless, randomised trials of biochemotherapy continue in order to see if subgroups of patients may benefit. An important issue is that of patient selection because of the toxicity associated with biochemotherapy. Most patients of good performance status, aged 70 years old or less, will be able to tolerate biochemotherapy.

Cerebral metastases

Brain metastases occur in 20–30% of patients with metastatic melanoma, and treatment has limited efficacy, with survival ranging from 3 to 6 months. A 20-year review from Duke University Medical Center included 702 patients with clinically significant brain metastases.[68] In this series, 178 patients were managed without antitumour therapy, 205 were treated with systemic chemotherapy and 139 underwent surgical excision, of whom 87 received postoperative radiotherapy. The most frequent modality of treatment was whole brain radiotherapy. Median survival was 39 days with chemotherapy and 120 days with radiotherapy. Surgery resulted in significantly longer survival than radiotherapy ($p < 0.0001$), but there was no advantage to postoperative radiotherapy (268 days) compared to surgery alone (195 days; $p = 0.9998$). The findings of this series were consistent with survival times based on a previous overview of the literature (Table 43.5). Furthermore, the survival benefit of surgical excision was consistent with a randomised study of 45 patients with solitary brain metastasis from solid tumours, including 3 patients with melanoma.[69] Overall survival was significantly longer with surgery + radiotherapy (40 weeks) compared to whole-brain radiotherapy alone (15 weeks; $p < 0.01$).

Based on these data, surgical resection of solitary brain metastasis in the absence of other visceral metastases is recommended. In addition, surgery may be

Table 43.5   Treatment of cerebral metastases of malignant melanoma

Therapeutic modality	Number	Median survival (range) (weeks)
No treatment	15	3 (<4–16)
Corticotherapy	17	6 (<4–16)
Surgery	119	20 (3–154)
Radiotherapy	308	13.4 (0.8–154)
Surgery + radiotherapy	192	28 (5–134)

considered for a solitary metastasis, especially in the posterior cranial fossa, associated with other visceral disease that is either indolent or responding to systemic therapy. Patients with multiple cerebral metastases or an operable metastasis concurrent with progressive disease at other sites should be treated with whole-brain radiotherapy.

VACCINE THERAPY

Vaccines use tumour-derived products to produce antitumour immune responses, which may be antibody and/or T-cell-mediated responses. Vaccine therapy for melanoma has been under evaluation for three decades. Vaccines may be autologous (requiring a tumour cell specimen to be processed for each patient) or allogenic (using antigens shared by many tumours). There are three broad categories of vaccine: cell vaccines, peptide vaccines and genetically modified vaccines.

Cell vaccines

In 1978, a randomised trial reported a non-significant reduction in recurrence rates after lymphadenectomy for nodal metastases using an allogenic vaccine.[70] This group have developed a polyvalent melanoma cell vaccine (CancerVax) that was anticipated to be more immunogenic. Phase II studies have demonstrated improved survival for patients treated with the vaccine (23 months) compared to historical control (7.5 months).[71] Subsequently, a randomised trial of BCG (bacille Calmette-Guérin) + CancerVax or placebo as post-surgical adjuvant treatment for stage IV melanoma has commenced.

Another polyvalent allogenic vaccine (Melacine) uses melanoma lysates and an adjuvant Detox (a 'detoxified' bacterial endotoxin).[72] Initially, this vaccine demonstrated 20% response rates (5% CR), but in multicentre studies the response rate fell to 8%, with 23% demonstrating stable disease for more than 6 months. The survival time for stable or responding patients was 23 months. A randomised comparison of Melacine + cyclophosphamide demonstrated no response advantage to the Dartmouth regimen, with survival of 12.1 months and 9.4 months, respectively.

An alternative strategy was the development of an autologous vaccine by modifying tumour cells with the hapten, dinitrophenyl.[73] Tumour responses were observed in 4 of 16 patients with lung metastases, but none of the other 64 patients.[74] This limited response was similar to the limited responses observed with autologous vaccines evaluated in the 1970s. It is possible that efficacy is limited by tumour burden and this type of vaccine may have a role in the adjuvant setting.

Peptide vaccines

Over recent years melanoma antigens recognised by T cells have been identified. These include tumour-specific antigens (MAGE, BAGE, CAGE proteins) and lineage-specific antigens (gp100, MART-1, tyrosinase). The identification of immunodominant peptides has formed the basis of many vaccines entering clinical trials in the late 1990s.

One group have treated patients with gp100 peptide in incomplete Freund's adjuvant.[75] Both modified and unmodified peptides were evaluated, together with modified peptide combined with high-dose IL-2. Objective clinical responses and T-cell responses were observed, as shown in Table 43.6. The observation of specific T-cell response in the absence of clinical response raises the question as to how tumour vaccines effect antitumour activity, and whether concurrent treatment with biological response modifiers, such as IL-2, is necessary for clinically effective treatment.

An alternative method to induce immune response to melanoma antigens is the use of pulsed dendritic cells. Dendritic cells are antigen-presenting cells that perform a central role in the induction of a primary T-cell response. One study treated 16 patients by injecting a non-involved inguinal node with dendritic cells cultured from blood pulsed with a cocktail of melanoma peptides or tumour lysate. Keyhole limpet haemocyanin was added to recruit T-helper cells and promote maturation of CTL. Five patients responded with 2 CRs; clinical responses were associated specific antigen responses. A second group treated 11 patients with dendritic cells pulsed with MAGE-3A1, tumour peptide and a recall antigen, tetanus toxoid or tuberculin.[76] Expansions of MAGE-3A1-specific CTL were induced in 8 patients and regression of metastases observed in 6 patients. Two patients had complete resolution of skin metastases. These studies suggest that

Table 43.6	Objective and T-cell responses to gp100 peptide vaccine[75]		
	Modified gp100 in IFA	Unmodified gp100 in IFA	Modified gp100 in IFA + IL-2
Number	11	9	19
Objective responses	0	1	8
Specific T-cell responses	10	2	3

IFA = incomplete Freund's adjuvant; IL-2 = interleukin-2.

Table 43.7 Studies using genetically modified autologous melanoma cell vaccines

Author	Genetic modification	Number	IgG response	CTL response	Clinical response
77	IFN-γ	13	8/13	–	2/13
78	IL-7	10	–	3/6	0
79	IFN-γ	12	–	–	0
80	GM-CSF	29 (21 completed vaccination)	11/16	11/16	1
81	IL-2	12	–	4/12	0

IgG = immunoglobulin G; CTL = cytotoxic T lymphocyte; IFN-γ = interferon-γ; IL-2 = interleukin-2; IL-7 = interleukin-7; GM-CSF = granulocyte–macrophage colony-stimulating factor.

pulsed dendritic cells may be effective in the management of advanced melanoma, but further studies are required.

Genetically modified vaccines

There are at least five studies reporting vaccination by autologous melanoma cells that have been genetically modified to produce cytokines.[77–81] These studies have used genetic modifications for IFN-γ, IL-2, IL-7 or GM-CSF (granulocyte–macrophage colony-stimulating factor) and have demonstrated both immunoglobulin and CTL responses (Table 43.7). In addition, some trials detected clinical responses while others observed disease stabilisation. Furthermore, these studies have demonstrated that vaccination with genetically modified autologous melanoma cells is safe. Consequently, further evaluation of this therapeutic strategy is justified.

CONCLUSIONS

Malignant melanoma is an increasingly common disease. The majority of patients present with early-stage disease and surgical excision results in cure rates of 90%. For patients at high risk of relapse after resection of a melanoma (stage IIB–III), adjuvant high-dose interferon may improve survival. Despite the consensus forming that such therapy should be adopted, many questions remain regarding the role of adjuvant interferon in the management of melanoma.

The prognosis for patients with metastatic melanoma remains poor. Currently, single agent DTIC is the gold standard treatment for patients with metastatic malignant melanoma. There is considerable enthusiasm for biochemotherapy despite the reality that randomised studies have not confirmed the gains observed in phase II trials. Nevertheless, trials should continue to explore the possibility that a small subset of patients may achieve durable responses. Future trials need to identify the characteristics of such patients, so that this treatment is limited to patients likely to benefit. In addition, trials need to examine the component parts of biochemotherapy to establish the optimal regimen. Increasing knowledge of tumour immunology is expanding the vaccine strategies under investigation. Vaccines have demonstrated induction of T-cell responses and objective responses. However, induction of CTL response does not consistently correlate directly with objective responses. It would seem likely that antitumour activity of vaccines will need to be better understood before a highly effective vaccine is developed.

In conclusion, clinicians treating patients with melanoma requiring adjuvant therapy or therapy for metastatic disease should be encouraged to enter patients in clinical trials whenever possible.

NURSING MANAGEMENT OF MALIGNANT MELANOMA

Dana Walker

INTRODUCTION

The established treatment of primary cutaneous melanoma, or skin or lymph node metastases is surgical excision. Chemotherapy has a role in stage IV disease, dacarbazine (DTIC) being the standard drug, which, since the advent of the 5HT3 antagonist is well tolerated, with a limited side-effect profile (see Medical Management section). However, at present, chemotherapy is palliative in intent, and no chemotherapy currently has a role in the adjuvant setting.[87]

As the incidence of malignant melanoma continues to rise, studies that use biological therapy in its treatment are increasing. Nurses will be caring for more patients receiving these agents and need to be able to effectively manage the side effects linked with these therapies. Two common areas are:

- as an adjuvant treatment for patients at high risk of relapse post-surgical resection of lymph node metastasis (adjuvant interferon)[88]
- in metastatic disease, whereby IFN-α and IL-2 are used in combination with chemotherapy (biochemotherapy).[89]

PATIENT ASSESSMENT

Biological agents such as INF-α and IL-2 have a unique profile of side effects differing from other anti-cancer agents. There is a group of side effects common to them both and also some individual to each agent (Table 43.8). All biological therapies are dose- and schedule-dependent: the higher the dose the more severe the side effects. Patients should be carefully screened for their suitability for treatment in relation

to performance status, extensive tumour involvement, medical history, physical examination and laboratory tests, before initiating treatment. Patients with a significant history of cardiac, renal, hepatic or pulmonary abnormality should not be considered as candidates for high-dose regimes.[90] Patients should also have an ECOG performance status of 2 or less, high-dose regimes being 0–1. The extent of tumour involvement should also be assessed and the presence of brain metastasis excluded.

PATIENT INFORMATION

Much of the use of biological agents in malignant melanoma is within the context of a clinical trial. Their role is still largely undefined and work is still being undertaken to find optimal doses and routes of administration that are clinically effective but less toxic. Patient information is critical for all patients with cancer, whatever treatments they are undergoing; however, it is vital that patients on trials are given enough accurate information and have a clear understanding of the goals of therapy and expected outcomes before treatment begins. Patients need to know the possible side effects and how these should be managed, as other sources such as the GP or district nurse may not have great experience for managing side effects from biological agents. They also need information on how to contact the relevant staff to report any problems experienced. This is particularly important when treatments are based in the community, such as IFN-α or subcutaneous (sc) IL-2 therapy. Patients and their families need teaching and support to enable them to self-administer these sc injections. It is important that written, verbal and even visual aids, such as videotapes, are given to the patient and the professionals in the community, to provide the support needed to facilitate self-administration.[91] (See also Ch. 5.)

MANAGEMENT OF SIDE EFFECTS

Flu–like syndrome

Flu-like syndrome (FLS) is an umbrella term used for the variety of symptoms that typically occur when using biological therapy. The major symptoms include fever, chills and rigors, headache and myalgia, arthralgia and fatigue. FLS is more severe following administration of the first dose, lessening in severity as treatment continues. Patients can develop tolerance to the symptoms (tachyphylaxis) with continued dosing (common when using IFN-α), finding symptoms disappear. However, patients should be warned that symptoms would probably return following restarting of the injections after a break from treatment

Table 43.8	Side effects of immunotherapy agents
Agent	**Common side effects**
Interferon	Flu-like symptoms
	Fatigue
	Anorexia/weight loss
	Alterations in laboratory values
	(haematology and liver function tests)
	Skin rash
	Injection site reactions
	Mental status changes
Interleukin-2	Flu-like symptoms
	Fatigue
	Anorexia
	Nausea and vomiting
	Mental status changes
	Diarrhoea
	Capillary leak syndrome
	Oedema and fluid retention
	Hypotension
	Oliguria
	Tachycardia
	Skin rash, erythema and desquamation
	Inflammatory reactions/induration at
	injection sites
	Weight gain
	Alterations in laboratory values
	(haematology, liver function tests)

(drug holiday), if severe toxicity has required it.[91,92] Nurses should ensure that patients are premedicated (Table 43.9) with an analgesic such as paracetamol, and continue to take medication until symptoms disappear.

Fever and rigors

The body's temperature is controlled by thermoregulatory receptors in the anterior hypothalmus that pick up deviations from a set normal temperature range (36.4–37.3°C). These receptors, through a feedback mechanism with the peripheral sensors, trigger heat-producing vasoconstriction and shivering or heat loss actions such as vasodilation and sweating.[93] Biological agents stimulate the release of endogenous pyrogenic cytokines, such as IL-1, IL-6 and tumour necrosis factor (TNF), which, along with infection, toxins or drugs, act on the thermoregulatory centres in the anterior hypo-thalamus, inducing prostaglandin release and causing the 'set' temperature norm to be increased. This results in fever, which can reach up to 40°C.[94,95] However, the raised 'set' temperature causes the body's feedback mechanism to think it is cold; therefore, it causes vaso-constriction actions such as involuntary muscle contraction, resulting in 'chills and rigors.'

Administering a premedication such as paracetamol will minimise the development of fever, chills and rigors as antipyretics act by blocking the endogenous pyrogen; therefore, the 'set' temperature range remains unchanged. When using IFN-α, the pre-medication can be given 1 hour before, although it is suggested that premedication with IL-2 should be commenced at least 8 hours prior to administration.[96] It is possible that, following the first dose or when using high-dose regimens of these agents, paracetamol alone will not be enough to prevent fever from developing. If fever experienced is severe, a non-steroidal anti-inflammatory drug (NSAIDs) may be used, such as naproxen, 250 mg twice daily, but with careful monitoring of renal function when using high-dose IL-2 therapy, as NSAIDs are also renal toxic. During episodes of fever, cool clothes and fan therapy can be applied. At the first sign of chills, patients should be kept warm using blankets; if a rigor develops, control of this can be gained by using 12.5–25 mg IM or IV pethidine, carefully monitoring respiratory rate. If this drug is ineffective, lorazepam can be used, again ensuring respiratory rate is not affected. Quick control ensures the patient's energy is conserved, quality of life is maintained and the patient is less likely to become severely fatigued.

Fatigue

Fatigue is a well-recognised condition of cancer patients undergoing chemotherapy or radiation therapy. It is also a very common side effect of biological therapy, especially when patients are receiving adjuvant therapy that potentially will continue over many months or years. It is a symptom that can disrupt physical, psychological and spiritual well-being.[97] It is important that patients on therapy receive quick and effective control of side effects such as FLS, as inadequate control of these symptoms will add to the patient's experience of fatigue. Patients should also be made aware of the causes of fatigue and advised on methods of energy conservation. It is also important that they are encouraged to maintain a level of activity, as there is evidence to suggest an improved overall functioning of patients on IFN-α.[98]

Capillary leak syndrome

A significant side effect of biological therapy, 'capillary' or 'vascular' leak syndrome is most commonly associated with high-dose IL-2 (Fig. 43.2). Hypotension and a decrease in systemic vascular resistance can be observed within 4 hours of administration of IL-2.[99]

Table 43.9	Management of side effects	
Drug steps	Dose	Comments
Paracetamol	500–1000 mg Continue 4 hourly as required within maximum dose of 4 g in 24 hours	Prophylactically IL-2 8 hours prior to administration
Naproxen	250–500 mg twice a day Add in if fever severe	Monitor renal function
Pethidine	12.5–25 mg IM or IV If rigors persisting >20 min	Can be repeated every 5 min with careful titration against respiratory rate and level of consciousness
Lorazepan	0.5–1 mg sublingual If rigors persisting post pethidine	Monitor respiratory rate and level of consciousness

a

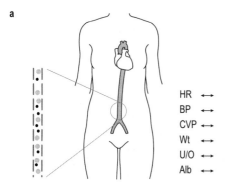

HR	↔
BP	↔
CVP	↔
Wt	↔
U/O	↔
Alb	↔

The walls of the capillaries are made up of a single layer of endothelial cells. The junctions between the cells permit the passage of small molecules, such as water and solutes, into the interstitium. The periluminal surface of all capillaries is surrounded by a basement membrane that provides additional support to the endothelial cells.

b

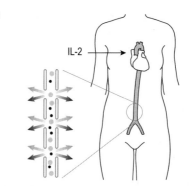

The administration of IL-2 affects the capillary endothelial layer making it more permeable. This may occur either as a direct effect of IL-2 or indirectly through the induction of other cytokines such as TNF and IFNg. As a result larger molecules, such as albumin, pass in to the interstitial fluid increasing its concentration and therefore more water and solutes are drawn into the interstitium.

c

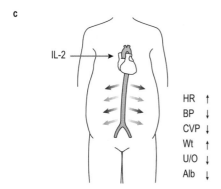

HR	↑
BP	↓
CVP	↓
Wt	↑
U/O	↓
Alb	↓

The efflux of fluid from the intravascular space to the interstitium results in hypovolaemia which leads to a rise in heart rate, fall in blood pressure and CVP and a decrease in urine output. The patient's weight increases and there is generalised oedema. The serum albumin level is depleted.

d

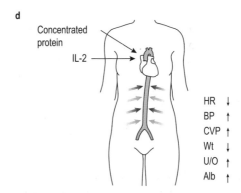

HR	↓
BP	↑
CVP	↑
Wt	↓
U/O	↑
Alb	↑

The intravenous administration of concentrated protein, such as 20% Human Serum Albumin, increases the concentration of the fluid in the intravascular space compared with that of the interstitial fluid. Water is therefore drawn back into the capillaries. As a consequence the circulatory volume rises and the patients vital signs return to normal. The urine output increases and the weight decreases.

Figure 43.2   Capillary leak syndrome.

The alteration in vascular resistance allows fluid to 'leak' from the capillaries into bodily tissues. This can rapidly lead to a fluid shift that gives rise to a generalised oedema, resulting in a weight gain that can be up to 10–15% of pretreatment body weight. It also leads to intravascular fluid depletion. Oliguria, increasing creatinine levels and tachycardia occur as compensatory measures to deal with this syndrome. Renal failure, pulmonary oedema and ascites can also occur if intervention to reverse this fluid shift is not instigated.

Management of this complex syndrome, which can lead to problems with all body systems, needs to be directed at correcting physiological changes quickly and effectively. Monitoring for these changes involves performing regular blood pressure (BP), pulse and central venous pressure (CVP) readings. A strict fluid balance should be maintained, with hourly recordings of urine output. Twice daily weights should be recorded. Careful fluid replacement, the administration of dopamine and other vasopressors should be used in an attempt to establish a haemodynamic balance despite ongoing capillary leak syndrome, so therapy can continue. Flow diagrams for the management of hypotension, fluid overload/weight gain and oliguria should be followed carefully (Figs 43.3–43.5).[100]

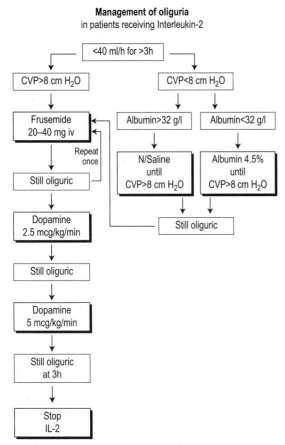

Figure 43.3   Management of oliguria in patients receiving interleukin-2 (IL-2). CVP = central venous pressure.

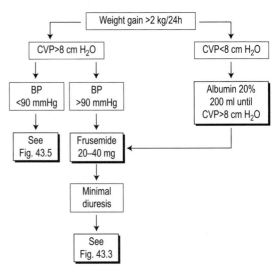

Figure 43.4   Management of fluid overload in patients receiving interleukin-2 (IL-2). CVP = central venous pressure; BP = blood pressure.

Skin toxicity

Dermatological changes from biological agents can be generalised or localised to the administration site. Again, severity relates to type of agent being used, frequency and intensity of dose. Common symptoms include generalised flushing, erythematous rash, dryness, flaking, swelling, pruritus and urticaria. Patients who have a history of skin conditions such as psoriasis may find these exacerbated. Hair thinning may occur, although total alopecia is rare unless using the agents in combination with chemotherapy agents. Patients should be advised to use a moisturiser on dry skin. This should be alcohol-free, fragrance-free and water-based, such as aqueous crème. A gentle non-drying soap or bath oil should be used for cleansing, advising patients to avoid hot showers and baths. If symptoms of pruritus develop, oral chlorphenamine (chlorpheniramine) can be taken, and bath preparations

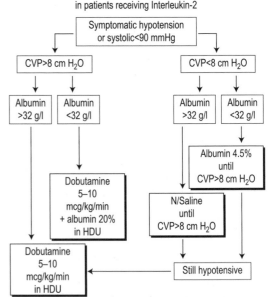

Figure 43.5   Management of hypotension in patients receiving interleukin-2 (IL-2). CVP = central venous pressure; HDU = High Dependency Unit.

Table 43.10   Skin toxicity

Toxicity	Intervention	Comments
Inflamed injection sites	Remove therapy from fridge 30 min prior to injection	
	Rotate injection sites	Use subcutaneous tissue of stomach and limbs
	Apply cold/hot packs to site post injection	Avoid injecting limb if lymph node dissection has been performed
	Apply topical non-steroidal creams	
	Apply topical lidocaine (lignocaine) gels	
Dry desquamation	Apply moisturiser – Diprobase or aqueous crème	
	Non-drying soap or oil in bath	Add to all washing/bathing water
	Tepid baths/showers	
	Avoid sun light	
Pruritus and erythema	Apply aqueous crème with menthol	
	Oral chlorphenamine (chlorpheniramine) 4–8 mg tds	Sedation from chlorphenamine (chlorpheniramine) may mask neurotoxicity
	Oatmeal baths	
	Wear light cotton clothing and avoid irritating fabrics	

containing oatmeal help to alleviate the itching. Wearing light cotton clothing and avoiding fabrics such as wool may also help.[101]

IL-2 can cause very painful inflamed injection site reactions, leaving 'nodules' under the skin for many weeks. IFN-α also causes soreness and irritation at the injection site, especially as it can be administered over a period of years. The skin toxicity can cause great distress and discomfort for the patient and needs to be taken seriously to prevent these symptoms having a detrimental effect on both body image and psychological well-being. Most importantly, patients need to be advised to remove the therapy from the fridge 30 min before administering, and to rotate the injection sites using legs, arms and stomach. Also using cool packs, aqueous menthol crème, topical NSAIDs and topical lidocaine (lignocaine) gel may also help relieve the discomfort experienced (Table 43.10).[102]

Other toxicities

Nurses caring for patients receiving these agents should also be aware of side effects that commonly occur when using high doses or when being combined with other anticancer therapies. Haematological toxicity, especially neutropenia and thrombocytopenia, can occur, as well as rises in liver function. These should be monitored closely, with breaks in treatment being introduced if toxicity is severe. Gastrointestinal toxicity, such as nausea and vomiting, stomatitis, diarrhoea and anorexia, can be severe. Central nervous system effects can result in mood changes such as depression, lethargy and confusion. Management of these side effects is addressed in the relevant sections within this book. However, medications or topical therapies that contain steroids should not be used when patients are receiving biological therapy, as steroids are immuno-suppressive and thought to work against biological agents that stimulate the immune system.

Finally, direct or indirect effects of interferon therapy may cause a temporary impotence or decreased libido, requiring sensitive assessment and intervention.[100] It is important that patients receiving these agents undergo regular assessment and toxicities should be checked against a toxicity tool such as the common toxicity criteria (CTC), which will identify when toxicity is severe enough to indicate reducing or stopping treatment.

References

1. Wingo P, Tong T, Bolden S. Cancer statistics. Cancer J Clin 1995.
2. CRC. Incidence –UK. CRC factsheet 1998; 1:1.
3. CRC. Mortality – UK. CRC cancer stats 2000.
4. Osterlind A, Tucker M, Stone B, et al. The Danish case control study of cutaneous malignant melanoma. Int J Cancer 1988; 42:319–324.
5. Elwood J, Jopson J. Melanoma and sun exposure. An overview of published studies. Int J Cancer 1997; 73:198–203.
6. MacKie R. The epidemiology of and screening for primary cutaneous malignant melanoma. In: MacKie R, Murray D, Rosin R, et al, eds. The effective management of malignant melanoma. UK Key Advances in Clinical

Practice Series. London: Aesculapius Medical Press; 2001:1–4.

7. Reintgen D, Kirkwood J. The adjuvant treatment of malignant melanoma. J Flor Med Assoc 1997; 84:147–152.

8. Agarwala S, Atkins M, Kirkwood J. Current approaches to advanced and high-risk melanoma. American Society of Clinical Oncology Educational Book Fall 1999; 1999:83–87.

9. Barth A, Wanek L, Morton D. Prognostic factors in 1521 melanoma patients with distant metastases. J Am Coll Surg 1995; 181:193–201.

10. Tomsu K, Van Eschen K, Lee M. Meta-analysis of median survival of patients with stage IV melanoma. Proc Am Soc Clin Oncol 1997; 16:1784.

11. Eton O, Legha S, Moon T, et al. Prognostic factors for survival of patients treated systemically for disseminated melanoma. J Clin Oncol 1998; 16:1103–1111.

12. Buer J, Probst M, Franzke A, et al. Elevated serum levels of S100 and survival in metastatic malignant melanoma. Br J Cancer 1997; 75:1373–1376.

13. Deichmann M, Benner A, Bock M, et al. S100-beta, melanoma-inhibiting activity, and lactate dehydrogenase discriminate progressive from nonprogressive American Joint Committee on Cancer stage IV melanoma. J Clin Oncol 1999; 17:1891–1896.

14. Damian D, Fulham M, Thompson E, et al. Positron emission tomography in the detection and management of metastatic melanoma. Melanoma Res 1996; 6:325–329.

15. Rinne D, Baum R, Hor G, et al. Primary staging and follow-up of high risk melanoma patients with whole-body ^{18}F-fluorodeoxyglucose positron emission tomography. Cancer 1998; 82:1664–1671.

16. Dietlein M, Krug B, Groth W, et al. Positron emission tomography using 18F-fluorodeoxyglucose in advanced stages of malignant melanoma: a comparison of ultrasonographic and radiological methods of diagnosis. Nucl Med Commun 1999; 20:255–261.

17. Hall P, Davalbhakta A. Scientific evidence and expert clinical opinion for the investigation and management of stage III malignant melanoma – surgical intervention. In: MacKie R, Murray D, Rosin R, et al, eds. The effective management of malignant melanoma. UK Key Advances in Clinical Practice series. London: Aesculapius Medical Press; 2001:51–64.

18. Hill G, Moss S, Golomb F, et al. DTIC and combination therapy for melanoma III. Surgical adjuvant study COG protocol 7040. Cancer 1981; 47:2556–2562.

19. Fisher RI, Terry WD, Hodes RJ, et al. Adjuvant immunotherapy or chemotherapy for malignant melanoma. Preliminary report of the National Cancer Institute randomized trial. Surg Clin North Am 1981; 61:1267–1277.

20. Veronesi U, Adamus J, Aubert C, et al. A randomised trial of adjuvant chemotherapy and immunotherapy in cutaneous melanoma. N Engl J Med 1982; 307:913–916.

21. Lejeune F, Macher E, Kleeberg U, et al. An assessment of DTIC versus levamisole or placebo in the treatment of high risk stage I patients after surgical removal of a primary melanoma of the skin: a phase III adjuvant study (EORTC 18761). Eur J Cancer 1988; 24:81–90.

22. Kirkwood J, Strawderman M, Ernstoff M, et al. Interferon alfa-2b adjuvant therapy of high-risk resected cutaneous melanoma: the Eastern Co-operative Oncology Group trial EST 1684. J Clin Oncol 1996; 14:7–17.

23. Cole B, Gelber R, Kirkwood J, et al. Quality of life adjusted survival analysis of interferon alpha 2b adjuvant treatment of high-risk resecteed cutaneous melanoma; an ECOG study. J Clin Oncol 1996; 14:2666–2673.

24. Kirkwood J, Ibrahim J, Sondak V, et al. Preliminary analysis of the E 1690/S 9111/C9190 Intergroup post-operative adjuvant trial of high- and low-dose IFNα2b (HDI and LDI) in high-risk primary or lymph node metastatic melanoma. Proc Am Soc Clin Oncol 1999; 18:537.

25. Pehamberger H, Soyer P, Steiner A, et al. Adjuvant interferon alfa-2a treatment in resected primary stage II cutaneous melanoma. J Clin Oncol 1998; 16:1425–1429.

26. Grob J, Dreno B, Salmoniere DL, et al. Randomised trial of interferon-α-2a as adjuvant therapy in resected primary melanoma thicker than 1.5 mm without clinically detectable lymph node metastases. Lancet 1985; 351:1905–1910.

27. Kirkwood JM, Manola J, Ibrahim J, et al. A pooled analysis of Eastern Cooperative Oncology Group and intergroup trials of adjuvant high-dose interferon for melanoma. Clin Cancer Res 2004; 10(5):1670–1677.

28. Comis R. DTIC (NSC-45388) in malignant melanoma: a perspective. Cancer Treat Rep 1976; 60:165–176.

29. Lee S, Betticher D, Thatcher N. Melanoma: chemotherapy. Br Med Bull 1995; 51:609–630.

30. Chowdhury S, Vaughan MM, Gore ME. New approaches to the systemic treatment of melanoma. Cancer Treat Rev 1999; 25(5):259–270.

31. Jacquillat C, Khayat D, Banzet P, et al. Final report of the French multicenter phase II study of the nitrosourea fotemustine in 153 evaluable patients with disseminated malignant melanoma including patients with cerebral metastases. Cancer 1990; 66:1873–1878.

32. Kleeberg U, Engel E, Israels P, et al. Palliative therapy of melanoma patients with fotemustine. Inverse relationship between tumour load and effectiveness. A multi-centre phase II trial of the EORTC-melanoma cooperative group (MCG). Melanoma Res 1995; 5:195–200.

33. Middleton M, Grob J, Aaronson N, et al. Randomised phase III study of temozolomide versus dacarbazine in the treatment of patients with advanced metastatic malignant melanoma. J Clin Oncol 2000; 18:158–166.

34. Legha S, Ring S, Papdopoulos N, et al. A phase II trial of taxol in metastatic melanoma. Cancer 1990; 65:2478–2481.

35. Einzig A, Hochster H, Wiernik P, et al. A phase II study of taxol in patients with malignant melanoma. Invest New Drugs 1991; 9:59–64.

36. Aamdal S, Wolff I, Kaplan S, et al. Docetaxel (Taxotere) in advanced malignant melanoma: a phase II study of the EORTC Early Clinical Trials Group. Eur J Cancer 1994; 30A:1061–1064.

37. Bedikian A, Weiss G, Legha S, et al. Phase II trial of docetaxel in patients with advanced cutaneous malignant melanoma previously untreated with chemotherapy. J Clin Oncol 1995; 13:2865–2867.

38. Einzig A, Schuchter L, Recio A, et al. Phase II trial of docetaxel (Taxotere) in patients with metastatic melanoma previously untreated with cytotoxic chemotherapy. Med Oncol 1996; 13:111–117.

39. Nathanson L, Kaufman S, Carey R. Vincristine-bleomycin-platinum (VBD): a high response rate regimen in metastatic melanoma. Proc Am Soc Clin Oncol 1980; 21:479.

40. Nathanson L, Kaufman S, Carey R. Vinblastine infusion, bleomycin, and cis-dichlorodiammine-platinum chemotherapy in metastatic melanoma. Cancer 1981; 48:1290–1298.

41. Luikart S, Kennealey G, Kirkwood J. Randomized phase III trial of vinblastine, bleomycin and cis-dichlorodiammine-platinum versus dacarbazine in malignant melanoma. J Clin Oncol 1984; 2:164–168.

42. Del Prete S, Maurer L, O'Donnell J, et al. Combination chemotherapy with cisplatin, carmustine, dacarbazine and tamoxifen metastatic melanoma. Cancer Treat Rep 1984; 68:1403–1405.

43. McClay E, McClay M-E. Systemic chemotherapy for the treatment of metastatic melanoma. Semin Oncol 1996; 23:744–753.

44. Chapman P, Einhorn L, Meyers M, et al. Phase III multicenter randomized trial of the Dartmouth regimen in patients with metastatic melanoma. J Clin Oncol 1999; 17:2745–2751.

45. Legha S. The role of interferon alfa in the treatment of metastatic melanoma. Semin Oncol 1997; 24:S4-24–31.

46. Rosenberg S, Yang J, Topalian S, et al. Treatment of 283 consecutive patients with metastatic melanoma or renal cell cancer using high-dose bolus interleukin 2. JAMA 1994; 271:907–913.

47. Atkins M, Lotze M, Wiernik P, et al. High-dose IL-2 therapy alone results in long-term durable complete responses in patients with metastatic melanoma. Proc Am Soc Clin Oncol 1997; 16:1780.

48. Allen I, Kupelnick B, Kumashiro M, et al. The combination of chemotherapy with IL-2 and αIFN is more active than chemotherapy or immunotherapy alone in patients with metastatic melanoma: a meta-analysis of 7711 patients with metastatic melanoma. Proc Am Soc Clin Oncol 1997; 16:1781.

49. Sparano J, Fisher R, Sunderland M, et al. Randomized phase III trial of treatment with high-dose interleukin-2 either alone or in combination with interferon alfa-2a in patients with advanced melanoma. J Clin Oncol 1993; 11:1969–1977.

50. Falkson C, Falkson G, Falkson H. Improved results with the addition of interferon alfa-2b to dacarbazine in the treatment of patients with metastatic malignant melanoma. J Clin Oncol 1991; 9:1403–1408.

51. Thomson D, Adena M, McLeod G, et al. Interferon-alpha 2a does not improve response or survival when combined with dacarbazine in metastatic maligant melanoma: results of a multi-institutional Australian randomized trial. Melanoma Res 1993; 3:133–138.

52. Bajetta E, Di Leo A, Zampino M, et al. Multicenter randomized trial of dacarbazine alone or in combination with two different doses and schedules of interferon alfa-2a in the treatment of advanced melanoma. J Clin Oncol 1994; 12:806–811.

53. Falkson C, Ibrahim J, Kirkwood J, et al. A randomised phase III trial of dacarbazine (DTIC) versus DTIC + interferon alfa2b (rIFN) versus DTIC + tamoxifen (TMX) versus DTIC + rIFN + TMX in metastatic melanoma: an ECOG trial. Proc Am Soc Clin Oncol 1996; 15:435.

54. Pyrhonen S, Hahka-Kemppinen M, Muhonen T. A promising interferon plus four-drug chemotherapy regimen for metastatic melanoma. J Clin Oncol 1992; 10:1919–1926.

55. Legha S, Ring S, Bedikian A, et al. Tamoxifen (T) added to a regimen of cisplatin (C), vinblastine (V), DTIC and alfa interferon (rIFN) in patients (pts) with metastatic melanoma (MM). Proc Am Soc Clin Oncol 1993; 12:388.

56. Schultz M, Poo W, Buzaid A. A phase II study of cisplatin (CDDP), dacarbazine (DTIC), carmustine (BCNU), tamoxifen (TM), and interferon-alpha 2B (alpha-rIFN) in metastatic melanoma. Proc Am Soc Clin Oncol 1993; 12:390.

57. Keiholz U, Scheibenbogen C, Stoelben E, et al. Immunotherapy of metastatic melanoma with interferon-alpha and interleukin-2: pattern of progression in responders and patients with stable disease with or without resection of individual lesions. Eur J Cancer 1994; 30A:955–958.

58. Hahka-Kemppinen M, Muhonen T, Virolainen M, et al. Response of subcutaneous and cutaneous metastases of malignant melanoma to combined cytostatic plus interferon therapy. Br J Dermatol 1995; 132:973–977.

59. Khayat D, Borel C, Tourani J, et al. Sequential chemoimmunotherapy with cisplatin, interleukin-2, and interferon alfa-2a for metastatic melanoma. J Clin Oncol 1993; 11:2173–2180.

60. Richards J, Mehta N, Ramming K, et al. Sequential chemoimmunotherapy in the treatment of metastatic melanoma. J Clin Oncol 1992; 10:1338–1343.

61. Richards JM, Gale D, Mehta N, et al. Combination of chemotherapy with interleukin-2 and interferon alfa

for the treatment of metastatic melanoma. J Clin Oncol 1999; 17:651–657.

62. Legha SS, Ring S, Bedikian A, et al. Treatment of metastatic melanoma with combined chemotherapy containing cisplatin, vinblastine and dacarbazine (CVD) and biotherapy using interleukin-2 and interferon-alpha. Ann Oncol 1996; 7:827–835.

63. Legha S, Ring S, Eton O, et al. Development of a biochemotherapy regimen with concurrent administration of cisplatin, vinblastine, dacarbazine, interferon alfa, and interleukin-2 for patients with metastatic melanoma. J Clin Oncol 1998; 16:1752–1759.

64. Keiholz U, Goey S, Punt C, et al. Interferon alfa-2a and interleukin-2 with or without cisplatin in metastatic melanoma: a randomized trial of the European Organization for Research and Treatment of Cancer Melanoma Cooperative Group. J Clin Oncol 1997; 15:2579–2588.

65. Johnston SR, Constenla DO, Moore J, et al. Randomized phase II trial of BCDT [carmustine (BCNU), cisplatin, dacarbazine (DTIC) and tamoxifen] with or without interferon alpha (IFN-alpha) and interleukin (IL-2) in patients with metastatic melanoma. Br J Cancer 1998; 77:1280–1286.

66. Sertoli M, Queirolo P, Bajetta E, et al. Multi-institutional phase II randomised trial of integrated therapy with cisplatin, dacarbazine, vindesine, subcutaneous interleukin-2, interferon alpha2a and tamoxifen in metastatic melanoma. BREMIM (Biological Response Modifiers in Melanoma). Melanoma Res 1999; 9:503–509.

67. Rosenberg S, Yang J, Schwartzentruber D, et al. Prospective randomized trial of the treatment of patients with metastatic melanoma using chemotherapy with cisplatin, dacarbazine and tamoxifen alone or in combination with interleukin-2 and interferon alfa-2b. J Clin Oncol 1999; 17:968–975.

68. Sampson J, Carter J, Friedman A, et al. Demographics, prognosis, and therapy in 702 patients with brain metastases from malignant melanoma. J Neurosurg 1998; 88:11–20.

69. Patchell R, Tibbs P, Walsh J, et al. A randomized trial of surgery in the treatment of single metastases to the brain. N Engl J Med 1990; 322:494–500.

70. Morton D, Eilber F, Holmes E, et al. Preliminary results of a randomised trial of adjuvant immunotherapy in patients with malignant melanoma who have lymph node metastases. Aust NZ J Surg 1978; 48:49–52.

71. Chan A, Morton D. Active immunotherapy with allogeneic tumour cell vaccines: Present status. Semin Oncol 1998; 25:611–622.

72. Mitchell M. Perspective on allogenic melanoma lysates in active specific immunotherapy. Semin Oncol 1998; 15:623–635.

73. Berd D, Kairys J, Dunton C, et al. Autologous, hapten-modified vaccine as a treatment for human cancers. Semin Oncol 1998; 25:646–653.

74. Berd D, Maguire H, Bloome E, et al. Regression of lung metastases after immunotherapy with autologous DNP modified melanoma vaccine. Proc Am Soc Clin Oncol 1998; 17:434.

75. Rosenberg S, Yang J, Schwartzentruber D, et al. Immunologic and therapeutic evaluation of a synthetic peptide vaccine for the treatment of patients with metastatic melanoma. Nature Med 1998; 4:321–327.

76. Thurner B, Haendle I, Roder C, et al. Vaccination with Mage-3A1 peptide-pulsed mature monocyte-derived dendritic cells expands specific cytotoxic T cells and induces regression of some metastases in advanced stage IV melanoma. J Exp Med 1999; 190:1669–1678.

77. Abdel-Wahab Z, Weltz C, Hester D, et al. A phase I clinical trial of immunotherapy with interferon-gamma gene-modified autologous melanoma cells: monitoring the humoral immune response. Cancer 1997; 80:401–412.

78. Moller P, Sun Y, Dorbic T, et al. Vaccination with IL-7 gene modified autologous melanoma cells can enhance the anti-melanoma lytic activity in peripheral blood of patients with a good clinical performance status: a clinical phase I study. Br J Cancer 1998; 77:1907–1916.

79. Nemunaitis J, Bohart C, Fong T, et al. Phase I trial of retroviral vector-mediated interferon (IFN)-gamma gene transfer into autologous tumor cells in patients with metastatic melanoma. Cancer Gene Ther 1998; 5:292–300.

80. Soiffer R, Lynch T, Mihm M, et al. Vaccination with irradiated autologous melanoma cells engineered to secrete human granulocyte-macrophage colony-stimulating factor generated potent antitumor immunity in patients with metastatic melanoma. Proc Natl Acad Sci 1998; 95:13141–13146.

81. Palmer K, Moore J, Everard M, et al. Gene therapy with autologous, interleukin 2-secreting tumor cells in patients with malignant melanoma. Human Gene Therapy 1999; 10:1261–1268.

82. Rusthoven J, Quirt I, Iscoe N, et al. Randomized, double-blind, placebo-controlled trial comparing the response rates of carmustine, dacarbazine, and cisplatin with and without tamoxifen in patients with metastatic melanoma. J Clin Oncol 1996; 14:2083–2090.

83. Sileni V, Nortilli R, Medici M, et al. BCNU (B), cisplatin (C), dacarbazine (D) and tamoxifen (T) (BCDT) in metastatic melanoma (MM): results of a randomised phase II study. Proc Am Soc Clin Oncol 1997; 16:1782.

84. Middleton M, Lorigan P, Owen J, et al. Dacarbazine, BCNU, cisplatin and tamoxifen (DCBT) versus dacarbazine and interferon (DI) in advanced melanoma, interim results of a randomised phase III study. Proc Am Soc Clin Oncol 1998; 17:1958.

85. Kirkwood J, Ernstoff M, Giuliano A, et al. Interferon α-2a and dacarbazine in melanoma. J Natl Cancer Inst 1990; 82:1062–1063.

86. Keiholz U, Punt C, Gore M, et al. Dacarbazine, cisplatin and interferon alpha with or without interleukin-2 in advanced melanoma: interim analysis of EORTC trial 18951. Proc Am Soc Clin Oncol 1999; 18:2043.

87. Veronesi U, Adamus J, Aubert C, et al. A randomised trial of adjuvant chemotherapy and immunotherapy in cutaneous melanoma. N Engl J Med 1982; 307:913–916.

88. Kirkwood J, Strawderman M, Ernstoff M, et al. Interferon alpha-2b adjuvant therapy of high-risk recepted cutaneous melanoma: the Easter Cooperative Oncology Group trial EST 1684. J Clin Oncol 1996; 14:7–17.

89. Allen I, Kupelnick B, Kumashio M, et al. The combination of chemotherapy with IL-2 and IFN alpha-2b is more active than chemotherapy or immunotherapy alone in patients with metastatic melanoma; a meta-analysis of 7711 patients with metastatic melanoma. Proc Am Soc Clin Oncol 1997; 16:1781.

90. Kammula US, White DE, Rosenberg SA. Trends in the safety of high dose bolus interleukin-2 administration in patients with metastatic cancer. Cancer 1998; 83:797–805.

91. Sandstrom SK. Nursing management of patients receiving biological therapy. Semin Oncol Nurs 1996; 12:152–162.

92. Schering –Plough Ltd. Interferon therapy. Burgess Hill: Schering Health Care Limited.

93. Dinarello CA, Cannon JG, Wolff S. New concepts on the pathogenesis of fever. Rev Infect Dis 1988; 10:168–189.

94. Holtzclaw BJ. Shivering, a clinical nursing problem. Nurs Clin North Am 1990; 25:977–986.

95. Hauber D. The flu-like syndrome. In: Reiger RT, ed. Biotherapy: a comprehensive overview. Boston: Jones and Barlett; 1995:243–258.

96. Chiron Therapeutics. Proleukin (aldesleukin) for the treatment of patients with metastatic melanoma and metastatic renal cell carcinoma: supplemental biologic licence application 1998. Available online at www.chiron.com/products/index.html

97. Skalla KA, Reiger PT. Fatigue. In: In: Reiger RT, ed. Biotherapy: a comprehensive overview. Boston: Jones and Barlett; 1995:221–242.

98. Davis C. Interferon induced fatigue. Oncol Nurs Bull 1997; 1:4–5.

99. Lee RE, Lotze MT, Skibber JM, et al. Cardiorespiratory effects of immunotherapy with interleukin-2. J Clin Oncol 1989; 7:7–20.

100. Moore J. Practical aspects of delivering cytokines, In: Gore ME, Riches P, eds. Immunotherapy in cancer. Chichester: John Wiley and Sons, 1996; 12:278–280.

101. Skalla K. The interferons. Semin Oncol Nurs 1996; 12:97–105.

102. Chiron Therapeutics. Proleukin (aldesleukin). A patient guide to treatment 2003.

103. Wheatley K, Ives N, Hancock B, et al. Does adjuvant interferon-alpha for high-risk melanoma provide a worthwhile benefit? A meta-analysis of the randomised trials. Cancer Treat Rev 2003; 29(4): 241–252.

Chapter **44**

Bone and soft tissue sarcoma

MEDICAL CARE FOR PATIENTS WITH BONE AND SOFT TISSUE SARCOMA

Alistair Ring and Andrew Webb

INTRODUCTION

Sarcomas are malignant neoplasms derived from mesenchymal connective tissue. The tissue of origin may be bone or soft tissue such as fat, peripheral neural tissue, blood vessels, smooth or striated muscle. Any part of the body can be affected, but about half of sarcomas occur in the limbs, with other common sites including the retroperitoneum, mediastinum and uterus.

EPIDEMIOLOGY

Bone and soft tissue sarcomas represent less than 1% of all new cancer diagnoses. In 1998 there were 860 deaths from bone and soft tissue sarcomas in England and Wales, and about 1200 new cases are diagnosed annually.[1] Overall, sarcomas are more common in men, but sex and age incidences vary depending on histological subtype.

AETIOLOGY

The aetiology of most sarcomas is not known, although genetic factors, previous irradiation and occupational exposure can all play a part.

Inherited cancer syndromes

Sarcomas are seen more commonly in a number of inherited cancer syndromes (Box 44.1).[2-5]

Ionising radiation

Ionising radiation is known to be capable of inducing bone and soft tissue sarcomas.[6] Radiotherapy is probably responsible for less than 5% of all sarcomas.[7]

Box 44.1   Inherited cancer syndromes

Neurofibromatosis
Basal cell naevus syndrome
Tuberous sclerosis
Werner's syndrome
Intestinal polyposis
Gardner's syndrome
Li-Fraumeni syndrome
Inherited retinoblastoma

However, the risk increases with higher doses, and if treatment is given in childhood.[8-10]

Occupational exposure

Exposure to industrial chemicals, including phenoxyacetic acids in herbicides and chlorophenol preservatives, may increase the risk of sarcoma.[11,12] There is also a specific association linking hepatic angiosarcoma with chronic exposure to vinyl chloride.[13]

SARCOMA CLASSIFICATION/PATHOLOGY

The classification of sarcomas is complex, and all histology should be reviewed by a pathologist with expertise in the identification of sarcomas using immunohistochemical techniques. Assessment should include some designation of grade, as determined by cellular and nuclear pleomorphism, mitotic activity, presence of necrosis and degree of differentiation. Further information can be gained from cytogenetic analysis, as distinct chromosomal translocations can be identified in myxoid liposarcoma, synovial sarcoma and Ewing's sarcoma.[14-16]

Existing histological classifications are purely descriptive, based on line of differentiation, and have limited clinical use. For the purposes of this review, sarcomas will be divided into the following five headings:

- soft tissue sarcomas
- bone-derived sarcomas
- Ewing's sarcoma and primitive neuroectodermal tumours (PNETs)
- rhabdomyosarcomas
- gastrointestinal stromal tumours (GISTs).

SOFT TISSUE SARCOMAS
Classification

The following tumours are included in the soft tissue category, categorised according to the normal tumours that they mimic:

Most frequent
- Fibrosarcoma
- Malignant fibrous histiocytoma
- Leiomyosarcoma
- Liposarcoma

Less frequent
- Alveolar soft-part sarcoma
- Angiosarcoma
- Clear cell sarcoma
- Epithelioid sarcoma

- Extraskeletal chondrosarcoma/osteosarcoma
- Haemangiopericytoma
- Peripheral nerve sheath tumour
- Synovial sarcoma
- Sarcoma not otherwise specified (NOS)

Clinical features

Patients with peripheral lesions usually present with a painless swelling which has been enlarging over the preceding weeks or months. Less commonly, they present with pain due to local invasion or with symptoms due to direct pressure on adjacent structures. Approximately 60% of sarcomas occur in the extremities, the majority in the lower limbs above the knee. Other sites include the head and neck region (9%) and trunk (31%). Within the trunk, the majority of lesions occur in the retroperitoneum, with the remainder in the mediastinum, chest and abdominal walls.[5] Intra-abdominal lesions can remain asymptomatic until well established, and present with pain or symptoms of bowel obstruction. Growth of sarcomas is usually by direct extension along tissue planes. Distant metastases (particularly to the lung) are common at presentation.[17]

Diagnosis and staging investigations

The diagnostic method of choice is a core needle or 'tru-cut' biopsy, which provides sufficient tissue for an accurate diagnosis in 90% of patients. Open biopsy is sometimes necessary and should be carefully planned so that the wound resulting from the biopsy can be resected later as part of a wide excision. Poorly planned biopsies can compromise definitive surgical procedures and result in tumour fungation.

Adequate staging requires evaluation of both the primary lesion and sites of potential metastases (Table 44.1). Evaluation of the primary site should determine the tumour size, compartmental borders and relationship to neurovascular structures, in order to facilitate surgical planning. This is often possible by computed tomography (CT) for visceral sites, although magnetic resonance imaging (MRI) may be necessary where the limbs are involved. The most common site of metastases is the lungs and these are best evaluated by CT scanning. Fluorodeoxyglucose positron emission tomography (FDG PET) scanning can successfully identify primary, recurrent and metastatic sarcomas, but has not proved superior to conventional imaging techniques.[18]

Staging systems

The AJCC/UICC (American Joint Committee Cancer/ Union Internationale Contre le Cancer) staging system is used for all sarcomas of soft tissues except childhood rhabdomyosarcomas.[19] However, there is evidence that this system does not correlate well with prognosis, since histological grade and tumour size are equally important determinants of distant metastases and survival. Therefore, a modified staging system has been proposed at the Royal Marsden Hospital which adds more weight to primary tumour size[20] (Tables 44.2 and 44.3).

Management plan

Surgery

Surgical resection remains the mainstay of treatment in soft tissue sarcoma. There is a high local recurrence rate after surgery, which can be reduced by ensuring wide excision margins. However, the need for adequate clearance has to be balanced against the need to preserve function. When the limbs are involved, the procedure of choice is a functional compartmentectomy. This requires the excision of all involved muscles, but with preservation of at least one functional muscle in the group.

Table 44.1   Investigations indicated by tumour type

Investigation	Soft tissue sarcoma	Osteosarcoma	PNET/ Ewing's sarcoma	Rhabdomyosarcoma	GIST
CT/MRI primary site	Yes	Yes	Yes	Yes	Yes
CXR/CT thorax	Yes	Yes	Yes	Yes	Yes
Isotope bone scan	No	Yes	Yes	No	No
Bone marrow aspirate/trephine	No	No	Yes	Yes	No
CT brain	No	No	No	Consider if head/neck primary site	No

PNET = primitive neuroectodermal tumours; GIST = gastrointestinal stromal tumours; CT = computed tomography; MRI = magnetic resonance imaging; CXR = chest X-ray.

Table 44.2 Tumour–node–metastasis (TNM) staging definitions

	AJCC/UICC staging	Modified Marsden staging
G (Histological grade)	G1 Well differentiated G2 Moderately differentiated G3 Poorly differentiated G4 Undifferentiated	As for AJCC/UICC
T (Primary tumour)	T1 < 5 cm T2 > 5 cm	T1 <5 cm T2 5–10 cm T3 10–15 cm T4 >15 cm
N (Lymph nodes)	N0 No lymph node involvement N1 Regional nodes involved	As for AJCC/UICC
M (Distant metastases)	M0 No distant metastases M1 Distant metastases	As for AJCC/UICC

AJCC = American Joint Committee Cancer; UICC = Union Internationale Contre le Cancer.

Radiotherapy

Radiotherapy for soft tissue sarcomas is used in the adjuvant, neoadjuvant and palliative settings.

Adjuvant radiotherapy Historical data show that if limb-sparing surgery is used, local control rates may be as low as 10–50%.[21,22] The addition of postoperative radiotherapy (with or without chemotherapy) can increase local control rates to more than 75%.[23,24] However, which subgroups of patients are most likely to benefit is unclear.[24,25] At present, adjuvant radiotherapy should be considered in all grade II and III tumours, and in low-grade tumours with positive excision margins. Treatment is given to the original tumour volume plus wide margins or the entire muscle compartment. High doses are used: 50 Gy with a boost of 10 Gy to the tumour bed is a common schedule. Radiotherapy can also be used to treat local recurrence when previous radiotherapy has not been given.

Neoadjuvant radiotherapy Neoadjuvant radiotherapy may be used prior to surgery in order to downstage large tumours which would otherwise be inoperable.

Palliative radiotherapy Palliative radiotherapy may be required for symptom relief in metastatic disease, often for bone or nodal metastases.

Chemotherapy

The mainstays of systemic treatment for soft tissue sarcoma remain doxorubicin or ifosfamide-containing regimens.

Adjuvant Chemotherapy in the adjuvant setting with or without radiotherapy remains controversial.

Trials are hampered by inadequate patient numbers and heterogeneity of tumour size, grade, type and site. A meta-analysis from 1997 does show a significant improvement in recurrence rates and recurrence-free survival with doxorubicin-based adjuvant treatment, but there was no overall survival benefit. However, there was a trend suggesting that patients with extremity tumours were more likely to benefit from chemotherapy.[26] Evidence to support this comes from the Italian Sarcoma Group, who conducted a study of 104 patients with large (>5 cm), high-grade, extremity or limb girdle tumours. This study used aggressive combination ifosfamide and epirubicin therapy and demonstrated both a disease-free and overall survival advantage.[27]

For most patients there is uncertainty as to the benefit of adjuvant chemotherapy and they should be

Table 44.3 Soft tissue staging systems

Stage	AJCC/UICC	Modified Marsden
IA	G1 T1	G1 T1
IB	G1 T2	G1 T2, G2 T1
IIA	G2 T1	G1 T3, G2 T2, G3 T1
IIB	G2 T2	G1 T4, G2 T3, G3 T2
IIIA	G3 T1	G2 T4, G3 T3
IIIB	G3 T2	G3 T4
IVA	G1-3, T1-2, N1	G1-3, T1-4, N1
IVB	G1-3, T1-2, N0-1, M1	G1-3, T1-4, N0-1, M1

AJCC = American Joint Committee Cancer; UICC = Union Internationale Contre le Cancer.

considered for entry into ongoing randomised controlled trials investigating this question. However adjuvant chemotherapy should be considered when:

1. there is residual disease following surgery, which cannot be re-excised
2. adjuvant radiotherapy is not possible, e.g. due to proximity to the spinal cord
3. there is chemosensitive disease, e.g. synovial sarcoma
4. the risk of relapse is high, such as in young patients with large high-grade tumours.

In this setting, combination therapy with ifosfamide 9 g/m^2 and doxorubicin 60 mg/m^2 should be used, as response to individual drugs cannot be assessed.

Neoadjuvant The neoadjuvant modality of choice in soft tissue sarcoma is radiotherapy. However, in potentially chemosensitive disease, or where radiotherapy is not possible, aggressive combination chemotherapy with ifosfamide 9 g/m^2 and doxorubicin 60 mg/m^2 may sufficiently reduce tumour size to make surgery possible.

Palliative The majority of chemotherapy given for soft tissue sarcoma is given in a palliative setting. No trials have been performed comparing palliative chemotherapy with best supportive care, so the magnitude of the survival benefit with chemotherapy is unknown. Therefore, quality of life issues are important determinants of the timing and schedule of treatment. Initial unrandomised studies of ifosfamide $(5–8 \text{ g/m}^2)$ showed response rates of 38–67%.[28,29] However, a subsequent randomised EORTC (European Organisation for Research and Treatment of Cancer) phase II study found a response rate of 25% to ifosfamide 5 g/m^2 in previously untreated patients.[30]

Doxorubicin is also an active single agent in soft tissue sarcomas, with response rates reported to be between 15 and 30%. A dose–response relationship has been observed with a dose rate of 60–70 mg/m^2 (once every 3 weeks) being superior to a dose rate of 50 mg/m^2 or less.[31–33] In the future, pegylated liposomal doxorubicin may replace doxorubicin, as equivalent activity but an improved toxicity profile has been demonstrated in a randomised trial.[34] Dacarbazine (DTIC) $(1.2 \text{ g/m}^2$ 3 weekly) has been shown to achieve single agent response rates of 18%.[35] Docetaxel 100 mg/m^2 has also demonstrated activity in advanced soft tissue sarcoma, with a response rate of 17% in previously treated patients.[36] Although single agents have consistently been shown to achieve response rates of up to 20%, complete responses are very uncommon.

An EORTC study of combination ifosfamide (5 g/m^2) and doxorubicin (50 mg/m^2) in previously untreated patients reported a response rate of 35%.[37] However, when compared with doxorubicin alone in a subsequent phase III study, there was no significant difference in response rate between the combination and single agent regimens.[38] An Intergroup phase III study compared doxorubicin (60 mg/m^2) and DTIC (1 g/m^2) with or without ifosfamide (7.5 g/m^2) and mesna (the MAID regimen.) Although the response rate and duration of response were significantly improved for the three-drug arm, myelosuppression (including fatal sepsis) was also more common.[39] Improved response rates may not translate into a survival advantage, and therefore in the palliative setting less toxic sequential single agent therapy may be preferable to maximise control of symptoms. Combination chemotherapy may be indicated in patients with rapidly progressive disease in whom there would be little time to assess response to individual agents. Under these cirumstances, the protocol used is ifosfamide 9 g/m^2 and doxorubicin 60 mg/m^2. All other patients in the palliative setting should be treated with sequential single agents.

The two most commonly used single agent schedules are:

- single agent doxorubicin 75 mg/m^2 or
- single agent ifosfamide 9 g/m^2 over 3 days.

The choice of initial agent will depend on a number of factors:

1. Ease of administration: most centres prefer single agent doxorubicin as first-line treatment, as this can be given on a day unit.
2. Cardiac status: patients with impaired left ventricular function (either due to previous anthracycline or prior cardiac condition) are not suitable for doxorubicin.
3. Renal function: patients with glomerular filtration rate less than 60 ml/min are not suitable for ifosfamide.

Monitoring treatment The aim is to give a cycle of treatment once every 3 weeks to a total of six cycles. Response to treatment should be assessed regularly (every two–three cycles) by clinical measurement or suitable imaging modalities in order to avoid undue toxicity. Close attention should be paid to symptom response, as the ultimate aim of treatment is palliation. If disease is stable or improved and the treatment tolerated, chemotherapy should be continued. If disease progression occurs, then the alternative agent may be considered. Renal and cardiac function should be monitored to avoid major toxicities.

Further chemotherapy When disease progression has occurred with both ifosfamide and doxorubicin, or treatment has had to cease due to toxicity, patients of good performance status may be considered for experimental studies, including phase I trials.

Pulmonary metastectomy

The lung is the most frequent site of metastasis from soft tissue sarcomas. Given the relative insensitivity of sarcomas to chemotherapy, fit patients with potentially resectable pulmonary metastases should be referred to a thoracic surgeon. Favourable prognostic features include a long disease-free interval, less than 10 metastases and grade I and II tumours. Overall the 5-year postmetastasectomy survival rate is 25–40%.[40,41]

Prognosis

The prognosis of soft tissue sarcoma depends on a number of factors, as the tumours represent a heterogeneous group:

- Stage is the main determinant of prognosis. Staging takes into account tumour size, nodal involvement, presence of metastases and histological grade.
- Tumour site: inaccessible tumours are less likely to be surgically resectable and radiotherapy doses may be limited by overlying tissue.
- Age >60 years carries a worse prognosis.
- Histological subtype may be an important prognostic and predictive factor. In a univariate analysis of 2185 patients with advanced soft tissue sarcoma treated with anthracycline-based chemotherapy, patients with synovial sarcomas and liposarcomas had a better overall survival than other cell types.[42]

About 50% of patients have high-grade sarcomas, and of these 50% will die from distant metastases. From the 1997 meta-analysis of patients undergoing adjuvant treatment for resected soft tissue sarcomas, the overall 5-year survival is 60–70%.[26] When metastatic disease has occurred the prognosis is poor, and the 5-year survival rates are less than 10%. (See also Ch. 1.)

BONE-DERIVED SARCOMAS

Classification

Osteosarcoma

This tumour usually arises in the epiphyseal region and consists of malignant osteoblasts that make osteoid.

Other primary sarcomas of bone

These include angiosarcomas, chondrosarcomas, giant cell tumours, malignant fibrous histiocytomas and spindle cell tumours.

Clinical features

Osteosarcomas are the most common primary malignant bone tumours. They usually occur during adolescence, but may occur in older patients and can be associated with Paget's disease or previous radiotherapy. The bones of the knee joint and proximal humerus are the most common sites of disease.[43] Patients present with pain and swelling at these sites, and clinical examination reveals a firm mass attached to the underlying bone. The lungs, pleura and bones are the most common sites of metastatic disease.

Diagnostic and staging investigations

These are shown in Table 44.1.

Staging system

The bone sarcoma staging sytem is shown in Table 44.4.[19]

Management plan

Surgery and chemotherapy

Limb-sparing surgery employing bone grafts or prostheses is currently possible in 70–90% of cases. It is now standard practice to give primary chemotherapy prior to surgery. This has the advantage of giving early systemic treatment, allowing time for manufacture of the prosthesis and allowing more limited surgery if tumour shrinkage occurs. The impact of adjuvant chemotherapy was demonstrated in randomised clinical trials more then 10 years ago; the chance of cure was increased from less than 20% to more than 60% with the use of pre- and postoperative chemotherapy.[44] The most active drugs in osteosarcoma are cisplatin, doxorubicin and methotrexate. Many of the initial studies of neoadjuvant and adjuvant chemotherapy included high-dose methotrexate as a standard component of the chemotherapy regimen.

Table 44.4 Bone sarcoma staging system

Stage	Grade	Tumour	Node	Metastasis
Stage IA	G1,G2	T1	N0	M0
Stage IB	G1,G2	T2	N0	M0
Stage IIA	G3,G4	T1	N0	M0
Stage IIB	G3,G4	T2	N0	M0
Stage III	Not defined			
Stage IVA	Any G	Any T	N1	M0
Stage IVB	Any G	Any T	Any N	M1

T1 = tumour confined to cortex, T2 = tumour invades beyond the cortex.

However, the First European Osteosarcoma Intergroup study found that three cycles pre- and postoperatively of cisplatin (100 mg/m^2) and doxorubicin (75 mg/m^2) led to better 5-year disease free-survival than the same duration regimen incorporating methotrexate (8 g/m^2).[45] In a subsequent European Osteosarcoma Intergroup study, the two-drug regimen was compared with the T10 multi-drug regimen which incorporates preoperative vincristine (1.5 mg/m^2), methotrexate (8 g/m^2) and doxorubicin (75 mg/m^2), and postoperative vincristine (1.2 mg/m^2), methotrexate (8 g/m^2), bleomycin (15 mg/m^2), cyclophosphamide (600 mg/m^2), doxorubicin (75 mg/m^2) and dactinomycin (0.6 mg/m^2). There was no significant difference in overall 5-year survival between the two groups, but the two-drug regimen was shorter and better tolerated.[46]

Therefore, the standard neoadjuvant protocol at the Royal Marsden Hospital is cisplatin 100 mg/m^2 and doxorubicin 75 mg/m^2. Treatment is given once every 3 weeks for a total of three cycles prior to surgery. Following surgery, the sensitivity to preoperative chemotherapy can be assessed. If total or subtotal tumour necrosis greater than 90% is identified in the resected specimen, then this is highly predictive of survival,[46] and a further three cycles of cisplatin/doxorubicin should be given. The most appropriate course of action if suboptimal necrosis occurs remains controversial. The value of changing to alternative chemotherapy in this situation is unproven, and our practice is to continue the same chemotherapy postoperatively.

Patients who present with metastatic disease may derive palliative benefit from the same standard regimen involving cisplatin/doxorubicin.

Radiotherapy

Radiotherapy is no longer routinely used as primary treatment in osteosarcoma. It can be used when the adequacy of local surgery is limited by anatomical site or when surgery is not feasible. Unfortunately, local radiotherapy rarely provides lasting control of the primary or local recurrence, although palliative radiotherapy is of great value in treating painful bony metastases.

Pulmonary metastatectomy

Patients who develop pulmonary metastases are still potentially curable by surgery. When metastases are detected, it is reasonable to treat the patient with chemotherapy for 2–3 months. If no further metastases have developed, then metastatectomy can be undertaken. This approach avoids thoracotomy in patients with chemotherapy-insensitive disease who are likely to progress rapidly anyway. Survival is influenced by the number of metastases and the length of the disease-free interval. Only a small proportion of patients are suitable for surgery; of those undergoing surgery, 5-year survival is 20–40%.[41,47]

Prognosis

For patients with localised osteosarcoma treated with combined surgery and chemotherapy, the overall survival rate at 5 years is 20–80%.[48] The most important prognostic variable is the degree of tumour necrosis following preoperative chemotherapy. When relapse occurs, the most important prognostic factor is whether complete resection of all recurrent disease is possible. After complete resection of metastatic pulmonary tumours, the 5-year survival rate is still 20–40%,[41,47] although the prognosis is worse if bone metastases or local recurrence occur.

EWING'S SARCOMA AND PRIMITIVE NEUROECTODERMAL TUMOURS

Classification

This closely related group of tumours includes bone and extraskeletal Ewing's sarcoma, PNETs and Askin's tumour (a characteristic PNET arising in the thorax). They are characterised by sheets of tightly packed small, round, blue cells. Although the tumours in this group can be differentiated by immunochemical techniques, they share a common chromosomal translocation t(11;22)(q24;12).[14] Therefore, they probably represent different stages of neural differentiation.

Clinical features

Ewing's sarcoma presents in adolescence with pain and swelling in the affected areas. The bones of the pelvis and knee joint are the commonest sites of involvement. Fever and weight loss also occur, particularly with large metastatic tumours. PNETs are derived almost exclusively from soft tissues: these, and the rare extraskeletal Ewings sarcoma, present with similar symptoms to soft tissue sarcomas. The commonest soft tissue sites are the trunk, extremities and retroperitoneum. These tumours grow rapidly and metastasise early to the bone, bone marrow and lungs.

Diagnosis and staging investigations

These are shown in Table 44.1.

Staging system

The same staging system as for sarcomas of bone (see Table 44.4), but all tumours are classified as G4 because they are all histologically aggressive.

Management plan

The high sensitivity of these tumours to chemotherapy means that the therapeutic goal should always be curative. Local treatment alone is associated with cure in only 10–20% of cases; therefore, all patients should receive early systemic chemotherapy to treat micrometastatic disease. The treatment strategy comprises induction chemotherapy, resection or radiotherapy of site of primary disease and maintenance chemotherapy.

Induction chemotherapy

Many drugs are active against Ewing's sarcoma and PNETs, but ifosfamide and doxorubicin have long been regarded as the most effective agents.[49] Major multicentre trials have attempted to identify the optimum combinations of drugs. The first US Intergroup Ewing's Sarcoma Study (IESS 1) found that the addition of doxorubicin (60 mg/m^2) to vincristine (1.5 mg/m^2), dactinomycin (15 µg/kg/day for 5 days) and cyclophosphamide (500 mg/m^2) increased the 5-year relapse-free survival from 24% to 60%.[50] In IESS 2, two schedules of VACA (vincristine, Adriamycin (doxorubicin), cyclophosphamide and actinomycin D (dactinomycin)) were compared. Increased dose intensity with all of the doxorubicin given early in the treatment improved 5-year disease-free survival (48 to 68%) and overall survival (63 to 77%) ($p = 0.02$ and 0.05, respectively).[51] The UK Children's Cancer Study Group (UKCCSG) ET1 trial treated patients with metastatic and non-metastatic Ewing's tumour with VAC and VAdriaC (vincristine, Adriamycin (doxorubicin) and cyclophosphamide) and radiotherapy. In ET2, cyclophosphamide was substituted with ifosfamide, and when the two trials were compared event-free survival was 36% vs 61% in favour of regimens including ifosfamide.[52]

Therefore, a standard induction chemotherapy is six cycles of IVAD (ifosfamide 9 g/m^2, vincristine 1.4 mg/m^2 and Adriamycin 60 mg/m^2) administered over 3 days. The Euro-Ewing's 99 study investigates the addition of etoposide to this induction regimen. Induction on this study, therefore, involves six cycles of VIDE (vincristine 1.5 mg/m^2, ifosfamide 9 g/m^2, doxorubicin 60 mg/m^2 and etoposide 450 mg/m^2).

Treatment of primary disease site

Following six cycles of induction chemotherapy, wide surgical excision should be performed. Radiotherapy should be given if surgery is not possible for anatomical or functional reasons, or if there are positive excision margins following surgery. Patients not suitable for surgery should be considered for concomitant chemoirradiation. In this schedule, maintenance chemotherapy is given at the same time as a course of radiotherapy, although radiotherapy is omitted on the days when chemotherapy is actually being administered to reduce toxicity.

Maintenance chemotherapy

The choice of maintenance treatment depends on a risk assessment based on histological response to preoperative treatment and the presence of metastatic disease after induction.

- For good prognosis disease (no metastatic disease and greater than 90% necrosis after induction chemotherapy) standard maintenance is with VAC (vincristine 1.5 mg/m^2, actinomycin D (dactinomycin) 0.75 mg/m^2 D1+2 and cyclophosphamide 1.5 g/m^2 D1–3) or VAI (vincristine, actinomycin D (dactinomycin) and ifosfamide 3g/m^2). The Euro-Ewing's 99 study is comparing these two schedules in a randomised manner.
- For poor-risk disease (metastatic disease or less than 90% necrosis following induction chemotherapy), standard chemotherapy is also with VAC or VAI, but recently high-dose chemotherapy has yielded promising results. Therefore, Euro-Ewing's 99 is also investigating the role of high-dose treatment with peripheral stem cell rescue in this subset of patients.

Whole lung radiotherapy

Patients with pulmonary metastases should undergo low-dose whole lung irradiation even if complete resolution of pulmonary metastatic disease has been achieved with chemotherapy.

Second-line chemotherapy

Patients who relapse after such combination treatments should be considered for further surgery or radiotherapy. Second-line chemotherapy can sometimes produce responses, but these are normally short-lived. The current second-line schedule used at the Royal Marsden Hospital is a combination of weekly cisplatin (70 mg/m^2 on days 1, 8, 15, 29, 36 and 43) and oral etoposide (50 mg daily on days 1–15 and 29–43.) If patients respond to this regimen, they can continue oral etoposide at the same dose (21 days of a 28-day cycle for up to four cycles).

Prognosis

Patients with localised disease at presentation treated with radiotherapy and multiagent chemotherapy have an overall 5-year survival rate of up to 60% in many large studies.[53,54] Patients presenting with pulmonary metastases may still have a 30% 5-year disease-free survival with intensive treatment.[55]

Poor prognostic factors include:

- less than 90% necrosis following primary chemotherapy
- bone or bone marrow involvement
- large tumour size
- unresectable tumours
- fever, anaemia or high lactate dehydrogenase (LDH) at presentation.

RHABDOMYOSARCOMAS

Classification

Rhabdomyosarcomas are thought to arise from primitive mesenchymal cells with the capacity for rhabdomyoblastic development. Histologically, embryonal and alveolar variants are recognised. Embryonal rhabdomyosarcomas account for 60% of cases and are usually seen in children. The alveolar subtype occurs in adolescents and young adults.

Clinical features

These tumours can arise anywhere in the body where mesenchymal tissue is present; a third of cases are also associated with congenital malformations. Embryonal tumours usually occur in the head and neck region or genitourinary tract. The embryonal botyroid variant is usually seen as a polypoid growth in hollow organs such as the vagina or bladder. It is very uncommon for these tumours to occur in adults. The symptoms at presentation depend on tumour site and depth of invasion. Swelling is a common complaint, but local symptoms such as proptosis, vaginal bleeding and dysuria also occur. They spread rapidly by local invasion into neighbouring organs and may also metastasise to lymph nodes, bone, bone marrow and lungs. Spread to the meninges and brain is common where the primary lesion is in the head or neck.[56]

Diagnosis and staging investigations

These are shown in Table 44.1.

Staging systems

There are several staging systems for rhabdomyosarcomas. The most widely used are the preoperative TNM-UICC system (Table 44.5) and the postoperative Intergroup Rhabdomyosarcoma Study (IRS) system (Table 44.6).

Management plan

The particular sites at which rhabdomyosarcomas occur mean that there are important anatomical, functional and cosmetic issues that have to be taken into

Table 44.5   TNM-UICC staging system

Stage	Description
Stage I	Tumour limited to the organ or tissue of origin (T1, N0, M0)
Stage II	Tumour invading adjacent organ(s) or tissue(s) and/or with adjacent malignant effusion (T2, N0, M0)
Stage III	Regional lymph node metastases (Any T, N1, M0)
Stage IV	Distant metastases (Any T, Any N, M1)

account when planning treatment. Rhabdomyosarcoma is an aggressive disease in adults and multiple treatment modalities are employed. Treatment usually begins with combination chemotherapy, followed by local treatment with surgery and/or radiotherapy.

Chemotherapy

Combination chemotherapy for childhood rhabdomyosarcomas is based on the SIOP (International Society for Paediatric Oncology) and Intergroup Rhabdomyosarcoma studies.[57,58] Patients older than 18 years old are not eligible for these studies. However, given the rarity of this disease in adults and the paucity of data, treatment programmes are based on these studies on an individual basis.

These studies stratify patients according to risk, and because age is a risk factor, adult patients can be presumed to fall into the high-risk categories. High-risk paediatric patients are treated with combinations of ifosfamide or cyclophosphamide, vincristine and dactinomycin or etoposide. In adults, a reasonable approach would be to give VAC or IVA, or to substitute an anthracycline for the dactinomycin, and administer IVAD (ifosfamide 9 g/m², doxorubicin 60 mg/m² and vincristine 1.4 mg/m²).

Table 44.6   IRS (post-operative) staging system

Stage	Description
Stage I	Completely resected local disease
Stage IIA	Microscopic residual disease after surgery
Stage IIB	Regional lymph nodes without residual disease
Stage IIC	Regional lymph nodes, with residual disease and/or histological involvement of the most distant regional nodes
Stage III	Gross residual disease after surgery
Stage IV	Distant metastases

Surgery

Surgery usually follows initial chemotherapy. Wide local excision is advocated in the case of extremity tumours; however, there are often important functional and practical limitations with disease elsewhere. Surgery is rarely indicated in orbital tumours, and can rarely be radical in other head and neck or parameningeal sites. There is a high risk of lymph node metastases in rhabdomyosarcoma; therefore, particular attention should be paid to thorough preoperative staging. Some surgeons advocate local lymph node sampling or dissection if involvement is suspected.

Radiotherapy

Radiotherapy should be considered when definitive surgery is not possible following primary chemotherapy or when there is microscopic or gross residual disease following surgery. Therefore, parameningeal, intracranial and orbital tumours often require radiotherapy. Doses of up to 40–50 Gy are often used to ensure local disease control.

Prognosis

The most important determinant of prognosis is disease extent following surgery. Most of the data available are for children, who have a better prognosis than adults.

Poor prognostic factors:

- parameningeal sites
- tumour >5 cm
- age more than 10 years old
- lymph node metastases
- unresectable
- poor response to neoadjuvant chemotherapy
- alveolar histology.

GASTROINTESTINAL STROMAL TUMOUR

Classification

GISTs are rare non-epithelial malignant tumours of the gastrointestinal tract, which, for the purposes of classification, fall into a separate group to gastrointestinal adenocarcinomas and sarcomas. They are thought to arise from the mesenchymal cells of the gastrointestinal tract, and overexpression of CD117, the c-kit receptor, is common.[59,60]

Clinical features

These rare tumours present as an abdominal mass or with abdominal pain. Less commonly, tumour complications such as bowel obstruction or gastrointestinal haemorrhage occur. The most common primary sites are the stomach and small bowel, with the large bowel occasionally being involved. Their malignant potential is difficult to predict and is best estimated by simultaneous evaluation of a number of clinical and pathological features. Local recurrences are common and the liver is the most common site of metastatic disease.[60]

Diagnosis and staging investigations

These are shown in Table 44.1.

Management plan

Historically, the mainstay of treatment has been complete surgical resection, which is curative in a proportion of patients.[61,62] However, local recurrences are common following surgery, and up to half of patients may present with metastatic disease.[62] Conventional cytotoxic chemotherapy and radiotherapy are not particularly effective treatment strategies. However, the recognition that the proto-oncogene *c-kit* is frequently upregulated in GI stromal tumours has suggested an alternative approach to treatment: *c-kit* encodes a transmembrane tyrosine kinase receptor, and the agent STI571 (imatinib or Glivec) is capable of inhibiting the tyrosine kinase activity of this receptor. In a European trial of 36 patients with gastrointestinal stromal tumours, oral imatinib (dose range 400–1000 mg daily) inhibited tumour growth in 32 patients, with partial responses being observed in 19 patients.[63] In a US study, a further 36 patients with gastrointestinal stromal tumours were treated with oral imatinib (dose range 400–600 mg daily). Nineteen partial responses were observed, and disease progression occurred in 4 patients.[64] These impressive phase I data are awaiting confirmation in randomised clinical trials.

Prognosis

In a series of 200 patients seen over 16 years at the Memorial Sloan-Kettering Hospital, 46% had primary disease alone at presentation, and 47% had metastatic disease (7% had isolated local recurrence.) In patients with no metastases who underwent complete resection of gross primary disease, the 5-year survival rate was 54%. Survival was predicted by tumour size, but not by microscopic resection margins.[62] How the development of imatinib will impact on long-term prognosis is not yet known.

NURSING FOR PATIENTS WITH BONE AND SOFT TISSUE SARCOMA

David Brighton

INTRODUCTION

Care of the patient undergoing chemotherapy for sarcoma presents a number of unique problems and issues. The relative rarity of sarcoma makes it difficult for staff not working in sarcoma units to be familiar with the disease and its treatment. Chemotherapy is also not usually the main treatment for patients with sarcoma. Chemotherapy will usually be given in combination with surgery, radiotherapy or with palliative intent. Patients will usually fall into three main groups:

- patients with chemotherapy-sensitive disease who will have chemotherapy to reduce the tumour mass prior to surgery
- patients who have had surgery or radiotherapy and are having chemotherapy as adjuvant treatment
- patients who are having chemotherapy to control metastatic or inoperable disease.

Surgery is often the first mode of treatment for sarcoma patients. Staff not directly providing surgical treatment and care may still need to be able to assist in the physical and psychological rehabilitation of the patient during chemotherapy treatment. This will be especially true for patients who may have had extensive muscle mass removal, large-volume disease debulking or amputation. Relatively straightforward surgical intervention may be undertaken within a sarcoma unit, but patients may also come from specialist orthopaedic centres having had very complicated surgery and prosthetic implants. In these circumstances, assessment and rehabilitation of patients may be as important as the assessment and care for the chemotherapy aspects of their treatment.

SPECIFIC SKILLS

Management of side effects

Side effects are inevitable for sarcoma chemotherapy. Successful management starts with monitoring, surveillance and preventative action. As well as the normal side effects of nausea, bone marrow depression and alopecia, there are a number of specific side effects for drugs. Ifosfamide is one of the main treatment drugs for sarcoma and has a number of unique side effects.

Neurological toxicity

Neurological toxicity is a well-documented problem with ifosfamide administration. Patients can become confused, drowsy, aphasic and in extreme cases lapse into unconsciousness. This may be compounded if the patient spends much of the admission asleep or exhibiting signs of profound tiredness. The limitation on mobility due to intravenous (IV) pumps may mean that many patients do little more than sleep during their admission for chemotherapy. Observation and supervision of the patient's neurological status, self-care activity, nutritional intake and compliance with medication may be necessary. This should be done as far as possible to maintain the independence and decision-making of the patient. (See also Chs 27 and 34.)

Haemorrhagic cystitis

Ifosfamide is associated with haemorrhagic cystitis. This is caused by acrolein, one of the breakdown products. Treatment involves forced hydration of 3 litres per 24 hours with the addition of mesna. Mesna binds to acrolein and helps to reduce the possibility of haemorrhagic cystitis. It also produces a false-positive reading on urinalysis for ketones, which is monitored in every specimen to ensure that sufficient mesna is being administered. Urinalysis is also used to detect blood, as urinalysis will detect microscopic haematuria prior to it being visible.

Late adolescent and young adult patients – caring for young adult patients with cancer

Cancer is generally a disease of the elderly, but sarcomas are also relatively common in children and young adults. Young adult patients face treatment at a time when they are still developing their own roles and personal maturation. The majority of this section is used to examine some of the unique issues of caring for young adult patients with cancer.

The role of the family in young adult patients

For young adult patients, the family may have a greater role to play than would immediately be assumed. Health carers sometimes underestimate the importance of the family in supporting young adults through treatment. The patient may have begun an independent lifestyle away from parents or siblings, but the family may re-emerge as the most enabling influence for the patient trying to manage the illness experience.[65] In addition to this, young adults may exhibit needs which would be normally associated with a much younger age group. Patients may revert to being more dependent than their physical maturation would suggest. This can often be exacerbated in the presence of treatments or physical changes that reduce their ability to manage their own lives, care for themselves or make decisions about their care. Any physical inability may also be traumatic for young patients who have had no reason to consider disability as part of their self-concept. Physical changes, such as amputation, can also lead to a delay in the patient asserting independence from the family.[65]

There are a number of needs for patients with cancer. When faced with problems, it is this network of significant people that is sought out to provide support. The family may be the main source of care and support for a young adult patient, especially if they have not established relationships that are able to provide the deep level of support that may be needed. Support during treatment for sarcoma may extend across a number of different fields. Physical assistance with tasks or activities may be required if the patient has had physical changes in ability due to surgery or lacks the energy or concentration levels required. Psychological support may also be required to help patients come to terms with the life-threatening nature of their disease. It will often be the parents of a young patient who are providing the majority of support for the patient. It may be the role of the healthcare team to help support the family members and ensure that they have access to the resources needed to adequately support the patient. This may include community care resources, information or a point of contact to share concerns.[66]

Diagnosis – finding zebras

There is a medical motto: 'If you hear hooves, think horses, not zebras'. It is more likely that a patient who presents with a lump will have a soft tissue injury than a sarcoma and some young adult patients may have faced delay in having their sarcoma diagnosed. Sarcoma is relatively rare and a diagnosis of cancer in a young adult is usually not the first thought on the minds of general practitioners.

The rarity of sarcoma can place burdens on the patient beyond the disease and the treatment. Patients talk about the 'loneliness' of having a cancer that no one else seems to have and no one knows about. There is also the issue of having to act as an informer or information resource when others do not know about the disease. This can extend to family, friends and work colleagues as well as health professionals who are unfamiliar with sarcoma.[67] Patients often express a wish to talk to someone who has had a similar treatment to what is being planned for them. This can be problematic for the patient with sarcoma due to the

differences in presentation and problems faced by different patients, but also the relatively small population of patients accessible at a given time. Many patients do take comfort from meeting other people with a similar diagnosis and may make contact through the internet utilising email mailing lists or groups. A quick search using the web search tool Google reveals a number of these. The Association of Cancer Online Resources (ACOR) (see Useful Addresses) have probably the most extensive mailing lists for cancer patients and have lists devoted to many of the classifications of sarcoma (and other types of cancer). Many patients find these very supportive, but should be advised to approach web resources with a degree of caution. Treatments in different centres can be very different and this can cause some confusion for patients. The majority of patients using these groups are also from the USA, where the health system is organised and delivered differently to the UK. Although the likelihood of negative effects from contact should be low, due the level of control offered by ACOR lists, patients should be aware of risks on other internet resources, notably unsolicited emails (spam), fraud, inappropriate content or abusive messages. (See Useful Addresses for alternative mailing lists and Ch. 5.)

Peer reintegration

The reintegration of young adult patients back into their normal peer group can also be difficult. First, they may have restrictions on their ability to maintain previous activities due to the disease or treatment. This is compounded by the need for a 72-hour admission with continuous IV treatment every 21 days and the periods dealing with the side effects, fatigue and lethargy of the treatment. Patients also cite hair loss as having an impact on their social pattern, not just as a physical change from treatment.[68]

Patients may also have difficulty in finding acceptance from friends who have not had to cope with a serious life-threatening illness in the past and they often have to initiate discussion of their illness, as friends would be uncomfortable doing this.[66] Very few young adults or adolescents are comfortable visiting in a hospital or 'sick' environment and many will actively avoid it. Making these issues known to patients may give them the opportunity to begin to think about the problems they will face and practice methods to deal with them in a safe environment.

Young patients – staff coping

A diagnosis of sarcoma places enormous burden on the friends and family and the young patient with sarcoma. It may also be difficult for healthcare professionals to cope with the demands of caring for a patient who may be the age of themselves, their sibling or their child. As an individual and a team, all who come into contact with young patients face the difficulty of their own emotions. This includes nurses, doctors and allied health staff, but also the ancillary workers. A recent study at the Royal Marsden NHS Trust[69] highlighted the role and involvement that porters, domestic and other staff have with patients. Many of them rightly value the input they can have into the treatment and care of patients. Many patients also value ancillary staff as people to talk to who know the organisation but are not taken up in treatment activities. With this involvement comes the risk of emotional upset if the patient does not do well from treatment. Reported ways of coping with this risk included avoiding conversation and contact with patients or moving on to other jobs or work areas periodically. The issues in coping with the patient involvement are the same for nurses, doctors and allied health staff, but these staff groups should find it more difficult to avoid contact with patients. Some of the ways to help support staff who care for young adult patients who may be emotionally taxing are:

- acknowledging that caring for patients can be emotionally draining

- forewarning new staff on the unit that it is helpful to think about their own emotional responses and coping skills
- maintaining communication and support to allow the team members to discuss any problems they are facing when caring for patients
- communicating any significant changes in condition or treatment to avoid 'shocks' to staff who may not have been in contact with the patient for a period
- acknowledging the sense of loss and grief within the team when a patient dies.

SUMMARY

Patients having treatment for sarcoma share many of the concerns of other cancer patients regarding prognosis and treatment issues but, additionally, may have physical problems caused by the disease or treatment. The higher proportion of younger patients with sarcoma places additional demands on staff and provides the opportunity to care using a wider range of skills. Much of the care will be centred on the administration of treatment, but the supportive and rehabilitative aspects of care are also important to help the patient come to terms with his own unique situation.

References

1. Office for National Statistics. Mortality statistics, United Kingdom, 1998.
2. Usui M, Ishii S, Yamawaki S, et al. The occurrence of soft tissue sarcomas in three siblings with Werner's syndrome. Cancer 1984; 54(11):2580–2586.
3. McAdam WA, Goligher JC. The occurrence of desmoids in patients with familial polyposis coli. Br J Surg 1970; 57(8):618–631.
4. Jensen RD, Miller RW. Retinoblastoma: epidemiologic characteristics. N Engl J Med 1971; 285(6):307–311.
5. Brennan MF, Alektiar KM, Maki RG. Sarcomas of soft tissue and bone. In: DeVita VT, Helman S, Rosenberg SA, eds. Cancer: principles and practice of oncology. 6th edn. Philadelphia: Lippincott, Williams and Wilkins; 2001:1841–1891.
6. Arlen M, Higinbotham NL, Huvos AG, et al. Radiation-induced sarcoma of bone. Cancer 1971; 28(5):1087–1099.
7. Souba WW, McKenna RJ Jr, Meis J, Benjamin R, et al. Radiation-induced sarcomas of the chest wall. Cancer 1986; 57(3):610–615.
8. Strong LC, Herson J, Osborne BM, et al. Risk of radiation-related subsequent malignant tumors in survivors of Ewing's sarcoma. J Natl Cancer Inst 1979; 62(6):1401–1406.
9. Kim JH, Chu FC, Woodard HQ, et al. Radiation-induced soft-tissue and bone sarcoma. Radiology 1978; 129(2):501–508.
10. Hatfield PM, Schulz MD. Postirradiation sarcoma. Including 5 cases after X-ray therapy of breast carcinoma. Radiology 1970; 96(3):593–602.
11. Kogevinas M, Kauppinen T, Winkelmann R, et al. Soft tissue sarcoma and non-Hodgkin's lymphoma in workers exposed to phenoxy herbicides, chlorophenols, and dioxins: two nested case–control studies. Epidemiology 1995; 6(4):396–402.
12. Lynge E. Cancer incidence in Danish phenoxy herbicide workers, 1947–1993. Environ Health Perspect 1998; 106(Suppl 2):683–688.
13. Locker GY, Doroshow JH, Zwelling LA, et al. The clinical features of hepatic angiosarcoma: a report of four cases and a review of the English literature. Medicine (Baltimore) 1979; 58(1):48–64.
14. Turc-Carel C, Philip I, Berger MP, et al. [Chromosomal translocation (11; 22) in cell lines of Ewing's sarcoma]. C R Seances Acad Sci III 1983; 296(23):1101–1103.
15. Turc-Carel C, Limon J, Dal Cin P, et al. Cytogenetic studies of adipose tissue tumors. II. Recurrent reciprocal translocation t(12;16)(q13;p11) in myxoid liposarcomas. Cancer Genet Cytogenet 1986; 23(4):291–299.

16. Turc-Carel C, Dal Cin P, Limon J, et al. Translocation X;18 in synovial sarcoma. Cancer Genet Cytogenet 1986; 23(1):93.

17. Lawrence W Jr, Donegan WL, Natarajan N, et al. Adult soft tissue sarcomas. A pattern of care survey of the American College of Surgeons. Ann Surg 1987; 205(4):349–359.

18. Lucas JD, O'Doherty MJ, Wong JC, et al. Evaluation of fluorodeoxyglucose positron emission tomography in the management of soft-tissue sarcomas. J Bone Joint Surg Br 1998; 80(3):441–447.

19. Musculoskeletal sites. In: Fleming ID, ed. American Joint Committee on Cancer Staging Manual. 5th edn. Philadelphia: Lippinicott-Raven; 1997:149–155.

20. Ramanathan RC, A'Hern R, Fisher C, et al. Modified staging system for extremity soft tissue sarcomas. Ann Surg Oncol 1999; 6(1):57–69.

21. Cantin J, McNeer GP, Chu FC, et al. The problem of local recurrence after treatment of soft tissue sarcoma. Ann Surg 1968; 168(1):47–53.

22. Gerner RE, Moore GE, Pickren JW. Soft tissue sarcomas. Ann Surg 1975; 181(6):803–808.

23. Lindberg RD, Martin RG, Romsdahl MM, et al. Conservative surgery and postoperative radiotherapy in 300 adults with soft-tissue sarcomas. Cancer 1981; 47(10):2391–2397.

24. Yang JC, Chang AE, Baker AR, et al. Randomized prospective study of the benefit of adjuvant radiation therapy in the treatment of soft tissue sarcomas of the extremity. J Clin Oncol 1998; 16(1):197–203.

25. Alektiar KM, Leung D, Zelefsky MJ, et al. Adjuvant radiation for stage II-B soft tissue sarcoma of the extremity. J Clin Oncol 2002; 20(6):1643–1650.

26. Adjuvant chemotherapy for localised resectable soft-tissue sarcoma of adults: meta-analysis of individual data. Sarcoma Meta-analysis Collaboration. Lancet 1997; 350(9092):1647–1654.

27. Fruscati S, Gherlinzoni F, Antonio PD, et al. Maintenance of efficacy of adjuvant chemotherapy in soft tissue sarcomas of the extremities, update of a randomised trial. Proc Am Soc Clin Oncol 1999:2108.

28. Stuart-Harris RC, Harper PG, Parsons CA, et al. High-dose alkylation therapy using ifosfamide infusion with mesna in the treatment of adult advanced soft-tissue sarcoma. Cancer Chemother Pharmacol 1983; 11(2):69–72.

29. Hoefer-Janker H, Scheef W, Gunther U, et al. [Experience with fractionate massive-dose Ifosfamid therapy of generalized malignant tumors]. Med Welt 1975; 26(20):972–979.

30. Bramwell VH, Mouridsen HT, Santoro A, et al. Cyclophosphamide versus ifosfamide: final report of a randomized phase II trial in adult soft tissue sarcomas. Eur J Cancer Clin Oncol 1987; 23(3):311–321.

31. O'Bryan RM, Baker LH, Gottlieb JE, et al. Dose response evaluation of adriamycin in human neoplasia. Cancer 1977; 39(5):1940–1948.

32. Mouridsen HT, Bastholt L, Somers R, et al. Adriamycin versus epirubicin in advanced soft tissue sarcomas. A randomized phase II/phase III study of the EORTC Soft Tissue and Bone Sarcoma Group. Eur J Cancer Clin Oncol 1987; 23(10):1477–1483.

33. Schoenfeld DA, Rosenbaum C, Horton J, et al. A comparison of adriamycin versus vincristine and adriamycin, and cyclophosphamide versus vincristine, actinomycin-D, and cyclophosphamide for advanced sarcoma. Cancer 1982; 50(12):2757–2562.

34. Judson I, Radford JA, Harris M, et al. Randomised phase II trial of pegylated liposomal doxorubicin (DOXIL/CAELYX) versus doxorubicin in the treatment of advanced or metastatic soft tissue sarcoma: a study by the EORTC Soft Tissue and Bone Sarcoma Group. Eur J Cancer 2001; 37(7):870–877.

35. Buesa JM, Mouridsen HT, van Oosterom AT, et al. High-dose DTIC in advanced soft-tissue sarcomas in the adult. A phase II study of the E.O.R.T.C. Soft Tissue and Bone Sarcoma Group. Ann Oncol 1991; 2(4):307–309.

36. van Hoesel QG, Verweij J, Catimel G, et al. Phase II study with docetaxel (Taxotere) in advanced soft tissue sarcomas of the adult. EORTC Soft Tissue and Bone Sarcoma Group. Ann Oncol 1994; 5(6):539–542.

37. Schutte J, Mouridsen HT, Steward W, et al. Ifosfamide plus doxorubicin in previously untreated patients with advanced soft-tissue sarcoma. Cancer Chemother Pharmacol 1993; 31(Suppl 2):S204–209.

38. Santoro A, Tursz T, Mouridsen H, et al. Doxorubicin versus CYVADIC versus doxorubicin plus ifosfamide in first-line treatment of advanced soft tissue sarcomas: a randomized study of the European Organization for Research and Treatment of Cancer Soft Tissue and Bone Sarcoma Group. J Clin Oncol 1995; 13(7):1537–1545.

39. Antman K, Crowley J, Balcerzak SP, et al. An intergroup phase III randomized study of doxorubicin and dacarbazine with or without ifosfamide and mesna in advanced soft tissue and bone sarcomas. J Clin Oncol 1993; 11(7):1276–1285.

40. van Geel AN, Pastorino U, Jauch KW, et al. Surgical treatment of lung metastases: The European Organization for Research and Treatment of Cancer-Soft Tissue and Bone Sarcoma Group study of 255 patients. Cancer 1996; 77(4):675–682.

41. Pastorino U, Valente M, Gasparini M, et al. Lung resection for metastatic sarcomas: total survival from primary treatment. J Surg Oncol 1989; 40(4):275–280.

42. Van Glabbeke M, van Oosterom AT, Oosterhuis JW, et al. Prognostic factors for the outcome of chemotherapy in advanced soft tissue sarcoma: an analysis of 2,185 patients treated with anthracycline-containing first-line regimens – a European Organization for Research and Treatment of Cancer Soft Tissue and Bone Sarcoma Group Study. J Clin Oncol 1999; 17(1):150–157.

43. Dahlin DC. Osteosarcoma of bone and a consideration of prognostic variables. Cancer Treat Rep 1978; 62(2):189–192.

44. Eilber F, Giuliano A, Eckardt J, et al. Adjuvant chemotherapy for osteosarcoma: a randomized prospective trial. J Clin Oncol 1987; 5(1):21–26.

45. Bramwell VH, Burgers M, Sneath R, et al. A comparison of two short intensive adjuvant chemotherapy regimens in operable osteosarcoma of limbs in children and young adults: the first study of the European Osteosarcoma Intergroup. J Clin Oncol 1992; 10(10):1579–1591.

46. Souhami RL, Craft AW, Van der Eijken JW, et al. Randomised trial of two regimens of chemotherapy in operable osteosarcoma: a study of the European Osteosarcoma Intergroup. Lancet 1997; 350(9082):911–917.

47. Ward WG, Mikaelian K, Dorey F, et al. Pulmonary metastases of stage IIB extremity osteosarcoma and subsequent pulmonary metastases. J Clin Oncol 1994; 12(9):1849–1858.

48. Davis AM, Bell RS, Goodwin PJ. Prognostic factors in osteosarcoma: a critical review. J Clin Oncol 1994; 12(2):423–431.

49. Oldham RK, Pomeroy TC. Treatment of Ewing's sarcoma with adriamycin (NSC-123127). Cancer Chemother Rep 1972; 56(5):635–639.

50. Nesbit ME Jr, Gehan EA, Burgert EO Jr, et al. Multimodal therapy for the management of primary, nonmetastatic Ewing's sarcoma of bone: a long-term follow-up of the First Intergroup study. J Clin Oncol 1990; 8(10):1664–674.

51. Burgert EO Jr, Nesbit ME, Garnsey LA, et al. Multimodal therapy for the management of nonpelvic, localized Ewing's sarcoma of bone: intergroup study IESS-II. J Clin Oncol 1990; 8(9):1514–1524.

52. Craft A, Cotterill S, Malcolm A, et al. Ifosfamide-containing chemotherapy in Ewing's sarcoma: The Second United Kingdom Children's Cancer Study Group and the Medical Research Council Ewing's Tumor Study. J Clin Oncol 1998; 16(11):3628–3633.

53. Bacci G, Ferrari S, Bertoni F, et al. Neoadjuvant chemotherapy for peripheral malignant neuroectodermal tumor of bone: recent experience at the istituto rizzoli. J Clin Oncol 2000; 18(4):885–892.

54. Bacci G, Picci P, Ferrari S, et al. Neoadjuvant chemotherapy for Ewing's sarcoma of bone: no benefit observed after adding ifosfamide and etoposide to vincristine, actinomycin, cyclophosphamide, and doxorubicin in the maintenance phase – results of two sequential studies. Cancer 1998; 82(6):1174–1183.

55. Paulussen M, Ahrens S, Craft AW, et al. Ewing's tumors with primary lung metastases: survival analysis of 114 (European Intergroup) Cooperative Ewing's Sarcoma Studies patients. J Clin Oncol 1998; 16(9):3044–3052.

56. Flamant F, Habrand J-L, Lacombe MJ, et al. Malignant mesenchymal tumours in childhood. In: Peckham M, Pinedo H, Veronesi U, eds. Oxford textbook of oncology. Oxford: Oxford University Press; 1995:1939–1953.

57. Flamant F, Rodary C, Rey A, et al. Treatment of non-metastatic rhabdomyosarcomas in childhood and adolescence. Results of the second study of the International Society of Paediatric Oncology: MMT84. Eur J Cancer 1998; 34(7):1050–1062.

58. Baker KS, Anderson JR, Link MP, et al. Benefit of intensified therapy for patients with local or regional embryonal rhabdomyosarcoma: results from the Intergroup Rhabdomyosarcoma Study IV. J Clin Oncol 2000; 18(12):2427–2434.

59. Longley BJ, Reguera MJ, Ma Y. Classes of c-KIT activating mutations: proposed mechanisms of action and implications for disease classification and therapy. Leuk Res 2001; 25(7):571–576.

60. Strickland L, Letson GD, Muro-Cacho CA. Gastrointestinal stromal tumors. Cancer Control 2001; 8(3):252–261.

61. Hillemanns M, Pasold S, Bottcher K, et al. [Prognostic factors of gastrointestinal stromal tumors of the stomach]. Verh Dtsch Ges Pathol 1998; 82:261–266.

62. DeMatteo RP, Lewis JJ, Leung D, et al. Two hundred gastrointestinal stromal tumors: recurrence patterns and prognostic factors for survival. Ann Surg 2000; 231(1):51–58.

63. van Oosterom AT, Judson I, Verweij J, et al. Safety and efficacy of imatinib (STI571) in metastatic gastrointestinal stromal tumours: a phase I study. Lancet 2001; 358(9291):1421–1423.

64. Blanke CD, von Mehren MM, Joensuu H, et al. Evaluation of the safety and efficacy of an oral molecularly-targeted therapy, STI 571, in patients with unresectable or metastatic gastrointestinal stromal tumours, expressing c-kit. Proc Am Soc Clin Oncol 2001:1.

65. Tebbi CK, Mallon JC. Long-term psychosocial outcome among cancer amputees in adolescence and early adulthood. J Psychosoc Oncol 1987; 5:69–82.

66. Lynam MJ. Supporting one another: the nature of family work when a young adult has cancer. J Advanced Nurs 1995; 22(1):116–125.

67. http://www.boston.com/globe/search/stories/ health/health_sense/062899.htm – article on orphan diseases from the Boston Globe: 'Orphan diseases leave patients on their own,' by Judy Foreman. Boston Globe 28 July 1999:C01.

68. Novakovic B, Fears TR, Wexler LH, et al. Experiences of cancer in children and adolescents. Cancer Nurs 1996; 19(1):54–59.

69. Mack H, Froggatt K, McClinton P. "A small cog in a large wheel": an exploratory study into the experiences of porters, ward clerks and domestics working in an English Cancer Centre. Eur J Oncol Nurs 2003; 7(3):153–161.

USEFUL ADDRESSES

Association of Cancer Online Resources (ACOR): http://www.acor.org/mailing.html

Alternative list of mailing lists: http://www.cancersource.com/community/boards/index.cfm

Chapter **45**

Central nervous system tumours

MEDICAL CARE FOR PATIENTS WITH CENTRAL HNERVOUS SYSTEM TUMOURS

Sally Trent

INCIDENCE

Primary intracranial neoplasms of the central nervous system (CNS) are rare and represent 2–5% of all tumours. The age-adjusted incidence ranges from 5.9 to 12.6 cases per 100 000 population per year.[1–4]

Of this group of tumours, neuroepithelial tumours constitute the largest histological group of primary brain tumours (40%) (Table 45.1). Some studies have suggested an increasing incidence of glial tumours, particularly in the older population; however this trend probably represents more frequent diagnosis, which has accompanied increasing availability of computed tomography (CT) and magnetic resonance imaging (MRI).[5]

Primary cerebral lymphoma represents only 1% of primary intracranial tumours. Its incidence has increased in both men and women of all ages. This increase preceded the onset of the acquired immune deficiency syndrome (AIDS) epidemic.[6–8]

AGE AND SEX DISTRIBUTION

The incidence of malignant gliomas and meningiomas rises with age, with a peak at 65–75 years old for malignant gliomas and even older for meningiomas. Medulloblastomas, primitive neuroectodermal tumours, and pilocytic astrocytomas are mostly seen in children but also occur in adults at a reducing frequency. Pineal and suprasellar germ cell tumours have a specific age distribution, with a peak incidence in children and young adults. There is a slight male predominance in neuroepithelial tumours, whereas meningiomas are more common in women than in men.

Table 45.1 CNS tumour distribution

Tumour	Frequency
Neuroepithelial tumours	40%
Tumours of peripheral nerve	8%
Meningeal tumours	25%
Lymphomas and haemopoietic neoplasms	5%
Germ cell tumours	1%
Tumours of the sellar region	1%
Metastatic tumours	20%

IMAGING

Patients with symptoms suggestive of a brain tumour should have a screening test to establish the presence of a lesion. This consists of a CT scan or MRI of the brain. Additional non-invasive tests such as plain skull radiography, an electroencephalogram (EEG) and psychometric evaluation are rarely necessary.

Computed tomography scanning

The features of supratentorial tumours are localised swelling of the brain with associated peritumoural oedema and compression of the ventricular system, as well as midline shift. On unenhanced CT scan, meningiomas, lymphomas and some metastases (such as melanoma) are usually hyperdense, while gliomas, ependymomas, and most metastases are iso- or hypodense and can often be recognised as tumour masses by contrasting them with surrounding low-density oedema. Tumour calcification is seen in approximately 10% of gliomas and 50% of oligodendrogliomas. Following injection of iodinated contrast, the degree of contrast enhancement in gliomas usually correlates with the degree of malignancy. Over 85% of high-grade gliomas, as well as meningiomas and metastases, show enhancement, whereas only a minority of lower-grade tumours enhance.

Magnetic resonance imaging

MRI has better contrast discrimination and is superior to CT in defining tumour extent, particularly in unenhancing low-grade tumours. Lesions in the middle and posterior fossae or in the spinal canal are demonstrated more readily as the lack of signal from bone obviates bone-induced artefacts. Cerebrospinal fluid (CSF) spaces, major blood vessels and grey and white matter can all be visualised. Pathological changes such as haemorrhage can be diagnosed, although calcification and bone changes are seen less well than on CT. Demyelination, ischaemic areas and low-grade gliomas, often not demonstrated by CT, are generally well shown by MRI.

CLINICAL MANIFESTATIONS OF BRAIN TUMOURS

Cerebral tumours may present with symptoms of raised intracranial pressure, headache and vomiting. The headache is often bifrontal or occipital, and is most noticeable in the morning. The fundi need to be assessed for evidence of papilloedema. Alterations of brain function, causing mental deterioration and change in personality, are slow in onset and are more obvious to relatives than to the patient. Epilepsy is a common presenting feature of brain tumours. These may be either focal or as generalised seizures.

Specific clinical syndromes

Cerebral hemisphere tumours

Frontal lobe tumours commonly cause personality change together with impairment of intellectual function and epilepsy. Dysphasia occurs if the dominant left hemisphere is affected. Temporal lobe tumours may be associated with hemiparesis, homonymous hemianopia, temporal lobe epilepsy and dysphasia with dominant hemisphere tumour. Involvement of the parietal sensory cortex causes neglect of the contralateral side of the body and inattention. Right parietal lobe tumours cause diminished ability to orientate the body image and impaired left/right discrimination, in addition to possible motor impairment, receptive as well as expressive dysphasia may occur in dominant hemisphere involvement. Occipital tumours may lead to homonymous hemianopia.

Midline and third ventricle region tumours

Gliomas in the optic chiasma or hypothalamus occurring in children or adolescents may impair growth or lead to precocious puberty and disturbances of temperature and appetite control as well as failure of vision. Tumours in this area may cause interruption of CSF circulation, leading to the development of hydrocephalus. Tumours affecting the thalamus and basal ganglia tend to cause contralateral motor and sensory deficit and occasional impairment of consciousness.

Posterior fossa tumours

Brainstem Brainstem tumours cause low cranial nerve palsies associated with varying degrees of disturbance of long tract function and ataxia. Hydrocephalus is unusual.

Cerebellum and fourth ventricle Tumours of the cerebellar hemispheres give rise to both ataxia and nystagmus.

Obstructive hydrocephalus is common and may be associated with symptoms of neck stiffness due to herniation of the cerebellar tonsils.

Cranial nerve tumours

Eighth nerve neurilemmoma, the most common of intrinsic nerve sheath tumours, usually presents with progressive unilateral deafness. Expansion into the cerebello-pontine angle may cause ataxia and involvement of the trigeminal and facial nerves.

Pituitary and suprasellar tumours

Non-functioning pituitary adenomas and craniopharyngiomas present with either visual disturbance (typically bitemporal hemianopia) or pituitary failure. Functioning pituitary adenomas present with specific endocrine disturbance. Hydrocephalus may be caused by obstruction of the ventricular system at the foramen of Monro.

TUMOURS OF NEUROEPITHELIAL ORIGIN

Table 45.2 gives the types and frequency of neuroepithelial tumours.

Gliomas

Gliomas are tumours of neuroepithelial origin, comprising astrocytomas, oligodendrogliomas and ependymomas. Mixed forms such as oligoastrocytomas occur. Tumours are graded on the basis of histological features and placed into the WHO classification system.[9] The grade relates to the biological behaviour of the tumours, ranging from malignancy grade I (the least biologically aggressive) to grade IV (the most malignant). This histologically based grading scheme is of prognostic relevance. Patients with pilocytic astrocytomas (grade I) have a very good prognosis, the average survival of patients with a diffuse astrocytoma (grade II) is around 7 years,[10,11] whereas patients with

Table 45.2   Types and frequency of neuroepithelial tumours

Tumour	WHO grade	Frequency
Astrocytic tumours		
Pilocytic astrocytoma	I	
Diffuse astrocytoma	II	15%
Anaplastic astrocytoma	III	
Glioblastoma	IV	50%
Oligodendroglial tumours		
Oligodendroglioma	II	1–5%
Anaplastic oligodendroglioma	III	
Ependymal tumours		
Ependymoma	II	6%
Anaplastic ependymoma	III	
Choroid plexus tumours		
Neuroblastic tumours		<1%
Olfactory neuroblastoma (Aesthesioneuroblastoma)	II–III	
Olfactory neuroepithelioma	IV	
Neuroblastomas of the adrenal gland and sympathetic nervous system	IV	
Pineal parenchymal tumours		<1%
Pineocytoma	II	
Pineoblastoma	IV	
Embryonal tumours		1.7%
Ependymoblastoma	IV	
Medulloblastoma	IV	
Supratentorial primitive neuroectodermal tumours (PNETs)	IV	
Neuroblastoma	IV	
Ganglioneuroblastoma	IV	

anaplastic astrocytomas have a median survival half that time.[12-14] Glioblastoma patients have a very poor prognosis, with average survival reported between 9 and 11 months.[13-15] For clinical purposes, gliomas are broadly divided into two groups. Grade I and II are grouped together as low-grade gliomas, whereas grade III and IV gliomas are categorised as high-grade tumours.

Low-grade gliomas

Astrocytomas

The pilocytic astrocytomas (grade I) are the least malignant and occur mainly in the **posterior fossa in** children. These tumours rarely progress to more malignant tumours. This contrasts with the adult diffuse astrocytomas (grade II) that often progress or transform to high-grade gliomas. Grade II tumours have a peak age of incidence between 25 and 50 years old.

Oligodendrogliomas

Oligodendrogliomas occur mainly in the cerebral hemispheres of adults. They are believed to be derived from oligodendrocytes, and are classified as WHO grade II tumours. These tumours are relatively indolent, although they usually recur at the primary site and may display a tendency for subependymal spread with <5% incidence of CSF seeding.

Ependymomas

Ependymomas arise at ependymal surfaces of both the supra- and infratentorial ventricular system and are commonest glioma of the spinal cord. Ependymomas in children are typically located in the posterior fossa, whereas in adults they frequently occur in a supratentorial location.

Management of low-grade gliomas

Surgery In selected patients with low-grade glioma, surgery offers the possibility of cure; however, this must not be pursued at the expense of unacceptable neurological deficit. Pilocytic astrocytomas in children and adults may be well circumscribed and amenable to curative complete surgical excision.[16]

Histological diagnosis of lesions which are poorly circumscribed or in a functional significant region may be obtained with either CT- or MRI-directed stereotactic biopsy. This technique carries a low risk of serious morbidity and mortality (1–2%), with a 93% chance of obtaining a definite histological diagnosis.[17]

Unlike astrocytomas or oligodendrogliomas, a complete macroscopic excision of ependymomas should be attempted, tempered by the risks of serious morbidity.[18-20] The extent of surgical resection of ependymomas and histological grade are the key determinants of survival.[21-24] Removal of posterior fossa ependymomas also re-establishes the flow of CSF. The role of second-look surgery to excise residual ependymoma is currently under evaluation.

Radiotherapy

Astrocytoma and oligodendroglioma Early retrospective studies of postoperative radiotherapy in the treatment of patients with incompletely excised astrocytoma and oligodendroglioma suggested a survival benefit for patients treated with radiation.[25-27] However, a prospective randomised trial of the European Organisation for Research and Treatment of Cancer (EORTC), did not show improved survival in patients receiving immediate, compared to delayed radiotherapy.[28] Currently, there is no evidence that delaying surgery or radiotherapy to the time of tumour progression is detrimental. A parallel randomised study assessing the effect of dose found no survival difference between patients receiving 45 Gy and 59 Gy.[29] On present evidence, radiotherapy is reserved for patients with progressive disease, with the aim of treatment being to stabilise or improve the neurological deficit caused by the tumour. A reduction in the frequency of convulsions, which often accompany the presentation of low-grade tumours, may occur. The recommended radiation dose is 45–55 Gy at 1.6–1.8 Gy per fraction, and the treatment should be restricted to the tumour and a surrounding margin of normal tissue.

Ependymoma Localised irradiation should be delivered to the site of disease following both complete or incomplete surgical excision of ependymomas.

Prognosis Age, performance status,[11] the extent of disease[29] and histology[30] are prognostic factors for survival in astrocytoma and oligodendroglioma. The reported 10-year survival rate for patients with pilocytic astrocytoma is 70–90%. Median survival for patients with diffuse astrocytomas is 6–10 years and mixed oligoastrocytomas and grade II oligodendrogliomas 8–13 years.[11,29-31] The overall 5-year survival of selected patients with cranial ependymoma is 50–60% and progression-free survival is approximately 10% less. In some reports the prognosis is related to the histological grade and the extent of surgical resection, particularly in grade II tumours.[32] Nevertheless, 30% of patients with incompletely excised ependymomas, particularly of low grade, remain alive without evidence of tumour progression at 5 years.[21,23]

Astrocytomas frequently transform to high-grade gliomas and management at the time of recurrent disease or malignant transformation is along the lines of management of either primary or recurrent malignant glioma, depending on previous therapy. The prognosis at that time is determined by performance status, age and tumour histology, although it is marginally better for patients with transformed malignant gliomas compared to recurrent primary malignant gliomas.[33,34] The prognosis of transformed anaplastic astrocytoma is similar to anaplastic astrocytoma de novo.[35]

High-grade gliomas

Anaplastic astrocytomas (WHO grade III) and glioblastomas (WHO grade IV) for clinical purposes are grouped together as high-grade gliomas. Glioblastomas are the most common form of astrocytic tumour. They may develop from a previously diagnosed astrocytoma or they develop de novo.[12] Clinical and molecular data support the hypothesis that these tumours may develop by different pathways.[36–38] Glioblastomas have a peak incidence between 45 and 70 years old.

Presentation and diagnosis of high-grade gliomas

The presenting features fit into the pattern described for cerebral tumours. The diagnosis is established by imaging followed by histological verification. The tumour mass of high-grade gliomas is generally inhomogeneous on CT scan, with variable enhancement after intravenous contrast and extensive peritumoural oedema.

Management of high-grade gliomas

The median survival of patients with high-grade astrocytomas is 9–12 months, therefore management of all recently diagnosed patients should include intensive psychological, physical and practical support. Corticosteroids are commonly used and are effective in reducing the symptoms of raised intracranial pressure and occasionally improve focal neurological deficit. They should be titrated to the lowest dose effective for symptom relief.

Prognosis   Age (<40, 40–60, >60 years old), performance status (Karnofsky performance status (KPS) <40%, 40–70%, >70%) and histology (anaplastic astrocytoma vs glioblastoma multiforme) have been identified in well conducted randomised studies as the most important independent prognostic factors for survival,[13,14,39] and should be considered in each individual before recommending treatment (Table 45.3). The limited usefulness and toxicity of antitumour therapy means that active treatment should be reserved for patients with reasonable life expectancy who are

Table 45.3   Prognostic factors in high-grade glioma[39]

Prognostic factor		18-month survival		
Age (years old)				
<40		64%		
40–60		20%		
>60		8%		
Histology				
Anaplastic astrocytoma		64%		
Glioblastoma		15%		
KPS	Age	<40	40–60	>60
70–100%		71%	25%	15%
40–60%		44%	15%	6%
20–30%		–	10%	0%

KPS = Karnofsky performance status.

likely to retain good quality of life. Patients with unfavourable life expectancy should be offered either symptomatic care alone, or symptomatic treatment together with hypofractionated palliative radiotherapy, depending on the wishes of the patient and their carers.

Surgery   High-grade gliomas are diffusely invasive tumours and complete surgical resection is not possible. There is considerable debate as to whether tumour debulking prolongs survival in patients with high-grade gliomas. Randomised studies addressing this question have not been conducted. Reports supporting extensive tumour resection being associated with prolonged survival are available,[40–43] but it is not clear as to whether it is undefined factors influencing tumour resectability or the tumour debulking itself which determines the outcome. However, there is general agreement that in patients with mass effect it may provide effective palliation.

Radiotherapy   Radiotherapy has an established role in the management of patients with high-grade astrocytoma. In randomised studies it was shown to prolong survival.[44,45] Normal function prior to radiotherapy is usually maintained until tumour progression and functional deficits improve in a third and stabilise in half of the treated patients.[46]

The mainstay of treatment is irradiation of the tumour, as defined by enhanced CT or MRI, with a 3–5 cm margin. The optimal total dose is 55–60 Gy, in doses of 1.7–2 Gy per fraction. A 3–5 cm margin around the tumour is required, as in pathological studies, tumour cells are frequently seen beyond the enhancing CT margin and occasionally beyond the region of suspected oedema.[47] However, at time of recurrence, the commonest site of recurrence is at or near the primary tumour site or as an extension of the pre-existing residual mass. This suggests that treatment failure is due to poor local control of the main tumour mass.

Modification of radiotherapy – unconventional fractionation
For patients with any of the following adverse factors – poor prognosis as defined by age and performance status, expected median survival of less that 6 months or severe disability – a 6-week course of radical radiotherapy is not appropriate. Shorter, palliative radiotherapy schedules have been explored in this group (30 Gy in 6 fractions, 30 Gy in 10 fractions, 45 Gy in 20 fractions).[48,49] In selected patients, the outcome following hypofractionated palliative irradiation is a median survival of 4–6 months. This is associated with an apparent neurological improvement in approximately one-third of treated patients.[48] However, palliative hypofractionated regimens have not been formally tested in a randomised setting against either supportive care alone or a conventional 6-week course of daily radiotherapy.

Chemotherapy – adjuvant chemotherapy The most active agents in high-grade gliomas are nitrosoureas; these agents readily cross the blood–brain barrier (BBB). They are given either as a single agent, carmustine (BCNU), or in combination chemotherapy with other agents that are know to cross the BBB, procarbazine, lomustine (CCNU) and vincristine (PCV regimen).[50] At present there is little evidence that combination chemotherapy is any more effective than single agents alone.

Following completion of radiotherapy, adjuvant chemotherapy is not routinely used in the management of patients with malignant glioma. Two small randomised trials, BTCG[51] and EORTC,[52] demonstrated a marginal survival benefit in favour of nitrosourea-containing chemotherapy. A meta-analysis, based on selected published trials, calculated that adjuvant chemotherapy increased survival from 43% to 53% at 12 months and from 16% to 25% at 24 months.[53] However, the largest randomised trial comparing adjuvant PCV chemotherapy to radiotherapy alone, carried out by the Medical Research Council (MRC) Brain Tumour Working Party, failed to show a survival benefit for adjuvant PCV chemotherapy (Table 45.4).[54] There is little information on the effect of adjuvant treatment on quality of life.

Management of recurrent disease Prognosis at the time of recurrence is limited and is again determined by age, performance status and histology.[33,34] Management of patients with recurrent malignant glioma must be aimed at palliation, with improvement in function and quality of life. Patients with severe disability, those with rapidly progressive disease without discernible progression-free interval and the elderly have a median life expectancy measured in weeks and issues of care are of primary importance.

Further surgery or reirradiation is rarely indicated at the time of recurrence. The most frequently employed palliative treatment is chemotherapy in the form of a nitrosourea-containing regimen. Response rates of 20–40% have been reported; however, these were based on studies performed prior to the introduction of CT scanning.[55–57] The chemoresponsiveness of recurrent tumours to other single agent cytotoxics is poor (e.g. complete and partial responses have been reported for etoposide (9%), Adriamycin (7%), carboplatin (9%) and cisplatin (7%)). A large phase II study

Table 45.4 Adjuvant treatment of glioma

Study	Regimen	Median survival (months)
Green et al[51]	XRT + methylprednisolone	9.4
	XRT + BCNU	11.5
	XRT + procarbazine	9.9
	XRT + BCNU + methylprednisolone	9.4
Hildebrand et al[52]	XRT	10.4
	XRT + dibromodulcitol + BCNU	13
MRC[54]	XRT	9.5
	XRT + PCV	10
Meta-analysis[53]	XRT	9.4
	XRT + chemotherapy	12

BCNU = carmustine (BCNU); XRT = radiotherapy; PCV = procarbazine + lomustine (CCNU) + vincristine regimen; MRC = Medical Research Council.

of favourable prognosis patients with recurrent anaplastic astrocytoma reported a response rate of 34% in those treated with an oral alkylating agent temozolomide, with a median time to progression (TTP) of 5.4 months.[58] There is no comparative response rate and TTP data for anaplastic astrocytoma treated with nitrosoureas, although it is recognised that the response rate in patients with anaplastic astrocytoma is higher than in patients with glioblastoma.[59] Currently, temozolomide is recommended as second-line chemotherapy.

Anaplastic oligodendroglioma

The anaplastic oligodendroglioma variant is uniquely chemoresponsive, with durable response rates of 75% reported.[60] The role of adjuvant chemotherapy is being considered in randomised trials. Outside clinical trials there are three alternative approaches following surgery – conventional radiotherapy alone, radiotherapy combined with chemotherapy either in neoadjuvant or adjuvant setting and chemotherapy alone. Nitrosourea-containing chemotherapy is an effective treatment at the time of recurrence.

Medulloblastoma

Medulloblastoma is part of the spectrum of primitive neuroectodermal tumours (PNETs) that include pineoblastoma, ependymoblastoma, medulloblastoma and other supratentorial PNETs. This is a rare tumour, representing only 2–6% of intracranial tumours in adults. The peak age of incidence is in childhood. Histologically, adult medulloblastoma is identical to the childhood variant and is a highly cellular, malignant invasive tumour. The tumours correspond to WHO grade IV malignancy, and the commonest site of PNET is in the posterior fossa. Due to a tendency to penetrate the ependymal surface, they are associated with a high risk of seeding through the subarachnoid space. The most frequent site for supratentorial PNETs is the pineal region (described as pineoblastoma), although the tumours can present in other locations.

Clinical presentation and diagnosis

Medulloblastomas, which arise in the posterior fossa, often present with a combination of symptoms, including raised intracranial pressure (usually due to obstruction of CSF flow through the fourth ventricle), cerebellar signs and, occasionally, brainstem cranial nerve palsies. A CT scan may demonstrate hydrocephalus and a hyperdense and homogeneously enhancing posterior fossa mass with distortion of the fourth ventricle. The differential diagnosis lies between medulloblastoma, ependymoma, glioma and solitary cerebellar metastasis. Lateral tumours may resemble meningioma. MRI improves the diagnostic accuracy and better delineates the tumour extension, particularly to the upper cervical cord. Supratentorial PNETs present with features of hemispheric tumours or pineal tumours (pineoblastoma).

Staging investigations should include an MRI of the craniospinal axis to detect occult spinal seeding, ideally performed prior to surgery and CSF cytology for the presence of malignant cells.

Treatment

Surgery   The principal prognostic factors for disease control and survival are the extent of residual disease after surgery and the presence of disseminated disease;[61] therefore, the aim of resection is to obtain complete tumour removal. This is best achieved via a posterior fossa craniectomy, avoiding disruption of the ependymal surface which would increase this risk of seeding through the subarachnoid space.

Radiotherapy   Regardless of the extent of tumour resection, postoperative radiotherapy is indicated in all patients. The whole craniospinal axis should be irradiated. The conventional whole brain dose is 35 Gy in 19–21 fractions and the whole spine dose 35 Gy in 20–25 fractions with a posterior fossa boost to a total dose of 55 Gy. Isolated spinal seeding should be treated with a radiotherapy boost to a small volume to the level of spinal cord tolerance.

Chemotherapy   Randomised trials assessing the role of adjuvant chemotherapy in adults have not been undertaken. Indications for chemotherapy in adults following radiotherapy have been extrapolated from data from randomised trials in children.[62,63] The only proven conventional regimen consists of weekly vincristine (1–1.5 mg/m^2) during radiotherapy, followed after a break of 1 month by lomustine (CCNU) (100 mg/m^2 orally) given every 6 weeks, with vincristine (1.4 mg/m^2 intravenously) on days 1, 8 and 15 of each cycle. More recent regimens containing cisplatin, vincristine and CCNU,[64] under trial in childhood medulloblastoma, have not been systematically evaluated in adults.

Prognosis   The extent of surgical excision and the presence of residual or metastatic disease are the most important prognostic factor for survival. The commonest site of recurrence is either within the posterior fossa or in other CNS sites. Up to 10% of recurrences occur outside the CNS. Recurrent tumours remain chemoresponsive, although they are rarely curable by chemotherapy. Active regimens include those used in the adjuvant setting. Isolated recurrence at the primary site can be treated by local excision and/or localised stereotactic irradiation.

Pineal tumours

Pineal tumours comprise 1% of all intracranial neoplasms; over half of these tumours are pineal germ cell tumours (germinoma and non-germinomatous germ cell tumours). Pineal parenchymal tumours (pineocytoma, pineoblastoma), glial tumours and benign cysts are less common.

Germ cell tumours are most frequent between 15 and 25 years of age, with germinomas and non-germinomatous germ cell tumours showing a male predominance. The tumour may infiltrate the ventricular space, causing seeding through the CSF.

Pineoblastomas (WHO grade IV) are malignant embryonal neoplasms, showing many histological features in common with PNET medulloblastomas. They are more frequent in childhood and may spread through the CSF.

Pineocytomas (WHO grade II) occur from childhood through to adult life; they are often well circumscribed, with varying degrees of a lobular structure.

Clinical presentation

Symptoms and signs of hydrocephalus are the commonest presenting features of pineal tumours, due to their close proximity to the third ventricle and the aqueduct. Other presenting features reflect the involvement of adjacent structures, such as the midbrain, hypothalamus and the brainstem.

Pineal germ cell tumours may secrete α-fetoprotein (AFP) and human chorionic gonadotrophin (β-hCG) into the CSF and systemic circulation. β-hCG levels may be elevated in either non-germinomas or germinomas, whereas elevated AFP is specific for non-germinomatous tumours containing yolk-sac elements.

Diagnosis and staging

Most pineal region tumours appear as enhancing masses of varying size in the pineal region, with possible hydrocephalus. It is difficult to differentiate between types of tumours on the basis of imaging.

In the absence of raised intracranial pressure, cytological examination of CSF is mandatory and is a predictor of CSF seeding. The CSF and peripheral blood should be assayed for AFP and β-HCG in patients with undiagnosed pineal tumours and those with verified germ cell tumours. In germ cell tumours and pineoblastomas, the spinal subarachnoid space should be assessed with a spinal MRI for the presence of occult metastases.

Surgery

If technically feasible, an endoscopic third ventriculostomy will provide relief of obstructive hydrocephalus, a CSF sample for analysis and may allow access for direct biopsy at the same procedure.[65,66] Alternatively, frame-based stereotactic biopsy may be used to obtain histological diagnosis.[67,68] Teratomas and pineocytomas are amenable to open surgical resection (or debulking), either by the supracerebellar infratentorial route, or via an occipital craniotomy with the patient in the sitting position.

Radiotherapy and chemotherapy

Germinoma Germinomas are radiosensitive tumours and therefore the dose of curative radiotherapy need not exceed 40 Gy to the primary site.[69,70]

The extent of irradiation and the role of chemotherapy continue to be debated. Patients treated with whole brain irradiation alone have a 10–20% risk or developing spinal metastases; this is reduced to <10% in patients treated with craniospinal radiotherapy.[71] The precise risk of spinal relapse after whole brain radiotherapy alone in patients with negative staging is likely to be less than 10%.[72]

Germinomas are responsive to cisplatin- or carboplatin-containing chemotherapy[73] but, if used alone, a high relapse rate is observed, making it an inappropriate sole treatment.[74] Chemotherapy has been employed in an attempt to modify both the radiation dose and the extent of irradiation, therefore reducing toxicity.[72,75] Although reports of primary chemotherapy followed by localised irradiation are encouraging,[72] there is no clear evidence that this approach reduces the risk of seeding.[76,77]

The current reasonable and safe treatment policy for patients with cranial germinoma is craniospinal irradiation to a dose of 24–30 Gy to whole brain and spinal cord (given in 20–25 fractions). The primary tumour site is treated with boost irradiation to a total dose of 40 Gy. In children with incomplete spinal growth and in young women where the ovaries are in the exit beam of the spinal field, spinal irradiation can be avoided, if there is a low risk of seeding. Craniospinal irradiation should always be employed in the presence of positive CSF cytology and occasionally following major surgical interference, when the risk of seeding may be higher. The treatment of verified germinoma with radiotherapy alone results in excellent cure rates, with a 5-year survival of 90–100%.

Non-germinoma The use of either radiotherapy or chemotherapy alone in the treatment of cranial teratomas is associated with a high relapse rate and a low survival.[74,78-81] Therefore, a policy of primary chemotherapy followed by craniospinal irradiation to a dose of 30 Gy and a boost to the primary site to a total dose of 50–55 Gy[81] is recommended. In patients with residual masses in the pineal region, surgical resection can be considered, providing it can be performed without major morbidity. The 5-year survival following a policy of primary chemotherapy, radiotherapy and selective surgery is 50–70%.

Pineoblastomas   Pineoblastomas, as PNETs, are treated with radiotherapy along similar lines to the treatment of medulloblastomas.

Pineocytomas   The majority of pineocytomas are localised indolent tumours, requiring surgical intervention only for enlarging or symptomatic tumours. For patients with progressive unresectable disease, local radiotherapy may improve long-term disease control and survival.[82-84]

Mixed pineocytoma/pineoblastoma   The biological behaviour of these tumours is poorly understood. Although the perception is that they are indolent localised tumours, they carry an undefined risk of CSF seeding. They are usually managed in the same way as pineoblastoma.

Primary cerebral lymphoma

Primary cerebral lymphoma accounts for 1–5% of intracranial tumours in adults and occurs in the fourth and fifth decade. It is a non-Hodgkin's lymphoma confined to the CNS and can be associated with immune deficiency following organ transplantation and in AIDS, when it presents in a younger age group. The incidence of sporadic primary cerebral lymphoma appears to be rising.[6-8]

Pathology
The predominant subtype is a diffuse, large B-cell lymphoma of intermediate and high-grade histology. T-cell tumours comprise <5% of cases. The tumours have a tendency for subependymal and leptomeningeal spread and distant seeding, particularly through the CSF. Ocular involvement, with infiltration of the vitreous and retina occurs in 40% of patients at presentation.

Clinical presentation and diagnosis
The presentation is similar to that of other primary intracranial tumours, although clinical deterioration tends to be faster, with a median duration of symptoms of 3 months. In 5–10% of patients, a history of uveitis may precede other neurological symptoms. CT findings are of single or multiple periventricular, iso- or hyperdense masses, often with uniform enhancement and frequent evidence of subependymal spread. The MRI features are equivalent and may mimic the radiological appearance of multiple sclerosis.

Staging investigations should include CSF cytology and ophthalmological examination. In HIV-negative patients the likelihood of lymphoma outside the CNS is small, and a CT scan of chest and abdomen or bone marrow examination is only indicated in the presence of systemic symptoms.

Surgery
Biopsy should be performed in suspected cases for diagnostic purposes; there is no role for extensive debulking. A rapid response to corticosteroids is often observed and this may cause diagnostic difficulties, as previously radiologically identifiable lesions may disappear. A short withdrawal of steroids may be required to allow reappearance of the lesions and image-directed biopsy for diagnosis.

Radiotherapy
Radiation produces both radiological and clinical responses. It prolongs survival and usually produces functional improvement or stabilisation of neurological deficit. There are no prospective studies evaluating radiation dose; however, retrospective data suggest need for doses >50 Gy. The widely accepted current practice is whole-brain irradiation to a dose of 40 Gy, followed by a boost to 15–20 Gy to the primary tumour site (with a margin) using 1.6–1.8 Gy per fraction. Spinal irradiation is recommended in patients with positive CSF cytology. Radiotherapy alone results in a median survival of 10–18 months.[71,85] Age and performance status are the primary determinants of prognosis.[85] Five-year survival in patients aged <60 years old with KPS >60 is 50–60%, although this may not be durable.

Chemotherapy
Primary cerebral lymphoma is responsive to chemotherapy, including high-dose methotrexate and conventional lymphoma regimens such as CHOP (cyclophosphamide, doxorubicin, vincristine, prednisone) or MACOP-B (methotrexate, doxorubicin, cyclophosphamide, vincristine, prednisone, bleomycin) and others. The addition of CHOP chemotherapy

either before[86] or after radiotherapy[87] is not associated with survival benefit compared to radiotherapy alone. The failure of conventional chemotherapy is considered to be due to poor penetration of drugs across an intact BBB. An approach adopted to overcome this problem has included administration of agents which cross the BBB, such as high-dose methotrexate.[88,89] Both prospective and retrospective studies suggest that the addition of high-dose methotrexate to chemotherapy regimens is associated with improvement in outcome, both in terms of median survival ($\geq$24 months) and long-term survival (52% vs 26% at 2 years).[90,91] However, in the absence of randomised studies, it is not clear to what extent the favourable results of combined treatment approaches are due to patient selection. The combination of chemotherapy and radiotherapy is associated with considerable delayed morbidity, particularly in the form of dementia and the risk of long-term sequelae increases with age.

Patients under 60 years of age with good performance status should be offered primary chemotherapy followed by radiotherapy. A number of chemotherapy regimens, including high-dose methotrexate, have been tested with similar outcome.[89,92,93] Trials currently underway investigate the potential for treatment with reduced dose of radiotherapy and potential for avoiding irradiation. This represents experimental therapy, and the long-term efficacy of this approach is not known.

Patients aged >60 years old, particularly those with marked disability, have poor outcome following intensive treatment and the options lie between palliative radiotherapy alone or primary chemotherapy alone.

Meningioma

Meningiomas are tumours arising in the meninges; they represent 13–26% of primary intracranial tumours, occurring more commonly in middle-aged and elderly patients, and show a marked female predominance. The majority of meningiomas occur within the intracranial, orbital and intravertebral cavities. Patients with neurofibromatosis type 2 (NF2) and members of some other non-NF2 familial syndromes may develop multiple meningiomas, often early in life.[94]

Histologically, meningiomas may be divided into subtypes, WHO grades I–III.[95] The majority of meningioma subtypes are graded as WHO grade I. Others, such as the choroid and clear cell types,[96,97] are associated with more frequent recurrence and are classified as WHO grade II. Tumours showing a papillary

Table 45.5 Meningothelial tumours

Tumours of meningothelial cells	WHO grade
Meningioma	I
Clear cell	II
Chordoid	II
Atypical	II
Papillary	III
Rhabdoid	III
Anaplastic meningioma	III

growth pattern or containing areas of rhabdoid cells are classified as papillary and rhabdoid meningiomas, respectively. They have been documented to behave in a very aggressive fashion and are classified as WHO grade III.[95] Tumours with frankly malignant cytology are classified as anaplastic (malignant) meningiomas, grade III (Table 45.5).[98] Atypical meningiomas constitute less than 7% of meningiomas, whereas anaplastic variants are even more unusual. Both atypical and anaplastic meningiomas are more common in men.[98–101]

Clinical presentation
Presenting symptoms will vary according to the site of the meningioma. Meningiomas occurring in the supratentorial compartment are relatively asymptomatic until a late stage and may be quite large at presentation, whereas those occurring at a more critical site tend to present earlier.

Both MRI and CT should be used to image meningiomas. MRI can better delineate the tumours, particularly in the temporal and the posterior fossae; however, bone changes with bone invasion or hyperostosis are best seen on CT.

Treatment
Symptomatic benign meningiomas should be treated by complete excision alone, providing it can be achieved with minimal morbidity. Local control rates following complete surgical excision are 70–95%. Postoperative radiotherapy is recommended in patients with incompletely excised tumours at time of progression or at time of recurrence. Retrospective studies comparing partial excision alone with partial excision and radiotherapy demonstrated that adjuvant radiotherapy halved the recurrence rate to 10–20%.[101,102] WHO grades II and III meningiomas should be completely excised where possible and adjuvant postoperative radiotherapy is recommended in all. Despite aggressive treatment with surgery

and radiotherapy, anaplastic meningiomas have a poor prognosis, with a median survival of 1–3 years.[103]

Craniopharyngioma

Craniopharyngiomas are benign neoplasms occurring in the suprasellar or, less frequently, the sella region and account for 2–9% of intracranial tumours. They arise from epithelial rests associated with Rathke's pouch. Approximately half of them occur in childhood, with a second, smaller peak of incidence at 50–60 years old.

Clinical presentation and investigations

Presenting clinical features include endocrine, visual and mental disturbances, as well as features of raised intracranial pressure. In children, growth retardation, due to growth hormone deficiency, is the most frequent endocrine presentation. Pituitary involvement in adults frequently leads to hypopituitarism. Up to 75–85% of patients will have evidence of compression of the optic chiasm, optic nerve or optic tract at presentation.[104,105] Raised intracranial pressure is usually due to hydrocephalus caused by the obstruction of CSF flow at the foramen of Monro.

CT or MRI scans are frequently diagnostic and show a partly cystic and partly solid suprasellar mass; calcification in the cyst wall is only visible on CT. There may be a considerable variation in size at presentation.

The natural history of craniopharyngioma varies from a benign to a rapidly progressive and destructive tumour, causing damage to the surrounding structures.

Treatment

The low morbidity and good long-term results of limited surgery followed by radiotherapy favour this approach in the majority of patients. Ten-year survival following such a policy is between 70 and 90% and late effects are minimal. Total excision is best reserved for young children, where radiotherapy may result in unacceptable late damage, and for patients with recurrent tumours following radiotherapy. Radical surgery carries a significant mortality related to tumour size and long-term morbidity and is also dependent on tumour size and relationship to the hypothalamus.[106] The reported recurrence rate following apparent complete tumour removal varies from 20 to 30% of surviving patients.[107–110] Instillation of radioactive colloidal chromic phosphate [P32] into cystic craniopharyngiomas should be reserved for patients with recurrent cystic craniopharyngiomas that have not been controlled with conventional radiotherapy.

Surgery   In the presence of hydrocephalus, urgent surgical intervention by CSF diversion or direct tumour decompression is required. This may be achieved with stereotactic cyst aspiration, or more radical tumour removal can be carried out through a transcranial route. The tumour is often firmly adherent to surrounding neural structures, particularly the hypothalamus, and radical attempts at removal lead to hypothalamic damage and consequent postoperative morbidity.[106,110–113] Partial excision to relieve the effect of the tumour mass followed by adjuvant radiotherapy avoids surgical morbidity and does not compromise tumour control rate or survival. Review of reported cases in the literature suggests a recurrence rate of 17% with a 5-year survival of 80–100% and a 10-year survival of 70–90%[114] with limited morbidity.

Panhypopituitarism due to the combination of tumour-induced damage, surgery and radiation is frequent and patients must have regular endocrine assessment.[115,116]

Pituitary adenoma

Pituitary adenomas are benign, slowly growing tumours arising from the cells of the anterior pituitary. The primary treatment is surgical, either via a transsphenoidal approach[117,118] or, occasionally, via a craniotomy. The aim of surgery is complete removal of tumour and decompression of the optic chiasm. Following surgery alone, tumour control rate ranges from 60 to 90% and is related to the extent of tumour resection.[119–121] Radiotherapy is recommended as primary treatment in patients not suitable for surgery, or patients with acromegaly, Cushing's disease and Nelson's syndrome (and other secreting adenomas) where endocrine control is not obtained by surgery.

Debate continues about the timing of radiotherapy in patients with residual non-functioning adenoma following surgery. Immediate postoperative radiotherapy is associated with a low risk of subsequent recurrence; however, the indolent natural history means that some patients may avoid the need for irradiation. A policy of observation requires close surveillance with regular ophthalmological assessment, and scans and may require second surgical intervention. There is no role for chemotherapy in pituitary adenomas.

Medical treatment

Dopamine agonists (bromocriptine or cabergoline) are the mainstay of treatment of prolactinoma. They may also reduce growth hormone secretion in acromegaly. Somatostatin analogues are used in the treatment of acromegaly and may have an additional growth inhibitory effect.

NURSING CARE FOR PATIENTS RECEIVING CHEMOTHERAPY FOR CENTRAL NERVOUS SYSTEM TUMOURS

Douglas Guerrero

INTRODUCTION

Primary CNS tumours represent a major challenge to all healthcare professionals. For doctors, the challenges are mainly those of providing the most appropriate therapy, which prolongs the patient's survival and minimises the unpleasant side effects of treatment. For nurses, the challenges are often those of support and care. Support and care when expertly delivered is complex and demanding, which only experienced nurses with knowledge and expertise within a given speciality can truly provide. As such, the role of nurses in the care of this group of patients is not to be underestimated.

TUMOURS

Primary CNS tumours range from relatively chemosensitive tumours such as primary CNS lymphomas to highly chemoresistant tumours such as the high-grade gliomas. Currently for most patients with primary CNS tumours, chemotherapy is not the first medical treatment option. This is because many CNS tumours, in particular high-grade gliomas (the most common primary CNS tumour), are not curable and chemotherapy treatment can only provide palliation and limited prolongation of survival. It is therefore important that any benefit that the chemotherapy can provide in respect of prolongation of survival is not outweighed by treatment toxicity to the patient. Therefore, often, when caring for this group of patients, the emphasis is on care and support and the maintenance of the individual's quality of life.[122]

As an expert practitioner, the nurse has a responsibility in understanding the benefits as well as the side effects of the chemotherapy regimen that has been proposed to the patient. The nurse needs to be familiar with issues such as drug action, the effect of the chemotherapy (not just on the tumour but also on normal tissue), the different types of chemotherapy agents available as well as the expected outcome to the patient in respect of quality of life.[123] All these factors are important in order to provide patients with realistic information and plan the best care and support possible. Such nursing expertise and knowledge will ensure that patients are at all times given realistic hope and education, allowing them to understand how best to manage their illness. (See also Ch. 7.)

CHEMOTHERAPY – LIMITATIONS AND DELIVERY

In the case of CNS tumours, chemotherapy often consists of a combination of cytotoxic drugs. Combination chemotherapy is important, as this ensure that a cocktail of medication is delivered to the tumour, causing interference at different stages of the cell cycle.

The brain is well protected by the BBB, which can preclude relevant penetration of the cytotoxic drugs to the tumour. The BBB is formed by tight junctions between endothelial cells and ensures a constant chemical environment in the brain as well as preventing harmful exogenous substances from entering the CNS. Of relevance is that many cancer drugs are hydrophilic (water soluble), whereas the cell membrane is composed of fatty substances.[123] Chemotherapeutic agents need to be lipophilic (fat soluble), so as to be able to penetrate the BBB effectively.

In cancer therapy, the route of drug administration is dependent on many factors, such as the stability, size, molecular charge and sclerosant characteristic (hardening effects) of the drug.[124] Although the oral route (in some cancers) is often used infrequently because of the fear of poor patient compliance and uncertain absorption, it is nevertheless often used in neuro-oncology, particularly in the treatment of patients with high-grade glioma as the emphasis for this group of patients is on care and support.[122] This reduces the necessity for hospital admission.

For other tumours such as primary CNS lymphomas, germinomas and primitive neuroectodermal tumours, which generally carry a more favourable prognosis, cytotoxic treatment entails regular planned admissions to hospital for intravenous drug administration as well as more complex pretreatment investigations.

INVESTIGATIONS

All patients undergoing chemotherapy will require full blood count and chemistry prior to each treatment. The patient's height and weight also need to be measured so as to determine the body surface area for drug dosage calculation. In neuro-oncology, patients should be weighed prior to each chemotherapy cycle. This is important, particularly for those patients on steroids who may have body weight changes that may necessitate drug dosage alteration.[123]

Some chemotherapy may require more specific investigations. For example, patients requiring platinum-based chemotherapy will require an EDTA (ethylene diamene tetra-acetic acid) test, undertaken prior to commencement of treatment, to assess their renal function. Baseline imaging, i.e. CT or MRI, is generally undertaken prior to treatment. This often acts as a baseline for future assessment of the radiological response of the tumour to treatment.[125]

PROVISION OF INFORMATION

It is important that all patients are provided with clear information in respect of any proposed chemotherapy treatment. This information should not just be given verbally but, whenever possible, supplemented with specific written material.

Some patients with CNS tumours may have (depending on tumour location) specific cognitive problems. Thus, it is advisable that, whenever possible, their partner or an appropriate member of the family/friend is available when treatment options are being discussed. Patients must not feel that they should consent to undertake treatment on their first visit. The nurse, therefore, has an important role as the patient's adviser, often clarifying issues of concern and at times explaining medical jargon. The provision of a telephone contact number for the patient often helps to reassure them and allow them to further discuss any issues that may be worrying them.[122] (See also Ch. 5.)

Where clinical trials are considered, the benefits as well as any expected risk should be made clear to the patient. Patients should also be told that their refusal to enter a trial would not jeopardise any future treatment. This may appear to be trivial, but some patients worry that by refusing to enter a trial they may be receiving suboptimal medical treatment and care. (See also Ch. 9.)

Fertility issues should always be discussed with the patient.[123] At times, professionals may not rank fertility issues high on their list of concern; this is generally true when dealing with patients with high-grade glioma, who generally have a poor prognosis. However, many patients are young, wanting to have more children or to start a family, and some may get distraught when told that certain cytotoxic drugs may be gonadotoxic in nature. (See also Ch. 32.)

EXPERT NURSING CARE

The concept of expert nursing practice can at times be difficult to explain in ways that may not be trivialised as simple by others. Often, what are considered to be simple nursing actions are in reality expert nursing practice, a result of educational knowledge and personal experience within a specialty. Expert nursing

practice is what provides a significant difference to the individual patient's experience of the illness and is as a result of that special relationship between the nurse and the patient.[126] An analogy would be that the experienced nurse specialist can see the whole elephant. A novice nurse needs to work her way up the elephant's trunk before realising what she is seeing. Therefore, by seeing the whole picture, the expert nurse can zoom in directly on the specific needs of that individual patient.

Expert nursing practice is paramount, as being a patient is often a frightening experience. Individuals often feel vulnerable and at times may not fully comprehend the enormity of the situation.[127] It is therefore imperative that the expert practitioner not only provides education, support and care to the patient and the family but also, very importantly, ensures that all professionals understand the complexities of care brought on by the tumour and its treatment. In the context of CNS tumours, particularly for those patients with high-grade gliomas, expert nursing care may at times usurp medical treatment as the best available option in the maintenance of the patient's quality of life.

SIDE EFFECTS OF CHEMOTHERAPY

Side effects of chemotherapy can be numerous. The nurse needs to ensure that patients and families, as well as community colleagues, are aware of any potential treatment-related problems. Contact telephone numbers should be provided and patients often need reassurance that what they may be experiencing may be attributed to the chemotherapy and not the tumour. For example, most patients undergoing chemotherapy feel fatigued and exhausted. Telling the patient that fatigue during chemotherapy is to be expected and experienced by most people is reassuring them that this is normal and that nothing sinister is occurring.

Gastrointestinal

Nausea and vomiting is the most common side effect of chemotherapy. Appropriate antiemetics should be provided. Some patients with CNS tumours may have swallowing problems, and there is often a concern in respect of fluid aspiration. Referral to the dietician may ensure that the patient maintains an adequate dietary intake. At times, non-pharmacological interventions may be appropriate.

Some chemotherapy agents can give rise to constipation. Referral to the dietician and advice on diet and fluids as well as the use of appropriate laxatives is important. (See also Ch. 17.)

Oral hygiene is paramount. Chemotherapy may give rise to mucositis and those patients on steroids are also more prone to oral candidiasis.[128] The nurse should regularly examine the patient's oral cavity and the use of appropriate oral care agents may help minimise superimposed infection. Mucositis can be very painful, as well as exacerbate anorexia. (See also Chs 18 and 19.)

Haematological

Because of the risk of bone marrow suppression, appropriate nadir count, dependent on the chemotherapeutic agent, needs to be undertaken. Bone marrow suppression can often delay chemotherapy courses. Professionals may not appreciate the psychological impact that this may have on the patient. To some patients, delay in treatment or reduction of the drug dosage indicates an opportunity for the tumour to continue growing. The nurse must comprehend such fears and explain to patients the rationale behind such medical actions. (See also Chs 20–22.)

Hair loss

Most patients with CNS tumours would have already undergone radiotherapy treatment prior to chemotherapy. As such, they would have already experienced a certain degree of hair loss.[123] Unlike radiotherapy, in the case of chemotherapy treatment,

the patient can be reassured that the hair will grow back again. Treatment-induced alopecia can be very distressing and patients should be referred for psychological care if and when required. (See also Ch. 23.)

Neurotoxicity

Most patients with CNS tumours will already have some degree of neurological deficits. As such, added neurotoxicity as a consequence of cytotoxic chemotherapy can be devastating and may further affect the patient's quality of life. This should be recognised and appropriate support and counselling provided when and as required. (See also Ch. 27.)

CONCLUSION

Of all professionals, nurses provide the most intense and continuous contribution to patients with CNS tumours and their families. The nurse's involvement in care is not limited and sporadic but continuous, from histological diagnosis throughout the illness trajectory and well into family support during bereavement. This is particularly the case when caring for the patient with high-grade glioma, for whom care issues are paramount and for whom chemotherapy treatment is generally palliative in nature.

References

1. Barker D, Weller R, Garfield J. Epidemiology of primary tumours of the brain and spinal cord: a regional survey in southern England. J Neurol Neurosurg Psychiatry 1976; 39:290–296.

2. Fogelholm R, Uutela T, Murros K. Epidemiology of central nervous system neoplasms. A regional survey in Central Finland. Acta Neurol Scand 1984; 69(3):129–136.

3. Velema JP, Walker AM. The age curve of nervous system tumour incidence in adults: common shape but changing levels by sex, race and geographical location, Int J Epidemiol 1987; 16(2):177–183.

4. Helseth A, Langmark F, Mork SJ. Neoplasms of the central nervous system in Norway. II. Descriptive epidemiology of intracranial neoplasms 1955–1984. APMIS 1988; 96(12):1066–1074.

5. Bohnen NI, Kurland LT. Epidemiology of brain tumors. In: Vecht CJ, ed. Neuro-oncology; Part I. Brain tumors: principles of biology, diagnosis and therapy. Series 23 edn. Amsterdam: Elsevier, 1997:139–166. (Vinken PJ, Bruyn GW, eds, Handbook of clinical neurology, Vol Neuro-oncology, Part I.)

6. Eby M, Grufferman S, Flannelly CM. Increasing incidence of primary brain lymphoma in the US. Cancer 1988; 62:2461–2462.

7. Lutz JM, Coleman MP. Trends in primary cerebral lymphoma, Br J Cancer 1994; 70:716–718.

8. Cote TR, Manns A, Hardy CR, et al. Epidemiology of brain lymphoma among people with or without acquired immunodeficiency syndrome. AIDS/Cancer Study Group, J Natl Cancer Inst 1996; 88(10):675–679.

9. Kleihues P, Cavenee WK, eds. World Health Organization classification of tumours: Vol. 1, Pathology and genetics of tumours of the nervous system. Lyon: IARC Press; 2000.

10. McCormack BM, Miller DC, Budzilovich GN, et al. Treatment and survival of low-grade astrocytoma in adults – 1977–1988. Neurosurgery 1992; 31(4):636–642; discussion 642.

11. Lote K, Egeland T, Hager B, et al. Survival, prognostic factors, and therapeutic efficacy in low-grade glioma: a retrospective study in 379 patients, J Clin Oncol 1997; 15(9):3129–3140.

12. Winger MJ, Macdonald DR, Cairncross JG. Supratentorial anaplastic gliomas in adults. The prognostic importance of extent of resection and prior low-grade glioma. J Neurosurg 1989; 71(4):487–493.

13. Curran WJ, Scott CB, Horton J, et al. Recursive partitioning analysis of prognostic factors in three Radiation Therapy Oncology Group Malignant Glioma Trials. J Natl Cancer Inst 1993; 85:704–710.

14. Scott CB, Scarantino C, Urtasun R, et al. Validation and predictive power of Radiation Therapy Oncology

Group (RTOG) recursive partitioning analysis classes for malignant glioma patients: a report using RTOG 90-06. Int J Radiat Oncol Biol Phys 1998; 40(1):51–55.

15. Simpson JR, Horton J, Scott C, et al. Influence of location and extent of surgical resection on survival of patients with glioblastoma multiforme: results of three consecutive Radiation Therapy Oncology Group (RTOG) clinical trials. Int J Radiat Oncol Biol Phys 1993; 26(2):239–244.

16. Dirven CMF, Mooij JJA, Molenaar WM. Cerebellar pilocytic astrocytoma: a treatment protocol based upon analysis of 73 cases and a review of the literature. Child's Nerv Syst 1997; 13(1):17–23.

17. Thomas DGT, Nouby RM. Experience in 300 cases of CT directed stereotactic surgery for lesion biopsy and aspiration of haematoma. Br J Neurosurg 1989; 3:321–326.

18. Ernestus RI, Wilcke O, Schroder R. Supratentorial ependymomas in childhood: clinicopathological findings and prognosis, Acta Neurochir Wien 1991; 111(3-4):96–102.

19. Rousseau P, Habrand JL, Sarrazin D, et al. Treatment of intracranial ependymomas of children: review of a 15-year experience. Int J Radiat Oncol Biol Phys 1994; 28(2):381–386.

20. Sutton L, Goldwein J, Perilongo G. Prognostic factors in childhood ependymomas. Paediatr Neurosurg 1991;16:57–65.

21. Vanuytsel LJ, Bessell EM, Ashley SE, et al. Intracranial ependymoma: long term results of a policy of surgery and radiotherapy. Int J Radiat Oncol Biol Phys 1992; 23(2):313–319.

22. Robertson PL, Zeltzer PM, Boyett JM, et al. Survival and prognostic factors following radiation therapy and chemotherapy for ependymomas in children: a report of the Children's Cancer Group, J Neurosurg 1998; 88(4):695–703.

23. Schild SE, Nisi K, Scheithauer BW, et al. The results of radiotherapy for ependymomas: the Mayo Clinic experience. Int J Radiat Oncol Biol Phys 1998; 42(5):953–958.

24. Perilongo G, Massimino M, Sotti G, et al. Analyses of prognostic factors in a retrospective review of 92 children with ependymoma: Italian Pediatric Neuro-oncology Group. Med Pediatr Oncol 1997; 29(2):79–85.

25. Fazekas JT. Treatment of grades I and II brain astrocytomas. The role of radiotherapy. Int J Radiat Oncol Biol Phys 1977; 2(7–8):661–666.

26. Shaw EG, Daumas Duport C, Scheithauer BW, et al. Radiation therapy in the management of low grade supratentorial astrocytomas. J Neurosurg 1989; 70(6):853–861.

27. Shaw EG, Scheithauer BW, Gilbertson DT, et al. Postoperative radiotherapy of supratentorial low-grade gliomas. Int J Radiat Oncol Biol Phys 1989; 16(3):663–668.

28. Karim ABMF, Cornu P, Bleehen N, et al. Immediate postoperative radiotherapy in low grade glioma improves progression free survival, but not overall survival: preliminary results of EORTC/MRC randomized phase III study (Proc ASCO 34) J Clin Oncol 1998; 17:400a.

29. Karim AB, Maat B, Hatlevoll R, et al. A randomized trial on dose-response in radiation therapy of low-grade cerebral glioma: European Organization for Research and Treatment of Cancer (EORTC) Study 22844. Int J Radiat Oncol Biol Phys 1996; 36(3):549–556.

30. Leighton C, Fisher B, Bauman G, et al. Supratentorial low-grade glioma in adults: an analysis of prognostic factors and timing of radiation [see comments]. J Clin Oncol 1997; 15(4):1294–1301.

31. Scerrati M, Roselli R, Iacoangeli M, et al. Prognostic factors in low grade (WHO grade II) gliomas of the cerebral hemispheres: the role of surgery. J Neurol Neurosurg Psychiatry 1996; 61(3):291–296.

32. Horn B, Heideman R, Geyer R, et al. A multi-institutional retrospective study of intracranial ependymoma in children: identification of risk factors. J Pediatr Hematol Oncol 1999; 21(3):203–211.

33. Wong E, Hess K, Gleason M, et al. Outcomes and prognostic factors in recurrent glioma patients enrolled onto phase II clinical trials. J Clin Oncol 1999; 17:2572–2578.

34. Rajan B, Ross G, Lim CC, et al. Survival in patients with recurrent glioma as a measure of treatment efficacy: prognostic factors following nitrosourea chemotherapy. Eur J Cancer 1994; 12(15):1809–1815.

35. Dropcho EJ, Soong SJ. The prognostic impact of prior low grade histology in patients with anaplastic gliomas: a case–control study. Neurology 1996; 47:684–690.

36. James CD, Carlbom E, Dumanski JP, et al. Clonal genomic alterations in glioma malignancy stages. Cancer Res 1988; 48(19):5546–5551.

37. von Deimling A, von Ammon K, Schoenfeld D, et al. Subsets of glioblastoma multiforme defined by molecular genetic analysis. Brain Pathol 1993; 3(1):19–26.

38. Ichimura K, Bondesson-Bolin M, Goike HM, et al. Deregulation of the p14ARF/MDM2/p53 pathway is a prerequisite for human astrocytic gliomas with G1/S transition control abnormalities. Cancer Res 2000; 60(2):417–424.

39. Chang CH, Horton J, Schoenfeld D, et al. Comparison of postoperative radiotherapy and combined postoperative radiotherapy and chemotherapy in the multidisciplinary management of malignant gliomas. A joint Radiation Therapy Oncology Group and Eastern Cooperative Oncology Group study. Cancer 1983; 52(6):997–1007.

40. Ammirati M, Vick N, Liao YL, et al. Effect of the extent of surgical resection on survival and quality of life in patients with supratentorial glioblastomas and anaplastic astrocytomas. Neurosurgery 1987; 21(2):201–206.

41. Berger MS, Deliganis AV, Dobbins J, et al. The effect of extent of resection on recurrence in patients with low grade cerebral hemisphere gliomas [see comments]. Cancer 1994; 74(6):1784–1791.

42. Nazzaro JM, Neuwelt EA. The role of surgery in the management of supratentorial intermediate and high-grade astrocytomas in adults [see comments]. J Neurosurg 1990; 73(3):331–344.

43. Quigley MR, Maroon JC. The relationship between survival and the extent of the resection in patients with supratentorial malignant gliomas. Neurosurgery 1991; 29(3):385–389.

44. Walker MD, Alexander E Jr, Hunt WE, et al. Evaluation of BCNU and/or radiotherapy in the treatment of anaplastic gliomas. A cooperative clinical trial. J Neurosurg 1978; 49(3):333–343.

45. Kristiansen K, Hagen S, Kollevold T, et al. Combined modality therapy of operated astrocytomas grade III and IV. Confirmation of the value of postoperative irradiation and lack of potentiation of bleomycin on survival time: a prospective multicenter trial of the Scandinavian Glioblastoma Study Group. Cancer 1981; 47(4):649–652.

46. Nelson DF, Diener West M, Weinstein AS, et al. A randomised comparison of misonidazole sensitised radiotherapy plus BCNU and radiotherapy plus BCNU for treatment of malignant glioma after surgery: final report of an RTOG Study. Int J Radiat Oncol Biol Phys 1986; 12(10):1793–1800.

47. Burger PC, Heinz ER, Shibata T, et al. Topographic anatomy and CT correlations in the untreated glioblastoma multiforme. J Neurosurg 1988; 68(5):698–704.

48. Thomas R, James N, Guerrero D, et al. Hypofractionated radiotherapy as palliative treatment in poor prognosis patients with high grade glioma. Radiother Oncol 1994; 33(2):113–116.

49. Bauman GS, Gaspar LE, Fisher BJ, et al. A prospective study of short course radiotherapy in poor prognosis glioblastoma multiforme. Int J Radiat Oncol Biol Phys 1994; 29:835–839.

50. Forsyth PA, Cairncross JG. Chemotherapy for malignant gliomas. Baillière's Clin Neurol 1996; 5(2):371–393.

51. Green SB, Byar DP, Walker MD, et al. Comparisons of carmustine, procarbazine, and high dose methylprednisolone as additions to surgery and radiotherapy of the treatment of malignant glioma. Cancer Treat Rep 1983; 67(2):121–132.

52. Hildebrand J, Sahmoud T, Mignolet F, et al. Adjuvant therapy with dibromodulcitol and BCNU increases survival of adults with malignant gliomas: EORTC brain tumour group. Neurology 1994; 44:1479–1483.

53. Fine HA, Dear KB, Loeffler JS, et al. Meta analysis of radiation therapy with and without adjuvant chemotherapy for malignant gliomas in adults. Cancer 1993; 71:2585–2597.

54. Brada M, Thomas D, Bleehan N, et al. Medical Research Council (MRC) randomised trial of adjuvant chemotherapy in high grade glioma (HGG) BR05. J Clin Oncol (Proc ASCO) 1998; 17:400a.

55. Levin VA, Crafts DC, Wilson CB, et al. BCNU (NSC-409962) and procarbazine (NSC-77213) treatment for malignant brain tumors. Cancer Treat Rep 1976; 60(3):243–249.

56. Levin VA, Wilson CB, Crafts DC, et al. Nitrosourea chemotherapy for primary malignant gliomas. Cancer Treat Rep 1976; 60(6):719–724.

57. Wilson CB, Gutin P, Boldrey EB, et al. Single-agent chemotherapy of brain tumors. A five-year review. Arch Neurol 1976; 33(11):739–744.

58. Yung W, Prados M, Yaya-Tur R, et al. Multicenter phase II trial of temozolomide in patients with anaplastic astrocytoma or anaplastic oligoastrocytoma at first relapse. J Clin Oncol 1999; 17:2762.

59. Hildebrand J, De Witte O, Sahmoud T. Response of recurrent glioblastoma and anaplastic astrocytoma to dibromodulcitol, BCNU and procarbazine – a phase-II study. J Neurooncol 1998; 37(2):155–160.

60. Cairncross G, Macdonald D, Ludwin S, et al. Chemotherapy for anaplastic oligodendroglioma. National Cancer Institute of Canada Clinical Trials Group. J Clin Oncol 1994; 12(10):2013–2021.

61. Zeltzer PM, Boyett JM, Finlay JL, et al. Metastasis stage, adjuvant treatment, and residual tumor are prognostic factors for medulloblastoma in children: conclusions from the Children's Cancer Group 921 randomized phase III study. J Clin Oncol 1999; 17(3):832–845.

62. Evans A, Jenkin D, Sposto R, et al. Results of a prospective randomised trial of radiation therapy with and without CCNU, vincristine and prednisone. J Neurosurg 1990; 72:572–582.

63. Tait DM, Thornton Jones H, Bloom HJ, et al. Adjuvant chemotherapy for medulloblastoma: the first multi-centre control trial of the International Society of Paediatric Oncology (SIOP I). Eur J Cancer 1990; 26(4):464–469.

64. Packer R, Goldwein, Nicholson J, et al. Treatment of children with medulloblastomas with reduced-dose craniospinal radiation therapy and adjuvant chemotherapy: a children's cancer group study. J Clin Oncol 1999; 17:2127.

65. Ferrer E, Santamarta D, Garcia Fructuoso G, et al. Neuroendoscopic management of pineal region tumours. Acta Neurochir Wien 1997; 139(1):12–20.

66. Gaab MR, Schroeder HW. Neuroendoscopic approach to intraventricular lesions. J Neurosurg 1998; 88(3):496–505.

67. Apuzzo ML, Chandrasoma PT, Cohen D, et al. Computed imaging stereotaxy: experience and perspective related to 500 procedures applied to brain masses. Neurosurgery 1987; 20(6):930–937.

68. Wild AM, Xuereb JH, Marks PV, et al. Computerized tomographic stereotaxy in the management of 200 consecutive intracranial mass lesions. Analysis of indications, benefits and outcome. Br J Neurosurg 1990; 4(5):407–415.

69. Shibamoto Y, Takahashi M, Abe M. Reduction of the radiation dose for intracranial germinoma: a prospective study. Br J Cancer 1994; 70:984–989.

70. Hardenbergh PH, Golden J, Billet A, et al. Intracranial germinoma: the case for lower dose radiation therapy. Int J Radiat Oncol Biol Phys 1997; 39(2):419–426.

71. Brada M, Rajan B. Spinal seeding in cranial germinoma [letter]. Br J Cancer 1990; 61(2):339–340.

72. Bouffet E, Baranzelli MC, Patte C, et al. Combined treatment modality for intracranial germinomas: results of a multicentre SFOP experience. Societe Francaise d'Oncologie Pediatrique. Br J Cancer 1999; 79(7–8):1199–1204.

73. Allen JC, DaRossa RC, Donahue B, et al. A phase II trial of preirradiation carboplatin in newly diagnosed germinoma of the central nervous system. Cancer 1994; 74(3):940–944.

74. Balmaceda C, Heller G, Rosenblum M, et al. Chemotherapy without irradiation. A novel approach for newly diagnosed CNS germ cell tumors: results of an international cooperative trial. J Clin Oncol 1996; 14(11):2908–2915.

75. Buckner JC, Peethambaram PP, Smithson WA, et al. Phase II trial of primary chemotherapy followed by reduced-dose radiation for CNS germ cell tumors. J Clin Oncol 1999; 17(3):933–940.

76. Aoyama H, Shirato H, Kakuto Y, et al. Pathologically-proven intracranial germinoma treated with radiation therapy [published erratum appears in Radiother Oncol 1999; 50(2):241] Radiother Oncol 1998; 47(2):201–205.

77. Haddock MG, Schild SE, Scheithauer BW, et al. Radiation therapy for histologically confirmed primary central nervous system germinoma. Int J Radiat Oncol Biol Phys 1997; 38(5):915–923.

78. Dearnaley DP, A'Hern RP, Whittaker S, et al. Pineal and CNS germ cell tumours: Royal Marsden Hospital experience 1962–1987. Int J Radiat Oncol Biol Phys 1990; 18:773–781.

79. Schild SE, Scheithauer BW, Haddock MG, et al. Histologically confirmed pineal tumors and other germ cell tumors of the brain. Cancer 1996; 78(12):2564–2571.

80. Sawamura Y, Ikeda J, Shirato H, et al. Germ cell tumours of the central nervous system: treatment consideration based on 111 cases and their long-term clinical outcomes. Eur J Cancer 1998; 34(1):104–110.

81. Baranzelli MC, Patte C, Bouffet E, et al. An attempt to treat pediatric intracranial alphaFP and betaHCG secreting germ cell tumors with chemotherapy alone. SFOP experience with 18 cases. Societe Francaise d'Oncologie Pediatrique. J Neurooncol 1998; 37(3):229–239.

82. Discalfani A, Hudgins RJ, Edwards MSB. Pineocytomas. Cancer 1989; 63:302–304.

83. Schild SE, Scheithauer BW, Schomberg PJ, et al. Pineal parenchymal tumors: clinical, pathologic, and therapeutic aspects. Cancer 1993; 72(3):870–880.

84. Kurisaka M, Arisawa M, Mori T, et al. Combination chemotherapy (cisplatin, vinblastin) and low-dose irradiation in the treatment of pineal parenchymal cell tumors. Childs Nerv Syst 1998; 14(10):564–569.

85. Nelson DF, Martz KL, Bonner H, et al. Non Hodgkin's lymphoma of the brain: can high dose, large volume radiation therapy improve survival? Report on a prospective trial by the Radiation Therapy Oncology Group (RTOG): RTOG 8315. Int J Radiat Oncol Biol Phys 1992; 23:9–17.

86. O'Neill BP, O'Fallon JR, Earle JD, et al. Primary central nervous system non Hodgkin's lymphoma: survival advantages with combined initial therapy? Int J Radiat Oncol Biol Phys 1995; 33:663–673.

87. Mead G, Bleehen N, Gregor A, et al. Medical Research Council (MRC) randomized trial of adjuvant chemotherapy in primary CNS lymphoma (PCL)-BR06. ASCO. Los Angeles: American Society of Clinical Oncology; 1998:401a.

88. De Angelis LM, Yahalom J, Thaler HT, et al. Combined modality therapy for primary CNS lymphoma. J Clin Oncol 1992; 10(4):635–643.

89. Bessell EM, Graus F, Punt JAG, et al. Primary non Hodgkin's lymphoma of the CNS treated with BVAM or CHOD/BVAM chemotherapy before radiotherapy. J Clin Oncol 1996; 14(3):945–954.

90. Reni M, Ferreri AJ, Garancini MP, et al. Therapeutic management of primary central nervous system lymphoma in immunocompetent patients: results of a critical review of the literature. Ann Oncol 1997; 8(3):227–234.

91. Blay JY, Conroy T, Chevreau C, et al. High-dose methotrexate for the treatment of primary cerebral lymphomas: analysis of survival and late neurologic toxicity in a retrospective series. J Clin Oncol 1998; 16(3):864–871.

92. Brada M. Central nervous system lymphomas: progress in chemotherapy and radiotherapy [editorial; comment]. Int J Radiat Oncol Biol Phys 1995; 33(3):769–771.

93. Brada M, Hjiyiannakis P, Hines R, et al. Short intensive primary chemotherapy and radiotherapy in sporadic primary CNS lymphoma (PCL). Int J Radiat Oncol Biol Phys 1998; 40(5):1157–1162.

94. Wellenreuther R, Kraus JA, Lenartz D, et al. Analysis of the neurofibromatosis 2 gene reveals molecular variants of meningioma. Am J Pathol 1995; 146(4):827–832.

95. Louis DH, Budka H, von Deimling A. Meningiomas. In: Kleihues P, Cavenee WK, eds. World Health Organization Classification of Tumours. In: Sobin L, ed. Vol. 1, Pathology and genetics of tumours of the nervous system. Lyon: IARC Press; 2000.

96. Zorludemir S, Scheithauer BW, Hirose T, et al. Clear cell meningioma. A clinicopathologic study of a potentially aggressive variant of meningioma. Am J Surg Pathol 1995; 19(5):493–505.

97. Kepes JJ, Chen WY, Connors MH, et al. "Chordoid" meningeal tumors in young individuals with peritumoral lymphoplasmacellular infiltrates causing systemic manifestations of the Castleman syndrome. A report of seven cases. Cancer 1988; 62(2):391–406.

98. Perry A, Stafford SL, Scheithauer BW, et al. Meningioma grading: an analysis of histologic parameters. Am J Surg Pathol 1997; 21(12):1455–1465.

99. Perry A, Scheithauer BW, Stafford SL, et al. "Malignancy" in meningiomas: a clinicopathologic study of 116 patients, with grading implications. Cancer 1999; 85(9):2046–2056.

100. Jaaskelainen J, Haltia M, Servo A. Atypical and anaplastic meningiomas: radiology, surgery, radiotherapy, and outcome. Surg Neurol 1986; 25(3):233–242.

101. Barbaro NM, Gutin PH, Wilson CB, et al. Radiation therapy in the treatment of partially resected meningiomas. Neurosurgery 1987; 20(4):525–528.

102. Taylor BW Jr, Marcus RB Jr, Friedman WA, et al. The meningioma controversy: postoperative radiation therapy. Int J Radiat Oncol Biol Phys 1988; 15(2):299–304.

103. Glaholm J, Bloom HJG, Crow JH. The role of radiotherapy in the management of intracranial meningiomas: The Royal Marsden Hospital experience with 186 patients. Int J Radiat Oncol Biol Phys 1990; 18:755–761.

104. Wen B, Hussey D, Staples J, et al. A comparison of the roles of surgery and radiation therapy in the management of craniopharyngiomas. Int J Radiat Oncol Biol Phys 1989; 16:17–24.

105. Rajan B, Ashley S, Gorman C, et al. Craniopharyngioma – a long term results following limited surgery and radiotherapy. Radiother Oncol 1993; 26(1):1–10.

106. De Vile CJ, Grant DB, Kendall BE, et al. Management of childhood craniopharyngioma: can the morbidity of radical surgery be predicted?, J Neurosurg 1996; 85(1):73–81.

107. Amacher AL. Craniopharyngioma: the controversy regarding radiotherapy. Child's Brain 1980; 6:57–64.

108. Danoff BF, Cowchock S, Kramer S. Childhood craniopharyngioma: survival, local control, endocrine and neurologic function following radiotherapy. Int J Radiat Oncol Biol Phys 1983; 9:171–175.

109. Symon L, Sprich W. Radical excision of craniopharyngioma. Results in 20 patients. J Neurosurg 1985; 62(2):174–181.

110. Fahlbusch R, Honegger J, Paulus W, et al. Surgical treatment of craniopharyngiomas: experience with 168 patients. J Neurosurg 1999; 90(2):237–250.

111. Al-Mefty O, Hassounha M, Weaver P. Microsurgery for giant craniopharyngiomas in children. Neurosurgery 1988; 33:1026–1029.

112. Hoffman HJ, Silva de M, Humphreys RP, et al. Aggressive surgical management of craniopharyngiomas in children. J Neurosurg 1992; 76:47–52.

113. Yasargil M, Curic M, Kis M, et al. Total removal of craniopharyngiomas. Approaches and long term results in 144 patients. J Neurosurg 1990; 73:3–11.

114. Brada M, Thomas DG. Craniopharyngioma revisited. Int J Radiat Oncol Biol Phys 1993; 27(2):471–475.

115. Honegger J, Buchfelder M, Fahlbusch R. Surgical treatment of craniopharyngiomas: endocrinological results. J Neurosurg 1999; 90(2):251–257.

116. Thomsett MJ, Conte FA, Kaplan SL, et al. Endocrine and neurologic outcome in childhood craniopharyngioma: review of effect of treatment in 42 patients. J Pediatr 1980; 97(5):728–735.

117. Andrews DW. Pituitary adenomas. Curr Opin Oncol 1997; 9(1):55–60.

118. Fahlbusch R, Buchfelder M. Transsphenoidal surgery of parasellar pituitary adenomas. Acta Neurochir Wien 1988; 92(1–4):93–99.

119. Fahlbusch R, Honegger J, Buchfelder M. Evidence supporting surgery as treatment of choice for acromegaly. J Endocrinol 1997; 155(Suppl 1):S53–55.

120. el Mahdy W, Powell M. Transsphenoidal management of 28 symptomatic Rathke's cleft cysts, with special reference to visual and hormonal recovery. Neurosurgery 1998; 42(1):7–16.

121. Massoud AF, Powell M, Williams RA, et al. Transsphenoidal surgery for pituitary tumours. Arch Dis Child 1997; 76(5):398–404.

122. Brada M, Guerrero D. One model of follow up care. In: Davies E, Hopkin A, eds. Improving care for patients with malignant cerebral glioma. London: Royal College of Physicians Research Unit; 1998:93–98.

123. Guerrero D, Sardell S, Hines F. Chemotherapy. In: Guerrero D, ed. Neuro-oncology for nurses. London: Whurr; 1998:179–200.

124. Steward WP, Cassidy J, Kaye SB. Principles of chemotherapy. In: Price P, Sikora K, Halnan KE, eds. Treatment of cancer. London: Chapman and Hall Medical; 1995:91–108.

125. Britton J, Ng V. Clinical neuro-imaging. In: Guerrero D, ed. Neuro-oncology for nurses. London: Whurr; 1998:81–123.

126. Benner P. From novice to expert. Excellence and power in clinical nursing practice. California: Addison-Wesley; 1984.

127. Guerrero D. Neuro-oncology: a clinical nurse specialist perspective. Int J Palliat Nurs 2002; 8(1):28–29.

128. Porter HJ. Mouth care. In: Mallett J, Dougherty L, eds. Manual of clinical nursing procedures. London: Blackwell Science; 2000:360–367.

Chapter 46

Lymphoma

CHAPTER CONTENTS

MEDICAL CARE FOR PATIENTS WITH LYMPHOMA

Ian Chau and David Cunningham

HODGKIN'S DISEASE

Epidemiology

Hodgkin's disease (HD) is an uncommon malignant lymphoma, with around 1200 new cases a year in England and Wales accounting for about 0.5% of all cancers. It was estimated to cause 340 deaths in 2000.[1] Worldwide, it was estimated to have about 62 000 new cases of HD in 2000 and 25 000 deaths.[2] In developed countries, Hodgkin's disease typically has a bimodal age distribution, with a peak in young adults aged 15–30 years old and a further peak above age 60 years old.

Histology

In the World Health Organisation (WHO) classification of tumours of haematopoietic and lymphoid tissue,[3] Hodgkin's lymphoma or Hodgkin's disease has been divided into:

1. Nodular lymphocyte predominant Hodgkin's lymphoma (NLPHL).
2. Classical Hodgkin's lymphoma. This has been subdivided into:

   - nodular sclerosing Hodgkin's lymphoma (NSHL)
   - lymphocyte rich classical Hodgkin's lymphoma (LRHL)
   - mixed cellularity Hodgkin's lymphoma (MCHL)
   - lymphocyte depleted Hodgkin's lymphoma (LDHL).

HD is characterised by its unique cellular composition, with a minority of neoplastic cells (Reed–Sternberg cells and their variants) in an inflammatory background. NLPHL and classical Hodgkin's lymphoma differ in their clinical features and behaviour and in their morphology, immunophenotype and immunoglobulin transcription of the neoplastic cells as well as in the composition of their cellular background.

Clinical features

Patients may present with painless enlarged lymph node(s). They may have associated systemic symptoms such as fever, night sweat and weight loss of more than 10%. Some patients may notice itching and abdominal pain. Physical examination may reveal single or multiple palpable lymphadenopathy, hepatomegaly and splenomegaly. Table 46.1 shows the frequency of histological subtypes.

Nodular lymphocyte predominant Hodgkin's lymphoma

NLPHL has been recognised as an uncommon indolent disease seen more frequently in males and has a tendency to present with limited nodal disease and infrequent constitutional symptoms. Median age of presentation is in the mid-thirties. It usually involves peripheral lymph nodes with sparing of mediastinum. About 80% of patients would have stage I or II at time of diagnosis.

Nodular sclerosing Hodgkin's lymphoma

NSHL is most common in adolescents and young adults, but can occur at any age. The mediastinum and other supradiaphragmatic sites are commonly involved.

Mixed cellularity Hodgkin's lymphoma

MCHL lacks the early adult peak of NSHL. Involvement of mediastinum is less common than NSHL, whereas abdominal lymph nodes and splenic involvement are more frequent.

Lymphocyte depleted Hodgkin's lymphoma

LDHL is the least common variant of HD. It occurs most in older people and in patients infected with

human immunodeficiency virus (HIV) and in non-industrialised countries. It frequently presents with abdominal lymphadenopathy and spleen, liver and bone marrow involvement, without peripheral lymphadenopathy. Stage is usually advanced at diagnosis.

Lymphocyte rich Hodgkin's lymphoma

Patients tend to have early stage disease and lack bulky disease or B symptoms. Mediastinal disease is less frequent and LRHL occurs predominantly in males.

Staging

One of the most important prognostic and therapeutic considerations for HD is the initial staging of patients at presentation. The Cotswold modification of the Ann Arbor classification is the most widely used.[4] Table 46.2 shows the Ann Arbor classification. Clinical stage (CS) refers to the stage of disease based on physical examination and imaging technique, whereas pathological stage (PS) is determined by additional invasive procedures such as laparotomy and bone marrow biopsy. Systemic symptoms of fever (>38°C), unexplained

Table 46.2   Staging classification

Stage	Description
I	Involvement of a single lymph node region or lymphoid structure (spleen, thymus, Waldeyer's ring), or involvement of a single extralymphatic site (I_E)
II	Involvement of two or more lymph node regions on the same side of the diaphragm, which may be accompanied by localised contiguous involvement of an extralymphatic organ or site (II_E)
III	Involvement of lymph node regions on both sides of the diaphragm, which may also be accompanied involvement (III_S) or by localised contiguous involvement of an extralymphatic organ or site (III_E)
IV	Diffuse of disseminated involvement of one or more extralymphatic organs or tissues, with or without associated lymph node involvement

Source: adapted from Aisenberg.[19]
Notes:
Stage III may be subdivided into III_1, to designate involvement of only to upper abdominal nodes ± spleen, and III_2 to designate involvement of the para-aortic and/or pelvic nodes.
Bulky mediastinal mass (>1/3 maximum chest diameter or a lymphoid mass >10 cm in diameter) may be designated by the subscript X.

Table 46.1   Frequency of histological subtypes in Hodgkin's disease

Histological subtypes	Frequency of cases (%)
Nodular sclerosing	60–80
Mixed cellularity	15
Lymphocyte rich	5
Lymphocyte depleted	<1
Nodular lymphocyte predominant	2–8

weight loss (>10% body weight) in the preceding 6 months and sweating are known as B symptoms. The absence or presence of these symptoms will denote a suffix (letters A or B, respectively) to the staging. Table 46.3 shows the initial staging investigations for Hodgkin's disease and non-Hodgkin's lymphoma (NHL).

Computed tomography (CT) can more precisely identify mediastinal, pericardial, pleural, lung and chest wall disease compared with chest X-ray. In addition, CT is capable of identifying upper abdominal lymph nodes as well as large hepatic and splenic lesions. It is useful in monitoring treatment response. However, CT fails to detect occult Hodgkin's disease in the upper abdominal lymph nodes or in the spleen, which may occur in 20–25% of patients.

Lymphangiography was introduced more than 40 years ago to assist in the diagnosis and treatment of HD. It involves cannulation of the lymphatic vessels of the dorsum of each foot, followed by the injection of an iodine-based radio-opaque dye. Opacification of lymph nodes remains for 1 year or more in most patients, thereby facilitating disease assessment before, during and after treatment. However, the procedure has largely been abandoned and replaced by CT, which is non-invasive.

Positron emission tomography (PET) with the glucose analogue 2-(fluorine-18)-fluoro-2-deoxy-D-glucose (^{18}F-FDG) can detect both nodal and extranodal sites of disease, reveal the activity or lack of activity of residual masses and provide evidence of recurrence. PET imaging is a useful supplementary investigation in the management of lymphomas, providing a non-invasive means of evaluating potential sites of active disease and complementing CT in the assessment of lymphomas.

Table 46.3	Initial investigations for Hodgkin's disease and non-Hodgkin's lymphoma
Investigation	Description
Laboratory tests	
Haematology	Full blood count
	Erythrocyte sedimentation rate (ESR)
Biochemistry	Renal function
	Liver function test
	Calcium/phosphate
	Lactate dehydrogenase
	β_2-microglobulin
	Immunoglobulins and paraproteins
Imaging	Chest X-ray
	Computer tomography of chest, abdomen and pelvis
	Magnetic resonance imaging (more relevant in NHL)
	Positron emission tomography (useful adjunct, but investigational)
	Lymphangiogram (rarely performed nowadays)
Histopathology review	Bone marrow trephine and aspirate (not necessary in stage I and IIA HD)
	Lumbar puncture-indicated in the following situations:
	1. Immunoblastic lymphoma, lymphoblastic lymphoma, Burkitt's, Burkitt-like lymphoma
	2. Diffuse large cell lymphoma involving a high-risk site
	3. Clinical evidence of central nervous system infiltration

HD = Hodgkin's disease; NHL = non-Hodgkin's lymphoma.

Treatment of Hodgkin's disease

Early stage Hodgkin's disease

Early stage HD is defined as lymph node involvement limited to one side of the diaphragm, i.e. Ann Arbor stage I or II in an asymptomatic patient. Patients with bulky mediastinal mass are not considered to have early stage disease, although the definition of bulky disease varies. It has been taken as more than 5–10 cm, or expressed as a ratio of the mass to the maximum intrathoracic diameter $\geq 1/3$.

Several therapeutic strategies have been pursued for early stage HD. Whereas the focus of treatment between 1960 and 1985 was the improvement of overall survival (OS), the success of treatment has prompted research to improve disease-free survival and salvage therapy for relapses between 1985 and 1995. Long-term complications from curative treatment for HD have also become apparent in this time period. Since 1995, attention has been directed towards minimal treatment without compromising cure and quality of life.

Single modality radiotherapy Radiotherapy (RT) has a long history of success in curative treatment of early stage disease. In the 1950s, patients received irradiation directed to involved and contiguously involved lymph nodes. Some patients achieved cure, but many relapsed outside the radiation field. Later, extended field RT has been reported to achieve less treatment failure compared to involved field RT. Extended field RT refers to:

- Subtotal lymphoid irradiation (STLI), including mantle field (cervical, axillary, mediastinal and hilar lymph nodes); upper abdominal and para-aortic lymph nodes; and spleen or splenic bed following splenectomy.

- Total lymphoid irradiation (TLI), including the addition of pelvic lymph nodes to the STLI field.

The effectiveness of extended field RT against involved field RT has been confirmed in a recent meta-analysis of 23 randomised trials involving 3888 patients. Extended field RT was associated with fewer treatment failures, reducing the risk of resistant or recurrent disease by more than one-third (p <0.00001).[5] However, OS between these two groups of patients was not different, due to the excellent ability to salvage patients with combination chemotherapy after radiation failures.

Combined modality therapy   The aims of combined modality therapy (CMT) are:

- to improve results with radiation therapy, especially in patients with poor prognostic factors
- to substitute for extended radiotherapy and associated morbidity and mortality
- to eliminate need for laparotomy staging.

Following the introduction of the MOPP regimen (mechlorethamine, vincristine, procarbazine and prednisolone) for advanced Hodgkin's disease, investigators have incorporated a full course of active combination chemotherapy to radiotherapy in early stage HD (see Appendix 1 and Appendix 2). Improved freedom from progression in favour of CMT has been consistent in several studies, but freedom from progression advantage has not been shown to translate into an OS benefit. These observations have been confirmed in a recent meta-analysis in which CMT decreased the risk of failure by 50% compared with RT alone, with no improvement in survival.[5] These conflicting results are probably related to the fact that patients who develop recurrences after single modality RT benefit from salvage chemotherapy and this neutralises the advantage of introducing chemotherapy at an earlier stage in CMT. In addition, with longer follow-up evaluation, increased mortality from other complications has been realised for patients who received CMT with an alkylating agent-based regimen at diagnosis. ABVD (doxorubicin, bleomycin, vinblastine and dacarbazine) is a non-cross-resistant regimen to MOPP which has now been established as standard therapy in advanced HD and its use has also been explored in early disease.[6]

Current strategies in early stage HD aim to define an optimal combination of chemotherapy and irradiation that further reduces late effects without compromising cure rates. Recent studies have confirmed that when CMT is used, shorter duration of chemotherapy may be as effective as long courses of chemotherapy and STLI confers no additional advantage over involved field RT. Moreover, the need of staging laparotomy has been reduced by the use of a systemic approach. Four courses of ABVD chemotherapy are sufficient when combined with involved field RT. Whether the duration of chemotherapy can be shortened further without compromising cure rate is currently under intense research.

Advanced stage Hodgkin's disease

Induction therapy   Advanced stage disease is defined as Ann Arbor bulky stage IIA, stage IIB, III or IV disease. The introduction of MOPP remains a landmark in the treatment of advanced stage HD.[7] It was the first regimen to effect cure, with 48% alive at 15 years, but it has significant short- and long-term toxicity. ABVD was developed by Bonadonna and colleagues to be a non-cross-resistant and less toxic regimen than MOPP.[8] It is not associated with an increased risk of leukaemia or a loss of fertility. It has also been combined with MOPP in an alternating schedule based on the hypothesis that it would result in less cross-resistance and was found to be superior to MOPP alone.[9] However, ABVD is now considered as standard treatment for untreated HD based on superior complete remission rate (82% vs 67%; $p = 0.006$) and 5-year failure-free survival (61% vs 50%) over MOPP in a randomised trial of 361 patients coordinated by the Cancer and Leukemia Group B (CALGB).[10] After 14 years of follow-up, no OS advantage ($p = 0.35$) was demonstrated with ABVD, although it continued to have a higher rate of failure-free survival ($p = 0.03$), reflecting the ability of salvage therapy to prolong survival.[11] In this study, alternating MOPP–ABVD conferred no advantage in efficacy compared to ABVD, but was more toxic. In another study coordinated by CALGB, 856 patients were randomised to 8–10 cycles of ABVD or MOPP/ABV hybrid regimen.[12] No significant differences in failure-free survival and OS were seen, but a greater number of treatment-related mortality was seen in the hybrid arm compared with ABVD. Clinically significant acute pulmonary and haematological toxicity were more common with MOPP/ABV ($p = 0.060$ and 0.001, respectively). There was no difference in cardiac toxicity. There were 24 deaths attributed to initial treatment: 9 with ABVD and 15 with MOPP/ABV ($p = 0.057$). In addition, there was an excess of second malignancies in the hybrid arm. There have been 18 second malignancies associated with ABVD and 28 associated with MOPP/ABV ($p = 0.13$). Thirteen patients have developed myelodysplastic syndrome or acute leukemia: 11 were initially treated with MOPP/ABV, and two were initially treated with ABVD but subsequently received MOPP-containing regimens and radiotherapy before developing leukemia ($p = 0.011$). At present, ABVD should remain as reference treatment for advanced Hodgkin's disease to which new treatment is compared. (See also Chs 28 and 32.)

Dose intensification in advanced stage Hodgkin's disease

In order to improve treatment results in patients with advanced HD, new regimens have been developed based on escalation of total dose of the putatively most effective cytotoxic drug and/or an increase in dose intensity. Two examples of such development are Stanford V and BEACOPP. Stanford V (doxorubicin, vinblastine, mechlorethamine, vincristine, bleomycin, etoposide and prednisolone) was developed on the hypothesis that the duration of chemotherapy could be shortened through a combination of dose intensification and the judicious use of radiotherapy, without compromising efficacy. Chemotherapy is given for 12 weeks, followed by 36 Gy consolidation RT to initial disease sites of 5 cm or more or macroscopic splenic disease. The treatment approach was designed to preserve fertility and minimise secondary leukaemia. BEACOPP (bleomycin, etoposide, doxorubicin, cyclophosphamide, vincristine, procarbazine and prednisolone) was designed on the hypothesis that moderate increase in drug dose would bring improved efficacy. The doses of doxorubicin and cyclophosphamide are escalated with the addition of etoposide to the regimen. This is made possible by the use of granulocyte colony-stimulating factor (G-CSF). In addition, the treatment interval can also be shortened from 4 to 3 weeks. Both Stanford V and BEACOPP can induce remission rates as high as 90% with a 5-year freedom from progression rate of 87–89%, although long-term cure rates are still awaited.[13-15] There is a lack of randomised data demonstrating efficacy with Stanford V at the moment. Baseline BEACOPP and escalated BEACOPP have been evaluated within a randomised study of 1180 patients comparing with ABVD/COPP (cyclophosphamide, vincristine, prednisolone and procarbazine). Both baseline and escalated BEACOPP showed a superior complete remission rate, failure-free, progression-free and overall survival compared with ABVD/COPP.[13] However, the acute toxicity with escalated BEACOPP is severe and there is increased incidence of early myelodysplasia and secondary leukaemia estimated at 2.5% at 5 years.

Adjuvant radiotherapy in advanced stage disease

The role of adjuvant radiotherapy in advanced stage HD remains controversial. There are many theoretical reasons for adding radiation therapy to chemotherapy in the treatment of advanced HD. The majority of relapses after chemotherapy occur at sites of initial disease, particularly nodal sites and sites of bulky tumour. Adjuvant irradiation markedly reduces the frequency of these recurrences and converts some partial responses to durable complete responses. However, with increasing awareness of secondary cancer risk associated with irradiation, this issue needs to be addressed in large randomised trials with long follow-up. A recent meta-analysis has confirmed improved disease control, with a nearly 40% reduction in treatment failures in favour of RT in trials that compared additional RT vs no RT. However, no beneficial effect on survival could be identified by additional RT. Interestingly, the OS showed a significant benefit for patients who received chemotherapy alone. This was mainly due to higher hazard for HD-unrelated fatal events in patients who received additional RT.[16] It therefore appears that the addition of RT in patients with advanced stage HD overall has a significantly inferior long-term survival outcome than chemotherapy alone if chemotherapy is given over an appropriate number of cycles. Moreover, as this meta-analysis only included trials conducted between 1972 and 1988 with 10 years of follow-up, the full impact of the newly introduced polychemotherapy regimens cannot be assessed yet. However, it can be reasonably assumed that these newer regimens may be more effective in terms of tumour control than the regimens used in the trials analysed in this meta-analysis, and hence the beneficial effects for radiotherapy may diminish further. However, improvement of radiation technique in the last two decades for HD may diminish the incidence of long-term complications of radiation therapy. These issues are being addressed in large ongoing randomised studies, and longer follow-up may answer the role of adjuvant radiotherapy in advanced HD.

Salvage therapy

Salvage for relapse after radiation therapy in early stage disease For patients with early stage disease who relapse after radiation treatment, salvage chemotherapy provides equivalent survival to patients receiving chemotherapy alone for advanced stage disease. Important poor prognostic variables in radiation failures include:

- advanced stage
- unfavourable histology (mixed cellularity or lymphocyte depletion)
- advanced age.

ABVD exhibits the same superiority over MOPP for radiation recurrence as it does in initial treatment of advanced disease.

Salvage for relapse after primary chemotherapy in advanced or bulky disease Chemotherapy failures can be divided into three groups with varying prognosis. For patients who have received a COPP or MOPP variant regimen, ABVD salvage therapy is moderately efficacious in achieving a second complete remission. However, long-term results experienced by these patients are dismal. Etoposide and platinum-based chemotherapy have also been used with low probability of long-term cure in conventional dose. Success of salvage treatment depends on:

- age
- performance status
- chemosensitivity
- remission duration.

High-dose chemotherapy with haemopoietic transplantation Two randomised trials have been reported in relapsed HD. The British National Lymphoma Investigation study randomised patients with high-risk HD (i.e. induction failure; relapse within 1 year of MOPP-type chemotherapy; failure after second or subsequent line of chemotherapy, irrespective of duration of remission) between BEAM (carmustine, etoposide, cytarabine and melphalan) + autologous bone marrow transplantation with the same drugs at lower doses not requiring bone marrow rescue (mini-BEAM). Three-year event-free survivals were 53% in BEAM and autograft and 10% in the mini-BEAM arm. No OS difference was observed, and these results were sustained at 5-year update. The apparent discrepancy between event-free and overall survival can partly be explained by the patients in the mini-BEAM arm being salvaged by an autologous bone marrow transplant at the time of relapse.[17]

A German Hodgkin's disease study group has also reported a study randomising 161 patients to a sequence of 2 cycles of Dexa-BEAM (dexamethasone, carmustine, etoposide, cytarabine and melphalan) chemotherapy followed by either 2 further cycles of Dexa-BEAM or an autologous transplant using BEAM chemotherapy. Again, time to treatment failure at 3 years favours the transplant arm (55% transplant arm vs 34% Dexa-BEAM only; $p = 0.019$) but no OS has been seen because of further treatment in the relapsed patients in the Dexa-BEAM arm.[18]

Late complications

Unfortunately, although the recent advances in radiotherapy and chemotherapy result in a high rate of cure, the price of late complications has only been realised recently following prolonged follow-up of these patients. Indeed, 15 years after diagnosis, the mortality from causes other than HD exceeds that due to HD. Few additional HD-related deaths occur beyond 15 years, whereas late treatment-related deaths are still accumulating. Table 46.4 shows the increased risk of developing long-term complications and second cancers.[19–21]

Splenectomy
It has been recognised that staging laparotomy and splenectomy are not without risk. The procedure carries a mortality of 0.7% and an incidence of significant or severe complications of approximately 12.8%.[22] In addition, patients are at long-term risk of overwhelming life-threatening sepsis for *Streptococcus pneumoniae*, *Haemophilus influenzae* and *Neisseria meningitidis*. Our current lymphoma unit guidelines recommend penicillin prophylaxis and immunisation against *S. pneumoniae*, *H. influenzae* and *N. meningitidis* C, as well as yearly influenza immunisation.

Fertility
Patients who have undergone chemotherapy and radiotherapy at a young age may have compromised fertility. Sperm cryopreservation is standard for young men prior to sterilising chemotherapy and irradiation. It is routine, inexpensive and technically undemanding, but has many shortcomings in practice. It cannot be used for preadolescents. Fertile men sometimes have difficulty producing a specimen under the stress of recent cancer diagnosis and may produce inferior specimens because of pyrexia or other disease-associated effects. The female equivalent of sperm banking is oocyte cryopreservation, but this is not yet a routine procedure. Frozen embryo banking to store surplus embryos after in-vitro fertilisation avoids the need to collect more fresh oocytes.

Second malignancy
Acute non-lymphocytic leukaemia Acute non-lymphocytic leukaemia (ANLL) was the first neoplasm noted following HD therapy. Chromosome 5 and 7 deletions are characteristic, and approximately half are preceded by myelodysplastic syndrome (MDS). The entire class of alkylating agent is leukaemogenic: cyclophosphamide is significantly less so than mechlorethamine, chlorambucil, mephalan, lomustine and thiotepa. The leukaemia risk is linearly related to total alkylating dose. In addition, drug-induced ANLL is also related to age at time of treatment, with 3 to 4 times increased cumulative leukaemia risk in patients who are 40 years old or older. However, this may reflect the increasing baseline (general population) incidence of ANLL with advancing age.

After administration of MOPP, the first cases appear several years after treatment, reach a peak in the second half of the decade, decline in the first half

Table 46.4   Long term complications from treatment of Hodgkin's disease

	Stanford[20]			Joint Centre[21]		
	Patients		Deaths	Patients		Deaths
	No.	%	%	No.	%	%
Total patients	2498	100		794	100	
Total deaths	754	30.2	100	124	15.6	100
Hodgkin's disease	333	13.3	44	56	7.0	45
Second malignancy	160	6.5	21	36	4.5	29
Cardiovascular	117	4.8	16	15	1.9	12
Pulmonary	50	2.0	7	1	0.1	1
Infectious	31	1.3	4	8	1.0	6
Accidental	14	0.6	2	3	0.4	2
Others	49	2.0	7	4	0.5	3

Site of type	Relative risk	Absolute excess risk (per 10 000 patients per year)
All malignancies	3.5	56.2
ANLL	70.8	15.5
NHL	18.6	10.7
Solid tumours	2.4	29.3
Lung	4.2	13.5
Breast	2.5	11.3
Gastrointestinal	2.5	5.8
Sarcoma	7.0	1.0
Thyroid	4.7	0.5
Melanoma	4.2	1.6

Source: adapted from Aisenberg.[19]
ANLL = acute non-lymphoblastic lymphoma; NHL = non-Hodgkin's lymphoma.

of the second decade, with few cases beyond the second decade. The leukaemia risk after a single course of MOPP is modest (2–3% at 10–15 years). Addition of involved field RT increases the risk over MOPP alone by little if at all, but combined modality treatment with aggressive extended field irradiation results in a 3× increase (6–9% at 10–15 years) in the risk of developing ANLL. Additional courses of alkylating agent chemotherapy increase the risk further (10–15%) and the cumulative risks are multiplied further in individuals aged 40 and older (reviewed by Aisenberg[19]).

The leukaemia risk after ABVD, either alone or combined with extensive irradiation, is much less than that following MOPP (15 years cumulative risk of 0.7% and 9.5%, respectively). Although ANLL is observed after radiation therapy alone, the relative risk is much less than that following alkylating agents.

Secondary non–Hodgkin's lymphoma   The relationship of secondary NHL to preceding HD is complex and poorly understood. Relative risks are high, with absolute risks similar to ANLL. Increasing age at HD treatment is a potent predictor of secondary NHL risk,

as it is of ANLL. The great majority of NHL after HD treatment is of intermediate or high-grade histology.

Second solid tumours   Second solid neoplasms are major obstacles to the cured HD patients. Because the population risk of these solid tumours (lung, breast, gastrointestinal tract) is much higher, modest increases in relative risk lead to major absolute risk. Therefore, although relative risks for ANLL and NHL are far greater, the cumulative risks of solid tumours are greater than ANLL and NHL combined. Furthermore, while the excess risks of ANLL and NHL are largely dissipated by the middle of the second decade after treatment, the solid cancer risk continues well into the third decade with no indication of when, if ever, the risk abates.

Irradiation has been implicated as the major carcinogen, with approximately two-thirds (65–90%) of second solid tumours arising within or at the edge of treatment fields. The role of chemotherapy as an independent contributor to second solid tumour remains controversial and available data suggest that ABVD and MOPP are equally culpable (reviewed by Aisenberg[19]).

Cardiac complications

Cardiac complications account for a quarter of the mortality from causes other than HD itself and 2–5% of mortality in the entire HD population. Again, although the relative risk of cardiac death is modest, because the background population risk is high, the absolute risk of cardiac death is high. This is mostly related to mantle field RT. Radiation damage to coronary arteries causes myocardial infarction (MI). Radiation injury to the rest of the heart can cause pericardial disease, diffuse myocardial disease (pancarditis and cardiomyopathy), valvular defects and conduction abnormalities. Whereas the risk of cardiac deaths from causes other than MI is markedly diminished with modern radiation techniques and the availability of chemotherapy as a viable treatment alternative, MI deaths have not been substantially reduced.

Doxorubicin has been responsible for only sporadic deaths in patients who enter treatment with satisfactory cardiac function, and medium-term follow-up (10 years) has not revealed any excessive cases of congestive cardiac failure or cardiac deaths.

Pulmonary toxicity

Pulmonary toxicity could be related to radiation pneumonitis or preparative regimens for high-dose therapy (carmustine, total body irradiation, cytarabine). Radiation pneumonitis occurs in 20% of patients after mantle field RT, but related to dose, fractionation and volume of lung irradiated. Bleomycin-related mortality after 6 cycles of ABVD chemotherapy is estimated at 1–3%.

Prognostic factors

An international prognostic score (IPS) has been developed in advanced HD based on 1618 patients treated with doxorubicin-containing or MOPP-type chemotherapy.[23] The final prognostic model incorporates seven prognostic factors:

1. serum albumin <4 g/dl
2. haemoglobin <10.5 g/dl
3. male sex
4. stage IV disease
5. aged 45 years old or over
6. white cell count ≥15 000/ml
7. lymphocyte count <600/ml.

This prognostic score predicts freedom from progression and overall survival. A score of 3 or more represents a moderately high risk, with an expected 5-year freedom from progression of disease of 55% and OS of 70%. A score of 4 or more is associated with 5-year freedom from progression rate of 47% and an OS of 59%. Thus, there is no distinct group of patients with advanced HD that can be identified as being at very high risk.

However, IPS was derived from patients treated in the MOPP/ABVD and ABVD era. More effective regimens such as BEACOPP may allow patients in high-risk groups to experience similar outcome to those in low-risk groups, and therefore IPS may lose its prognostic value.

NON-HODGKIN'S LYMPHOMA

Epidemiology

Non-Hodgkin's lymphoma (NHL) is increasing in incidence in recent decades. It is the most common malignancy among the leukaemias and lymphomas, with 8000 new cases in the United Kingdom causing an estimated 4500 deaths in 2000. Worldwide, it is estimated there were about 287 000 new cases of NHL in 2000 and 160 000 deaths.[2]

Histology

The current WHO classification divides NHL subtypes according to the putative cell of origin. Table 46.5 shows the histology subtypes according to the WHO classification,[3] Revised European and American Lymphoma (REAL) calssification[24] and Working Formulation.[25] Table 46.6 shows the frequency of selected histological subtypes.[26]

Aggressive non–Hodgkin's lymphomas

International prognostic index

Although many patients with aggressive NHL are cured by combination chemotherapy, the remainder are not cured and ultimately die of their disease. The Ann Arbor classification does not consistently distinguish between patients with different long-term prognoses. The international Non-Hodgkin's Lymphoma Prognostic Factors Project evaluated 2031 patients of all ages treated with doxorubicin containing combination chemotherapy regimens.[27] The five pretreatment characteristics that independently predicted poor prognosis were:

- age >60 years old
- tumour stage III or IV
- performance status ≥ 2
- serum lactate dehydrogenase (LDH) >1 × normal
- more than one extranodal sites of disease.

Patients are then assigned to one of four risk groups on the basis of their number of presenting risk factors:

- low risk   0 or 1
- low intermediate risk   2

Table 46.5   Classification of NHL World Health Organisation (WHO)[3] / Revised European and American Lymphoma (REAL) classification[24] and Working Formulation (WF)[25] equivalent

WHO classification	REAL classification (WF equivalent)
B-cell neoplasms	**B-cell neoplasms**
Precursor B-cell neoplasms	*Precursor B-cell neoplasms*
Precursor B-lymphoblastic leukaemia/lymphoma (precursor B-cell acute lymphoblastic leukaemia)	1. Precursor B-lymphoblastic leukaemia/lymphoma (I)
Mature (peripheral) B-cell neoplasms	*Peripheral B-cell neoplasms*
B-cell chronic lymphocytic leukaemia/ small lymphocytic lymphoma	1. B-cell CLL/prolymphocytic leukaemia/small lymphocytic lymphoma (A)
B-cell prolymphocytic leukaemia	
Lymphoplasmacytic lymphoma/Waldenström macroglobulinemia	2. Lymphoplasmacytid lymphoma/immunocytoma (A)
Splenic marginal zone B-cell lymphoma (+/− villous lymphocytes)	3. Mantle cell lymphoma (E)
Hairy cell leukaemia	4. Follicle centre lymphoma, follicular
Plasma cell myeloma/plasmacytoma	Cytological grades: I (small cell) (B)
Extranodal marginal zone B-cell lymphoma of MALT type	II (mixed cell) (C)
Nodal marginal zone B-cell lymphoma (+/− monocytoid B cells)	III (large cell) (D)
Follicular lymphoma	5. Marginal zone B-cell lymphoma (A–C)
	Extranodal (MALT ± monocytoid B cells) (U)
Grade 1, 0–5 centroblasts/hpf	6. Splenic marginal zone lymphoma (A)
Grade 2, 6–15 centroblasts/hpf	7. Hairy cell leukaemia (U)
Grade 3, >15 centroblasts/hpf	8. Plasmacytoma/myeloma (U)
Grade 3a, >15 centroblasts – centrocytes present	9. Diffuse large B-cell lymphoma (F,G)
Grade 3b, centroblasts in solid sheets – no centrocyte	10. Burkitt's lymphoma (J)
Mantle cell lymphoma	11. High-grade B-cell lymphoma, Burkitt-type (U)
Diffuse large B-cell lymphoma	
Mediastinal large B-cell lymphoma	**T-cell and putative NK-cell neoplasms**
Primary effusion lymphoma	
Burkitt's lymphoma	*Precursor T-cell neoplasm*
Intravascular large B cell lymphoma	1. Precursor T-lymphoblastic lymphoma/leukaemia (I)
T-cell and NK-cell neoplasms	
Precursor T-cell neoplasm	*Peripheral T-cell and NK-cell neoplasms*
Precursor T-lymphoblastic lymphoma/leukaemia (precursor T-cell acute lymphoblastic leukaemia)	T-cell CLL / prolymphocytic leukaemia (A)
Mature (peripheral) T-cell neoplasms	2. Large granular lymphocyte leukaemia (A)
T-cell prolymphocytic leukaemia	3. Mycosis fungoides /Sézary syndrome (U)
	4. Peripheral T-cell lymphomas, unspecified (F,G,H)
T-cell large granular lymphocytic leukaemia	5. Adult T-cell lymphoma/leukaemia (U)
Aggressive NK-cell leukaemia	6. Angioimmunoblastic T-cell lymphoma (F,H)
Adult T-cell lymphoma/leukaemia (HTLV1+)	7. Angiocentric lymphoma (E–H)
Extranodal NK/T-cell lymphoma, nasal type	
Enteropathy-type T-cell lymphoma	8. Intestinal T-cell lymphoma (± enteropathy) (E–H)
Hepatosplenic gamma-delta T-cell lymphoma	
Subcutaneous panniculitis-like T-cell lymphoma	9. Anaplastic large cell lymphoma (T/null) (G,H)
Blastic NK-cell lymphoma	
Mycosis fungoides/Sézary syndrome	
Angioimmunoblastic T-cell lymphoma	
Peripheral T-cell lymphoma, unspecified	
Anaplastic large cell lymphoma	

Letters in parentheses refer to classification according to Working Formulation.

Table 46.6 Frequency of selected histological subtypes of non-Hodgkin's lymphoma

Histological subtypes	Frequency of cases (%)
Diffuse large B-cell	31
Follicular	22
Small lymphocytic	6
Mantle cell	6
Peripheral T-cell	6
Margin zone B-cell, MALT type	5
Primary mediastinal large B-cell	2
Anaplastic large T-/null-cell	2
Lymphoblastic (T/B cell)	2
Burkitt-like	2
Marginal zone B-cell, nodal type	1
Lymphoplasmacytic	1
Burkitt's	<1

Source: adapted from Armitage et al.[26]

- high intermediate risk   3
- high risk   4 or 5

An age-adjusted international prognostic index (IPI) for patients less than 60 years old has also been developed, including tumour stage, performance status and LDH level. Patients are again assigned to one of four risk groups:

- low risk   0
- low intermediate risk   1
- high intermediate risk   2
- high risk   3

Clinical features

Diffuse large B–cell non–Hodgkin's lymphomas Diffuse large B-cell non-Hodgkin's lymphomas (DLBCLs) are composed of different histological subtypes and are heterogeneous in their morphological, genetic and clinical presentation. They are composed of large B cells with vesicular nuclei, prominent nucleoli, often basophilic cytoplasm and a moderate to high proliferation fraction. Tumour cells are SIg^+, CIg^+, B-cell associated antigens$^+$, $CD45^+$, $CD5^+$ and $CD10^+$. Patients present with a rapidly enlarging nodal or extranodal mass or masses. Up to 40% of the cases are extranodal and all body sites may be involved. Localised disease occurs in 30% of the cases and some of these cases are frequently associated with large tumour masses, particularly the mediastinum and abdomen.

Burkitt's lymphomas Burkitt's lymphoma is composed of monomorphic, medium-sized cells with round nuclei, multiple nucleoli and relatively abundant basophilic cytoplasm. This tumour has an extremely high rate of proliferation. Tumour cells are $SIgM^+$, B-cell associated antigen$^+$, $CD5^-$ and $CD10^+$. Most patients present with abdominal tumour involving the caecum and mesentery, but in rare cases the tumour may involve the ovaries, breasts or testes. Bone marrow and/or central nervous system (CNS) involvement are associated with poor outcome.

Lymphoblastic lymphoma Lymphoblastic lymphoma has two phenotypes – T cells and B cells. The T-cell phenotype is generally a disease of adolescent or young adult males, comprising 40% of childhood lymphoma and <5% of adult lymphomas. B-cell lymphoblastic lymphoma is a rare tumour, comprising <1% of all NHLs and is mostly seen in elderly patients as a transformation of an unknown indolent B-cell lymphoma. Lymphoblastic lymphomas are composed of lymphoblasts slightly larger than small lymphocytes. Mitosis is frequent. The T-cell phenotype expresses CD7, CD3 and other T-cell antigens variably. Patients usually present with a rapidly enlarging mediastinal mass. Bone marrow or CNS involvement or both are associated with poor outcome. Patients may have nodal localisation only, particularly in the mediastinum or a nodal mass with bone marrow and/or CNS localisation.

Anaplastic large cell non–Hodgkin's lymphomas These lymphomas are composed of large cells expressing $CD30^+$, $CD45^+$, EMA^+, $CD15^-$, $CD3^\pm$, $Alk1^+$ and variable for T-cell associated antigens. There are two clinical forms of anaplastic large cell NHL:

- a systemic form that may involve lymph nodes or extranodal sites, including skin
- a primary cutaneous form that may spontaneously regress.

Anasplatic T- or NK (natural killer)-cell lymphomas are mostly seen in young adult patients. The systemic form appears to behave like other large cell lymphomas.

Peripheral T–cell lymphoma and natural killer cell lymphoma These lymphomas, which contain a mixture of small and large atypical cells, are heterogeneic and difficult to describe and classify. Distinct clinical syndromes such as hepatosplenic T-cell lymphoma, nasal NK-cell lymphoma, angioimmunoblastic T-cell lymphoma, angiocentric lymphoma and intestinal T-cell lymphoma have been described.

Patients with an unspecified subtype usually have disseminated disease with involvement of lymph nodes, skin, liver, spleen or other extranodal sites. B symptoms are frequent. Patients with angioimmunoblastic T-cell lymphomas usually present with generalised lymph node involvement, fever, skin rash and polyclonal hypergammaglobulinaemia. NK-cell lymphomas are rare and present with involvement of extranodal sites, such as nose, palate and skin. Intestinal T-cell lymphoma occurs in adults after a history of gluten-sensitive enteropathy, but also occasionally as the primary event.

Mantle cell lymphoma   The tumour is composed exclusively of small to medium-sized lymphoid cells with dispersed chromatin, scant pale cytoplasm and inconspicuous nucleoli. Tumour cells are SIgM$^+$, usually IgD$^+$, B-cell associated antigen$^+$, CD5$^+$, CD10$^-$, CD23$^-$ and CD43$^+$. It occurs more frequently in older adults, with predominance in men. Disease is usually widespread at the time of diagnosis, with involvement of lymph nodes, spleen, bone marrow, peripheral blood and extranodal sites, especially the gastrointestinal tract (lymphomatous polyposis). The clinical course is initially moderately aggressive but becomes progressively more aggressive with the inefficacy of treatment.

Clinical management

Diffuse large B–cell non–Hodgkin's lymphoma   This consists of a diverse group of diseases, which have in common an aggressive clinical behaviour leading to rapid clinical deterioration. However, chemosensitivity of DLBCL renders approximately 40–50% of patients curable. Sixty to seventy per cent of DLBCL patients who reach complete response (CR) may be cured, as opposed to almost none not in CR. The ultimate goal of treatment must therefore be to achieve CR.

Induction treatment   Patients with early stage disease (stage I or II non-bulky, without adverse prognostic factors) have a much better outcome than patients with advanced stage disease. In a randomised trial by Southwest Oncology Group (SWOG) comparing 8 cycles of CHOP (cyclophosphamide, doxorubicin, vincristine and prednisolone) with 3 cycles of CHOP followed by involved field RT in 401 stage I and II patients, the latter produced superior 5-year progression-free survival (64% vs 77%, respectively; p = 0.03) and OS (72% vs 82%, respectively; p = 0.02).[28] However, on longer follow-up, 5-year estimates of OS and progression-free survival did not differ; the survival curves of the treatment arms overlapped. The treatment advantage for CHOP and involved field radiotherapy for the first 7–9 years is diminished because of excess late relapses and deaths due to lymphoma occurring between years 5–10 in that arm.[29] In a second randomised study by the Eastern Cooperative Oncology Group (ECOG), 345 eligible patients with untreated bulky or extranodal stage I and stage II disease were randomly assigned to either 8 cycles of CHOP or 8 cycles of CHOP followed by consolidation radiotherapy. Again, the addition of radiotherapy resulted in a superior disease-free survival, but no OS advantage.[30] For patients with non-bulky stage I or II disease, short-course chemotherapy with an anthracycline-containing regimen followed by involved field RT is now recommended.

For advanced disease (bulky stage II, stage III or IV), CHOP represented the cornerstone therapy for advanced aggressive NHL. Approximately 30–40% of patients with advanced disease enjoy long-term disease-free survival with CHOP therapy. Second- and third-generation regimens were developed to try to improve on the results achieved by CHOP. Agents such as methotrexate, cytarabine, bleomycin or etoposide were added and weekly intensive regimens were developed with impressive results in phase II studies. However, a large phase III randomised 4-arm trial comparing CHOP with M-BACOD, ProMACE/CytaBOM and MACOP-B was performed.[31] In essence, no regimens appeared to be more effective than CHOP. Therefore, CHOP remains as the gold standard treatment in patients with DLBCL.

The management of elderly patients with DLBCL requires special consideration because of the increased risk of toxicity and death from treatment and disease. However, the results from two recent studies have challenged the role of CHOP given every 3 weeks as the standard of care for the elderly patients with DLBCL. A French study organised by Groupe d'Etude des Lymphomes de l'Adulte (GELA) investigated the addition of rituximab to CHOP,[32] whereas the German High Grade Non-Hodgkin's Lymphoma Study Group investigated dose-intensified CHOP by recycling CHOP at standard doses every 2 weeks with G-CSF support (CHOP-14).[33]

Rituximab is a chimeric anti-CD20 antibody containing human immunoglobulin G (IgG) lambda and kappa constant regions with murine variable regions. Rituximab and CHOP chemotherapy have non-overlapping toxic effects, with some evidence of in-vitro synergy. This combination has been tested in chemotherapy-naive or previously treated patients. A response rate of 95% has been reported in indolent B-cell lymphoma[34] and 94% in aggressive NHL.[35] In the GELA study, 400 patients aged 60–80 years old were randomly assigned to receive 8 cycles of CHOP every 3 weeks (197 patients) or 8 cycles of CHOP plus rituximab (202 patients).[32] CHOP and rituximab is associated with significantly better complete response rate (76% vs 63%; p = 0.005), event-free (p <0.001) and OS (p = 0.007) compared to CHOP alone. Although patients with low and high IPI appeared to benefit from the addition of rituximab to CHOP in this trial, patients with low IPI appeared to benefit more. No significant increase in adverse effects was seen with the addition of rituximab.

Another strategy to improve on the results of CHOP in aggressive NHL is through enhancing the intensity of chemotherapy. One approach to achieve this is to shorten the treatment intervals in an effective regimen. In the German NHL-B2 study, a full dose of cytotoxic drugs used in CHOP-21 is given at 14-day therapy interval (CHOP-14) with GCSF support.[33] Patients were randomly assigned to CHOP-21 (n = 152) or CHOP-14 (n = 153). The dose intensities for both cyclophosphamide and doxorubicin were 93%. Complete remission rate was significantly better for CHOP-14 compared with CHOP-21 (77% vs 63.2%; p = 0.009). This effect was particularly pronounced in patients with elevated LDH (70.4% vs 48.6%). Time to treatment failure and OS were significantly prolonged with CHOP-14 (p = 0.05 and p = 0.04, respectively). However, only 21% of patients in this trial had a high IPI (age-adjusted IPI 2 and 3) as opposed to 60% of patients in the GELA study.

Specific extranodal sites of disease may require special consideration. Certain disease sites constitute for high-risk CNS involvement, either at initial presentation or at relapse. These sites include orbital disease (43%), testes (40%), peripheral blood (33%), bone (29%), nasal/paranasal sinuses (23%) and bone marrow (20%). Cerebrospinal fluid (CSF) examination should be part of the staging for patients with these disease sites and prophylactic intrathecal chemotherapy should be given in conjunction with the initial chemotherapy and radiotherapy programme. (See also Ch. 2 for information regarding intrathecal chemotherapy.)

Salvage treatment Patients who do not go into complete remission with initial induction therapy or relapse at a later time need additional therapy for their NHL. The Parma trial has firmly established the role of high-dose chemotherapy followed by autologous bone marrow transplantation in patients with chemotherapy-sensitive relapsed NHL. Both event-free and overall survival were improved by high-dose chemotherapy.[36] IPI appears to correlate with survival in patients with aggressive lymphoma in relapse. Several randomised trials have tested the role of high-dose chemotherapy and autograft in patients in first remission.[37–39] It appears that benefits are confined in several subgroups:

- high risk or high intermediate risk patients, according to age-adjusted IPI
- patients who achieve at least a partial response

- patients who receive a full course as opposed to an abbreviated course of induction chemotherapy before autograft.

As supportive care for high-dose chemotherapy and stem cell transplantation improves, treatment-related mortality becomes less frequent. Currently, treatment-related mortality for autograft is less than 5%. An increasing number of patients are being considered for autograft and age is less frequently used as a sole discriminating factor.

For patients who are not candidates for transplantation, several salvage chemotherapy regimens have reported modest response rates, but poor long-term survival. Platinum-containing regimens such as DHAP (dexamethasone, cytarabine and cisplatin),[40] ESHAP (etoposide, methylprednisolone, cytarabine and cisplatin)[41] and EPIC (etoposide, prednisolone, ifosfamide and cisplatin/carboplatin)[42] were developed in the 1980s to be non-cross-resistant to doxorubicin-containing regimens used in front-line therapy. In one long-term follow-up study, DHAP produced a response rate (RR) of 43% in relapsed or primary refractory NHL patients, with median survival of 6 months and 3- and 5-year survival rates at 18% and 7%, respectively. ESHAP, on the other hand, produced an RR of 56% and median survival of 14 months with 3- and 5-year survival rates at 31% and 22%, respectively.[43]

Burkitt's and Burkitt–like lymphomas The most important issue about managing Burkitt's lymphoma is that it is among the most rapidly growing of human tumours. Some Burkitt-like lymphomas have a high, essentially 100%, proliferative index. The rapid growth rate is certainly the reason that patients with these tumours usually succumb within a matter of months if left untreated. This, coupled to the high rate of apoptosis, also explains the frequent complication of acute renal failure that is present at the time of diagnosis in patients with heavy tumour burdens. The extremely high sensitivity of these rapidly proliferative tumours to chemotherapy also results in a high potential for metabolic and renal problems in patients with substantial tumour burden.

Two important principles of managing Burkitt's and Burkitt-like lymphoma are:

1. Patients must be assessed as rapidly as possible, so that definitive therapy can be instituted at the earliest time.
2. During the initial few days of chemotherapy, careful management to avoid precipitation of acute oliguric renal failure is essential. The key to this is hydration and the use of allopurinol.

The primary therapeutic modality is combination chemotherapy. Adjuvant radiotherapy has not shown any additional advantages. Several clinical trials have demonstrated excellent overall results for children and adults with Burkitt's and Burkitt-like lymphomas. Many regimens have been developed from paediatric regimens. Multiple effective drugs (i.e. >5) are necessary to the achievement of such excellent results in all patients except those with the most limited disease.

CODOX-M (cyclophosphamide, vincristine, doxorubicin and high-dose methotrexate)/IVAC (ifosfamide, etoposide and high-dose cytarabine) is an alternating non-cross-resistant regimen developed at the National Cancer Institute (NCI) in the USA. In a multicentre study coordinated by NCI, involving 91 adults and children, high-risk patients (defined as either bulky disease ≥10 cm diameter, serum LDH ≥ 1× normal, Ann Arbor stage III or IV or performance status ≥1) were given 4 cycles of alternating CODOX-M and IVAC. Low-risk patients were given 3 cycles of CODOX-M only. An event-free survival (EFS) of 85% was achieved,[44-46] compared with 55% for those treated with CODOX-M alone.[44] No differences in the effectiveness of this therapy were seen between adults and children.[45] Relapses were rarely seen beyond 2 years. Notably, some patients (17%) in this study had large cell lymphoma and not Burkitt's lymphoma.

In another multicentre phase II study recruiting patients from the UK, Italy, Poland and Australasia, CODOX-M/IVAC produced an EFS of 69.2% and OS of 75% at 1 year.[47] Even for high-risk patients, the EFS was 65% and OS was 70% at 1 year. More encouragingly, no relapses or disease-related deaths occurred beyond 2 years.

The main toxicity seen with this regimen was neutropenia, although its duration was significantly shortened with the use of G-CSF. Duration of thrombocytopenia was also prolonged when G-CSF was used; 57% of patients experienced mild to severe peripheral neuropathy, more often seen in adults.[45] Interestingly, an unusual, acute onset, severe atypical neuropathy was evident, which was related to the use of colony-stimulating factors and cycle 1 (CODOX-M) cumulative vincristine dose. The majority of patients received GM-CSF (granulocyte–macrophage colony-stimulating factor).[48] This neuropathy was characterised by excruciating, constant pain confined to the lower limbs, especially the soles of the feet, accompanied by severe motor neuropathy.

With the high cure rate, long-term complications from this treatment regimen will need to be quantified. One hundred and sixty-two patients were treated with NCI protocols between 1973 and 1993. Of these patients, 103 received CODOX-M alone and 21

received alternating CODOX-M/IVAC (except those with limited or completely resected disease, where CODOX-M alone was given). Eighty-six patients were assessed for late effects of their treatment.[49] Left ventricular dysfunction was detected in 14% of patients and half of these patients were symptomatic. These patients had received a cumulative doxorubicin dose of 200–560 mg/m². Two patients (2.3%) developed a second cancer. Twenty-three patients reported pregnancies after completing therapy and 9 out of 18 men who showed azoospermia or oligospermia after therapy completion, later fathered children. Other observed major late effects, including seizures, leukomalacia, hypopituitarism, hypothyroidism and hypogonadism, followed irradiation. Radiotherapy contributed to the highest risk of late effects, with extensive surgery as the second most important risk factor. The results of this study showed that CODOX-M/IVAC has a much lower tendency to induce second malignancies or impair fertility than regimens used in Hodgkin's disease and suggest that chemotherapy alone is less likely to induce major late effects than combined modality therapy.

Similar efficacy results have been achieved with other short, intensive regimens. The French Pediatric Oncology Society developed a six-drug induction regimen based on high-dose fractionated cyclophosphamide, high-dose methotrexate and continuous infused cytarabine. In a randomised study of 216 children, EFS of 89% was seen with no difference in EFS between short (4 months) and long (7 months) course treatment.[50] When the identical or similar protocol was used in 65 adults, 3-year EFS of 71% and OS of 74% were seen.[51] Other regimens developed by the Berlin–Frankfurt–Munster (BFM) Group and NCI of Italy, again including high-dose methotrexate and intravenous/intrathecal cytarabine, produced EFS in excess of 80% in the paediatric population.[52,53] The schedule developed by the Italian NCI was only a short 45-day intensive treatment programme, with comparable results to other regimens.[52]

Intrathecal therapy is needed to prevent the development of CNS disease which, although uncommon at presentation, has a high likelihood of subsequent development in the absence of CNS prophylaxis. Therefore, everyone, except those with completely resected, small-volume gastrointestinal disease, should receive intrathecal drugs with cytarabine and methotrexate. No CNS irradiation has been shown to be effective in this setting, but RT adds to significant CNS toxicity in conjunction with high-dose S-phase agents.

Lymphoblastic lymphoma Lymphoblastic lymphoma is a very rapidly growing tumour, although the fraction of cells in the S phase is lower than that of

Burkitt's lymphoma. It frequently presents in the anterior superior mediastinum, with the potential for tracheal, bronchial or oesophageal obstruction, as well as the development of pleural and pericardial effusions. Therefore, it requires rapid assessment and early initiation of therapy.

Combination chemotherapy is the mainstay treatment and adjuvant radiation after an optimal chemotherapy regimen has not produced additional benefits. Response to therapy is almost universal, with many patients having a significant response to corticosteroid alone. In the paediatric population, patients with extensive lymphoblastic lymphoma have a better outcome when receiving treatment based on acute lymphoblastic lymphoma therapy such as the LSA_2L_2 protocol (Fig. 46.1) than patients treated with a 4-drug regimen containing cyclophosphamide, vincristine, prednisolone and methotrexate. In adult patients, many oncologists treat with drug combinations used for 'diffuse aggressive lymphomas': namely, CHOP or its variants. Results of treatment are considerably worse in adults than in children. However, these may not necessarily reflect the choice of drugs in the treatment regimen alone, but that adult patients may have a different spectrum of subtypes of lymphoblastic lymphoma. At our institution, we are currently using a modified LSA_2L_2 protocol with autologous transplantation for newly diagnosed lymphoblastic lymphoma.

Mantle cell lymphoma　Mantle cell lymphoma (MCL) seems to have the worst characteristics of aggressive and indolent lymphomas. The clinical course is fairly aggressive and the disease appears to be incurable with conventional therapy. The median survival time of patients with mantle cell lymphoma has ranged between 2.5 and 4 years in most series. However, these studies have only included small numbers of patients, as mantle cell lymphoma is relatively uncommon. Patients with mantle cell lymphoma have a pattern of continuous relapse after initial therapy, similar to that seen with low-grade lymphomas, but these relapses occur earlier than in low-grade lymphoma, with a pattern more similar to that of lymphoma of intermediate or high grade. There is no definite evidence of a significantly cured proportion. Although no survival advantage emerges from any chemotherapy regimens, CHOP is generally thought to be associated with better response rate. Furthermore, standard salvage chemotherapy regimens are not curative in the setting of relapse. Purine analogues, such as fludarabine, produced a response rate of 41% in patients with untreated MCL, which was not superior to CHOP or CVP (cyclophosphamide, vincristine and prednisolone)-like regimens.[54] Fludarabine only produced partial responses in recurrent disease and the responses are usually short-lived.

Several groups of investigators have used conventional chemotherapy regimens to induce a complete or partial response, and follow that response with further intensive chemotherapy and autologous stem cell rescue. However, as in management of many patients with follicular lymphomas, standard chemotherapy regimens do not often render the blood or bone marrow

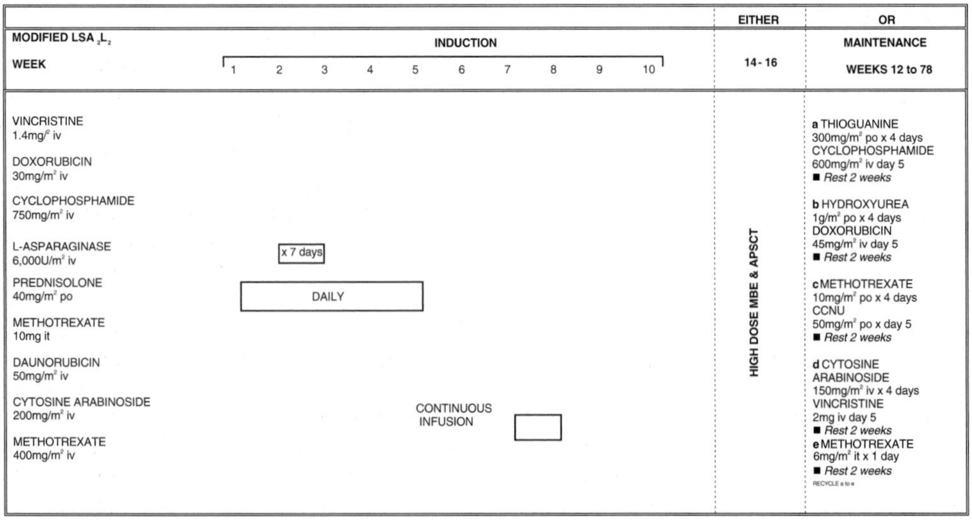

Figure 46.1　The LSA_2L_2 protocol: MBE = mephalan, BCNU and etoposide; APSCT = autologous peripheral stem cell transplantation; iv = intravenous; po = oral.

free of submicroscopic involvement by mantle cell lymphoma. Therefore, many patients who undergo high-dose chemotherapy with stem cell support have recurrence of the disease, because the patient's own stem cells are contaminated with malignant cells. Therefore, outside randomised clinical trials, the following strategy may be used:

- patients with localised disease may be treated with involved field RT
- elderly patients without adverse prognostic parameters may be treated with chlorambucil or CVP initially or after disease progression
- patients with adverse prognostic parameters should be treated with CHOP
- young patients may be treated with CHOP and consolidated with high-dose therapy and autologous stem cell transplantation in the event of good responses.

Rituximab has also been shown to induce a high response rate in MCL when combined with CHOP, but relapses are frequent as patients are not consolidated with high-dose chemotherapy.[55] Studies evaluating rituximab and CHOP followed by autograft have shown some early promising results.

Indolent non–Hodgkin's lymphoma

The largest category under indolent lymphomas is follicular lymphoma. Approximately 10–20% of patients have localised disease and these patients can be cured with irradiation alone. However, most patients with follicular lymphoma present with disseminated disease, including bone marrow involvement. However many patients can be asymptomatic at the time of diagnosis. Deferral of treatment or the 'watch and wait' policy in asymptomatic patients with extensive disease does not alter the survival of these patients. Conversely, the administration of intensive therapy from the outset may improve the disease-free survival but has not been shown to offer a survival advantage to date. A 'watch and wait' policy can be adopted unless patients have systemic symptoms, compromised vital organs, painful lymph nodes or bone marrow failure.

Chemotherapy

In induction chemotherapy, although improved response rates can be seen with more intensive regimens, no survival advantage has been demonstrated, so the most convenient and tolerable regimens should be used: i.e. single alkylating agents such as chlorambucil or CVP. Addition of doxorubicin (CHOP regimen), improves CR rates without influencing survival.

Purine nucleoside analogues such as fludarabine and cladribine have been evaluated extensively in indolent lymphoma. Both drugs can induce remission rates of between 70 and 80% in previously untreated patients with advanced stage follicular lymphoma. Fludarabine has been compared in a randomised trial with CVP. Although fludarabine resulted in higher complete and overall response rates compared with CVP, no progression-free or overall survival differences were seen. Fludarabine has also been combined with other drugs such as doxorubicin, mitoxantrone (mitozantrone), cyclophosphamide or steroids with encouraging response rates.

Biological therapy

Interferon   One of the therapeutic challenges of follicular lymphoma is to maintain remission; hence, various maintenance or consolidation therapies have been devised. Alpha-interferon (IFN) has been tested either in combination with cytotoxic drugs as induction therapy and/or used in isolation as maintenance therapy. As first-line treatment, addition of IFN to alkylating agents did not impact on outcome, whereas when added to CVP, an improvement of freedom from relapse was observed with IFN. When interferon was added to CHOP given as 4-weekly cycle, a prolonged time to treatment failure and disease-free survival was seen, but not a statistically significant difference in OS compared to CHOP alone.[56] Maintenance therapy with IFN has also been addressed in eight randomised trials. Overall, maintenance treatment in responding patients probably delays relapse. However, this needs to be balanced with tolerance to IFN and quality of life of the patients.[57]

Rituximab   Monoclonal antibodies target specific cellular populations based on the recognition of cell surface markers or antigens. Lymphomas present a natural target for antibody therapy because of their clonal nature. Once the antibody is injected, the recipient's own immune system is mobilised to exert a cytotoxic effect on the tumour cells via complement-dependent cytotoxicity and/or antibody-dependent, cell-mediated cytotoxicity. The CD20 antigen has been studied most widely. It is expressed on the cell surface in 90% of B-cell lymphomas. It is not shed into the circulation, nor does it circulate as a free protein.

Rituximab is used for treatment of patients with relapsed or refractory low-grade and follicular CD20+ B-cell lymphoma. A dose of 375 mg/m^2 rituximab given weekly for 4 weeks is now considered standard dose and schedule.[58] Response rate is between 40 and 60%, with a median duration of response of 6–8 months. More importantly, even patients who have been pretreated extensively with cytotoxic drugs, those who relapse after myeloablative chemotherapy and those with bulky disease can respond. Patients can also be retreated and still show a response. Of interest, the median time to progression for retreated patients can be considerably longer than those treated with first course of rituximab.[59] Therefore, prior treatment with rituximab does not induce resistance to subsequent treatment, nor does efficacy decline. Moreover, it may delay patients from receiving cytotoxic treatment, potentially reducing the risk of long-term complications such as myelodysplasia associated with alkylating agents.

Very few haematological toxic effects are associated with rituximab. Non-haematological toxicities are mainly infusion-associated, including fevers, asthenia, chills, rash, urticaria, bronchospasm, hypotension and dyspnoea. Infusion-related reactions can be treated with stopping the infusion, using paracetamol and H_1 antagonist, and reinstituting the infusion at a slower rate when symptoms subside. The infusion-related reaction appears to lessen substantially following the first cycle of treatment and no increased rate of infection or immunological compromise has been observed.

Rituximab plus chemotherapy Rituximab and CHOP chemotherapy have non-overlapping toxic effects, with some evidence of in-vitro synergy. This combination has been tested in chemotherapy-naive patients and a response rate of 95% has been reported.[34] Further randomised studies are being conducted comparing CHOP or CVP with or without rituximab in both high-grade and low-grade NHL.

Radiolabelled anti-CD20 monoclonal antibodies

Indolent lymphomas are known to be radiosensitive, and in limited-stage indolent lymphoma, external beam radiation can be a potentially curative treatment modality. The concept of radiolabelled antibodies is that the monoclonal antibody will guide to a specific target – i.e. the antigen that the antibody has been generated from – and minimise damage to healthy surrounding tissue. Two radiolabelled anti-CD20 monoclonal antibodies have reached advanced clinical development – yttrium-90 (Y-90) labelled ibritumomab and iodine-131 (I-131) labelled tositumomab.

Both Y-90 and I-131 emit beta radiation, which is discharged over 1–5 mm. In addition, I-131 emits gamma rays, which spread over several feet and through body tissues. This poses a risk to family members and healthcare professionals and may require hospitalisation. However, recent data suggest that I-131 tositumomab can be safely administered on an outpatient basis.[60] Y-90, however, is not useful for imaging; thus, ibritumomab needs to be conjugated to indium 111

(In-111) as a surrogate to determine biodistribution for calculating dosimetry and pharmacokinetics.

The treatment schedules of both radiolabelled antibodies can be characterised by a 'cold' phase and a 'hot' phase, separated by approximately 1 week. For ibritumomab, rituximab is typically given on days 1 and 8 with Y-90 ibritumomab given on day 8. For tositumomab, unlabelled or 'cold' tositumomab is given on day 1, then both cold and I-131 tositumomab are given on the same day, between days 8 and 14.

Y-90 ibritumomab has been tested in a randomised phase III trial against rituximab in patients with relapsed or refractory low-grade follicular, or transformed B-cell NHL. One hundred and forty-three patients were randomly assigned to receive a single dose of Y-90 ibritumomab 0.4 mCi/kg or rituximab 375 mg/m² weekly for four doses.[61] Statistically significant higher complete and overall response rates were seen with Y-90 ibritumomab. This did not translate to prolonged time to progression, although the study was powered to show difference in response rates only. In another study evaluating Y-90 ibritumomab in patients with follicular lymphoma refractory to rituximab, an objective response rate of 74% was found.[62] Subsequent chemotherapy regimens were also found to be well tolerated after Y-90 ibritumomab, even with autologous stem cell transplantation.[63]

Based on the fact that patients' duration of response becomes progressively shorter with each subsequent line of treatment for indolent lymphoma,[64] I-131 tositumomab was tested in a pivotal study in 60 patients using patients as their own control.[65] In this study, the median duration of response was significantly longer with I-131 toxitumomab compared to that seen after the individual patient's last chemotherapy regimen. I-131 tositumomab was concluded to be an efficacious treatment.

For both ibritumomab and tositumomab, the most common acute toxicity seen is infusion-related reaction similar to that seen with rituximab. However, the main toxicity seen with these radiolabelled anti-CD20 antibodies is haematological, especially thrombocytopenia. Patients included in their studies were required to have less than 25% of bone marrow involvement with lymphoma. Haematological toxicity tends to occur later than typically encountered with chemotherapy – approximately 5–7 weeks after treatment – and requires 2–4 weeks recovery. Potential long-term complications include myelodysplasia or acute leukaemia and hypothyroidism resulting from I-131 tositumomab. Although the incidences of myelodysplasia/ acute leukaemia in patients treated with radiolabelled anti-CD20 antibodies are no higher than anticipated in this patient population who has been multiply pretreated often with alkalyting agents, long-term monitoring will be required to accurately quantify the risk.

Mucosa–associated lymphoid tissue lymphoma

Mucosa-associated lymphoid tissue (MALT) lymphoma is included in the WHO classification as extranodal marginal zone B-cell lymphoma. It is positive for CD19, CD20 and CD22 and negative for CD5 and CD23. MALT lymphomas typically arise in the mucosal lymphoid tissue or glandular epithelium, such as the stomach, salivary glands, lungs or thyroid, with gastrointestinal tract involvement being the most common presentation. Bacterial infection with *Helicobacter pylori* is associated with 92% of gastric MALT lymphomas. MALT lymphoma is usually a very indolent disease and often remains localised for a prolonged period of time. Overall survival rates range from 80% to 95% at 5 years. Eradication of *H. pylori* with antibiotics and proton pump inhibitors can be used as the sole initial treatment for localised gastric MALT lymphomas. More interestingly, responses can be delayed as long as 18 months after completion of antibiotic therapy. Endoscopic and endosonographic surveillance is therefore required to document true response rates. In case of unsuccessful *H. pylori* eradication, a second-line anti-*Helicobacter* therapy should be attempted. Recurrence may occur either with or without *H. pylori* reinfection. No treatment guidelines exist for management of patients after antibiotics failure or in those where evidence of *H. pylori* infection has not been found. Chemotherapy with single agent chlorambucil has been tested, but efficacy data are scanty. Local radiotherapy has been used, although data are again lacking. Encouraging results, however, have been reported, with 100% biopsy-confirmed CR.[66] Rituximab has been evaluated by the International Extranodal Lymphoma Study Group, with a response rate of 73%.[67]

Outside the stomach, the most frequent sites of MALT lymphoma are in the head and neck region and ocular adnexa. Disseminated disease appears to be more common in non-gastrointestinal MALT lymphoma. However, despite presenting with stage IV disease in approximately 25% of cases, non-gastric MALT lymphoma usually has an indolent course, with a 5-year survival of about 90%. Optimal management in these patients remains to be defined and no survival advantage is apparent with any type of therapy.

NURSING CARE FOR PATIENTS WITH LYMPHOMA

Tracey Murray

INTRODUCTION

The term 'lymphoma' encompasses a hotchpotch of conditions with very different morphological appearance and behaviour and a clinical outcome that varies from a benign indolent course to a rapidly progressing disease with a prognosis from weeks to years.[68] Understanding the challenges associated with this diverse group such as the classification,[69,70] staging, molecular biology[71] and prognostic indices[72–74] will aid cancer nurses in providing the most up-to-date and accurate education to patients and their families regarding prognosis and treatment for this malignacy.[71]

IMPACT OF THE DIAGNOSIS AND TREATMENT ON THE PATIENT AND FAMILY

A diagnosis of any cancer arouses fear in many patients, with punitive notions of a 'fight' or 'crusade' against a 'killer' disease and of people becoming cancer 'victims'.[75] Accurate diagnosis and staging is essential if patients are to be given correct information that may help allay their fears, as cure is attainable for most patients with Hodgkin's disease and a considerable proportion of patients with high-grade NHL. However, for the large majority of patients with indolent or low-grade NHL, cure is currently not possible.[76]

Chemotherapy regimens and their associated side effects vary considerably between each of the lymphomas classified according to the WHO criteria.[69,70] Treatment may consist of 1-, 2-, 3- or 4-weekly intravenous chemotherapy, tablet-only chemotherapy, continuous infusions, antibody treatments and high-dose chemotherapy with peripheral blood stem cell return. The treatment pathway should be determined within a multidisciplinary team (MDT)[77,78] approach to care. This ensures that each team member applies specialised knowledge and skills collectively to provide quality care.[79]

Many cancer patients are admitted to hospital for the diagnosis and initial phase of their treatment and, once stabilised, manage their symptoms and ongoing treatment at home.[80] For most patients with lymphoma, however; diagnosis and treatment will both commence and continue in the outpatient setting. Outpatient-based treatment represents a model of care delivery, with the onus on the patient and family.[80] A central role of the cancer nurse caring for this group of patients is therefore to ensure that they are provided with the knowledge, skills and power to perform the role of an autonomous self-manager of their illness and its treatment.[80]

Alternatively, a small group of patients with more aggressive forms of lymphoma will require intensive chemotherapy that necessitates a protracted period of stay in hospital in an isolated environment. Campbell's study[81] demonstrated patients' concerns regarding their experience in the isolation environment of 'being shut in', 'coping with the experience', 'being alone' and 'maintaining contact with the outside world'. Patients within this study described 'developing relationships with health professionals' as an essential and positive part of the cancer experience. This illustrates the need for alternative levels of support and education compared to the patient receiving outpatient chemotherapy.

Lymphoma affects both males and females, and the older and younger age populations. Generalised potential side effects of chemotherapy will be similar for all groups, but to the individual patient there will be an enhanced emphasis on some side effects. Hence, holistic assessment, patient-centred care planning and astute anticipation of potential untoward effects of treatment for each individual comprise a central role for the nurse.[82]

HOLISTIC ASSESSMENT OF THE PATIENT WITH LYMPHOMA

Cure rates and long-term survival in this patient population is high; however, this is counterbalanced by the administration of treatment that is often more aggressive than the chemotherapy treatment for other cancer diagnoses.[83] The impact of the diagnosis and treatment for this patient group is likely to affect their quality of life (QOL) in all four domains of physical, psychological, social and spiritual well-being and may include some of the following factors.

Physical effects

Short-term side effects are likely to include nausea and vomiting, fatigue, alopecia, peripheral neuropathy, gastrointestinal disturbances and lowering of the blood counts. Long-term side effects such as second malignancies,[84,85] infertility and sexuality problems[86,87] and pulmonary and cardiac toxicity[88] will need serious consideration when decisions are made regarding treatment choices. Cure rates have improved greatly over the past decade and the emphasis on current

treatment and clinical trials is to try and reduce the impact of these side effects while maintaining a positive outcome.

Psychological effects

Psychological effects may include anxiety and depression, caused by the impact of the disease and treatment and its intrusion upon normal lifestyles; drug therapy, such as steroids; and fear of recurrence when treatment is completed.[85,88]

Social effects

The impact of attending the hospital for treatment and its impending effects, such as fatigue, protection from infection (including avoiding crowded places) and changes in diet and eating habits, are all likely to impact on the individual's attendance at school, university or work, relationships with friends and partners and leisure-time activities. This may lead to further psychological distress from isolation, loneliness and anxiety related to financial worries.[85,88,89]

Spiritual effects

The most poorly assessed of the four domains of QOL,[90] spiritual distress may be characterised by questioning one's faith or whole outlook on life,

Table 46.7 Strategies to improve the patient's quality of life (QOL)

QOL domian	Services the lymphoma patient on chemotherapy may require to maintain QOL
Physical	Wig specialist; assessment for appropriate intravenous access, i.e. cannula or indwelling central venous device; physiotherapist; occupational therapist; district nurse; oral hygienist; social services; massage and relaxation; symptom control
Psychological	Psychiatrist/counsellor; support groups; massage and relaxation therapy; 'look good feel better'; Patient Advice and Liaison Support (PALS)
Social	Social services/benefits agency; pharmacy for pre-paid prescription forms; support group; PALS; 'look good feel better'; wig specialist; dietician
Spiritual	Hospital chaplain/priest; psychological support/counselling; massage and relaxation; support groups

relationships with others, a need to give and receive love, having hope and living with a cancer diagnosis.[89,90]

STRATEGIES TO IMPROVE QUALITY OF LIFE

Side effects of chemotherapy will vary, depending on the regimen being administered. The nurse will need a sound knowledge base of the different regimens used in order to ensure that the patient is fully aware of the potential side effects of the treatment. This will allow education and initiation of preventative strategies such as antiemetics, fertility preservation, tumour lysis syndrome prevention and oral hygiene and will ensure the patient is fully informed to consent to the treatment and is prepared for the role of self-manager of their care.

The nurse's role is pivotal in assessing all aspects of QOL for the individual, resulting in a personalised plan of care. This central role as a member of the MDT ensures appropriate referral to other services that enable all four domains of the patients QOL to be cared for (Table 46.7).

SURVIVING AFTER CHEMOTHERAPY IS COMPLETED

Survivorship studies highlight that the impact of the disease and its treatment does not stop with remission or cure but can continue for the foreseeable future.[83,85,88,89,91] Patients often feel more vulnerable and anxious when treatment is discontinued, as fear of recurrence becomes a more prominent issue and continuing symptoms are a reminder of the disease process. The cancer nurse caring for this patient group must be aware that these patients continue to require assessment, support and holistic care management in order that they do not feel abandoned when treatment is completed.[92]

References

1. Office for National Statistics. Cancer survival trends in England & Wales 1971–1995. Office for National Statistics; 1999.

2. Ferlay J, Bray F, Pisani P, et al. GLOBOCAN 2000 – Cancer incidence, mortality and prevalence worldwide, Version 1.0. IARC CancerBase No.5, Lyon: IARC Press; 2001.

3. Jaffe ES, Harris NL, Stein H, et al. World Health Organization classification of tumours. Pathology & genetics of tumours of haematopoietic and lymphoid tissues. WHO; 2001.

4. Lister TA, Crowther D, Sutcliffe SB, et al. Report of a committee convened to discuss the evaluation and staging of patients with Hodgkin's disease: Cotswolds meeting. J Clin Oncol 1989; 7:1630–1636.

5. Specht L, Gray RG, Clarke MJ, et al. Influence of more extensive radiotherapy and adjuvant chemotherapy on long-term outcome of early-stage Hodgkin's disease: a meta-analysis of 23 randomized trials involving 3,888 patients. International Hodgkin's Disease Collaborative Group. J Clin Oncol 1998; 16:830–843.

6. Rueda A, Alba E, Ribelles N, et al. Six cycles of ABVD in the treatment of stage I and II Hodgkin's lymphoma: a pilot study. J Clin Oncol 1997; 15:1118–1122.

7. Longo DL, Young RC, Wesley M, et al. Twenty years of MOPP therapy for Hodgkin's disease. J Clin Oncol 1986; 4:1295–1306.

8. Bonadonna G, Zucali R, Monfardini S, et al. Combination chemotherapy of Hodgkin's disease with adriamycin, bleomycin, vinblastine, and imidazole carboxamide versus MOPP. Cancer 1975; 36: 252–259.

9. Bonadonna G, Valagussa P, Santoro A. Alternating non-cross-resistant combination chemotherapy or MOPP in stage IV Hodgkin's disease. A report of 8-year results. Ann Intern Med 1986; 104:739–746.

10. Canellos GP, Anderson JR, Propert KJ, et al. Chemotherapy of advanced Hodgkin's disease with MOPP, ABVD, or MOPP alternating with ABVD. N Engl J Med 1992; 327:1478–1484.

11. Canellos GP, Niedzwiecki D. Long-term follow-up of Hodgkin's disease trial. N Engl J Med 2002; 346:1417–1418.

12. Duggan DB, Petroni GR, Johnson JL, et al. Randomized comparison of ABVD and MOPP/ABV hybrid for the treatment of advanced Hodgkin's disease: report of an Intergroup Trial. J Clin Oncol 2003; 21:607–614.

13. Diehl V, Franklin J, Paulus U, et al. BEACOPP chemotherapy with dose escalation in advanced Hodgkin's disease: final analysis of the German Hodgkin lymphoma study group HD9 randomized trial. Blood 2001; 98:3202.

14. Horning SJ, Williams J, Bartlett NL, et al. Assessment of the Stanford V regimen and consolidative radiotherapy for bulky and advanced Hodgkin's disease: Eastern Cooperative Oncology Group pilot study E1492. J Clin Oncol 2000; 18:972–980.

15. Horning SJ, Hoppe RT, Breslin S, et al. Stanford V and radiotherapy for locally extensive and advanced Hodgkin's disease: mature results of a prospective clinical trial. J Clin Oncol 2002; 20:630–637.

16. Loeffler M, Brosteanu O, Hasenclever D, et al. Meta-analysis of chemotherapy versus combined modality treatment trials in Hodgkin's disease. International Database on Hodgkin's Disease Overview Study Group. J Clin Oncol 1998; 16: 818–829.

17. Linch DC, Winfield D, Goldstone AH, et al. Dose intensification with autologous bone-marrow transplantation

in relapsed and resistant Hodgkin's disease: results of a BNLI randomised trial. Lancet 1993; 341:1051–1054.

18. Schmitz N, Pfistner B, Sextro M, et al. Aggressive conventional chemotherapy compared with high-dose chemotherapy with autologous haemopoietic stem-cell transplantation for relapsed chemosensitive Hodgkin's disease: a randomised trial. Lancet 2002; 359:2065–2071.

19. Aisenberg AC. Problems in Hodgkin's disease management. Blood 1999; 93:761–779.

20. Hoppe RT. Hodgkin's disease: complications of therapy and excess mortality. Ann Oncol 1997; 8(Suppl 1):115–118.

21. Mauch PM, Kalish LA, Marcus KC, et al. Long-term survival in Hodgkin's disease. Cancer J Sci Am 1995; 1:33.

22. Williams SF, Golomb HM. Perspective on staging approaches in the malignant lymphomas. Surg Gynecol Obstet 1986; 163:193–201.

23. Hasenclever D, Diehl V. A prognostic score for advanced Hodgkin's disease. International Prognostic Factors Project on Advanced Hodgkin's Disease. N Engl J Med 1998; 339:1506–1514.

24. Harris NL, Jaffe ES, Stein H, et al. A revised European–American classification of lymphoid neoplasms: a proposal from the International Lymphoma Study Group. Blood 1994; 84:1361–1392.

25. Rosenberg SA, Berard CW, Brown BW, et al. National Cancer Institute sponsored study of classifications of non-Hodgkin's lymphomas: summary and description of a working formulation for clinical usage. The Non-Hodgkin's Lymphoma Pathologic Classification Project. Cancer 1982; 49:2112–2135.

26. Armitage JO, Weisenburger DD. New approach to classifying non-Hodgkin's lymphomas: clinical features of the major histologic subtypes. Non-Hodgkin's Lymphoma Classification Project. J Clin Oncol 1998; 16:2780–2795.

27. The International Non-Hodgkin's Lymphoma Prognostic Factors Project. A predictive model for aggressive non-Hodgkin's lymphoma. N Engl J Med 1993; 329:987–994.

28. Miller TP, Dahlberg S, Cassady JR, et al. Chemotherapy alone compared with chemotherapy plus radiotherapy for localized intermediate- and high-grade non-Hodgkin's lymphoma. N Engl J Med 1998; 339:21–26.

29. Miller TP, LeBlanc M, Spier C, et al. CHOP alone compared to CHOP plus radiotherapy for early stage aggressive non-Hodgkin's lymphomas: update of the Southwest Oncology Group (SWOG) randomized trial. Blood 2001; 98:3024.

30. Horning SJ, Glick JH, Kim K, et al. Final report of E1484: CHOP v CHOP plus radiotherapy (RT) for limited stage diffuse aggressive lymphoma. Blood 2001; 98:3023.

31. Fisher RI, Gaynor ER, Dahlberg S, et al. Comparison of a standard regimen (CHOP) with three intensive chemotherapy regimens for advanced non-Hodgkin's lymphoma. N Engl J Med 1993; 328:1002–1006.

32. Coiffier B, Lepage E, Briere J, et al. CHOP chemotherapy plus rituximab compared with CHOP alone in elderly patients with diffuse large-B-cell lymphoma. N Engl J Med 2002; 346:235–242.

33. Pfreundschuh M, Trumper L, Kloess M, et al. 2-weekly chop (CHOP-14): the new standard regimen for patients with aggressive non-Hodgkin's lymphoma (NHL) > 60 years of age. Blood 2001; 98:3027.

34. Czuczman MS, Grillo-Lopez AJ, White CA, et al. Treatment of patients with low-grade B-cell lymphoma with the combination of chimeric anti-CD20 monoclonal antibody and CHOP chemotherapy. J Clin Oncol 1999; 17:268–276.

35. Vose JM, Link BK, Grossbard ML, et al. Phase II study of rituximab in combination with CHOP chemotherapy in patients with previously untreated, aggressive non-Hodgkin's lymphoma. J Clin Oncol 2001; 19:389–397.

36. Philip T, Guglielmi C, Hagenbeek A, et al. Autologous bone marrow transplantation as compared with salvage chemotherapy in relapses of chemotherapy-sensitive non-Hodgkin's lymphoma. N Engl J Med 1995; 333:1540–1545.

37. Gisselbrecht C, Lepage E, Molina T, et al. Shortened first-line high-dose chemotherapy for patients with poor-prognosis aggressive lymphoma. J Clin Oncol 2002; 20:2472–2479.

38. Haioun C, Lepage E, Gisselbrecht C, et al. Survival benefit of high-dose therapy in poor-risk aggressive non-Hodgkin's lymphoma: final analysis of the prospective LNH87-2 protocol – a groupe d'Etude des lymphomes de l'Adulte study. J Clin Oncol 2000; 18:3025–3030.

39. Santini G, Salvagno L, Leoni P, et al. VACOP-B versus VACOP-B plus autologous bone marrow transplantation for advanced diffuse non-Hodgkin's lymphoma: results of a prospective randomized trial by the non-Hodgkin's Lymphoma Cooperative Study Group. J Clin Oncol 1998; 16:2796–2802.

40. Velasquez WS, Cabanillas F, Salvador P, et al. Effective salvage therapy for lymphoma with cisplatin in combination with high-dose Ara-C and dexamethasone (DHAP). Blood 1988; 71:117–122.

41. Velasquez WS, McLaughlin P, Tucker S, et al. ESHAP – an effective chemotherapy regimen in refractory and relapsing lymphoma: a 4-year follow-up study. J Clin Oncol 1994; 12:1169–1176.

42. Hickish T, Roldan A, Cunningham D, et al. EPIC: an effective low toxicity regimen for relapsing lymphoma. Br J Cancer 1993; 68:599–604.

43. Rodriguez-Monge EJ, Cabanillas F. Long-term follow-up of platinum-based lymphoma salvage regimens. The M.D. Anderson Cancer Center experience. Hematol Oncol Clin North Am 1997; 11:937–947.

44. Bishop PC, Rao VK, Wilson WH. Burkitt's lymphoma: molecular pathogenesis and treatment. Cancer Invest 2000; 18:574–583.

45. Adde M, Shad A, Venzon D, et al. Additional chemotherapy agents improve treatment outcome for children and adults with advanced B-cell lymphomas. Semin Oncol 1998; 25:33–39.

46. Magrath I, Adde M, Shad A, et al. Adults and children with small non-cleaved-cell lymphoma have a similar excellent outcome when treated with the same chemotherapy regimen. J Clin Oncol 1996; 14:925–934.

47. Mead GM, Sydes MR, Walewski J, et al. An international evaluation of CODOX-M and CODOX-M alternating with IVAC in adult Burkitt's lymphoma: results of United Kingdom Lymphoma Group LY06 study. Ann Oncol 2002; 13:1264–1274.

48. Weintraub M, Adde MA, Venzon DJ, et al. Severe atypical neuropathy associated with administration of hematopoietic colony-stimulating factors and vincristine. J Clin Oncol 1996; 14:935–940.

49. Haddy TB, Adde MA, McCalla J, et al. Late effects in long-term survivors of high-grade non-Hodgkin's lymphomas. J Clin Oncol 1998; 16:2070–2079.

50. Patte C, Philip T, Rodary C, et al. High survival rate in advanced-stage B-cell lymphomas and leukemias without CNS involvement with a short intensive polychemotherapy: results from the French Pediatric Oncology Society of a randomized trial of 216 children. J Clin Oncol 1991; 9:123–132.

51. Soussain C, Patte C, Ostronoff M, et al. Small non-cleaved cell lymphoma and leukemia in adults. A retrospective study of 65 adults treated with the LMB pediatric protocols. Blood 1995; 85:664–674.

52. Spreafico F, Massimino M, Luksch R, et al. Intensive, very short-term chemotherapy for advanced Burkitt's lymphoma in children. J Clin Oncol 2002; 20:2783–2788.

53. Reiter A, Schrappe M, Parwaresch R, et al. Non-Hodgkin's lymphomas of childhood and adolescence: results of a treatment stratified for biologic subtypes and stage – a report of the Berlin–Frankfurt–Munster Group. J Clin Oncol 1995; 13:359–372.

54. Foran JM, Rohatiner AZ, Coiffier B, et al. Multicenter phase II study of fludarabine phosphate for patients with newly diagnosed lymphoplasmacytoid lymphoma, Waldenstrom's macroglobulinemia, and mantle-cell lymphoma. J Clin Oncol 1999; 17:546–553.

55. Howard OM, Gribben JG, Neuberg DS, et al. Rituximab and CHOP induction therapy for newly diagnosed mantle-cell lymphoma: molecular complete responses are not predictive of progression-free survival. J Clin Oncol 2002; 20:1288–1294.

56. Smalley RV, Weller E, Hawkins MJ, et al. Final analysis of the ECOG I-COPA trial (E6484) in patients with non-Hodgkin's lymphoma treated with interferon alfa (IFN-alpha2a) plus an anthracycline-based induction regimen. Leukemia 2001; 15:1118–1122.

57. Soubeyran P, Debled M, Tchen N, et al. Follicular lymphomas – a review of treatment modalities. Crit Rev Oncol Hematol 2000; 35:13–32.

58. McLaughlin P, Grillo-Lopez AJ, Link BK, et al. Rituximab chimeric anti-CD20 monoclonal antibody therapy for relapsed indolent lymphoma: half of patients respond to a four-dose treatment program. J Clin Oncol 1998; 16:2825–2833.

59. Davis TA, Grillo-Lopez AJ, White CA, et al. Rituximab anti-CD20 monoclonal antibody therapy in non-Hodgkin's lymphoma: safety and efficacy of re-treatment. J Clin Oncol 2000; 18:3135–3143.

60. Rutar FJ, Augustine SC, Kaminski MS, et al. Feasibility and safety of outpatient Bexxar therapy (tositumomab and iodine I 131 tositumomab) for non-Hodgkin's lymphoma based on radiation doses to family members. Clin Lymphoma 2001; 2:164–172.

61. Witzig TE, Gordon LI, Cabanillas F, et al. Randomized controlled trial of yttrium-90-labeled ibritumomab tiuxetan radioimmunotherapy versus rituximab immunotherapy for patients with relapsed or refractory low-grade, follicular, or transformed B-cell non-Hodgkin's lymphoma. J Clin Oncol 2002; 20:2453–2463.

62. Witzig TE, Flinn IW, Gordon LI, et al. Treatment with ibritumomab tiuxetan radioimmunotherapy in patients with rituximab-refractory follicular non-Hodgkin's lymphoma. J Clin Oncol 2002; 20:3262–3269.

63. Ansell SM, Ristow KM, Habermann TM, et al. Subsequent chemotherapy regimens are well tolerated after radioimmunotherapy with yttrium-90 ibritumomab tiuxetan for non-Hodgkin's lymphoma. J Clin Oncol 2002; 20:3885–3890.

64. Gallagher CJ, Gregory WM, Jones AE, et al. Follicular lymphoma: prognostic factors for response and survival. J Clin Oncol 1986; 4:1470–1480.

65. Kaminski MS, Zelenetz AD, Press OW, et al. Pivotal study of iodine I 131 tositumomab for chemotherapy-refractory low-grade or transformed low-grade B-cell non-Hodgkin's lymphomas. J Clin Oncol 2001; 19:3918–3928.

66. Schechter NR, Portlock CS, Yahalom J. Treatment of mucosa-associated lymphoid tissue lymphoma of the stomach with radiation alone. J Clin Oncol 1998; 16:1916–1921.

67. Conconi A, Thieblemont C, Martinelli G, et al. IELSG phase II study of rituximab in MALT lymphomas. Ann Oncol 2002; 13:81.

68. Mounter PJ, Lennard AL. Management of non-Hodgkin's lymphomas. Postgrad Med J 1999; 75:2–6.

69. Harris NL, Jaffe ES, Diebold J, et al. World Health Organisation classification of neoplastic diseases of the hematopoietic and lymphoid tissues: report of the Clinical Advisory Committee Meeting – Airlie House, Virginia, November 1997. J Clin Oncol 1999; 17(120):3835–3849.

70. Jaffe ES, Harris NL, Diebold, J et al. World Health Organization classification of neoplastic diseases of the hematopoietic and lymphoid tissues. A progress report. Am J Clin Pathol 1999; 111(Suppl 1):S8–S12.

71. Engstrom CA, Sarkodee-Adoo C. The molecular biology of lymphoma. Semin Oncol Nurs 1998; 14(4):256–261.

72. Shipp MA, Harrington DP, Anderson JR, et al. The non-Hodgkin's lymphoma prognostic factors project: a predictive model for aggressive non-Hodgkin's lymphoma. N Engl J Med 1993; 329(14):987–994.

73. Carde P, Hagenbeek A, Hayat M, et al. Clinical staging versus laparotomy and combined modality MOPP versus ABVD in early stage Hodgkin's disease; the H6 Twin Randomized Trials from the European Organization for Research and Treatment of Cancer Lymphoma Cooperative Group. J Clin Oncol 1993; 11:2258–2272.

74. Hasenclever D, Diehl V. A prognostic score for advanced Hodgkin's disease. N Engl J Med 1998; 339(21):1506–1514.

75. Sontang S. Illness as a metaphor aids and its metaphor. London: Penguin; 1991.

76. Voliotis D, Diehl V. Challenges in treating hematologic malignancies. Semin Oncol 2002; 29(3 Suppl 8):30–39.

77. Department of Health. The NHS Cancer Plan. London: HMSO; 2000.

78. Department of Health. Manual of Cancer Services Assessment Standards Consultation Document; 2000.

79. Krcmar CR. Cancer nursing as a speciality. In: Kearney N, Richardson A, Di Giulio P, eds. Cancer nursing practice: a textbook for the specialist nurse. London: Harcourt; 2000:1–18.

80. Ream E. Information for patients and families. In: Kearney N, Richardson A, Di Giulio P, eds. Cancer nursing practice: a textbook for the specialist nurse. London: Harcourt; 2000:135–160.

81. Campbell T. Feelings of oncology patients about being nursed in protective isolation as a consequence of cancer chemotherapy treatment. J Adv Nurs 1999; 30(2):439–447.

82. Boyle DA, Angert VJ. Lymphoma at the extremes of age. Semin Oncol Nurs 1998; 14(4):302–311.

83. Persson L, Hallberg IR. Acute leukaemia or highly malignant lymphoma patients' quality of life over two years: a pilot study Eur J Cancer Care 2001; 10:36–47.

84. Swerdlow AJ, Barber JA, Vaughan Hudson G, et al. Risk of second malignancy after Hodgkin's disease in a collaborative British cohort: the relation to age at treatment. J Clin Oncol 2000; 18(3):498–509.

85. Fernsler J, Fanuele J. Lymphomas: long-term sequelae and survivorship issues. Oncol Nurs Forum 1998; 14(4):321–328.

86. Schover LR. Sexuality and fertility after cancer. New York: John Wiley; 1997.

87. Thaler-DeMers D. Intimacy issues: sexuality, fertility and relationships. Semin Oncol Nurs 2001; 17(4):255–262.

88. Ganz PA. Late effects of cancer and its treatment. Semin Oncol Nurs 2001;17(4):241–248.

89. Ferrell BR, Dow KH, Leigh S, et al. Quality of life in long-term cancer survivors. Oncol Nurs Forum 1995; 22(60):915–922.

90. Pennell M, Corner J. Palliative care and cancer. In: Corner J, Bailey C, eds. Cancer nursing care in context. Oxford: Blackwell Science; 2001:527–529.

91. Wallwork L, Richardson A. Beyond cancer: changes, problems and needs expressed by adult lymphoma survivors attending an out-patients clinic. Eur J Cancer Care 1994; 3:122–132.

92. Mullan F. Seasons of survival: reflections of a physician with cancer. N Engl J Med 1985; 313(4): 270–273.

Appendix 1   Drug regimens for Hodgkin's disease

Drug regimen	Recommended dose (mg/m^2)	Route	Days
MOPP			
Mechlorethamine	6	IV	1,8
Vincristine	1.4	IV	1,8
Procarbazine	100	Oral	1–14
Prednisolone	40	Oral	1–14
Repeated on day 29			
COPP			
Cyclophosphamide	650	IV	1,8
Vincristine	1.4	IV	1,8
Procarbazine	100	Oral	1–14
Prednisolone	40	Oral	1–14
Repeated on day 29			
ChlVPP			
Chlorambucil	6	Oral	1–14
Vinblastine	6	IV	1,8
Procarbazine	100	Oral	1–14
Prednisolone	40	Oral	1–14
Repeated on day 29			
ABVD			
Doxorubicin	25	IV	1,15
Bleomycin	10,000 iu	IV	1,15
Vinblastine	6	IV	1,15
Dacarbazine	375	IV	1,15
Repeated on day 29			
VEEP			
Vincristine	1.4	IV	1,8
Epirubicin	50	IV	1
Etoposide	200 or	Oral	1–4
	100	IV	1–4
Prednisolone	100	Oral	1–8
Repeated on day 22			
Stanford V			
Doxorubicin	25	IV	1,15
Vinblastine	6	IV	1,15
Mechlorethamine	6	IV	1
Vincristine	1.4	IV	8,22
Bleomycin	5000 iu	IV	8,22
Etoposide	60	IV	15,16
Prednisolone	40	Oral	alt.days for 12 weeks[a]
Repeated on day 29			
BEACOPP (basic)			
Bleomycin	10,000 iu	IV	8
Etopside	100	IV	1–3
Doxorubicin	25	IV	1
Cyclophosphamide	650	IV	1
Vincristine	1.4	IV	8

Continued

Appendix 1   Drug regimens for Hodgkin's disease—cont'd

Drug regimen	Recommended dose (mg/m²)	Route	Days
Procarbazine	100	Oral	1–7
Prednisone	40	Oral	1–14
Repeated on day 22			
BEACOPP (escalated)			
Bleomycin	10,000 iu	IV	8
Etoposide	200	IV	1–3
Doxorubicin	35	IV	1
Cyclophosphamide	1200	IV	1
Vincristine	1.4	IV	1
Procarbazine	100	Oral	1–7
Prednisolone	40	Oral	1–14
Repeated on day 22			

[a]Tapered by 10 mg alternate days starting at week 10.

Appendix 2   Drug regimens for Non-Hodgkin's lymphoma

Drug regimen	Recommended dose (mg/m²)	Route	Days
Chlorambucil	10 mg od (fixed dose)	Oral	1–14
Repeated on day 29			
High-dose methylprednisolone	1.5 g od (fixed dose)	Oral	1–5
Repeated on day 29			
CVP			
Cyclophosphamide	750	IV	1
Vincristine	1.4	IV	1
Prednisolone	10	Oral	1–5
Repeated on day 22			
CHOP			
Cyclophosphamide	750	IV	1
Doxorubicin	50	IV	1
Vincristine	1.4	IV	1
Prednisolone	100 mg (fixed dose)	Oral	1–5
Repeated on day 22			
PMitCEBOM			
Prednisolone	50 mg (fixed dose)	Oral	1–14 (alternate days from week 5)
Cyclophosphamide	300	IV	1
Mitoxantrone (mitozantrone)	7	IV	1
Etoposide	150	IV	1
Bleomycin	10,000 iu	IV	8
Vincristine	1.4	IV	8
Methotrexate	100	IV	8
Repeated on day 15			

Appendix 2   Drug regimens for Non-Hodgkin's lymphoma—cont'd

Drug regimen	Recommended dose (mg/m²)	Route	Days
PACEBOM			
Prednisolone	50	Oral	1–14 (alternate days from week 5)
Cyclophosphamide	300	IV	1
Doxorubicin	35	IV	1
Etoposide	150	IV	1
Bleomycin	10,000 iu	IV	8
Vincristine	1.4	IV	8
Methotrexate	100	IV	8
Repeated on day 15			
EPIC			
Etoposide	100	IV	1–4
Prednisolone	100 mg (fixed dose)	Oral	1–5
Ifosfamide	1000	IV	1–5
Cisplatin	60	IV	10
Repeated on day 22			
DHAP			
Dexamethasone	40 mg (fixed dose)	Oral/IV	1–4
Cytarabine	2000	IV	2
Cisplatin	100	IV	1
Repeated on day 22 or 29			
FAD			
Fludarabine	25	IV	1–3
Doxorubicin	50	IV	1
Dexamethasone	20	Oral/IV	1–5
Repeated on day 29			
FMD			
Fludarabine	25	IV	1–3
Mitoxantrone (mitozantrone)	10	IV	1
Dexamethasone	20	Oral/IV	1–5
Repeated on day 29			
MACOP-B			
Methotrexate	400	IV	8,36,64
Doxorubicin	50	IV	1,15,29,43.57,71
Cyclophosphamide	350	IV	1,15,29,43.57,71
Vincristine	1.4	IV	8,22,36,50,64,78
Bleomycin	10,000 iu	IV	22,50,78
Prednisolone	60 mg (fixed dose)	Oral	1–70 then taper
DexaBEAM			
Dexamethasone	8 mg tds	Oral	1–10
BCNU	60	IV	2
Etoposide	75	IV	4–7
Cytarabine	200	IV	4–7
Melphalan	20	IV	3
Repeated on day 29			

Continued

Appendix 2   Drug regimens for Non-Hodgkin's lymphoma—cont'd

Drug regimen	Recommended dose (mg/m^2)	Route	Days
MiniBEAM			
BCNU	60	IV	1
Etoposide	75	IV	2–5
Cytarabine	200	IV	2–5
Mephalan	30	IV	6
Repeated after haematological recovery			
CODOX-M/IVAC			
Cycle A			
Cyclophosphamide	800	IV	1
	200	IV	2–5
Vincristine	1.5	IV	1,8,15
Doxorubicin	40	IV	1
Methotrexate	1.2 g	IV	10
Cytarabine	70 mg (fixed dose)	IT	1,3,(5)
Methotrexate	12 mg (fixed dose)	IT	15,(17)
Cycle B			
Ifosfamide	1.5	IV	1–5
Etoposide	60	IV	1–5
Cytarabine	4g	IV	1–2
Methotrexate	12	IT	5
Cytarabine	70	IT	(7,9)
			() additional IT therapy if CNS involvement

Chapter 47

Myeloma and the acute and chronic leukaemias

CHAPTER CONTENTS

MEDICAL CARE FOR PATIENTS WITH LEUKAEMIA

Jennifer Treleaven

ACUTE MYELOID LEUKAEMIA

Acute myeloid leukaemia (AML) is a heterogeneous, malignant disorder of the haemopoietic cells – those which give rise to cells found in the blood (red cells, white cells and platelets). The incidence rises with age, from 1 case per 100 000 individuals per year in childhood to 10/100 000/year in those over 70 years old; more than 50% of cases arise in people over the age of 60 years old and age is in itself a poor prognostic factor.

AML can be divided into seven main categories based on microscopic appearances (morphology) and the appearances when certain special stains are applied (cytochemistry; Sudan black, PAS (periodic acid–Schiff), etc.), as proposed by the French, American and British (FAB) group in 1976[1] (Box 47.1). More recently, immunophenotyping (classification of cells by the presence or absence of various surface antigens) and cytogenetics (presence or absence of certain chromosomal abnormalities) have allowed further identification and subclassification of leukaemia cells. Some of these subtypes may be associated with a particularly poor or particularly good outcome after chemotherapy alone. M5 (monoblastic leukaemia), for example, is associated with the presence of extramedullary disease and gum hypertrophy, which may represent an increased tumour load and hence render the disease less sensitive to the effects of chemotherapy. Other subtypes, for example M3 (promyelocytic leukaemia), are associated with a more favourable outcome, and in some series up to 90% of patients attain remission and more than 50% are disease-free 5 years from diagnosis after chemotherapy alone or after all-*trans* retinoic acid (ATRA) and chemotherapy, provided that they do not succumb to the problems associated with diffuse intravascular coagulation, which may occur during remission induction.[2,3]

The use of a stem cell transplantation procedure, which may be associated with a relatively high morbidity and mortality particularly in the allogeneic setting, is therefore usually not indicated for this particular subgroup of AML patients, and tends to be reserved for patients likely to have a particularly poor outlook with conventional therapy. Overall, however, the FAB classification has not been found to be significantly useful as a predictive factor for outcome after chemotherapy alone, or with allogeneic transplantation. However, cell surface immunophenotype and cytogenetic features may be of use to define the very poor risk leukaemias. For example, presence of both lymphoid and myeloid markers may be associated with a poorer outcome after treatment, as is the presence of abnormalities of chromosomes 5 and 7 (Box 47.2). In such cases, patients may lack any normal stem cells, and allogeneic stem cell transplantation may represent the only chance of effecting long-term disease-free survival.

Treatment of acute myeloid leukaemia

Overall, of patients aged 15–59 years old who entered a chemotherapy-only clinical trial in the mid to late 1990s, more than 50% were alive after 3 years, and 70–80% of those under 60 years old entered remission. Similar results were seen in children with AML.[4]

There have been few major changes in induction chemotherapy strategies over the past decade, and the best post-induction therapy for AML is yet to be clearly defined. However, over the years doses of the cytotoxic agents commonly used have been escalated, and cytotoxic drugs have been given in various combinations, which have resulted in more successful disease eradication. In the UK, for many years, the Medical Research Council (MRC) has been responsible for organising ongoing chemotherapy programmes or 'trials' both for AML and acute lymphoblastic leukaemia (ALL) in an effort to define a treatment approach most likely to eradicate the disease permanently, and also to define poor and good disease risk factors. For example, in the MRC AML 11 Trial, three induction schedules were compared (DAT vs ADE vs MAT) and DAT emerged as superior. A total of 3 vs 6 courses of treatment or the addition of interferon maintenance did not improve results. In the MRC

Box 47.1 FAB morphological classification of acute myeloid leukaemia (AML)

M0	AML without maturation
M1	AML with some maturation
M2	AML with more maturation – granules, Auer rods
M3	Acute hypergranular promyelocytic leukaemia; many Auer rods
M4	Acute myelomonocytic leukaemia
(M4 Eo)	Acute myelomonocytic leukaemia with eosinophilia
M5	Acute monocytic/monoblastic leukaemia
M6	Erythroleukaemia
M7	Acute megakaryoblastic leukaemia

Box 47.2 Prognostic features in acute myeloid leukaemia (AML)

Secondary leukaemia	Poor
Evolving after myelodysplastic syndromes	Poor
Relapsed disease	Poor
Complex chromosomal abnormalities	Poor
Involvement of chromosomes 5 and 7	Poor
M0, M6, M7	Poor
Older age at diagnosis	Poor
Presence of extramedullary disease	Poor
Biphenotypic disease	Poor
t(8;21), t(15;17), inv(16)	Good
M4 Eo and AML M3	Good

AML 10 Trial, data on 1711 patients with AML, aged up to 55 years old, were used to create a prognostic index for defining poor and good risk factors. Response after course 1 of chemotherapy and cytogenetics were strongly predictive of outcome. For patients with complete remission, partial remission and resistant disease, 5-year survival from the start of course 2 was 53%, 44% and 22% and relapse rates were 46%, 48% and 69%, respectively, and for patients with favourable, intermediate and adverse karyotypic abnormalities, survival was 72%, 43% and 17% and relapse rates were 34%, 51% and 75%, respectively (all p <0.0001). Patients with FAB type M3 but no cytogenetic t(15;17) also had a low relapse rate (29%). These three factors were combined to give three risk groups:

- good (favourable karyotype or M3, irrespective of response status or presence of additional abnormalities)
- standard (neither good nor poor)
- poor (adverse karyotype or resistant disease, and no good-risk features).

Survival for these three groups was 70%, 48% and 15%, respectively, and relapse rates were 33%, 50% and 78% (both p <0.0001).[5] Thus, patients with disease which merited a more aggressive treatment approach, such as a stem cell allograft, could be identified. Currently, the MRC AML 15 is underway, which aims to examine the role of the anti-CD33 immunoconjugate (Mylotarg) in induction and other chemotherapy.

Cytosine arabinoside (cytarabine) and the anthracycline daunorubicin are the mainstays of treatment,[5,6] and some of the newer anthracyclines such as mitoxantrone (mitozantrone) or idarubicin may provide additional benefit.[7] Many regimens have incorporated tioguanine and etoposide and, more recently, newer agents such as fludarabine have been combined with cytosine arabinoside. Patients require 3–5 cycles of treatment, the aim being to effect remission – normalisation of the peripheral blood count with less than 5% of blast cells in the marrow.

Use of high-dose cytarabine in combination with an anthracyline has been claimed to result in more durable remissions, although this is not necessarily the case in patients who are subsequently transplanted (see later). A recent report from the European Bone Marrow Transplant (EBMT) Working Party for Acute Leukaemia examined 1672 patients with AML in first remission who were reported to the Leukaemia Working Party and who were transplanted between 1980 and 1995. They were then analysed in terms of dose intensity of cytosine given during induction and consolidation: 846 patients underwent autologous,

and 826 allogeneic stem cell transplantation. The dose of cytosine used did not appear to influence relapse incidence and did not confer any advantage in terms of overall outcome in this study,[8] although some of the MRC data indicate that a post-induction course of high-dose cytosine may afford equivalent or improved disease-free survival than autologous stem cell transplantation in adults with AML.

As mentioned above, successful remission induction is strongly age-related, and becomes less common in patients above 50 years old. Without further chemotherapy, the median time to relapse for first remission patients is commonly less than 1 year. Both relapse and long-term survival probabilities can be considerably improved with additional 'consolidation' chemotherapy, usually given as two or three courses of sufficient intensity to produce pancytopenia. Maintenance chemotherapy – chemotherapy given for 2–3 years after induction and consolidation therapy is complete – has not generally been found to prolong remission in AML, a situation at variance from that seen with ALL. Relapse remains the major cause of treatment failure, after which the likelihood of attaining a second remission is approximately 50% and the probability of a prolonged remission is correspondingly reduced.

Allogeneic and autologous stem cell transplantation for acute myeloid leukaemia

Allogeneic stem cell transplantation (SCT) in first remission from an HLA (human leucocyte antigen) identical sibling may be the most successful approach to preventing leukaemia relapse and increasing the probability of long-term disease-free survival and potential cure in some patient groups. In this situation, 40–70% disease-free survival rates are to be anticipated. This approach is, however, limited by age constraints and the availability of a matched sibling donor. Only 10–15% of patients with a median age at presentation of approximately 50 years old are candidates for a matched sibling allograft, since there is only an approximately 1:4 chance of any sibling being a full HLA match. Also, the relatively high likelihood of treatment-related morbidity and mortality – infections, graft versus host disease (GvHD), pneumonitis – need to be taken into consideration when deciding if a patient is a suitable candidate for allo-SCT, and the UK MRC AML trial found that in children, patients over 35 years old and with good-risk disease there was no survival advantage, this being restricted to patients in the intermediate-risk group.[9]

Reasonably good survival rates have been reported for transplants from related partially HLA-matched donors, but for HLA-matched unrelated donors the survival is often less than 20%, perhaps reflecting the longer time taken to identify a suitable donor, the need for increased immunosuppression of the recipient and a consequently enhanced likelihood of disease relapse. However, the ESCT (European Stem Cell Transplant) Working party for Acute Leukaemia recently examined 170 patients who had relapsed after an allogenic transplant performed between 1978 and 1997 and found that provided relapse had occurred more than 292 days after the first transplant and provided that the patient was in remission when the second transplant took place, there was a 3-year leukaemia-free survival rate of 52%.[10]

In an attempt to reduce transplant-related toxicity, intensified GvHD prophylaxis using a combination of ciclosporin and methotrexate has been shown to reduce acute, but not chronic GvHD. This measure is, however, associated with an increased relapse rate, almost certainly because the graft versus leukaemia effect, known to be associated with the occurrence of GvHD, is reduced.[11]

Autologous stem cell transplantation

Autologous SCT may be effective for selected patients, but the early encouraging results have not been confirmed by large, randomised trials; although an improvement in disease-free survival was shown after autografting in the MRC AML 10 study, the autograft was given as additional treatment, which may have only been the equivalent of giving a further course of chemotherapy.[12] However, the same major drawback remains of the possible presence of minimal residual disease, even though the patient is in morphological and cytogenetic remission when the stem cells are harvested, and in the absence of the graft versus leukaemia effect associated with allogeneic SCT. The procedure is also associated with a treatment-related mortality of 7–10%, which may reduce any gain conferred over that to be expected after non-ablative chemotherapy.

In summary, age is a particularly poor prognostic factor in AML. It is still unclear from the various trials that have been carried out worldwide whether an SCT procedure confers any advantage over chemotherapy alone in patients under 60 years old who are standard risk, particularly when the hazards associated with allografting are taken into consideration. There are also still many questions concerning the most appropriate doses of the various chemotherapy agents, which agents are the most appropriate and the optimum number of courses of chemotherapy that will translate into an increased number of patients in all risk groups remaining in first remission.

THE MYELODYSPLASTIC SYNDROMES

The myelodysplastic syndromes (MDS) are microscopically classified as shown in Box 47.3. In patients of an appropriate age, allogeneic bone marrow transplantation is the treatment of choice since all of these syndromes eventually progress into AML, and treatment with chemotherapy alone is usually even more unsatisfactory than is the case with de-novo AML. However, stem cell transplantation is frequently not feasible in view of the fact that older patients who are not eligible for transplantation by virtue of their age tend to develop these conditions. The leukaemia cells frequently carry cytogenetic abnormalities associated with a poor prognosis, such as 5q- (see Box 47.2).

The generally accepted policy for the management of older patients with myelodysplasia is supportive therapy. However, the prognosis for the majority of patients is less than 1 year, and this has led to the trial of alternative strategies, especially in younger patients. Scoring systems have been developed to enable better prediction of outcome for an individual patient,[13] and, as with de-novo AML, factors known to affect prognosis include the presence of certain chromosomal abnormalities, the percentage of bone marrow blasts and the number of cytopenias. These systems now permit the evaluation of more aggressive therapies such as intensive chemotherapy and autologous and allogeneic transplantation.

Preliminary data with combination chemotherapy used in the myelodysplastic syndromes show rates of complete remission from 15% to 64%. Although experience with autologous SCT is limited, the ESCT Group have recently analysed the results on 79 patients reported to the registry of the Chronic Leukaemia Working Party.[14,15] The 2-year survival, disease-free survival and relapse rates for the 79 patients were 39%, 34% and 64%, respectively.

Allogeneic SCT offers a potential cure for younger patients with MDS. Data have been collected on 118 patients who underwent an unrelated allograft for MDS or secondary AML between 1986 and 1996.

Box 47.3	Myelodysplastic syndrome FAB classification

Refractory anaemia
Refractory anaemia with ring sideroblasts (RARS)
Refractory anaemia with excess of blasts (RAEB)
Chronic myelomonocytic leukaemia
Refractory anaemia with excess of blasts in transformation

Actuarial probability of survival at 2 years was 28%, relapse risk 35% and transplant-related mortality 58%. The latter was significantly influenced by the age of the patient, and relapse risk was influenced by disease stage. There was also evidence of a graft versus leukaemia effect in those patients who experienced GvHD, with a 24% relapse probability in patients with GvHD as opposed to 42% in those without, or with grade 1 only.[16]

A further study was conducted evaluating results after either allo-SCT or auto-SCT in 39 patients.[16] Twenty-eight of these with a donor were allografted in first complete remission – and had a 4-year disease-free survival (DFS) of 31%. Thirty-six patients received an autograft in first remission and had a DFS of 27% at 4 years.

In summary, MDS is commoner in older patients and is much more difficult to cure than is de-novo AML. Disease relapse after all treatment approaches is much commoner, and attempts are still ongoing to define the therapy most likely to result in cure.

ACUTE LYMPHOBLASTIC LEUKAEMIA

The FAB classification for ALL is depicted in Box 47.4. Most cases of adult and childhood ALL are morphologically either L1 or L2, with only approximately 2% being L3. In adults, acute lymphoblastic leukaemia carries a much poorer prognosis than is the case in childhood, with only approximately 20% of patients remaining disease-free after 5 years with chemotherapy alone. The reasons for this are not entirely clear, except for the fact that certain poor prognostic features, such as Philadelphia positivity, occur more commonly with advancing age. In children, however, a substantial proportion may expect to be cured with chemotherapy alone, provided that they do not fall into a 'poor-risk' group (Box 47.5). These include some chromosome abnormalities of the leukaemic cells, such as presence of the Philadelphia chromosome, presence of the B-cell phenotype (as opposed to pre-B), boys with very high white blood cell (WBC) counts at

Box 47.4	FAB classification of acute lymphoblastic leukaemia
L1	Small, round blast cells with little cytoplasm
L2	Bigger, more pleomorphic blasts with more cytoplasm
L3	Medium-sized blasts with intensely basophilic cytoplasm and marked vacuolation

Box 47.5	Prognostic factors in acute lymphoblastic leukaemia (ALL)	
Male sex		Poor
Initial white blood cells (WBCs)		
>100 × 10⁹/l		Poor
Bone marrow disease at day 15		Poor
Infants		Poor
Presence of chromosomes t9;22 and t4;11		Poor
Cell phenotype (B-cell ALL)		Poor
Extramedullary disease		Poor
Relapsed disease		Poor
Female sex		Good
Age 4–10 years		Good
CD10 positivity		Good
Prompt treatment response		Good

presentation and disease which has already relapsed after conventional chemotherapy. The proponents of aggressive chemotherapy alone claim that results from this are as good as those seen following bone marrow transplantation, in that the higher procedure-related mortality offsets the higher relapse rate after chemotherapy alone.

The progress made in the treatment of ALL reflects advances in the understanding of the biology and immunology of the disease, and the development of effective treatment strategies. In particular, recognition of different 'risk groups' has led to the development of more intensive treatment regimens for poor-risk patients, whereas the good-risk patients receive less toxic therapy to achieve cure.

The first documented success in treatment was published in 1948 when Farber et al used the antifolate agent aminopterin to produce short-lived responses in some children with ALL.[17] Subsequently, corticosteroids were used,[18] and they still remain one of the key drugs employed in remission induction. Between 1950 and 1960, other drugs were introduced, including vincristine, cyclophosphamide and 6-mercaptopurine.[19] Around this time, it was realised that the chance of achieving remission with a combination of drugs, e.g. vincristine and prednisolone, was greater than the sum of using each drug as a single agent (the phenomenon of synergism). From 1962 onwards, multi-agent combinations were introduced in an attempt to circumvent the problem of drug resistance. The success of the multi-drug approach in achieving long-term remission led to the concept of leukaemia relapse in patients who had been free of disease for several years. The central nervous system (CNS) as a site of relapse was recognised, occurring in 50–60% of patients, and prophylactic CNS-directed therapy was developed, employing craniospinal radiotherapy and intrathecal methotrexate. Pinkel[20] introduced the concept of 'total therapy', designed to treat ALL as a truly systemic disease with CNS-directed therapy employed for all patients regardless of whether CNS disease could be detected at presentation. This approach was the forerunner of the current treatment strategies, which include induction, consolidation and continuation phases of treatment.

For adult ALL patients entering first remission, who in general may be expected to fare worse than children, there is a treatment dilemma: provided they are reasonably fit and under the age of 55 years old, those with an HLA identical sibling have the option of an allogeneic stem cell transplant. The dilemma for these individuals is the contrasting outcome that allogeneic SCT offers in comparison with either continued chemotherapy or autologous transplantation: while the allograft has the best chance of curing the leukaemia, it also has the highest risk of early mortality. To date, all comparisons between allografting, autografting and chemotherapy are characterised by significant superiority of the antileukaemia effect of the allograft, but only small and usually non-significant differences in leukaemia-free survival.[21,22] One such study compared International Bone Marrow Transplant Registry (ISCTR) data for a large group of adults with ALL transplanted in first remission, with a German multicentre chemotherapy (CT) study of patients entering remission. The results showed a significantly lower relapse probability following SCT (32% vs 96%), but this benefit was offset by a high treatment-related mortality, resulting in no significant difference in disease-free survival between CT (47%) and SCT (51%). No prognostic factor predicted better outcome for one treatment vs the other.[23]

An alternative strategy is to use a 'total therapy' approach; adult patients with ALL achieving remission receive high-dose melphalan (HDM) followed by a G-CSF (granulocyte colony-stimulating factor)-mobilised peripheral blood stem cell autograft. Patients who subsequently relapse go on to receive an allograft from a matched or closely matched donor. Initial results show a very low procedure-related mortality and a projected disease-free survival of 68%.[24]

With children, the position is less clear regarding indications for transplantation. Overall, the disease carries a good prognosis with chemotherapy alone if certain specific risk factors are absent at diagnosis (see Box 47.5).

As data have accumulated on stem cell transplantation for ALL, it has now become possible to compare results of SCT series with those seen after chemotherapy alone. While SCT has a higher probability of curing poor-risk ALL, the higher procedure-related mortality has brought the disease-free survival into the same range as that achieved by chemotherapy alone. Thus, the place of SCT in ALL of childhood has remained controversial. Proponents of SCT emphasise the low chance of long-term survival following chemotherapy alone in relapsed ALL and in ALL presenting with poor prognosis features, whereas proponents of chemotherapy have drawn attention to the increasing success achieved with new, more intensive and better-designed protocols, which, it is claimed, may ultimately eliminate the need for SCT with a few exceptions. Currently, however, there may be more relapses in chemotherapy-treated patients and more treatment-related deaths in SCT patients, although the poor risk factors outlined in Box 47.5 may also have an influence on treatment outcome, and deaths after SCT do tend to plateau after about 5 years, whereas late relapses are more likely to go on happening in chemotherapy-only recipients. This is shown in one of the few published series of children treated with SCT in first complete remission (CR) for ALL with poor prognostic features. The MRC UKALL X trial compared SCT with a chemotherapy regimen for patients presenting with WBC >100 000 × 10^9/l.[24–26] Patients with HLA-DR matched siblings were eligible for SCT. There was no difference in DFS between patients treated with chemotherapy or SCT, but the relapse rate was higher in the chemotherapy group.

As many patients considered suitable for a bone marrow transplant have no HLA-compatible sibling donor, autografting in remission is commonly considered as an alternative, and as is the case with the other haematological malignancies, younger patients in first remission at the time of transplant tend to suffer less disease relapse and less toxicity than do those at more advanced stages of their disease. It may also well be the case that the use of 'maintenance' chemotherapy (daily 6-mercaptopurine, weekly methotrexate and monthly steroid and vincristine), following autologous stem cell transplantation, such as is given in the non-autologous setting in childhood ALL, results in a higher percentage of sustained remissions.[24]

Environmental and occupational causes of leukaemia

Although it is now possible to classify the acute leukaemias very accurately, the aetiology in most cases remains unclear. It is recognised that exposure to certain chemicals, drugs or radiation may cause leukaemic transformation to occur in later life. Examples include benzene and related compounds, some anticancer drugs and accidental exposure to ionising irradiation. Also, prior therapy with certain antineoplastic agents is associated with subsequent onset of myelodysplasia, and in particular, patients who have previously been treated with dual modality therapy for Hodgkin's disease have been noted to have a high incidence of secondary acute myeloid leukaemia. Viral agents have not been reliably linked to most types of human leukaemia except for the association of HTLV1 (human T-cell lymphotrophic virus 1) with adult T-lymphocytic lymphoid leukaemia, and in most cases the causes are likely to be multifactional.

Overall, which patients with acute leukaemia should be considered for stem cell transplantation ?

As with many such questions relating to indications for SCT, the answer is superficially simple but open to varied interpretation:

- 'good-risk' patients should not be considered for SCT in first remission
- conversely, 'poor-risk' patients should be considered for SCT in first remission
- any patient no longer in first remission should be considered for SCT.

Clearly, one of the major problems arises in arriving at tight definitions of good and poor risk above. In some cases, this is relatively straightforward and there is little variation between SCT centres. However, in other cases the prognostic features in question may be 'soft', and a decision may be swayed by other factors such as patient age, identity of donor, cytomegalovirus (CMV) status of patient and donor, general condition of the patient, patient and referring physician preference, etc.

In summary, individual patients may require careful consideration of risk/benefit issues, and repeated discussion between all parties may be necessary.

CHRONIC MYELOID LEUKAEMIA

Chronic myeloid leukaemia (CML) is a clonal disorder of the pluripotent stem cell. It is commonest in people who are 40–60 years of age and has an annual incidence of approximately 1/100 000. The disease is characterised by the presence of the Philadelphia (Ph) chromosome; chromosome 22 is shortened, secondary to a reciprocal translocation between chromosomes 9 and 22. In this translocation the Ableson proto-oncogene (ABL)

from the long arm of chromosome 9 is juxtaposed to the breakpoint cluster region (BCR) on chromosome 22 to form a chimeric BCR/ABL gene. This new gene transcribes an 8.5 kb messenger RNA (mRNA) instead of the normal 6 or 7 kb mRNA associated with ABL and is translated into a protein of 210 kDA (p210). Unlike the normal 145 kDA ABL product, the p210 protein has a much higher tyrosine kinase activity. This altered enzymatic activity, and evidence that the BCR/ABL product can transform haemopoietic cells strongly implicates its role in the genesis of CML.

CML usually follows a prolonged chronic phase (3–5 years) that eventually proceeds to accelerated phase and finally to a blastic transformation of acute leukaemia, which may be myeloid or lymphoid in type. No chemotherapy is curative, since only the blood count is suppressed without eradicating the Philadelphia positive cells. Alpha-interferon may effect haematologic remission in up to 70% of cases and complete suppression of the Philadelphia chromosome in up to 23% of cases.[27,28] Although this Ph negativity is not sustained in most cases, a number of trials are still in progress to assess whether survival is prolonged in those who have shown cytogenetic response.

Until recently, allogeneic SCT remained the only option affording possible cure, provided that the transplant is carried out while patients are in chronic phase of the disease, preferably within a year of diagnosis, or relapse risk is greatly increased. STI-571 (Gleevec) – see below – is currently under evaluation as a possible curative agent.

To reduce the chances of patients succumbing to transplant-related problems, attempts have been made to attenuate the course of GvHD by using T-cell depletion of donor marrow with or without additional ciclosporin and/or methotrexate. Very high rates of disease relapse were seen in the patients who had suffered no GvHD, again highlighting the concept of a graft versus leukaemia effect coexisting with GvHD.[29,30] It is possible, however, that more selective removal of cells such as the CD8-positive T lymphocytes that mediate GvHD will result in a reduction in GvHD without compromising the graft versus leukaemia effect.

Various conditioning regimens have been used prior to SCT, the best known of which is the Seattle combination of cyclophosphamide and total body irradiation (TBI). However, newer preparative regimens such as a combination of busulfan and cyclophosphamide have provided promising results.[31] Worldwide, the results of allografting in the chronic phase of CML show that approximately 50% of patients are long-term disease-free survivors. This is reduced to a 15–20% long-term survival for SCT in accelerated or blastic phase. Box 47.6 shows the features associated with a good oucome after SCT in CML.

The probability of relapse is about 10% and 45% for those transplanted in chronic and accelerated phases, respectively. Relapsed patients may receive a second transplant from the original donor. Another interesting approach used by some centres is treatment with donor-derived leucocytes harvested by leucapharesis and given with or without interferon. With such an approach, many patients have been restored to Ph negativity because of the presumed graft versus leukaemia effect of the donor lymphocytes.[32,33]

Bone marrow or PBSC (peripheral blood stem cell) autotransplantation in chronic phase has surprisingly led to persistent Ph negative haemopoiesis in some cases,[34,35] and such results may be improved in the future by in-vitro manipulations including long-term cell culture, or use of marrow treated with α-interferon before reinfusion, or the use of α-interferon to maintain Ph negativity. Using matched but unrelated donors, the incidence of graft failure and GvHD is greater, but a 2-year disease-free survival of about 40% has been achieved.

At diagnosis, peripheral blood as a source of haemopoietic stem cells for later use should be harvested and cryopreserved in all patients. If leucostasis is present, red cell transfusion should be avoided and urgent leucapheresis may be indicated.

If transfusion of blood products is necessary, all patients should receive CMV-negative, irradiated blood products in the anticipation that they may proceed to an SCT procedure at a later date.

New approaches in the treatment of chronic myeloid leukaemia

The signal transduction inhibitor 571 (STI-571), now known as Gleevec (imatinib) manufactured by Novartis, is a phenylaminopyrimidine derivative which may to be an important advance in the treatment of CML.[36-39] It is a tyrosine kinase inhibitor that acts on the ABL gene, which is located on chromosome 9 and contains a tyrosine kinase domain (see above). ATP (adenosine triphosphate) in its binding site in the kinase domain of the protein is able to phosphorylate tyrosine residues on selected substrates. The phosphorylated substrate then binds with other molecules and activates downstream pathways in leukaemogenesis. In CML, STI-571 occupies the ATP pocket in the BCR–ABL kinase domain and substrates cannot be phosphorylated. Clinical trials on this agent commenced in 1998, the drug initially being given to patients with interferon-resistant disease. Of those patients in the chronic phase of their disease, a substantial proportion entered haematological remission and a proportion also showed a cytogenetic response. For patients with more advanced disease the results were less impressive, although, overall, results seemed better than those achievable with any other agent available to treat CML. Various prospective clinical studies are now underway. Figures 47.1–47.3 illustrate the Ph chromosome and the actions of STI and its interaction with the Ph chromosome.

Doses higher than the usual 400 mg/day of imatinib may be more effective in either de-novo CML or when other treatment approaches have failed. Thirty-six patients with chronic phase CML unresponsive to interferon were treated with imatinib 400 mg twice daily. All 11 patients with active disease achieved complete haematologic response. Excluding patients with <35% Ph-positive metaphases before the start of therapy, 19/21 (90%) evaluable patients achieved a major cytogenetic response. Twenty-four of 27 (89%) evaluable patients achieved a complete cytogenetic response. Eighteen of 32 evaluable patients (56%) showed BCR–ABL/ABL percentage ratios <0.045%, including 13 (41%) with undetectable levels. With a median

---

Box 47.6 Factors positively influencing outcome after sibling or MUD allogeneic stem cell transplantation for CML

Chronic disease phase
Transplant within 1 year of diagnosis
Full donor/recipient histocompatibility
T-cell replete donor stem cells
Younger patient age
Younger donor age
Patient serologically negative for CMV

CML, chronic myeloid leukaemia; CMV, cytomegalovirus; MUD, matched unrelated donor.

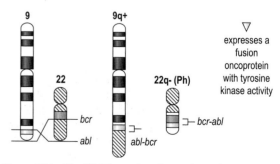

Figure 47.1 The t(9;22) translocation produces the Philadelphia (Ph) chromosome.

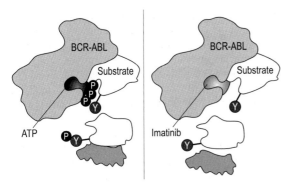

Figure 47.2 Competition for ATP binding.

follow-up of 15 months, all patients were alive in chronic phase. Toxicities were similar to those reported with standard dose; 71% of patients continue to receive ≥ 600 mg of imatinib daily. Thus, high-dose imatinib induces complete cytogenetic responses in most patients with chronic phase CML post-interferon failure. This is accompanied by a high rate of molecular remission.[39]

In another study, imatinib was compared with α-interferon combined with low-dose cytarabine in newly diagnosed chronic-phase CML. Randomly assigned 1106 patients received imatinib (553 patients) or α-interferon + low-dose cytarabine (553 patients). Crossover to the alternative group was allowed if stringent criteria defining treatment failure or intolerance were met. After a median follow-up of 19 months, the estimated rate of a major cytogenetic response was 87.1% in the imatinib group and 34.7% in the group given α-interferon + cytarabine (p <0.001). The estimated rates of complete cytogenetic response were 76.2% and 14.5%, respectively (p <0.001). At 18 months, the estimated rate of freedom from progression to accelerated-phase or blast-crisis CML was 96.7% in the imatinib group and 91.5% in the combination therapy group (p <0.001). Imatinib was better tolerated than combination therapy.[40]

Mini-autografting for chronic myeloid leukaemia in blast crisis

Experience with autografting in blast crisis has shown that the majority of patients are restored transiently to chronic phase. However, morbidity from the procedure is considerable and patients spend much of their remaining life in hospital. In an attempt to maximise quality of life, mini-autografting is a possibility and may keep patients out of hospital as much as possible.

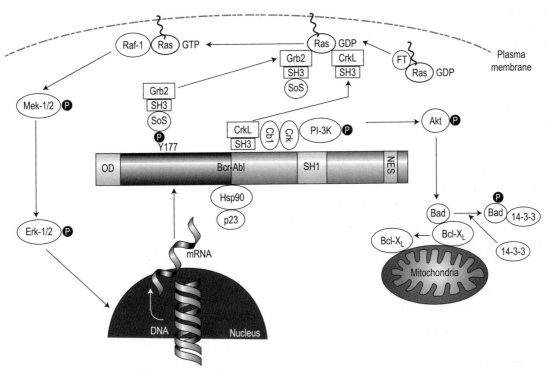

Figure 47.3 Interaction of the signal transduction inhibitor (STI) with the Ph chromosome.

CHRONIC LYMPHOCYTIC LEUKAEMIA

Chronic lymphocytic leukaemia (CLL) most commonly occurs in patients over the age of 60, but it is also found in the younger age groups. Men are more commonly affected than women and, although no predisposing causes have been identified such as prior exposure to irradiation, drugs or chemicals, there is some evidence that there may be a familial predisposition to the disease; many families have now been identified where either more than one closely related family member has the disease, or where members of successive generations develop the disease. Often when successive generations are involved, the disease is diagnosed at an earlier age in the ensuing generation, a phenomenon known as 'anticipation'. CLL is often entirely asymptomatic in its early stages, and a chance finding on blood testing for an unrelated reason. Alternatively, patients may notice an increase in the size of a group of lymph nodes or the spleen and seek advice for this reason. CLL is classified according to the situation with regard to peripheral blood appearances and number of clinical sites involved by disease (Tables 47.1 and 47.2).

Laboratory findings of CLL include a persistent lymphocytosis with lymphocytes which are monoclonal and which express a single immunoglobulin light-chain type on their surface. The lymphocytes are morphologically small, round and mature-looking with nuclei which contain chromatin clumps. Immunophenotyping shows surface immunoglobulin which is less dense than that found on normal B cells, and surface markers show the cells to be positive for CD5, CD23 and CD 25 and to form rosettes with mouse erythrocytes, although this latter test has now largely been abandoned. They are also negative for CD22 and 35.

Table 47.1   The Rai clinical staging system

Stage	Five-year survival	Clinical features
0	Approx. 98%	Lymphocytosis in blood and marrow only
I	Approx. 95%	Lymphocytosis + lymphadenopathy
II	Approx. 95%	Lymphocytosis + splenomegaly or hepatomegaly
III	Less than 5%	Lymphocytosis + anaemia (Hb <10 g/dl)
IV	0%	Lymphocytosis + thrombocytopenia (platelets $<100 \times 10^9$/l)

Table 47.2   The Binet clinical staging system

Stage	Clinical features
A	<3 involved sites, Hb >10 g/dl; platelets $>100 \times 10^9$/l
B	>3 sites involves, Hb >10 g/dl; platelets $>100 \times 10^9$/l
C	Hb <10 g/dl or platelets $<100 \times 10^9$/l

This pattern of positivity and negativity serves to distinguish CLL cells from those seen in some of the other B-cell lymphoid malignancies, including prolymphocytic leukaemia (PLL), hairy cell leukaemia (HCL), splenic lymphoma with villous lymphocytes (SLVL), mantle cell lymphoma (MCL) and follicular centre cell lymphoma (FCCL).

Chromosomal abnormalities in B–chronic lymphocytic leukaemia

These are common in CLL, but are often hard to define, as CLL cells are predominantly in the resting phase of the cell cycle and therefore difficult to induce to enter mitosis. The advent of sensitive detection methods such as fluorescent in-situ hybridisation (FISH), which can be used to detect changes during interphase, and optimisation of mitosis-induction protocols, has helped resolve these problems. The most common abnormalities are trisomy 12, which occurs in up to 34% of cases and is associated with progressive disease, and deletions or translocations of chromosome 13q14, which occur in approximately 40% of cases and are associated with a benign disease course. Other abnormalities occur less frequently and have different prognostic implications.

A great many patients enjoy a long survival with few symptoms or signs of evidence of disease progression. Overall, poor prognostic features in CLL may be summarised as in Box 47.7.

Infections are the major cause of death. The usual organisns are *Streptococcus pneumoniae*, *Staphylococcus aureus* and *Escherichia coli*. Since the introduction of the

Box 47.7	Poor prognostic features of chronic lymphocytic leukaemia

Lymphocyte count $>50 \times 10^9$/l
Lymphocyte doubling time <12 months
Greater than 15% prolymphocytes
Diffuse involvement of bone marrow
Karyotype abnormalities
Poor response to treatment

purine analogues into treatment (see below), opportunist infections with such agents as *Listeria monocytogenes* and *Pneumocystis carinii* have become much more common. Herpes zoster infections are also very common and occur in approximately 30% of patients at some time during their illness.

Rituximab

This is an anti-CD 20 monoclonal antibody which has been used to good effect to treat CD 20-expressing lymphomas and chronic lymphocytic leukaemia. It is often more effective in the treatment of CLL when used in combination with another agent such as steroids.[70]

Treatment

In the earlier stages of the disease, treatment is usually unnecessary and patients should just be monitored with regular 6-monthly or yearly blood tests and physical examination. The three most important factors affecting prognosis in CLL are tumour mass, rate of disease progression and response to chemotherapy. If the WBC count does become so high that the haemoglobin and platelet levels are compromised, or if the patient develops problems with splenomegaly or substantial lymph node enlargement necessitating treatment, chlorambucil has long been established as the initial treatment of choice, and is often given for a few days each month, sometimes with prednisolone, particularly if there is evidence of autoimmune disease (see below).

Combination chemotherapy involving an anthracycline, CHOP being the most commonly used, may prove effective for more advanced disease, or disease which is failing to respond to chlorambucil alone. However, other intensive regimens excluding an anthracycline have proven no more effective than chlorambucil and prednisolone alone, implying that anthracyclines may have a particular role to play in treatment.

Newer treatment purine analogue agents include fludarabine, pentostatin and cladribine and some monoclonal antibodies such as Campath-IH (alemtuzumab) which recognise the lymphoid cells.

Purine analogues

The most intensively investigated purine nucleoside analogues are very similar in structure but do not all act in precisely the same way and have been found to shown different clinical efficacies. Pentostatin (deoxycoformycin; DCF) is primarily an adenosine deaminase inhibitor. Cladribine (2-CdA) and fludarabine, however, have multiple inhibitory effects within the cell, not all of which have been fully characterised.

Fludarabine   Fludarabine is a purine analogue that is a water-soluble derivative of vidarabine. Given at doses of 25 mg/m²/day over 30 min for 5 days every 4 weeks, it is the most effective single agent known in CLL. Among previously untreated patients, the response rate has been as high as 79%,[41] with most responses being complete. It has also compared very favourably with CAP (chlorambucil, doxorubicin and prednisolone) and durations of remission have been significantly longer with fludarabine with less side effects.

Pentostatin   2-Deoxycoformycin is a purine analogue which comes from fermentation cultures of *Streptomyces antibioticus*. It is a potent adenosine deaminase inhibitor, resulting in inhibition of DNA replication and repair. It is effective against CLL, but less so than fludarabine and cladribine, being most effective in the treatment of HCL.

Cladribine   2-Chlorodeoxyadenosine is converted to its active triphosphate in cells with high levels of deoxycytidine kinase and low levels of 5'-nucleotidase activity. It was originally introduced as an immunosuppressant, but was subsequently shown to have antiproliferative activity against a wide variety of leukaemia cells. It has been shown to effect a response in the majority of CLLs requiring treatment, and responses last for up to 4 years in cases where complete remission has been attained.

Campath-IH

The Campath-1 antibodies were first produced in Cambridge by a research team led by Hermann Waldman in the late 1970s. These antibodies were selected because of their broad reactivity with normal and malignant cells due to the nature and distribution of the target antigen, CD 52. This antigen is expressed at a high density on most mature normal and malignant lymphocytes, but not on haemopoietic stem cells, and is not internalised in response to antibody binding. Once the Campath has bound to its target cells, cell death is effected by a combination of lysis by complement, antibody-dependent cellular cytotoxicity and apoptosis.

Use of Campath in patients with late-stage and refractory disease can cause profound lymphopenia and consequent immunosuppression. Opportunistic infections, including fungus, cytomegalovirus, *Pneumocystis* and herpes, are common. The DC 16+ natural killer cells are the first to recover after therapy, but complete immune reconstitution can take many months. Patients may also experience fever rigors, nausea and vomiting during and after infusion because of the release of inflammatory cytokines, including tumour necrosis factor, interleukins IL-6 and IL-10 and γ-interferon.

Campath-IH in CLL

- Most effective antibody in CLL
- Administration relatively straightforward
- Profound immunosuppression
- Life-threatening infective complications, which may be delayed
- Careful patient selection, prophylaxis and monitoring are essential.

Autologous and allogeneic stem cell transplantation
As a substantial number of patients are over 60 years of age at diagnosis, allogeneic SCT is an option which can only be offered to the minority. A number of centres have now carried out small numbers of allogeneic transplants, mainly using cyclophosphamide, busulfan or etoposide with or without TBI and ciclosporin and methotrexate as GvHD prophylaxis. Actuarial survival in one group of 25 patients at 5 years was 32%.[42] Another group looked at survival after allogeneic transplantation in 28 patients and found a progression-free survival at 66 months of 78% in chemosensitive patients, compared with 31% in those with refractory disease.[43]

Autologous SCT has been found to be safe and to induce long-lasting clinical and molecular remissions, which may improve the prognosis of some patients with CLL. Feasibility and efficacy appear to be best early in the course of the disease and it is still unclear whether such an approach can ever be curative.[44]

Minimal residual disease status (MRD) at the time of transplantation may also be important. In 14 patients who received an autograft, of whom 9 were MRD-negative and 5 MRD-positive, only 2 of the MRD-negative patients relapsed, whereas 4 of the 5 MRD-positive patients relapsed. Of another small group who underwent allografting, a similar outcome was observed; of those who cleared their MRD after transplantation, none had a clinical or MRD relapse at 43 months. From this study, it would therefore seem that the likelihood of achieving a sustained MRD-negative remission is greater in patients who have been allografted, although the increased transplant-related mortality occurring after allografting has to be taken into consideration.[45] Transplant procedures in CLL should, however, still be considered experimental and prospective patients should be entered into trials in an effort to improve upon patient numbers and to identify the most appropriate conditioning therapy, and GvHD prophylaxis.

MULTIPLE MYELOMA

This disease affects 5–10/100 000 people per year in the USA and European populations, and in the UK the annual incidence is approximately 40 per million, with about 2500 new cases per year. Approximately 50% of patients are over 60 years old at diagnosis and fewer than 2% are below 40 years old. Most cases present de novo, but a minority evolve from monoclonal gammopathy of undetermined significance (MGUS).

Clinical presentation

The most common presentations of myeloma include bone pain, recurrent or persistent infection, anaemia, renal impairment or a combination of these. Some patients are asymptomatic, abnormalities being identified on blood tests being carried out for other reasons. Box 47.8 shows some of the presenting features that require urgent investigation.

Box 47.9 shows the investigations which should be carried out at diagnosis.

Box 47.10 shows some other conditions where a paraprotein may be present.

The currently accepted criteria for distinguishing myeloma from MGUS are shown in Table 47.3.

Indications for starting therapy

Chemotherapy is indicated for management of symptomatic myeloma. Chemotherapy is not indicated for patients with MGUS or those with equivocal/indolent/smouldering myeloma. Patients with no symptoms, normal haemoglobin, calcium and renal function and no bone lesions may remain stable for a long period without treatment. Early intervention has shown no benefit.[46]

Patients who are asymptomatic but have radiological evidence of bone disease (at least one lytic lesion) are at

---

Box 47.8 Presenting features of multiple myeloma that require urgent investigation

- Symptoms of bone destruction
- Compromised immunity
- Impaired bone marrow function
- Persistent elevation of erythrocyte sedimentation rate (ESR)
- Increased plasma viscosity
- Impaired renal function
- Hypercalcaemia

Box 47.9   Investigations of multiple myeloma to be carried out at diagnosis

- Full blood count
- Serum urea, electrolytes and creatinine
- Serum calcium, albumin and uric acid
- Serum and concentrated urine electropheresis
- Immunofixation and quantification of serum paraprotein
- Quantification of urinary light-chain excretion
- Creatinine clearance
- Plasma viscosity
- X-rays of the skeleton (radionucleide bone scanning is not usually helpful)
- MRI, where spinal cord compression is suspected
- CT scanning if evaluating extramedullary disease
- Bone marrow aspirate
- Trephine biopsy
- β_2-microglobulin, LDH and CRP
- Cytogenetic studies on bone marrow

CT, computed tomography; MRI, magnetic resonance imaging; LDH, lactate dehydrogenase; CRP, C-reactive protein.

Box 47.10   Other conditions where a paraprotein may be present

- MGUS
- Primary amyloidosis
- B-cell non-Hodgkin's lymphoma
- Waldenström's macroglobulinaemia
- Chronic lymphocytic leukaemia
- Connective tissue disorders

MGUS = monoclonal gammopathy of undetermined significance.

recombinant human erythropoietin (EPO), as shown in two large placebo-controlled trials.[47,48]

Choice of initial chemotherapy

Choice of initial chemotherapy depends on factors such as age and performance status and on whether it is planned to proceed to stem cell collection and high-dose therapy (HDT).

Melphalan with or without prednisolone

Melphalan produces a partial remission (PR), defined as a greater than 50% reduction in paraprotein levels, in approximately 50% patients when administered at a dose of 6–8 mg/m^2/day. This may be improved with the addition of prednisolone 40–60 mg/day for 4–7 days at 4–6 week intervals.[49] However, MRC trials have shown no benefit from the addition of standard doses of corticosteroids to oral melphalan or to the ABCM combination chemotherapy regimen.[50] Most patients reach a stable plateau phase, defined as paraprotein level stable for at least 3 months and transfusion independence with minimal symptoms, which usually lasts 18–24 months before relapse. The median

high-risk of progression, as are those with no evidence of bone disease but with abnormal marrow appearances on magnetic resonance imaging (MRI) examination.

Anaemia

Anaemia is very common and usually improves with response to therapy. Red cell transfusion must be given with caution in patients with high paraprotein levels because of the risk of exacerbating hyperviscosity. Patients with myeloma may well respond to

Table 47.3   Criteria for distinguishing myeloma from MGUS

	Myeloma	MGUS
Bone marrow plasma cells	>10% on aspirate	<10% on aspirate
Serum paraprotein	Variable concentration in serum; no specific diagnostic levels	IgG usually<20 g/L IgA usually <10 g/L
Bence Jones proteinuria	>50% cases	Rare
Immune paresis	>95% cases	Rare
Lytic bone lesions	Often present	Absent
Symptoms	Frequent	Absent
Anaemia	Frequent	Absent
Hypercalcaemia	May be present	Absent
Abnormal renal function	May be present	Absent

MGUS, monoclonal gammopathy of undetermined significance; IgA, immunoglobulin A; IgG, immunoglobulin G.

duration of survival is between 2 and 4 years from diagnosis in most series.

Melphalan is thus the initial treatment of choice for most patients in whom HDT is not planned, and treatment should be continued to plateau phase (paraprotein level stable for 3 months) and then stopped. Since the evidence of benefit from steroids in standard doses is controversial, it is reasonable not to include prednisolone, particularly in patients at risk of steroid-related side effects.

Cyclophosphamide with or without prednisolone

Randomised trials have shown that cyclophosphamide (C) produces results similar to those of melphalan in terms of response rate and survival,[50] and there are no data from randomised controlled trials on the effect of adding prednisolone to cyclophosphamide.

Alkylator-based combination chemotherapy regimens

Various combination regimens have been used in at attempt to improve the outcome obtained with simple alkylating agents. These regimens generally include cyclophosphamide and melphalan with two or more of the following drugs: vincristine (V), Adriamycin (A), prednisolone (P) and BCNU (carmustine) (B). As with melphalan alone, regimens which include melphalan or nitrosoureas may prejudice subsequent stem cell harvesting. Over 20 randomised trials have been carried out comparing such regimens with melphalan or MP (melphalan + prednisone),[51] concluding that there was no survival benefit for patients receiving combination chemotherapy.

VAD and related regimens

VAD   VAD comprises vincristine and doxorubicin (Adriamycin) given by continuous 4-day infusion together with high-dose dexamethasone. In newly diagnosed patients, VAD is associated with a high response rate of 60–80% and a 10–25% CR rate.

VAD does not damage stem cells and is also suitable for patients with severe renal failure, as no dosage modification is required and toxicity is not increased. The disadvantages are the requirement for a central line for administration and the high incidence of steroid-related side effects. Remissions are not durable and there is no long-term survival advantage of VAD over MP or combination chemotherapy.

VAMP and C-VAMP   In these regimens, high-dose dexamethasone is replaced by intravenous methyprednisolone with a view to reducing steroid-related toxicity. C-VAMP includes weekly intravenous (IV) cyclophosphamide between courses of VAMP.

There have been no randomised trials comparing VAMP, C-VAMP and VAD. Overall response and CR rates appear similar. In a non-randomised study comparing VAMP and C-VAMP, C-VAMP was associated with a higher CR rate than VAMP (24% vs 8%),[52] whereas the CR rate with VAD has varied from 7% to 28% in different non-randomised series.

Oral idarubicin with dexamethasone   The introduction of oral idarubicin led to the development of a regimen in which idarubicin (Zavedos) is given daily for 4 days together with high-dose dexamethasone (Z-Dex). In a phase I/II study,[53] 80% of newly diagnosed patients responded with a CR rate of 7%. Responses appeared to be as rapid as those observed with VAD.

High–dose dexamethasone   Advantages of high-dose dexamethasone (HDD) include absence of myelotoxicity, suitability for use in renal failure and rapidity of response. A schedule of dexamethasone 40 mg daily for 4 days every 2 weeks until response occurs, then reducing to 4 weekly, is widely used.

High–dose therapy with autologous stem cell transplant
The past decade has seen increasing use of HDT in an attempt to improve disease control and prolong survival. HDT usually comprises HDM with or without other cytotoxic drugs or TBI, and requires stem cell support with peripheral blood progenitor cells or bone marrow. It is normally given after establishing initial responsiveness to VAD-based chemotherapy regimens. PBSC are usually harvested after mobilisation with a combination of chemotherapy and growth factors.

Most centres use intravenous alone at a dose of 200 mg/m², and some also give TBI, although toxicity increased with TBI with no survival benefit. Purging harvested stem cells with monoclonal antibodies and/or CD34⁺ stem cell selection does reduce marrow contamination with tumour cells, but there is no evidence that this reduces the risk of relapse.

The EBMT now holds data on over 8000 patients who have undergone autografting for myeloma.[54] Median overall and progression-free survivals are 50 and 26 months, respectively. Rates of relapse and progression are high, but a plateau appears to occur at about 8 years after autografting, such that a small proportion of patients remains alive and progression-free up to 14 years later.

Favourable prognostic features include good response to early treatment, young age and only one line of primary induction treatment. Karyotype abnormalities, particularly those involving chromosome 13, have also recently been found to have a negative impact;

> **Box 47.11   Poor prognostic features in multiple myeloma**
>
> High paraprotein levels
> Low haemoglobin
> Hypercalcaemia
> Advanced lytic bone lesions
> Abnormal renal function
> Hypoalbuminaemia
> High β_2-microglobulin
> Poor response to therapy
> Abnormalities of chromosome 13

FISH analysis identifies chromosomal abnormalities in most patients, the most frequent being translocations involving 14q and deletions of chromosome 13.[55] There is currently no evidence to support the use of tandem or double transplants outside of a clinical trial. Box 47.11 shows the poor prognostic features of myeloma.

Allogeneic transplantation in myeloma

The role of allogeneic SCT in multiple myeloma is controversial because of high transplant-related mortality (TRM) and significant relapse rates after transplantation. TRM is higher in male patients and in those transplanted late in the course of the disease.

Patients transplanted in first response have a 60% chance of entering CR, and the potential benefit of this outcome may justify the risks of allogeneic SCT in younger patients, particularly women. Patients relapsing after an allogeneic SCT have been shown to respond to donor lymphocyte infusions (DLI), whereas those with persistent disease may achieve a complete remission following DLI.[56]

By 1990, data on 90 patients had been reported to the EBMT.[57] In this early series, the overall long-term survival was 40%, and patients transplanted electively following first-line treatment fared much better than those transplanted later in the course of their disease. Long-term survival was most likely in those who experienced grade I GvHD rather than grades II, III or IV, and in those who were in complete remission after engraftment.[57]

The EBMT currently holds data on 1300 patients, gathered since 1983. Good prognostic features include female recipients, low β_2-microglobulin at diagnosis, good response to treatment and only one prior treatment regimen. The long-term actuarial survival was around 30%, with a median survival after stem cell transplant of around 1.5 years. The relapse rate approached 70%, with many very late relapses. TRM approached 50%.[58]

In a series of 41 myeloma patients allografted at the Royal Marsden Hospital from a matched sibling, between 1986 and the end of 2000, there is a 36% long-term disease-free survival, with the longest follow-up being 13 years and the shortest 2 years. Factors which predisposed negatively to outcome were a previous HDT-conditioned autograft and poor renal function. Good prognostic features included immunoglobulin G (IgG) subclass, lower dose of conditioning radiotherapy and no previous autograft. Other recognised good prognostic factors include good renal function, serum albumin above 30 g/L, chemosensitive disease and a good response of disease to transplant.

In the Seattle allograft experience, 80 patients were transplanted between 1987 and 1994, many with chemo-resistant disease or beyond first response.[59] Thirty-five died within 100 days, and 11 more died later. Risk factors for a poor outcome included transplantation more than 1 year from diagnosis, a male donor for a female patient, Durie stage III disease at transplant and more than 8 cycles of chemotherapy before transplant. Chemotherapy resistance was also important.

Recently 'low-intensity' or 'mini' allograft approaches have been developed which are associated with lower toxicity and TRM.[60] Such an approaches may increase the numbers of patients who are suitable for an allogeneic SCT, but as yet such procedures should be considered experimental.

Interferon

The interferons are a family of compounds produced by leucocytes, fibroblasts and T lymphocytes that have antiproliferative activity against viruses and human tumour cells. The therapeutic effects of α-interferon (IFN-α) have been assessed in myeloma patients at induction, plateau phase, following HDT and in patients with relapse/refractory disease, both as monotherapy and combined with chemotherapy.

IFN-α has been shown to have a role in multiple myeloma. Small, statistically significant increases in progression-free survival and overall survival of up to 6 months are identified in meta-analysis, most clearly observed for patients receiving maintenance therapy following chemotherapy or autologous transplant. However, only 5–10% of myeloma patients achieve a significant gain in survival from IFN-α.[61]

Bisphosphonates

Bone pain, hypercalcaemia and pathological fractures are a major cause of morbidity and mortality in patients with multiple myeloma. Randomised placebo-controlled studies with both pamidronate and clodronate have shown a significant benefit for bisphosphonate treatment.[62,63] Long-term therapy with bisphosphonates has been shown to reduce skeletal morbidity, improve quality of life and reduce the need for surgery and radiotherapy.

Zoledronate is a new, more potent bisphosphonate in vitro. It is given intravenously and requires only a 10-min infusion in comparison with 90 min for pamidronate. It is currently undergoing clinical trial evaluation. It has been shown to be more effective than pamidronate in the treatment of tumour-related hypercalcaemia, and to be as effective as pamidronate in reducing skeletal-related events in patients with osteolytic lesions due to myeloma or breast carcinoma.[64]

Long-term bisphosphonate therapy is recommended for all patients with myeloma whether or not bone lesions are evident, and both oral clodronate and IV pamidronate are effective. Caution is required when renal impairment is present.[65]

Relapsed/progressive disease

Early relapse carries a bad prognosis and is likely to respond poorly to most treatment approaches. Patients who relapse or progress after a long stable plateau phase are more likely to respond well to further treatment.

Current treatment options include:

- no further antineoplastic treatment
- melphalan with or without prednisolone
- weekly cyclophosphamide
- VAD and similar regimens with or without resistance modification agents (e.g. PSC 833)
- oral idarubicin alone or with steroid
- high-dose dexamethasone
- high-dose therapy with stem cell transplantation
- thalidomide
- hemibody irradiation.

If the patient was initially treated with MP and achieved stable plateau, a further response can be achieved in 50% of patients.[66] A second HDT may also be appropriate in selected patients who relapse after an initial autograft, and steroids alone may be beneficial in patients in second or later relapse or in patients who cannot tolerate chemotherapy.

Anti-angiogenesis agents such as thalidomide and its analogues (Celgene Corp) have been shown to be effective in refractory myeloma, and tolerance usually develops to most side effects, including somnolence. Doses may be increased slowly up to 800 mg daily, and responses may occur with as little as 50 mg/day. It may be given with dexamethasone, 40 mg for 4 days each month. Responses may be seen in up to 70% of patients where other therapies have failed, and the mode of action is not clearly understood but may relate more to the immunomodulatory effects of thalidomide rather than to any anti-angiogenic effect.[67,68]

Velcade (Bortezomib)

Tumours secrete factors that promote blood vessel formation known as angiogenesis, and a good blood supply is essential for tumour survival. Bortezomib-mediated proteasome inhibition blocks generation of angiogenic signals, thus leading to tumour cell death. The drug has been tried recently to treat myeloma patients, particularly those who have relapsed after other treatment approaches. It can induce a further remission in up to one third of patients, effect a good partial response in approximately one third, and is ineffective in about one third of patients. The main side-effect is painful neuropathy, which requires careful monitoring.[71,72]

Management of patients with renal failure

A degree of renal impairment occurs in up to 50% of patients with myeloma at some stage of the illness, and advanced renal failure requiring dialysis or other major intervention occurs in 3–12% of patients. A modest increase in the serum creatinine indicates a substantial degree of renal impairment. Urgent intervention is required to correct early renal impairment and prevent long-term renal damage.

The pathogenesis of renal failure in myeloma is multifactorial. Factors negatively influencing renal function include immunoglobulin deposition, particularly the light-chain component, causing proximal tubular damage and myeloma cast nephropathy. Dehydration, hypercalcaemia, hyperuricaemia, infection, nephrotoxic drugs, including non-steroidal anti-inflammatory drugs (NSAIDs) and some antibiotics, also play a role. Less frequently, amyloid, light-chain deposition and plasma cell infiltration may occur. Dialysis should be offered to patients where appropriate for the management of the renal failure, and the advice of a nephrologist should be sought when response to conservative measures is poor.

NEW APPROACHES IN THE TREATMENT OF HAEMATOLOGICAL MALIGNANCIES

1. Growth factors, such as G-CSF and GM-CSF (granulocyte–macrophage colony-stimulating factor), EPO and interleukin 6 (IL-6). Stem cell factor is being developed.

2. Improved supportive care: blood products, antibiotics, new antifungal agents (caspofungin and voriconazole) and antivirals (ribavirin).
3. New cytotoxic drugs: deoxycoformycin, 2-CdA, oral idarubicin.
4. 'Directed' agents such as tyrosine kinase inhibitors (STI-571 – Gleevec)
5. Monoclonal antibodies such as the anti-CD33 imatinib (Mylotarg), the pan-lymphocyte and monocyte antibody, Campath,

and the anti-CD20 monoclonal antibody Rituximab
6. Thalidomide in resistant/relapsed myeloma and other conditions. Velcade, a proteosome inhibitor, in relapsed myeloma.
7. Mini transplants, which rely on a graft versus tumour effect, rather than on the cytotoxic effects of the conditioning therapy for eradication of the malignant disease.
8. ATRA for AML M3, where the cells have retinoic acid receptors.

NURSING CARE FOR PATIENTS WITH LEUKAEMIA

Moira Stephens

INTRODUCTION

The leukaemias are a complex collection of haematological disorders first described in 1845 by Virchow, and comprise two main groups: the acute and the chronic leukaemias.

The nurse's role in caring for a patient with leukaemia may vary in detail, according to disease type and treatment, but in principle it is largely the same. Both medical and nursing supportive care of the leukaemic patient are major contributors to increased survival and quality of life.

CARING FOR THE PATIENT WITH LEUKAEMIA

Nursing care is centred on the following:

1. Providing information to the patient and family about diagnosis, the disease and treatment options at all times throughout the treatment trajectory.
2. Addressing anxiety issues, from diagnosis through all stages of treatment, as these may differ at varying stages of the trajectory.
3. The nursing management of disease-related complications:

   - thrombocytopenia (see Ch. 22)
   - anaemia (see Ch. 21)
   - neutropenia (see Ch. 20)
   - renal failure (see Ch. 24)
   - hyperleucocytosis and leucostasis
   - coagulopathies
   - extramedullary disease: e.g. CNS, splenic or skin infiltration.

4. The nursing management of treatment-related complications:

   - myelosuppression (see Chs 20, 21 and 22)
   - renal damage (see Ch. 24)
   - changes in mental status (see Ch. 27)
   - neuropathy (see Ch. 27)
   - cardiopulmonary toxicities (see Ch. 28)
   - gastrointestinal toxicities (see Ch. 17)
   - transplant-related complications (see Ch. 48)
   - fatigue (see Ch. 34).

SUPPORT RESOURCES

A variety of support networks exist for patients and their carers, consisting of written information, practical and financial support from organisations such as Cancer BACUP (see Useful Addresses) and the Leukaemia Care Society (see Useful Addresses). Organisations such as the EBMT (see Useful Addresses) and the British Society for Haematology provide information for healthcare workers.

Acute leukaemia is an aggressive disease; it is life threatening and is characterised by a rapid onset and quickly progresses to a fatal outcome if untreated. There two types of acute leukaemia – acute lymphoblastic leukaemia (ALL) and acute myeloid leukaemia (AML) – both have a number of subtypes. (See Medical Care section above.)

SYMPTOMS

The patient's journey often begins with complaints of fatigue due to anaemia, infections secondary to neutropenia or spontaneous bleeding or bruising due to thrombocytopenia. This symptomology is caused by the failure of the bone marrow to produce adequate numbers of fully functional normal haemopoietic cells due to the rapidly expanding leukaemic cell population. Other presenting symptoms may include nerve palsies, ataxia, headaches and visual disturbances, indicative of CNS involvement, more commonly with ALL. Lymphadenopathy, skin, testicular and other extramedullary involvement is also most commonly seen in ALL patients, but is also seen with some subtypes of AML (Fig. 47.4).

TRANSFER TO A SPECIALIST CENTRE

Immediately on diagnosis, either by the general practitioner (GP) or in a local hospital, the patient is often transferred to a specialist centre equipped to care for patients undergoing treatment for leukaemia. The impact of the rapid onset of the leukaemia and need for immediate treatment for the patient, perhaps in a centre some distance from home, must be taken into consideration in supporting the patient through their initial management.

DIAGNOSTIC INVESTIGATIONS AND TREATMENT

A number of diagnostic tests are undertaken, which will always include a bone marrow aspirate and trephine and a variety of blood tests. The patient, at this early stage, may also be extremely unwell, presenting in a state of sepsis or with bleeding and coagulation problems for example; therefore, in addition to coping with the diagnosis of a life-threatening disease, patients may be battling for survival. The nurse has an immense role in supporting the family as well as the patient through this initial period, assisting them to assimilate the information given to them. It is important to understand that although the patient may be extremely unwell, the underlying disease must be treated in order to arrest the septic or haemorrhagic process.

Knowledgeable nursing input may help the patient to consider the options for treatment and, at

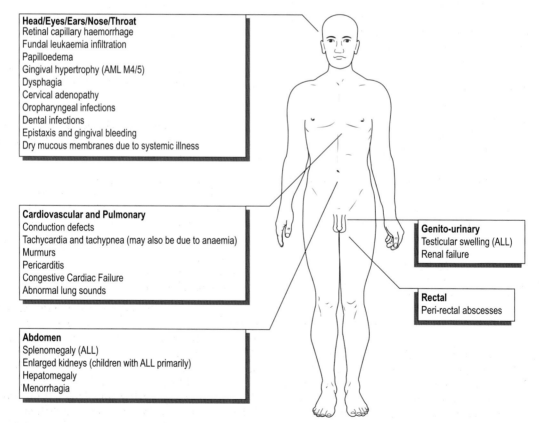

Head/Eyes/Ears/Nose/Throat
Retinal capillary haemorrhage
Fundal leukaemia infiltration
Papilloedema
Gingival hypertrophy (AML M4/5)
Dysphagia
Cervical adenopathy
Oropharyngeal infections
Dental infections
Epistaxis and gingival bleeding
Dry mucous membranes due to systemic illness

Cardiovascular and Pulmonary
Conduction defects
Tachycardia and tachypnea (may also be due to anaemia)
Murmurs
Pericarditis
Congestive Cardiac Failure
Abnormal lung sounds

Abdomen
Splenomegaly (ALL)
Enlarged kidneys (children with ALL primarily)
Hepatomegaly
Menorrhagia

Genito-urinary
Testicular swelling (ALL)
Renal failure

Rectal
Peri-rectal abscesses

Figure 47.4   Clinical features in acute leukaemias.

this stage, information and guidance are of immense value.

Treatment for leukaemia consists of a therapeutic package of a series of courses of chemotherapy which may include an SCT, using cells from either an autologous or allogeneic source. Following the initial course of induction chemotherapy, a further bone marrow aspirate is taken in order to establish that the regenerating bone marrow does not contain leukaemic cells. If this is the case, and the patient has not gone into remission, the patient will immediately undergo an alternative course of chemotherapy which prolongs the initial length of hospitalisation and period of neutropenia. (See also Ch. 48.)

This initial period of hospitalisation usually lasts for about 4 weeks, but may be prolonged for up to 12 weeks, depending on complications and response to treatment.

Acute myeloid leukaemia

Induction treatment
In AML, the initial induction course of intensive polychemotherapy and combines of an anthracycline such as daunorubicin, cytarabine (ara-C) and another agent such as etoposide (VP16) or tioguanine (thioguanine). Successful treatment depends on control of the bone marrow and extramedullary disease, as well as treating the presenting symptoms and complications.

Consolidation treatment
Further, consolidation, chemotherapy is given once remission has been established. Studies have shown that if further chemotherapy is not given, survival time is much shorter and most patients relapse within 6–8 months (1). SCT may be the treatment of choice in certain AML patients in first remission, but controversy exists whether further consolidation, maintenance, autologous or allogeneic transplant is the treatment of choice in first remission, in others (Fig. 47.5). (See Medical Care section above.)

Acute promyelocytic leukaemia
Acute promyelocytic leukaemia (APL), or AML FAB type 3 (AML-M3), is treated differently to other AMLs. It frequently presents with bleeding due to disseminating intravascular coagulation requiring urgent stabilisation with replacement coagulation factors, platelets and induction with all-*trans* retonic acid (ATRA, tretinoin), which promotes cell differentiation and reduces and, eventually, eradicates the APL blasts, which, in turn, arrests the coagulopathy. The introduction of ATRA has not only made treating AML-M3 much safer, but has, when given in combination with

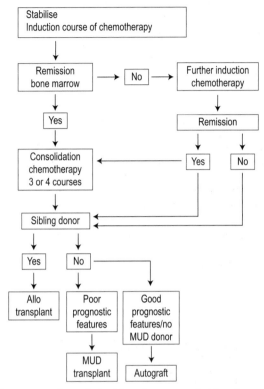

General algorithm of treatment decisions for patient with AML

Figure 47.5 General algorithm of treatment decisions for patient with acute myeloid leukaemia. MUD = matched unrelated donor.

induction and maintenance chemotherapy, improved survival and long-term remission rates. (See Medical Care section above.)

Acute lymphoblastic leukaemia

ALL is also treated using induction and consolidation therapy, followed by one or a combination of:

- long-term maintenance chemotherapy over 2–3 years
- autologous transplant
- allogeneic transplant.

Therapy choice is made depending on individual risk factors, putting the patient in a standard or high risk category. The initial induction therapy universally includes a combination of an anthracycline, such as doxorubicin, a corticosteroid and a vinca alkaloid, usually vincristine. Either prophylactic or treatment chemotherapy is given intrathecally, which is usually followed at a later date by cranial radiation, as the CNS may serve as a sanctuary site for lymphoblastic

**General algorithm of treatment decisions
for patient with ALL**

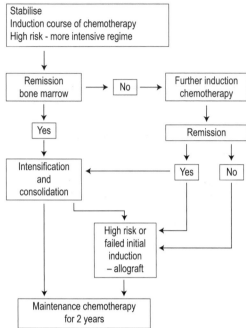

Figure 47.6 General algorithm of treatment decisions for patient with acute lymphoblastic leukaemia. GMALL = German Acute Lymphoblastic Lymphoma Protocol.

leukaemia. Fewer than 10% of adults present with CNS involvement, (2) but, if the CNS is not treated, 50–75% of adults will develop CNS involvement (2) (Fig. 47.6). (See Medical Care section above.)

Chronic myeloid leukaemia

CML may present in any one of three phases – chronic, accelerated and blastic – with their own presenting features.

Chronic phase
- Fatigue
- Night sweats
- Pallor
- Weight loss
- Sternal tenderness
- Abdominal discomfort, resulting from splenomegaly
- Anaemia
- Dyspnoea
- High WBC (>100 000/mm³)
- Mature and immature granulocytes predominate
- Hypercellular bone marrow

- 95% Philadelphia chromosome positivity on cytogenetic examination
- Median duration 3–5 years.

Accelerated phase
- All of the above
- Increased fatigue
- Increasing anaemia
- Thrombocytopenia
- Lymphadenopathy
- Generalised bony pain
- Recurrent splenomegaly
- Hepatomegaly
- Fever of unknown origin
- Thrombocytosis
- High WBC (maybe >100 000/mm³, with 15% blasts and thrombocytopenia)
- Leucocyte doubling time less than 20 days
- Failure to respond to therapy given in chronic phase
- Bone marrow shows increased blasts
- Median survival about 1 year.

Blastic phase
- All of the above
- Haemorrhagic complications, such as bleeding, cerebral or pulmonary haemorrhage
- Infections
- Two-thirds of blastic transformation is myeloid and then has features of AML
- One-third of blastic transformation is lymphoid and then has features of ALL
- Median survival less than 6 months.

The only curative option is allogeneic transplant. Patients with CML often present in chronic phase with little or no symptoms, having been diagnosed as part of a routine blood test. This must be taken into account as, unlike the acute leukaemias, the patient may have no knowledge of being ill and is suddenly undergoing a bone marrow biopsy and being tissue typed for a potential bone marrow transplant with their siblings.

Chronic lymphocytic leukaemia

CLL is diagnosed at a routine blood test in the 25% of patients who are asymptomatic. The incidence rises with increasing age and a small proportion are familial. Diagnosis is suspected if there is an unexplained lymphocytosis on the peripheral blood film.

The clinical features and expected survival are dependent on the stage. Treatment is largely aimed at alleviating symptoms using single agent chemotherapy such as chlorambucil or combination chemotherapy such as CVP or CHOP. Nucleoside analogues such as fludarabine, cladribine (2-CdA) and pentostatin are currently undergoing trials and studies are underway to ascertain the role of allogeneic and autologous transplant. (See Medical Care section above.)

NURSING CARE FOR PATIENTS WITH MYELOMA

Moira Stephens

INTRODUCTION

Although some patients may be asymptomatic, most patients present to their GP with a history of fatigue, weight loss, anorexia and repeated infection, sometimes with bone pain or a pathological fracture (Fig. 47.7). (See Medical Care section above.)

Myeloma is diagnosed according to the presence of minimum criteria and then staged according to Durie–Salmon staging.

DIAGNOSTIC INVESTIGATIONS

- Standard X-ray imaging of bones (skeletal survey)
- Bone marrow aspirate and biopsy
- Serum protein electrophoresis
- Serum immunoglobulin
- Free light-chain essay
- Full blood count, erythrocyte sedimentation rate (ESR)
- Serum urea and electrolytes; calcium
- Serum β_2-microglobulin

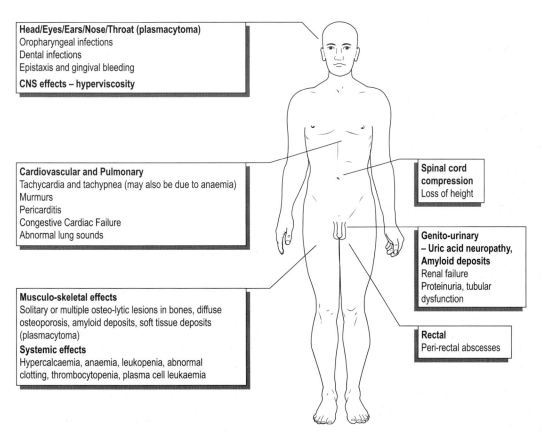

Head/Eyes/Ears/Nose/Throat (plasmacytoma)
Oropharyngeal infections
Dental infections
Epistaxis and gingival bleeding
CNS effects – hyperviscosity

Cardiovascular and Pulmonary
Tachycardia and tachypnea (may also be due to anaemia)
Murmurs
Pericarditis
Congestive Cardiac Failure
Abnormal lung sounds

Musculo-skeletal effects
Solitary or multiple osteo-lytic lesions in bones, diffuse osteoporosis, amyloid deposits, soft tissue deposits (plasmacytoma)
Systemic effects
Hypercalcaemia, anaemia, leukopenia, abnormal clotting, thrombocytopenia, plasma cell leukaemia

Spinal cord compression
Loss of height

Genito-urinary
– Uric acid neuropathy,
Amyloid deposits
Renal failure
Proteinuria, tubular dysfunction

Rectal
Peri-rectal abscesses

Figure 47.7 Clinical features in multiple myeloma.

Table 47.4 Standard therapies Adapted from Durie B. (2000) A concise review of disease and treatment of multiple myeloma. IMF, UK.

Regimen name	Composition	Treatment
MP	Melphalan ± prednisone	Oral – outpatient therapy
C week	Cyclophosphamide ± prednisone	Oral + IV – outpatient therapy
ABCM	Adriamycin, BCNU (carmustine), cyclophosphamide, melphalan	Oral + IV – in/outpatient therapy
VAD	Vincristine, Adriamycin, dexamethasone	Oral + IV – in/outpatient therapy
VAMP	Vincristine, Adriamycin, methylprednisolone	Oral + IV – in/outpatient therapy
C-VAMP	Cyclophosphamide + VAMP	Oral + IV – in/outpatient therapy
Z-Dex	Oral idarubicin + dexamethasone	Oral – outpatient therapy
High-dose melphalan	Up to 100 mg/m², with no stem cell rescue may occasionally be used	IV– inpatient
Autologous transplant	140–200 mg/m² of melphalan + high-dose methylprednisolone followed by autograft	IV – inpatient
Allogeneic transplant	High-dose melphalan + total body irradiation followed by allogeneic cells	IV – inpatient
Alpha-interferon	Traditionally used as maintenance therapy, but side effects may outweigh benefit	SC – outpatient

IV, intravenous; S/C, subcutaneous.

- Serum EPO level
- Urine – (free light chain, Bence Jones protein).

(See also Box 47.9.)

TREATMENT

Treatment modalities are aimed at symptom control as well as obtaining remission (Tables 47.4 and 47.5).

Myeloma is essentially incurable; however, in younger patients, allogeneic and autologous transplant performed early may offer a long-term remission. Survival essentially depends on stage at diagnosis and response to active treatment (Fig. 47.8).

THE NURSE'S ROLE

The nurse's role in caring for a patient with myeloma is centred on the following:

1. Providing information to the patient and family about diagnosis, the disease and treatment options.
2. Addressing anxiety issues, from diagnosis through all stages of treatment.
3. Disease-related complications:

   - thrombocytopenia (see Ch. 22)
   - anaemia (see Ch. 21)
   - neutropenia (see Ch. 20)

Table 47.5 Novel/trial therapies Adapted from Durie B. (2000) A concise review of disease and treatment of multiple myeloma. IMF, UK.

Therapy	Description
Thalidomide	Currently used in relapse, trials in use as maintenance and may be used as front-line therapy
IMiDs (immunomodulatory drugs): Revimid, Actimid	Thalidomide analogues – may be more potent, with fewer side effects
Proteasome inhibitors: bortezimib (Velcade or PS-341)	Phase III trials ongoing. Induces myeloma cell death
Arsenic trioxide (Trisenox)	Phase II trials ongoing. Inhibits myeloma cell growth and promotes cell death
Genasense (Bcl-2 antisense)	Phase II and III trials. Increases myeloma cell sensitivity to chemotherapy and cell death
Skeletal targeted radiotherapy: 166Ho-DOTMP	Used in conjunction with transplant. Myeloma cells are very radiosensitive
DNA vaccines	Patient's own immune system destroys the myeloma cell after antigens on myeloma cells have been encoded

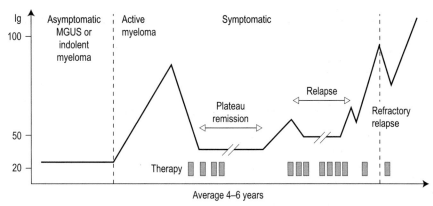

Figure 47.8 Disease phases. MGUS, monoclonal gammopathy of undetermined significance. Adapted from Durie B. (2000) A concise review of disease and treatment of multiple myeloma. IMF, UK.

- renal failure (see Ch. 24)
- hypercalcaemia
- spinal cord compression
- lytic bone lesions
- pathological fractures
- repeated infections (see Chs 13 and 20).

4. Treatment-related complications:

- myelosuppression (see Ch. 20)
- renal damage (see Ch. 24)
- changes in mental status (see Ch. 27)
- neuropathy status (see Ch. 27)
- cardiopulmonary tonicities status (see Ch. 28)
- gastrointestinal tonicities status (see Ch. 17)
- fatigue status (see Ch. 34).

SPINAL CORD COMPRESSION

Spinal cord compression may occur when there is degeneration of the spine causing verterbral collapse or due to the pressure of a plasmacytoma on the cord. Signs and symptoms are related to loss of sensory and motor function, leading to paralysis below the lesion. The diagnosis is confirmed by an MRI. Treatment is required urgently and may include surgical removal of the plasmacytoma, radiotherapy and steroids.

BONE DISEASE

Bone disease is one of the main features of myeloma and is manifested as lytic lesions, bone pain, osteoporosis, pathological fractures and hypercalcaemia. This is caused by myeloma cells proliferating uncontrollably, interacting with, and increasing, osteoclast activity. This will cause interaction with the bone marrow environment and skeletal destruction. These effects are a major cause of morbidity and mortality in patients with myeloma. The ribs, skull, long bones and spine are commonly affected and some patients lose 2–3 inches in height. Bisphosphonates have been shown to reduce bone pain, skeletal events and improve quality of life. Long-term bisphosphonate therapy is therefore recommended for all patients with myeloma requiring treatment for their disease (Fig. 47.9) .[69]

Bisphosphonates

Bisphosphonates work by inhibiting bone resorption, and thus treat hypercalcaemia, in addition to treating bone destruction (Fig. 47.10). They may have a direct antimyeloma effect. There are four types in use:

- clodronate   oral
- pamidronate   IV
- zoledronic acid   IV
- ibandronate   IV

(See Medical Care section above.)

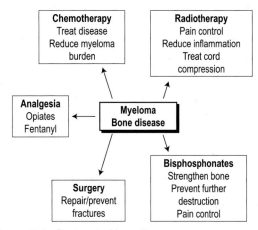

Figure 47.9   Treatment of bone disease.

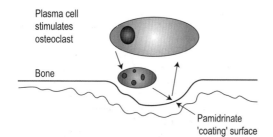

Figure 47.10 Bisphosphonate (pamidronate) action. Adapted from Durie B. (2000) A concise review of disease and treatment of multiple myeloma. IMF, UK.

SUPPORT

A variety of support networks exist for patients and their carers, consisting of written information, practical and financial support from organisations such as CancerBACUP (see Useful Addresses), the International Myeloma (see Useful Addresses) and the UK Myeloma Forum (see Useful Addresses); organisations such as EBMT (see Useful Addresses) provide information for healthcare workers.

References

1. Bennett JM, Catovsky D, Daniel MT, et al. Proposals for the classification of the acute leukaemias. French–American–British (FAB) co-operative group. Br J Haematol 1976; 33(4):451–458.

2. Degos L, Wang ZY. All trans retinoic acid in acute promyelocytic leukemia. Oncogene 2001; 20(49): 7140–7145.

3. Tallman M, Anderson J, Schiffer C, et al. All-transretinoic acid in acute promyelocytic leukemia. N Engl J Med 1997; 337(15):1021–1077.

4. Stevens RF, Hann I, Wheatley K. Marked improvements in outcome with chemotherapy alone in paediatric acute myeloid leukaemias. Results of the Medical Research Council's 10th AML trial. Br J Haematol 1998; 101:130–140.

5. Wheatley K, Burnett AK, Goldstone AH, et al. A simple, robust, validated and highly predictive index for the determination of risk-directed therapy in acute myeloid leukaemia derived from the MRC AML 10 trial. United Kingdom Medical Research Council's Adult and Childhood Leukaemia Working Parties. Br J Haematol 1999; 107(1):69–79.

6. Hann IM, Steven RF, Goldstone AH, et al. Randomised comparison of DAT versus ADE as induction chemotherapy in children and young adults with acute myeloid leukaemia. Results of the Medical Research Council's 10th AML trial (MRC AML 10) Blood 1997; 89:2311–2318.

7. Buchner T, Hiddemann W , Wormann B, et al. Double induction strategy for acute myeloid leukaemia: the effect of high-dose cytarabine with mitoxantrone instead of standard-dose cytarabine with daunorubicin and 6-thioguanine: a randomized trial by the German AML Co-operative Group. Blood 1999; 93(12):4116–4124.

8. Cahn JY, Labopin M, Sierra J, et al. No impact of high-dose cytarabine on the outcome of patients transplanted for acute myeloblastic leukaemia in first remission. Acute Leukaemia Working Party of the European Group for Blood and Marrow Transplantation (EBMT). Br J Haematol. 2000; 110:308–314.

9. Burnett AK, Wheatley K, Goldstone AH, et al. The value of allogeneic marrow transplant in patients with acute myeloid leukaemia at differing risk of relapse: results of the UK MRC AML 10 trial. Br J Haematol 2002; 118(2):385–400.

10. Bosi A, Laslo D, Labopin M, et al. Second allogeneic bone marrow transplantation in acute leukaemia: results of a survey by the European Cooperative Group for Blood and Marrow Transplantation. J Clin Oncol 2001; 19(16):3675–3684.

11. Apperley JF, Mauro FR, Goldman JM, et al. Bone marrow transplantation for chronic myeloid leukaemia in first chronic phase: importance of a graft-versus-leukaemia effect. Br J Haematol 1988; 69(2):239–245.

12. Burnett AK, Goldstone AH, Stevens RM, et al. Randomised comparison of addition of autologous bone marrow transplantation to intensive chemotherapy for acute myeloid leukaemia in first remission: results of MRC AML 10 trial. UK Medical Research Council Adult and Children's Leukaemia Working Parties. Lancet 1998; 351: 700–708.

13. Mufti GJ, Stevens JR, Oscier DG, et al. Myelodysplastic syndromes: a scoring system with prognostic significance. Br J Haematol 1985; 59:425–433.

14. De Witte T, Van Biezen A, Labopin M, et al. Autologous SCT for patients with myelodysplastic syndromes (MDS) or acute myeloid leukemia following MDS. Blood 1997; 90(10):3853–3857.

15. Arnold R, de Witte T, van Biezen A, et al. Unrelated bone marrow transplantation in patients with myelodysplastic syndromes and secondary acute myeloid leukaemia: an EBMT survey. European Blood and Marrow Transplantation Group. Bone Marrow Transpl 1998; 21(12):1213–1216.

16. De Witte T, Suciu S, Verhoef G, et al. Intensive chemotherapy followed by allogeneic or autologous stem cell transplantation for patients with myelodysplastic syndromes (MDSs) and acute myeloid leukaemia following MDS. Blood 2001; 98(8):2326–2331.

17. Farber S, Diamond RD, Mercer R. Temporary remissions in acute leukaemia in children produced by folic acid antagonist 4-aminoglutamic acid (aminopterin). N Engl J Med 1948; 238:787–793.

18. Pearson OH, Eliel LP. Use of pituitary adrenocorticotropic hormone (ACTH) and cortisone in lymphomas and leukaemia. J Am Med Assoc 1950; 144:1349–1353.

19. Frei E, Karon M, Levin RH, et al. The effectiveness of combinations of antileukaemia agents in inducing and maintaining remission in children with acute leukaemia. Blood 1965; 26:642–653.

20. Pinkel D. Five-year follow up of 'total therapy' of childhood lymphoblastic leukaemia. J Am Med Assoc 1971; 216:648–652.

21. Frassoni F, Labopin M, Gluckman E, et al. Results of allogeneic bone marrow transplantation for acute leukemia have improved in Europe with time – a report of the Acute Leukemia Working Party of the European Group for Blood and Marrow Transplantation (ESCT) Bone Marrow Transplant. 1996; 17:13–18.

22. Barrett AJ. Bone marrow transplantation for acute lymphoblastic leukaemia. In: Hoelzer D, ed. Acute lymphoblastic leukaemia. Baillière's Clinical Haematology, London: Baillière Tindall; 1994; 7:377–401.

23. Zhang MJ, Hoelzer D, Horowitz MM. Long-term follow-up of adults with acute lymphoblastic leukemia in first remission treated with chemotherapy or bone marrow transplantation. Ann Intern Med 1995; 123: 428–431.

24. Powles R, Mehta J, Singhal S, et al. Autologous bone marrow or peripheral blood stem cell transplantation followed by maintenance chemotherapy for adult acute lymphoblastic leukemia in first remission: 50 cases from a single centre. Bone Marrow Transplant 1995; 16:241–247.

25. Chessells JM, Bailey C, Richards SM. Intensification of treatment and survival in all children with lymphoblastic leukemia: results of UK Medical Research Council trial UKALL X. Lancet 1995; 345: 143–148.

26. Chessells JM, Bailey C, Wheeler K, et al. Bone marrow transplantation for high-risk childhood lymphoblastic leukemia in first remission experience in MRC UKALL X. Lancet 1992; 340:565–568.

27. Tura S, Baccarani M, Zuffa E, for the Italian Cooperative Study Group on Chronic Myeloid Leukemia. Interferon alfa-2a as compared with conventional chemotherapy for the treatment of chronic myeloid leukemia. N Engl J Med 1994; 330:820.

28. Allan NC, Richards SM, Shepherd PCA. UK Medical Research Council randomised multicentre trial of interferon-an1 for chronic myeloid leukemia: improved survival irrespective of cytogenetic response. Lancet 1995; 345:1392–1397.

29. Goldman JM, Gale RP, Horowitz MM, et al. Bone marrow transplantation for chronic myelogenous leukemia in chronic phase: increased risk of relapse associated with T-cell depletion. Ann Int Med 1988; 108: 806–814.

30. Apperley JF, Jones L, Hale G, et al. Bone marrow transplantation for patients with chronic myeloid leukaemia: T-cell depletion with Campath-1 reduce the incidence of graft-versus-host disease but may increase the risk of leukaemic relapse. Bone Marrow Transplant 1986; 1:199–204.

31. Clift RA, Buckner D, Thomas ED, et al. Marrow transplantation for chronic myeloid leukemia: a randomized study comparing cyclophosphamide and total body irradiation with busulphan and cyclophosphamide. Blood 1994; 84(6):2036–2043.

32. Barrett AJ, Malkovska V. Graft-versus-leukaemia: understanding and using the allo-immune response to treat haematological malignancies. Br J Haematol 1996; 93:754–761.

33. Mackinnon S, Papadopoulos EP, Carabasi MH, et al. Adoptive immunotherapy evaluating escalating doses of donor leukocytes for relapse of chronic myeloid leukemia following bone marrow transplantation: separation of graft-versus-leukemia responses from graft-versus-host disease. Blood 1995; 86:1261–1267.

34. Carella AM, Lerma E, Corsetti MT, et al. Autografting with Philadelphia chromosome-negative mobilized hematopoietic progenitor cells in chronic myeloid leukemia. Blood 1999; 1(5):1534–1539.

35. Carella AM, Cavaliere M, Lerma E, et al. Autologous peripheral hematopoietic stem cell transplantation for chronic myeloid leukaemia. Baillière's Best Practice Res Clin Haematol 1999; 12(1–2):209–217.

36. Thiesing JT, Ohno-Jones S, Kolibaba KS, et al. Efficacy of STI571, an abl tyrosine kinase inhibitor, in conjunction with other antileukemic agents against bcr-abl-positive cells. Blood 2000; 96:3195–3199.

37. Goldman JM. Tyrosine-kinase inhibition in treatment of chronic myeloid leukaemia. Lancet 2000; 355(9209):1031–1032.

38. Hehlmann R, Hochhaus A, Berger U, et al. Current trends in the management of chronic myelogenous leukemia. Ann Hematol 2000; 79(7):345–354.

39. Cortes J, Giles F, O'Brien S, et al. Result of high-dose imatinib mesylate in patients with Philadelphia chromosome-positive chronic myeloid leukemia after failure of interferon-α. Blood 2003.

40. O'Brien SG, Guilhot F, Larson RA, et al. Imatinib compared with interferon and low-dose cytarabine for newly diagnosed chronic-phase chronic myeloid leukemia. N Engl J Med 2003; 348(11): 1048–1050.

41. Keating MR, Kantarjian H, O'Brien S et al. Fludarabine: a new agent with marked cytoreductive activity in untreated CLL. J Clin Oncol 1991; 9:44–49.

42. Doney KC, Chauncey T, Appelbaum F. Allogeneic related donor hemopoietic stem cell transplantation for treatment of chronic lymphocytic leukemia. Bone Marrow Transpl 2002: 299(10):817–823.

43. Khouri IF, Keating MJ, Saliba RM, et al. Long-term follow up of patients with CLL treated with allogeneic

hempoietic transplantation. Cytotherapy 2002; 4(3):217–212.

44. Dreger P, Michallet M, Schmitz N. Stem-cell transplantation for chronic lymphocytic leukemia: the 1999 perspective. Ann Oncol 2000;11(Suppl 1):49–53.

45. Esteve J, Villamor N, Colomer D, et al. Stem cell transplantation for chronic lymphocytic leukemia: different outcome after autologous and allogeneic transplantation and correlation with minimal residual disease status. Leukemia 2001; 15(3):445–451.

46. Riccardi A, Mora O, Tinelli C, et al. Long-term survival of stage I multiple myeloma given chemotherapy just after diagnosis or at progression of the disease: a multicentre randomised study. Br J Cancer 2000; 82:1254–1260.

47. Glaspy J, Bukowski R, Steinberg D, et al. Impact of therapy with Epoietin Alfa on clinical outcomes of patients with nonmyeloid malignancies during cancer chemotherapy in community oncology practice. Procrit Study Group. J Clin Oncol 1997; 15:1218–1234.

48. Demetri G, Kris M, Wade J, et al for the Proctrit Study Group. Quality-of-life benefit in chemotherapy patients treated with Epoietin Alfa is independent of disease response or tumour type: results from a prospective community oncology study. J Clin Oncol 1998; 16:3412–3425.

49. Alexanian R, Haut A, Khan AU, et al. Treatment for multiple myeloma: combination chemotherapy with different melphalan dose regimens. J Am Med Assoc 1969; 208:1680–1685.

50. Medical Research Council's Working Party on Leukaemia in Adults. Report on the second myelomatosis trial after five years of follow-up. Br J Cancer 1980; 42:813–822.

51. Combination chemotherapy versus melphalan plus prednisone as treatment for multiple myeloma: an overview of 6,633 patients from 27 randomized trials. Myeloma Trialists' Collaborative Group. J Clin Oncol 1998; 16(12):3832–3842.

52. Raje N, Powles R, Kulkarni S, et al. A comparison of vincristine and doxorubicin infusional chemotherapy with methylprednisolone (VAMP) with the addition of weekly cyclophosphamide (C-VAMP) as induction treatment followed by autografting in previously untreated myeloma. Br J Haematol 1997; 97:153–160.

53. Cook G, Sharp RA, Tansey P, et al. A phase I/II trial of Z-Dex (oral idarubicin and dexamethasone), an oral equivalent of VAD, as initial therapy at diagnosis or progression in multiple myeloma. Br J Haematol 1996; 93:931–934.

54. Bjorkstrand B, Svensson H, Goldschmidt H, et al. Alpha-interferon maintenance treatment is associated with improved survival after high-dose treatment and autologous stem cell transplantation in patients with multiple myeloma: a retrospective registry study from the European Group for Blood and Marrow Transplantation (EBMT). Bone Marrow Transplant 2001; 27:511–515.

55. Desikan R, Barlogie B, Sawyer J, et al. Results of high-dose therapy for 1000 patients with multiple myeloma: durable complete remissions and superior survival in the absence of chromosome 13 abnormalities. Blood 2000; 95:4008–4010.

56. MacKinnon S. Who may benefit from donor leucocyte infusions after allogeneic stem cell transplantation? Br J Haematol 2000; 110(1):12–17.

57. Gahrton G, Tura S, Ljungman P, et al. Allogeneic bone marrow transplantation in multiple myeloma. European Group for Bone Marrow Transplantation. N Engl J Med 1991; 325(18):1267–1273.

58. Gahrton G, Svensson H, Cavo M, et al. Progress in allogenic bone marrow and peripheral blood stem cell transplantation for multiple myeloma: a comparison between transplants performed 1983–93 and 1994–98 at European Group for Blood and Marrow Transplantation centres. Br J Haematol 2001; 113:209–216.

59. Bensinger WI, Buckner D, Anasetti C, et al. Allogeneic marrow transplantation for multiple myeloma: an analysis of risk factors on outcome. Blood 1996; 88(7):2787–2798.

60. Craddock C, Bardy P, Kreiter S, et al. Short report: engraftment of T-cell-depleted allogeneic haematopoietic stem cells using a reduced intensity conditioning regimen. Br J Haematol 2000; 111:797–800.

61. Blade J, Esteve J. Viewpoint on the impact of interferon in the treatment of multiple myeloma: benefit for a small proportion of patients? Med Oncol 2000; 17:77–84.

62. Berenson JR, Lichtenstein A, Porter L, et al. Long-term pamidronate treatment of advanced multiple myeloma patients reduces skeletal events. Myeloma Aredia Study Group. J Clin Oncol 1998; 16:593–602.

63. McCloskey EV, MacLennan ICM, Drayson MT, et al. A randomised trial of the effect of clodronate on skeletal morbidity in multiple myeloma. Br J Haematol 1998; 100:317–325.

64. Berenson JR, Rosen LS, Howell A, et al. Zoledronic acid reduces skeletal-related events in patients with osteolytic metastases. Cancer 2001; 91:1191–1200.

65. Belch AR, Bergsagel DE, Wilson K, et al. Effect of daily etidronate on the osteolysis of multiple myeloma. J Clin Oncol 1991; 9:1397–1402.

66. Belch A, Shelley W, Bergsagel D, et al. A randomised trial of maintenance versus no maintenance melphalan and prednisone in responding multiple myeloma patients. Br J Cancer 1988; 57: 94–99.

67. Kyle RA, Rajkumar SV. Therapeutic application of thalidomide in multiple myeloma. Semin Oncol 2001; 28(6):583–587.

68. Barlogie B, Desikan R, Eddlemon P, et al. Extended survival in advanced and refractory multiple myeloma after single-agent thalidomide: identification of prognostic factors in a phase 2 study of 169 patients. Blood 2001; 98(2):492–494.

69. Guidelines on the diagnosis and management of multiple myeloma. Br J Haematol 2001; 115:522–540. http://www.ukmf.org.uk/guidelines/

70. Nabhan C, Patton D, Gordon L, et al. A pilot trial of rituximab and alemtuzumab combination therapy in patients with relapsed and/or refractory chronic lymphocytic leukemia (CLL). Leuk Lymphoma 2004; 45(11):2269–2273.

71. Richardson P, Barlogie B, Berenson J, et al. Phase II study of Velcade™ (Bortezomib) for injection in patients with relapsed and refractory multiple myeloma. Br J Haematol 2004; 127(2):165–172.

72. Jagannath S, Barlogie B, Berenson J, et al. Phase II multicentre randomised study of Velcade™ (Bortezomib) for injection in multiple myeloma patients relapsed after front-line therapy. N Engl J Med 2003; 348(26):2609–2617.

USEFUL ADDRESSES

Cancer BACUP:
www.cancerbacup.org.uk

The Leukaemia Care Society:
www.leukaemiacare.org

European Blood and Marrow Transplant Group (EBMT):
www.ebmt.org

The International Myeloma Forum:
www.myeloma.org.uk

The UK Myeloma Forum:
www.ukmf.org.uk

The British Society for Haematology
www.b-s-h.org.uk

Chapter **48**

High–dose chemotherapy and transplantation

Moira Stephens

INTRODUCTION

Haemopoietic stem cell transplantation (HSCT) is a treatment modality whereby very high doses of chemotherapy and/or radiotherapy are given to the patient with the aim of eradicating the disease and ablating the marrow. Haemopoietic stem cells, either from a donor (allogeneic transplant) or collected previously from the patient (autologous transplant) are then given to the patient intravenously. These infused stem cells then repopulate the marrow.

HSCT was introduced in the early 1960s through the pioneering work of individuals including Mathe, McFarland and Donnal Thomas. It has rapidly developed from an experimental procedure to an established treatment for a variety of serious disorders. The number of patients undergoing HSCT increased 10-fold during the 1980s, with a similar increase in the number of transplant centres. Treatment advances, successful recruitment of unrelated volunteer donors, and wider treatment and disease applications now offer this therapy to thousands who would otherwise die of their disease.[1]

Definitions

Ablative

An ablative treatment regimen consists of very high doses of chemotherapy and/or radiotherapy which effectively eradicates haemopoietic cell production in the bone marrow. With ablative treatment, such as total body irradiation (TBI) using a dose of 12.5 Gy or melphalan 200 mg/m^2, bone marrow function would not recover without the introduction of new stem cells through transplantation.

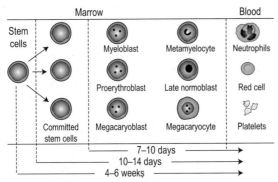

Figure 48.1   Haemopoiesis.

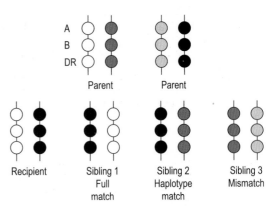

Figure 48.2   Major histocompatibility complex.

Haemopoietic stem cell population

Haemopoiesis, the production of blood cells, occurs mainly in the bone marrow. The pluripotent stem cell is produced by the bone marrow; it starts to mature, becoming a committed (to a blood cell line such as red cells, platelets, neutrophils or lymphocytes) stem cell (Fig. 48.1). These cells then continue to mature along their chosen cell paths, until they become fully functional blood cells circulating in the peripheral blood. As the stem cell is uncommitted, however, it has the potential to become any of the blood cells.

Haemopoietic stem cell transplantation

HSCT refers to any procedure that involves transplanting a haemopoietic cell population into a recipient (the patient), with the intent to repopulate or replace the haemopoietic system totally or partially for transient or permanent periods of time. Stem cells may be collected from the bone marrow, peripherally or from the umbilical cord blood. They may be autologous, from a sibling or from an unrelated donor.

Human leucocyte antigens

The human leucocyte antigen (HLA) or major histocompatibility complex (MHC) is the polymorphic gene cluster on chromosome 6 that codes for cell surface proteins involved in tissue recognition. It is the method of tissue typing to ascertain if a donor is immunologically 'matched' to the recipient. The gene complex is subdivided into two regions: class 1, the A, B and C loci; and class 2, the DR, DP and DQ loci. There are also other histocompatibility loci apart from the HLA system and these differences may contribute to the incidence of graft versus host disease (GvHD). Two siblings have a one in four chance of being HLA identical (Fig. 48.2).

Because the loci are close together on the MHC gene complex, each child inherits the HLA genes as a single haplotype from each parent. Siblings, therefore, are either fully matched, half (haplotype-matched) or not matched at all (mismatched). Parents can only be half matched to their siblings, unless they themselves share a haplotype (e.g. due to intermarriage).

Autologous transplantation

The patient's own haemopoietic stem cells are used for transplantation.

Allogeneic transplantation

In allogeneic transplantation, another individual, related or not, provides the haemopoietic stem cells for the transplant.

Syngeneic transplantation

An identical twin of the patient acts as the source for haemopoietic stem cells.

Matched unrelated donor transplantation or volunteer unrelated donor transplantation

In the case of a matched unrelated donor (MUD) transplant or a volunteer unrelated donor transplant, an unrelated volunteer donor who is HLA matched provides the haemopoietic stem cells.

Stem cell source

Stem cells may be collected in a variety of ways (Table 48.1):

- directly from the bone marrow
- from the peripheral veins following mobilisation of the stem cells by a growth factor such as granulocyte colony-stimulating factor (G-CSF), either used alone or in combination with chemotherapy

Table 48.1   Stem cell sources: indications, advantages and disadvantages

Source	Indications	Advantages	Disadvantages

Bone marrow	Autologous transplant
	Allogeneic transplant
	Syngeneic transplant
		Can be harvested on day of
		    transplant (for an allograft)
			Risks associated with general
			    anaesthetic, infection at harvest sites,
			    bacteraemia, fractured iliac crest or
			    sternum, haematomas, pain at
			    harvest sites.
			Usually involves an inpatient stay

Peripheral
blood
	Autologous transplant
	Allogeneic transplant
	Syngeneic transplant
	Donor lymphocyte
	    infusion
		Can be undertaken as an outpatient,
		More rapid engraftment of
		    neutrophils and platelets
			Growth factors ± chemotherapy
			    required to mobilise stem cells.
			May be an increased incidence of
			    chronic GvHD

Cord blood	Allogeneic transplant
	Syngeneic transplant
	Haplo-identical or
	    partially mismatched
	    transplant
		Relatively low levels of GvHD
		    despite use of mismatched grafts.
		Unrelated donor cells increasingly
		    available from cord blood banks
		    are additional source for small or
		    low weight children without siblings
			Only small numbers of cells in collections
			    (recipient cell dose is weight-related,
			    therefore not suitable for adults)

GvHD, graft versus host disease.

- from umbilical cord and placental blood – collected at the birth of a newborn infant.

Donor lymphocyte infusions

Donor lymphocyte infusions (DLI) refers to any situation where lymphocytes from a previous donor of haemopoietic stem cells are given to the same recipient with the intention to shift the balance between donor and recipient haemopoiesis towards donor type. This may be used in situations such as relapse following a sibling allograft or MUD transplants and works, in principle, by using the immune response of the graft versus tumour effect.

Allogeneic transplantation with reduced intensity conditioning

Also referred to as 'mini-transplants' or 'transplant-light', these transplants utilise reduced intensity conditioning (RIC) regimens and the immunological benefits of the graft versus tumour effect with the intention of reducing the risk of transplant-related mortality while not increasing the risk of relapse. Long-term results are yet unknown. Allo-HSCT with reduced conditioning may provide a potentially curative option for those not fit enough for conventional allogeneic transplantation.

RIC is, at present, an ill-defined procedure with varying regimens. Further research will hopefully establish the role and efficacy of mini transplants.

Rationale and indications for haemopoietic stem cell transplantation

The rationale of using HSCT takes into account the following:

1. The dose intensity of most chemotherapy agents is limited by dose-related marrow toxicity.
2. Haemopoietic stem cells reconstitute the patient's haemopoietic and immunological system after high-dose chemotherapy and/or TBI.

The rationale for supportive care during HSCT takes into account the following:

1. Resulting complications occur secondary to the effects of:

   - dose-intensive conditioning regimens such as infection, bleeding and organ toxicity
   - GvHD
   - supportive medications being used to treat transplant complications (e.g. amphotericin B)
   - treatment failure, e.g. relapse.

2. Supportive care techniques sustain the recipient until stabilised engraftment.[2]

A comparison of autologous and allogeneic haemopoietic stem cell transplantation is shown in Table 48.2.

New indications for transplantation have emerged, such as autoimmune disorders and amyloidosis for autologous and solid tumours for allogeneic

Table 48.2 Comparison of autologous and allogeneic haemopoietic stem cell transplantation

Parameter	Autologous	Allogeneic
Indications	Haematological malignancies and solid tumours. Possible role in autoimmune disorders. Future role in combination with gene therapy to treat genetic disorders, HIV, etc.	Haematological malignancies, aplastic anaemia, congenital bone marrow disorders, immune deficiency states, some inborn errors of metabolism
Stem cell source	Autologous marrow or peripheral stem cells	Marrow, peripheral blood, cord blood, family donors, unrelated donors, HLA-matched or partially matched
Preparative regimen	Primarily designed to provide intensive myeloablative treatment to eradicate malignant disease	Required to provide immunosuppression to allow engraftment. Intensive therapy for malignant disease
Post-transplant treatment	Supportive care, transfusions, growth factors, immune manipulation	Supportive care, transfusions, growth factors, immune manipulation, prophylaxis of GvHD
Infectious complication risk	Low – mainly in the early transplant period	High – sustained risk of infection for months or years
Major complications	Preparative regimen toxicity. Disease recurrence/progression. Treatment-related mortality usually <5%	Preparative regimen toxicity. Disease recurrence/progression. GvHD. Immune deficiency. Treatment-related mortality 5–35%, depending on many patient-, donor- and disease-related factors

GvHD, graft versus host disease (see the Graft versus host disease section for more information on GvHD); HIV, human immunodeficiency virus; HLA, human leucocyte antigen.

transplants; other indications, such as autologous transplants for breast cancer, have been challenged.

Indications for transplant procedures in adult malignant disease are shown in Table 48.3.

MANAGEMENT OF THE PATIENT

Management of a patient undergoing HSCT involves a number of phases. For the purposes of this chapter, they are delineated into steps:

1. Assessment
2. Education
3. Stem cell harvesting and cryopreservation
4. Conditioning therapy and transplant
5. Supportive care
6. Management of complications
7. Follow-up, rehabilitation and survivorship.

Table 48.3 Indications for transplant procedures (adult malignant disease)[3]

Disease	Disease status	Allogeneic		Autologous
		Sibling donor	Alternative donor	
AML	CR1, CR2 or 3, incipient relapse	Standard	Clinical protocol	Standard
	M3 molecular persistance	Standard	Clinical protocol	Not recommended
	M3 2nd molecular remission	Standard	Not recommended	Standard
	Relapse or refractory	Clinical protocol	Not recommended	Not recommended
ALL	CR1 (high risk), CR2, incipient relapse	Standard	Clinical protocol	Clinical protocol
	Relapse or refractory	Clinical protocol	Not recommended	Not recommended

Table 48.3 Indications for transplant procedures (adult malignant disease)[3]—cont'd

Disease	Disease status	Allogeneic		Autologous
		Sibling donor	Alternative donor	
CML	Chronic phase	Standard	Standard	Clinical protocol
	Advanced phase	Standard	Clinical protocol	Not recommended
	Blast crisis	Developmental	Not recommended	Not recommended
Myeloproliferative disorders (non-CML)		Clinical protocol	Developmental	Developemental
Myelodysplastic syndrome	RA, RARS, RAEB, CMMoL	Standard	Clinical protocol	Clinical protocol
	RAEBt, sAML in CR1 or CR2	Standard	Clinical protocol	Clinical protocol
	More advanced stages	Standard	Clinical protocol	Not recommended
CLL		Clinical protocol	Developmental	Clinical protocol
NHL:				
Lymphoblastic	As ALL	Clinical protocol	Developmental	Standard
High & intermediate grade	CR1	Not recommended	Not recommended	Standard
	Relapse, CR2, CR3	Clinical protocol	Clinical protocol	Standard
	Refractory	Clinical protocol	Not recommended	Not recommended
Low grade	CR1	Not recommended	Not recommended	Clinical protocol
	Relapse, CR2, CR3	Clinical protocol	Developmental	Standard
Hodgkin's disease	CR1	Not recommended	Not recommended	Clinical protocol
	1st relapse, CR2, CR3	Clinical protocol	Not recommended	Standard
	Refractory	Clinical protocol	Not recommended	Clinical protocol
Myeloma		Clinical protocol	Developmental	Standard
Solid tumours				
Breast cancer	Adjuvant and inflammatory	Not recommended	Not recommended	Clinical protocol
Breast cancer	Metastatic responding	Developmental	Not recommended	Clinical protocol
Germ cell tumours	Sensitive relapses	Not recommended	Not recommended	Standard
Germ cell tumours	Refractory	Not recommended	Not recommended	Clinical protocol
Ovarian cancer	MRD	Not recommended	Not recommended	Clinical protocol
Ovarian cancer	Refractory	Developmental	Not recommended	Not recommended
Glioma	Post-surgery	Not recommended	Not recommended	Developmental
Small cell lung cancer (limited/'good')	Upfront	Not recommended	Not recommended	Clinical protocol
Renal cell carcinoma	Metastatic	Clinical protocol	Not recommended	Not recommended
Amyloidosis (AL)		Developmental	Not recommended	Clinical protocol

AML, acute myeloid leukaemia, ALL, acute lymphoblastic leukaemia; CML, chronic myeloid leukaemia; CLL, chronic lymphocytic leukaemia; NHL, non-Hodgkin's lymphoma.

1. *Standard:* transplants categorised as standard are carried out in many centres in Europe, often without entering the patient into an institutional or national study. The results of such transplants are in general reasonably well defined and compare favourably (or are superior to) results of non-transplant treatment approaches. The term 'standard' has been incorporated in place of 'routine'.

2. *Clinical protocol:* the value of transplants for patients in these categories is not fully defined. Candidate patients are therefore offered the opportunity of undergoing allogeneic or autologous haemopoietic stem cell transplantation (HSCT) in the context of a clinical protocol that has been designed specifically to cover a series of patients who satisfy defined diagnostic criteria.

3. *Developmental:* transplants have been classified as developmental if there is little or no national or international experience with this particular type of transplant. In general, such transplants will involve single cases or small pilot series undertaken by transplant units with acknowledged special expertise in the management of that particular disease.

4. *Not generally recommended:* this category covers procedures contemplated for a disease in a phase or status in which patients are not conventionally treated by HSCT.

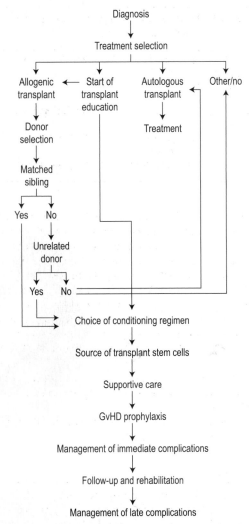

Figure 48.3 An algorithm for decision pathway for the clinical management of haemopoietic stem cell transplantation. GvHD, graft versus host disease (see the Graft versus host disease section for more information on GvHD).

An algorithm for decision pathway for the clinical management of HSCT is given in Figure 48.3.

Assessment

Assessment is an integral part of the decision process. It includes assessing risks concerning transplant-related mortality and risks concerning relapse of the disease. It is multifactorial, comprising patient-related, disease-related and donor-related factors. Factors that need to be considered include:

- Appropriateness of HSCT – guidelines for indication for HSCT according to disease type and disease status vary between countries and centres.

- Age – advancing age is usually associated with higher transplant-related toxicity and poorer long-term survival.[4,5]
- Performance status – poor performance status at the beginning of the transplant process increases transplant-related mortality, especially if due to active infection or acute medical problems. However, some disease-specific co-morbidity such as renal failure secondary to myeloma may not be a contraindication. Patients have been transplanted successfully in this situation.[6]
- Psychological assessment – this is useful in assessing not only the ability of the patient to undergo the transplant procedure but also the support the patient and family may need during and following transplant.
- Nutritional assessment – this helps to identify undernourished patients, who can then be helped to gain optimal weight prior to transplant. Patients who are likely to be at risk of excessive weight loss during transplant, when oral intake is compromised, may also be identified. This may enable pre-emptive steps, such as a PEG (percutaneous endoscopic gastrostomy) tube or a nasogastric tube being placed, prior to transplant.
- Dental assessment – this is an important part of pre-transplant assessment and dealing with potential sources of infection such as dental abscesses should be undertaken 2–3 weeks prior to transplant to allow adequate time for healing.

In addition, there should be a physical assessment, assessing organ function such as kidney, heart and lung function tests, screening tests (Table 48.4) and ensuring an adequate number of haemopoietic stem cells have been harvested to ensure engraftment in a timely manner.

Donor assessment

In addition to the screening tests of Table 48.4, the most important selection criteria in donor selection is HLA typing. If there is more than one matched donor (sibling or unrelated donor), selection will take into account:

- Minor histocompatability antigens – which help to determine the amount of GvHD.
- Cytomegalovirus (CMV) serology – especially important if the recipient is serologically CMV negative. The CMV-negative donor may be the preferred choice, as CMV infection is a significant source of morbidity post-transplantation.
- Age – young adult donors are thought to tolerate the procedure of marrow donation better than older people. There is also some evidence that the risk of treatment failure increases with advancing donor age.[7,8]

Table 48.4 Pretransplant investigations for haemopoietic stem cell transplant patients and donors

Patient	Donor
Essential investigations	
Blood group and antibody screen	Blood group and antibody screen
Coagulation studies	Coagulation studies
Full blood count	Full blood count
Bone marrow aspirate	Liver function tests
Creatinine clearance	Pregnancy test
Liver function tests	Urea, creatinine, electrolytes
Urea, creatinine and electrolytes	VDRL test
Toxoplasma titre	Viral serology:
Viral serology:	Cytomegalovirus
Cytomegalovirus	Epstein–Barr virus
Epstein–Barr virus	Hepatitis B
Hepatitis B	Hepatitis C
Hepatitis C	HIV
HIV	Herpes simplex virus
Herpes simplex virus	Varicella-zoster virus
Varicella-zoster virus	Chest X-ray
Chest X-ray	ECG
Echocardiogram or MUGA scan	
Lung function tests	
Dental examination	
Disease restaging	
Indicated under specific circumstances	
CT scan of paranasal sinuses	Cytogenetic studies
CT scan of chest	Bone marrow examination
Lumbar puncture	Echocardiogram or MUGA scan
Pregnancy test	Lung function tests
	Sickling tests
	Toxoplasma titre

CT, computed tomography; ECG, electrocardiography; HIV, human immunodeficiency virus; MUGA, multiple gated acquisition; VDRL, Venereal Disease Research Laboratory.

Table 48.5 The order of preference for allogeneic donors based on sex and parity

Order of preference of donor	Male patient	Female patient
First	Male donor	Nulliparous female donor
Second	Nulliparous female donor	Male donor
Third	Parous female donor	Parous female donor

- Blood group – ABO incompatibility may produce immune complications, such as haemolysis[9] and increased transfusion requirements.[10]
- Sex and parity (Table 48.5) – donor–recipient sex mismatch[11,12] and donor parity[11,13] (have been shown to be associated with increased risk of GvHD and treatment failure. (See the Graft versus host disease section for more information on GvHD.)
- Psychological assessment – donating bone marrow or peripheral stem cells involves undertaking a procedure with varying complications, including a small risk of death, with no benefit to the donor themselves. Sibling donors rarely refuse to donate marrow but there may be direct or indirect pressure from other family members and it is often very difficult for the potential donor to choose not to undergo stem cell harvesting. Unrelated, volunteer donors are assessed by the transplant registry and initially have no psychological pressure to donate. If the graft fails, however, or there is relapse, there may be pressure for the volunteer to donate again. Two of the largest registries (National Marrow Donor Program and the Anthony Nolan Bone Marrow Registry) prevent this by prohibiting direct contact between the volunteer donor and the transplant team.
- Physical assessment – donors need to be physically fit to undergo the procedure.

Education

Initial education and informing the patient and family about HSCT may start at diagnosis for some patients: for example, those with acute leukaemia. It always needs to commence, however, as soon as the decision to transplant is made. Comprehensive information, both written and verbal, must be provided by the transplant centre in order to prepare recipients and their care givers throughout the phases of HSCT and must include:

- information about the type of transplant
- potential physical and psychological short- and long-term complications of the procedure
- risks associated with not undergoing transplant
- alternative treatment options
- clear information about local policies and procedure.

In terms of general information about transplantation, an increasing number of written and electronic resources have emerged, including transplant patient's testimony, to help prepare patients, but this information does not negate the importance of individual patient focused education at the transplant centre. (See Ch. 5.)

Haemopoietic stem cell harvesting and cryopreservation

The method of collection for the two main sources of stem cells – marrow and peripheral stem cells – are principally the same for both allogeneic and autologous donors.

Bone marrow harvesting

Typically, the donor is admitted to hospital either on the day before or on the day of the donation. Donors normally stay in the hospital for 1 or 2 nights, as most receive general anaesthesia; however, in some centres the patient is recovered and discharged home on the same day, as the use of newer anaesthetics has made bone marrow donation possible as an outpatient procedure.

Bone marrow is removed from the iliac crests and, occasionally, from the sternum as well. Generally, four to eight small incisions are made in the area, and a large needle is inserted through these incisions 20–30 times to draw the marrow out of the bones. Usually, 500–1000 ml of the donor's marrow is taken. This marrow contains 3–5% of the donor's developing blood cells. Typically, the extraction process lasts about 1 hour.

Harvested bone marrow is then processed to remove blood and bone fragments. Marrow that is to be stored may be combined with the preservative dimethyl sulfoxide (DMSO) and placed in a freezer and stored in liquid nitrogen vapour at –130°C to –160°C. Using this technique, known as cryopreservation, stem cells can be preserved indefinitely.

Because only a small amount of marrow is removed, donating usually does not pose any significant problems for the donor. Within a few weeks, with normal haemopoeisis, the donor's body will have replaced the donated marrow. Soreness around the incisions may last for a few days, and donors often feel tired for some time. The time required for a donor to recover varies from person to person. Some are back to their usual routine in a day or two. Others may take several days or as long as a week, but rarely longer.

Donor complications   Although donor complications are uncommon and much effort is devoted to their prevention, they sometimes occur. Complications are easily treated with proper medical attention. Because incisions are made to extract the marrow, infection is a possibility. Blood loss can also occur. For this reason donors routinely store two units of their own blood beforehand to be given during and after the procedure. There may be psychological implications for sibling donors, as feelings such as guilt and a sense of responsibility for graft failure or GvHD, may ensue.

When autologous transplantation is planned, the procedures for harvesting marrow differ, depending on factors such as the patient's physical condition and the time between harvesting and transplantation. In general, harvesting procedures are similar to those for allogeneic and syngeneic donors. However, if purging (processing the marrow to eradicate any potential leukaemia cells) is to be done, up to 2 litres may be taken so that an adequate amount of marrow remains after purging. Removal of a larger amount of marrow requires a greater number of needle punctures and a longer period of time to collect the marrow. The marrow is stored until the time of transplantation.

Peripheral stem cells harvested by apheresis

In this procedure, blood is removed through an intravenous catheter or through a large vein in the arm and is run through a cell separator machine that removes stem cells. The rest of the blood is returned to the patient. Typically, apheresis takes 2–4 hours and is repeated an average of two to four times. There is usually no need for hospitalisation or anaesthesia. Stem cells collected by apheresis may be processed and cryopreserved in the same way as bone marrow. (See video footage on CD-ROM.)

Because 90% of stem cells live in the bone marrow, they need to be mobilised or moved into the peripheral blood. Mobilisation is usually undertaken in one of two ways:

- G-CSF alone, which involves administering a haemopoietic growth factor (G-CSF) for 3–4 days prior to the harvest at a dose of 5–16 mg/kg, once daily subcutaneously. The dose varies between centres.
- G-CSF and chemotherapy, where G-CSF is administered during the recovery period of either a conventional course of chemotherapy, or following a mobilisation dose of chemotherapy such as cyclophosphamide 2–4 mg/kg administered specifically for the purpose of stem cell harvesting.

Conditioning regimens and stem cell reinfusion

Conditioning is critical to the success of the HSCT. Conditioning serves two functions:

- its primary purpose is to destroy malignant cells throughout the body more effectively than through conventional treatment

- it destroys the cells of the immune system (immunosuppression) in patients undergoing allogeneic transplantation and therefore reduces the risk that the recipient will reject the graft.

The conditioning regimen sets the stage for potential cure and transplant-related complications. The ideal conditioning regimen eradicates malignant disease with tolerable side effects. In theory, optimal timing of the transplant needs to allow sufficient recovery from the last course of conventional chemotherapy, yet not allow relapse.

Conditioning regimens for HSCT vary according to the patient's disease and medical condition, and according to local protocols. All regimens, however, utilise agents, either singly or in combination, that provide disease eradication with or without immunosuppression (Table 48.6). High-dose chemotherapy may be given over a course of 1–6 days. If TBI is used, it may be given in one dose or in multiple doses over the course of several days (fractionated radiation therapy). Fractionated schedules appear to minimise the risk of side effects from the radiation.

Following the conditioning regimen, the patient receives the donated or autologous stem cells intravenously. The infusion of marrow or peripheral blood stem cells (PBSC) may be called the rescue process.

Stem cells are thawed and warmed to 37°C on the ward and given to patient via a syringe or as an infusion together with hydration.

Engraftment (blood cell production from transplanted stem cells) usually occurs within about 2–4 weeks following transplantation and is evidenced by rising blood counts. Prior to engraftment, the patient experiences severe pancytopenia and immunosuppression. Priorities of patient care at this time are focused on prevention of and early recognition and treatment of:

- infection
- bleeding
- GvHD
- veno-occlusive disease (VOD)
- other organ complications.

Complete recovery of immune function takes much longer, however – up to several months for autologous transplant recipients and 1–2 years for patients receiving allogeneic transplants. (See the Graft versus host disease section for more information on GvHD and the Rehabilitation and follow-up care section for vaccination and immunisation.)

Supportive care

Supportive care is an essential aspect of transplantation (Table 48.7). The goal of supportive care is to prevent or manage the side effects of high-dose chemotherapy and/or radiotherapy. The very high doses of radiation and chemotherapy required for HSCT cause transient and sometimes permanent damage to the mucosa of the oropharynx and gastrointestinal tract and organs such as lungs, liver and kidneys. Other organ systems may also be involved. In allogeneic transplant the immune system of the donor is transplanted and these transferred immunocompetent cells may also cause GvHD. An extended period of pancytopenia and impaired resistance to infections follows the conditioning. The accompanying persistent immunodeficiency may predispose to severe complications and infections. Therefore, transplant procedures should ideally be carried out only in transplant units where facilities are adequate and dedicated staff have been trained to deal with specific problems associated with transplant.[15] (See the Graft versus host disease section for more information on GvHD.)

Table 48.6   Conditioning regimen components used in near maximal doses[14]

Agents used primarily for immunosuppression	Agents used primarily for disease eradication	Agents used for both purposes
Antithymocyte globulin	Busulfan	Cyclophosphamide
Corticosteroids	Carboplatin	Melphalan
Fludarabine	Carmustine	Thiotepa
Total lymphocyte irradiation	Cytarabine	Total body irradiation (TBI)
Various monoclonal antibody preparations	Diaziquone	
	Etoposide	
	Mitoxantrone (mitozantrone)	
	Paclitaxel	

Table 48.7 Nursing management (may vary according to local practice)

	Management	Rationale
Assessment	4 hourly observation of temperature, pulse, respirations, BP	Signs of infection and sepsis or bleeding
	Daily skin assessment	Signs of infection, skin reactions
	Daily oral assessment	Signs and degree of mucosal breakdown, signs of infection, bleeding
	Fluid balance, daily weight	Assessment of hydration and renal function
Hygiene care	Daily shower	Reduce bacterial load
	Daily clothing change	
	Low bacterial diet	
Specific care	Physiotherapy – daily exercises as prescribed	Maintains muscle tone, assists cardiovascular system and reduces pulmonary complications
Psychological care	Supportive care offered and given as needed	Referral to psychological care as required
	Family/friend presence encouraged if appropriate	To reduce sense of isolation

MANAGEMENT OF COMPLICATIONS

Immunosuppression

One of the most serious effects of HSCT is immuno-suppression. Supportive care for immunosuppression usually includes a degree of protective isolation. Patients may stay in a single hospital room with HEPA air filtration and positive air pressure (indicated for patients undergoing allogeneic transplant), in single side rooms with no air filtration, in four bedded bays or in the patient's own home. Globally, practice varies according to local protocols and resources. There is no clear evidence to promote one environment over another; however, there is increasing evidence supporting the feasibility of outpatient HSCT.[16,17] Depending on the institution, medical staff and visitors entering the patient's room may be required to go through some preventative measures, ranging from thorough hand washing to putting on masks and gowns. Generally, patients may also start receiving antibiotics, antiviral agents and antifungal agents just before or soon after chemotherapy or radiotherapy as prophylaxis, but this varies in various centres. The most commonly used prophylactic antibiotic during the period of neutrope-nia is one of the quinolones, e.g. ciprofloxacin. It has been shown that the use of these agents in neutropenic patients reduces the risk for Gram-negative infections and the number of days with fever, but does not affect survival. Many centres are reluctant to use antibacterial prophylaxis due to the risk of developing resistance.

Antifungal prophylaxis with fluconazole 400 mg/day has been tested in randomised trials, 2 of which showed a reduced risk for invasive fungal infections

with some *Candida* species.[18,19] Patients undergoing allografts require prophylaxis against *Pneumocystis carinii* with either pentamidine or co-trimoxazole.

Antiviral prophylaxis may be indicated in herpes simplex seropositive patients. Intravenous immuno-globulin therapy is also used by some centres as a preventative measure against infection. In this treatment, antibodies are isolated from donor blood and administered to the patient. These protective measures are continued from the time the patient's own marrow is destroyed until the HSCT is immune competent. To reduce the severity of immunosuppression, patients may receive haemopoietic growth factors such as G-CSF or granulocyte–macrophage colony-stimulating factor (GM-CSF). The criteria for initiating treatment vary according to underlying disease, patient condition and the centre's own protocols. Growth factors administered after HSCT can speed engraftment, decrease the risk of infection and reduce the likelihood of graft failure.

Patients undergoing HSCT are at significant risk of developing infections for several months after transplantation. CMV, *Aspergillus* and *Pneumocystis carinii* are among the most important causes of life-threatening infections, including pneumonia. Many patients develop herpes zoster virus infections (shingles), and herpes simplex virus infections (cold sores and genital herpes) often become reactivated in patients who were previously infected with this virus.

Following allogeneic HSCT, the post-transplant period can be divided into three phases of infection risk:

- The pancytopenic, or aplastic phase. Neutropenia and damage to the body barriers through the conditioning regimen are the main infection risk factors, in addition to some macrophage, T-cell and NK-cell function depression.

- T-cell function depression characterises the second phase. This occurs during the time that acute GvHD is expected. The patient will receive immunosuppressive therapy, such as ciclosporin A, to prevent or control GvHD. In addition, there may be skin barrier breakdown: for example, through the use of central venous lines. There may also be a secondary neutropenia, and this phase may last for a few weeks or several months.
- The third phase may not develop in all patients or may last for many months or even years and is seen when there is B-cell dysfunction, often combined with T-cell dysfunction in chronic GvHD.

In autologous stem cell transplant, the initial 'at-risk' phase during the period of neutropenia is similar to patients undergoing allografts, except that these patients have better T-cell function. (See the Graft versus host disease section for more information on GvHD.)

Pyrexia of unknown origin occurs frequently post transplant, and differential diagnosis should include toxic reactions to other drugs, infection and GvHD. Bacterial infection with Gram-positive or Gram-negative bacteria due to neutropenia and breakdown of the natural barriers such as skin and mucosal surfaces is most common and must be promptly treated empirically with broad-spectrum antibiotics due to the risks of endotoxin release and ensuing septic shock. Diagnosis of fungal infection is not straightforward and many infections are confirmed at autopsy.[20] The reasons for poor diagnosis are numerous and include:

- lack of specific signs and symptoms of systemic fungal infection to differentiate them from bacterial and viral infections
- lack of a detectable serological response in immuno-compromised individuals
- unreliable isolation of fungi from clinical samples.[21]

Antifungal therapy is therefore often started based on the presence of unresolving pyrexia. Computed tomography (CT) scanning may be useful in diagnosing fungal pneumonia, in particular *Aspergillus*, as the characteristic 'halo' feature of this may be seen more easily on CT than X-ray. Viral infection may impact immediately post transplant, in particular human herpesvirus 6 and, a little later, CMV. Other herpes viri and adenovirus may also be seen at this stage. Hepatic–splenic candidiasis may be suspected in the presence of a rising neutrophil count and slightly raised liver function tests, particularly alkaline phosphatase. Abdominal ultrasound may be useful in assisting diagnosis. (For further information see Chs 13 and 20.)

Thrombocytopenia and bleeding

There are a number of possible reasons for an increased risk of bleeding post transplant. The most common is thrombocytopenia. Other complications are:

- platelet dysfunction
- coagulation disorders such as disseminated intravascular coagulation (DIC)
- autoimmune effects such as thrombotic thrombocytopenic purpura (TTP) (see the following section)
- erosion of a blood vessel.

Due to the release of endotoxins that increase platelet consumption, septic patients are at an increased risk of spontaneous bleeding.

Bleeding is frequently seen in the mucous membranes of the nose and mouth. It also may develop under the skin or, more seriously, in the gastrointestinal tract, central nervous system or lungs. Platelet transfusions are given if there is any evidence of bleeding and/or to maintain the platelet count at the minimum needed to prevent bleeding. This minimum varies in different centres; however, spontaneous bleeding may occur when the platelet count is lower than $100 \times 10^9/L$, and major haemorrhage is more likely when the platelet count is below $20 \times 10^9/L$;[22] however, the relationship between platelet count and bleeding varies among individuals.[23]

In addition to a full blood count to check platelet numbers, a coagulation screen should always be performed if the patient is bleeding or septic. Fresh frozen plasma (FFP) and/or cryoprecipitate may be given to correct clotting abnormalities. Septic patients may have DIC secondary to their sepsis, particularly if a Gram-negative sepsis.

All female patients pre transplant and pre chemotherapy require pharmacological cessation of menstruation to cover the period of thrombocytopenia, and this is continued until platelets are greater than $100 \times 10^9/L$. Norethisterone, 5 mg orally three times a day, is used and Cyclogest (progesterone) pessaries, one $\times$ 400 mg daily, is an alternative in those patients who can no longer take medications orally. Cyclogest may be increased to 400 mg twice a day if no response. (For further information on thrombocytopenia see Ch. 22.)

Anaemia

Because chemotherapy and radiotherapy also damage the bone marrow's ability to produce red blood cells (RBCs), patients usually require periodic blood product transfusions to treat anaemia. To reduce the risk of transfusion-induced GvHD, all donated blood products given to transplantation patients are irradiated. Irradiation destroys lymphocytes that might otherwise attack the patient's cells and cause transfusion-related GvHD. All patients should receive CMV-negative blood products until the patient's CMV status is known. Many centres provide leuco-depleted blood products, which some centres consider safe to give to autologous transplant patients. However, as there is a 0.01% risk of transmitting CMV, many centres continue to give CMV-negative blood products to CMV-negative allograft recipients. (For further information on anaemia see Ch. 21; see the Graft versus host disease section for more information on GvHD.)

Thrombotic thrombocytopenic purpura and haemolytic uraemic syndrome

TTP and haemolytic uraemic syndrome (HUS) are notably seen post-allogeneic SCT and share a common microvascular defect. This consists of platelet microthrombi partly occluding the vascular lumen of arterioles, capillaries and overlying proliferating endothelial cells. This leads to the formation of fragmented red cells and haemolysis. This is known as the TTP/HUS syndrome and is manifested by thrombocytopenia, anaemia and ischaemic manifestations in the affected organs (usually the kidney and brain). Consequently, neurological disturbances and renal failure may be present.

Several factors may contribute to the occurrence of the TTP/HUS syndrome, including:

- ciclosporin A
- GvHD
- TBI
- intensive conditioning chemotherapy
- infection.

Outlook even with appropriate treatment is poor.

In TTP alone, the primary event is thought to be platelet aggregation, which leads to the formation of generalised microvascular thrombotic lesions. There is widespread endothelial damage and release into the circulation of ultra-large multimeric forms of von Willebrand factor (VWF), which have been shown to induce endothelial cell apoptosis. The specific factor present in normal plasma that is beneficial to the patient is not known, but since some patients respond to infusions of normal plasma, it would imply that in TTP there is a deficiency of an unidentified plasma factor.

Treatment of TTP/HUS

- Initial treatment is usually with plasma exchange. The standard replacement fluid is FFP. Cryoprecipitate-poor plasma may be used in cases where regular FFP has failed. Cryoprecipitate-poor plasma is mostly depleted of VWF, fibrinogen, fibronectin and factor XIII, and since VWF is implicated in TTP, this may be relevant.
- Some studies have shown that plasma infusion alone, as opposed to plasma exchange, is as effective.
- Platelet transfusion is strongly contraindicated, and may contribute to death. It is thought that trans-fused platelets compound the micro aggregates already present.
- Defibrotide (an antithrombotic agent) may be given at a dose of 10 mg/kg/day.
- The benefit of glucocorticoids is unproven, but may help in some cases, especially if symptoms are mild.
- Vincristine injections of 1–2 mg per week may be beneficial, and the effect is thought to be secondary to an inhibition of platelet aggregation by vincristine.
- Splenectomy has proven beneficial in some cases resistant to plasma exchange.[24]

Graft versus host disease

GvHD is one of the most serious potential complications of allogeneic HSCT. It occurs when T cells in the donated marrow (the graft) identify the recipient's body (the host) as foreign and attack it. This situation is different from other types of organ transplantation (such as kidney or heart transplantation), in which the donated organ is rejected by the patient's immune system. Although the donated marrow can be rejected by whatever remains of the patient's original immune system, more often, it is the T lymphocytes produced by the new marrow that launch an attack against the patient. Without preventative measures, most patients undergoing allogeneic HSCT would develop GvHD.

Patients with mild forms of acute GvHD are likely to recover completely, but those with severe forms may die of complications of the disease. Several factors affect a patient's risk of developing GvHD:

- The most important factor is the degree of HLA matching: the more antigens that match, the lower the risk of GvHD. About 70% of patients who receive donor marrow with two mismatched antigens develop significant acute GvHD vs 40% of patients receiving HLA-identical marrow (Table 48.8).[24]
- Mild GvHD occurs in approximately 8% of patients after autologous HSCT; it is thought to be due to the presence of damaged thymocytes (immature T cells) and is thought to be underdiagnosed.

Table 48.8 Incidence of various types of graft versus host disease[24]

Type	Incidence
Matched sibling	40%
Matched unrelated	60%
Mismatched related	65–70%
Mismatched unrelated	>80%

- Age also affects the risk of GvHD, with older patients being more susceptible to the disease than younger ones.
- Recipients whose donor is of the opposite sex are more likely to develop GvHD than a recipient whose donor is of the same sex.
- Chronic GvHD, which affects at least one-third of allogeneic HSCT patients, develops most often in those who have had acute GvHD.

To reduce the risk of GvHD after transplantation, most patients routinely receive immunosuppressive therapy with ciclosporin and/or methotrexate, drugs that help suppress T lymphocytes. Combinations of drugs appear to be most effective. Another technique for preventing GvHD is T-cell depletion, which involves eliminating T lymphocytes in the donated marrow before it is given to the patient. The T cells are removed or destroyed by means of monoclonal antibodies or other processes. Although T-cell depletion appears to reduce the chance that a patient will develop severe GvHD, this technique has other associated risks. Graft failure may be more likely when T-cell depleted marrow is used, and leukaemia patients may be more likely to have a relapse.

Should GvHD occur despite efforts to prevent it, high-dose corticosteroids (such as prednisone) are given to relieve symptoms of the disease and to suppress T-cell activity. Patients may receive antithymocyte globulin, which acts against immature T cells (thymocytes), or monoclonal antibodies that are directed against T cells. Higher doses of ciclosporin can also be helpful.

Symptoms of GvHD can develop within days or as long as 3 years after transplantation. Generally, GvHD that develops within 3 months following transplantation is known as acute GvHD; when it develops later, it is called chronic GvHD. Because the time periods in which acute and chronic GvHD can develop overlap, these diseases are better identified by their symptoms, which are somewhat different for each type.

Clinical features of acute graft versus host disease
Skin A maculopapular rash first appears on the palms, soles and ear lobules and spreads to the trunk and chest (centripetal distribution). It may become confluent and painful. In severe cases, generalised erythroderma and bullae formation are seen. (See also Ch. 26.)

Genitourinary tract Clinical features are:

- Watery diarrhoea, which is greenish, mucoid and contains epithelial flecks (minced meat diarrhoea).
- Bleeding.
- Abdominal pain and ileus may develop.
- Stool volume may be large (5–10 litres per 24 hours) and should be recorded.
- Excessive protein leak and hypoalbuminaemia can develop.
- Upper gastrointestinal (GI) tract symptoms such as nausea, vomiting and dyspepsia in the absence of other causes indicate the possibility of upper GI acute GvHD, which may develop without the intestinal involvement. This is more common in the elderly population and has a tendency to evolve into chronic GvHD.
- Differential diagnosis includes chemotherapy- and radiotherapy-induced changes and infections.
- Histology of the GI tract shows crypt cell necrosis and cell dropout.[25]

(See also Ch. 17.)

Liver Clinical features in the liver manifest in the form of cholestasis (elevated bilirubin and alkaline phosphatase levels). Histologically, the damage is limited to bile ducts and canaliculi. In severe cases, syndrome of 'vanishing bile ducts' can develop. Differential diagnosis includes hepatic VOD and drug toxicity, including ciclosporin or methotrexate toxicity. Liver biopsy may be useful in some patients but may be risky.[26] (See also Ch. 30.)

The skin changes are generally the first to appear, followed by gut and liver manifestations. Median day of onset is 14–19 days after transplant. Occasional manifestations include thrombocytopenia, pulmonary dysfunction, haemolysis and microangiopathy. Occasionally, photophobia, haemorrhagic conjunctivitis and pseudomembrane formation and lagophthalmos can develop (Table 48.9).[26]

Chronic graft versus host disease
Chronic GvHD produces temporary darkening of the skin, and hardening and thickening of patches of skin and the layers of tissues under it. Occasionally, the liver, esophagus, and other parts of the GI tract are affected. Mucous membranes may become dry, and hair loss may occur. Bacterial infections and weight loss are common. As with acute GvHD, severe cases of chronic GvHD may be fatal.

Table 48.9 Simplified grading of acute graft versus host disease[d][26]

	Organ/extent of involvement		
Grade	Skin	Liver	Intestinal tract
I	Rash on < 50% skin	None	None
II	Rash on >50%	or bilirubin 2–3 mg/dl	or diarrhoea >500 ml per day[a] or persistent nausea[b]
III–IV[c]	Generalised erythroderma with bullous formation	or bilirubin >3 mg/dl	or diarrhoea >1000 ml/day

[a]Volume of diarrhoea applies to adults. For paediatric patients, the volume of diarrhoea should be based on body surface area.
[b]Persistent nausea with histological evidence of graft versus host disease (GvHD) in the stomach or duodenum.
[c]As suggested by this scheme, three severity grades may suffice:
- Grade I: favourable prognosis; does not require treatment.
- Grade II: moderately severe disease that requires treatment; usually consists of multi-organ involvement. Sometimes, patients with Grade III or IV skin toxicity without gastrointestinal (GI) tract or liver involvement will be graded as II; upper GI tract symptoms confirmed endoscopically as due to acute GvHD should be graded as II.
- Grade III: severe multi-organ disease.
- Grade IV: life-threatening or fatal condition.

Mortality is 40% in mild to moderate acute GVHD (grade I–II) and more than 80% in severe disease (grade III–IV).

Interestingly, many studies have shown that mild GVHD may be beneficial over the long term, perhaps because the activated graft cells may be better able to kill cancer cells (a so-called graft versus tumour effect). Leukaemia and lymphoma patients who develop mild GvHD may be less likely to have a relapse than patients who never have the reaction. For this reason, researchers are studying ways to introduce effects in autologous HSCT. There is limited evidence that the development of autologous GvHD has a graft versus tumour effect; however, there may be a spontaneous autologous graft versus myeloma effect and a graft versus leukaemia effect.[26]

Veno-occlusive disease

VOD is one consequence of toxic injury to the liver. It occurs mainly during the first 3 weeks post transplant and is characterised by:

- raised bilirubin
- right upper quadrant pain
- weight gain
- ascites

in the absence of other liver disease. Diagnosis relies on clinical criteria and is usually made if two of the above criteria are present, ultrasound and, where feasible, transjugular liver biopsy. Differential diagnosis may be infection, acute GvHD and drug toxicity.

The reported incidence ranges from 3 to 50% and the mortality rate from 0 to 90% (median 30%).[27]

Risk factors include:

- pre-transplant elevation of liver enzymes
- intensity of chemotherapy prior to transplant
- presence of active hepatocellular disease at the time of transplant
- type and intensity of conditioning regimen
- TBI dose and dose rate
- mismatched or unrelated donor allografts
- second transplant.

VOD can be mild or severe, with complete recovery or with rapidly progressive hepatic failure with encephalopathy and death, usually from multi-organ failure.

Management of VOD aims to maintain intravascular volume and renal perfusion without increasing extravascular fluid accumulation, but the optimum treatment is not clear. Trials using recombinant tissue plasminogen activator (rh-Tpa) together with low-dose heparin, defibrotide (antithrombotic agents), high-dose steroids and prostaglandin E_1 have all shown some benefit to varying degrees with associated varying toxicity. (See also Ch. 30.)

Central nervous system complications

Symptoms associated with the major central nervous system (CNS) complications after HSCT are often non-specific and make differential diagnosis difficult. Imaging using CT or magnetic resonance imaging (MRI) is helpful, and lumbar puncture should be performed if safe to do so. The major complications are listed below:

- Metabolic encephalopathy may be the result of multi-organ failure resulting from sepsis, severe GvHD or VOD, and symptoms vary from mild disturbances of the level of consciousness to coma.
- Leucoencephalopathy is a degenerative process and is most often seen in patients with acute lymphoblastic leukaemia (ALL) who have undergone a combination of TBI and intrathecal chemotherapy. It is more common in children than adults andmay present with lethargy, slurred speech, ataxia, seizures, confusion, dysphagia, spasticity and dementia. Imaging of the brain may show a decreased density and, later, destruction of the white matter, ventricular dilatation and calcification.[28]
- Drug-induced neurotoxicity.
- Infection due to viral, fungal or bacterial infection.
- Haemorrhage secondary to thrombocytopenia and/or coagulopathies.
- Thrombotic microangiopathy, most often in the presence of TTP.
- Relapse in the CNS.

(See also Ch. 27.)

Pulmonary complications

Overall, 40–60% of allograft recipients develop pneumonia or pulmonary disease at some time after HSCT. Among these, up to 40% will require intensive care, either on a transplant unit or a critical care unit, and 10% will die. Factors contributing to and causing pulmonary complications are toxicity from chemotherapy and radiotherapy and viral, bacterial or fungal infection.

- Idiopathic pneumonia syndrome accounts for half of the interstitial pneumonitis after transplant[27] and is diagnosed when no specific organism is recovered in bronchial washings or lung tissue biopsy. Symptoms may occur early (before 100 days) or late (after 100 days)[29] and are similar to those of acute respiratory distress syndrome (ARDS).
- Pulmonary oedema syndromes can occur immediately post transplant and may be secondary to sodium excess and cardiomyopathy, myocarditis and volume overload. Volume overload secondary to VOD may also contribute to pulmonary oedema.

- CMV pneumonia occurs in approximately 20% of allograft patients and is the leading cause of infectious pneumonia.
- Pulmonary GvHD tends to be chronic and progressive, with repeated infective episodes and may be complicated by bronchiolitis obliterans.[26]

(See also Ch. 29.)

Graft failure

Grafting is considered a failure when bone marrow function does not return or when it is lost after a period of recovery. However, the definition of graft failure is controversial and a distinction between graft failure and graft rejection may be useful:

- Graft failure is generally thought to have occurred if the granulocyte count is not sustained at >200/µl by day 21, or at the latest day 28. This may be evidenced by a failure of the blood counts to rise following transplantation.
- In graft rejection, the recipient's body rejects the donated marrow. This may be evidenced by an initial rise in blood counts following transplantation, followed by a fall in counts.

A number of factors may influence graft failure. Mechanisms involved in graft failure are not completely understood; however; at least five categories are recognised:

- in the allosensitised patient transplanted from an allogeneic donor
- in the patient transplanted from a histoincompatible donor
- in the patient transplanted with T-cell depleted stem cells
- in the patient transplanted with autologous stem cells
- in the patient with pre-existing marrow defects.[26]

Graft failure may also result:

- from a viral illness
- from the use of immunosuppressants (such as methotrexate)
- in leukaemia patients, associated with a recurrence of leukaemia, where the leukaemia cells may inhibit the growth of the transplanted cells
- (in some cases) for idiopathic reasons.

Graft rejection is a problem that is exclusive to allogeneic transplant recipients, whereas other types of graft failure may occur in patients receiving any type of transplant.

A number of factors may contribute to the risk of graft rejection: two of the most significant are the use of marrow with an imperfect HLA match and patients receiving T-cell depleted donor marrow. Graft rejection is also more common among patients who have not had TBI, because such patients may retain some immune activity after pre-transplantation conditioning with chemotherapy alone.

The implications of graft failure or graft rejection are that the patient remains inmmunosuppressed and at great risk of infection and bleeding. In other words, they may remain in a state of permanent bone marrow failure.

A top-up transplant of either donor cells or the patient's own cells may be given if available. Sibling donors are usually fairly easily available; however, unrelated donors are not and, for this reason, these transplant recipients have autologous cells harvested and stored, which may be given. Autologous transplant patients may not have been able to collect sufficient cells for a top-up transplant and this remains a problem.

Multi–organ failure

Patients undergoing transplantation have often received intensive chemotherapy as induction treatment for their disease. In undergoing transplantation, they receive high-dose chemo/radiotherapy as part of their conditioning regimen. In addition, they may receive immunosuppression to prevent and treat GvHD and antibacterial, antiviral and antifungal drugs, either as prophylaxis or treatment. All of these drug regimens are associated with multi-organ toxicity that, in combination with a critical event, such as septic shock, may precipitate multi-organ failure.

Gut toxicity

The mucosa of the gut is sensitive and, consequently, is directly affected by the effects of high-dose chemo/radiotherapy, infection and GvHD.

- Oral complications such as mucositis can cause pain, inflammation and ulceration, xerostomia, and infection that may be bacterial, fungal or viral in origin. (See also Ch. 18.)
- Nausea and vomiting may be caused by the conditioning regimen, GvHD or infection. (See also Ch. 16.)
- Diarrhoea occurs in 50–70% of transplant recipients[30] and may be due to treatment toxicity, infection or GvHD. It may be debilitating or even life-threatening, resulting in massive losses of fluid and electrolytes. Intravenous hydration, electrolyte replacement, treatment of underlying cause and antidiarrhoeal

agents such as loperamide and codeine phosphate comprise a standard management plan. Octreotide has sometimes been found to be effective in controlling diarrhoea resulting from GvHD or high-dose therapy.[31]

(See also Ch. 17.)

Nutritional needs

Adequate nutrition is vitally important for HSCT patients. GvHD, chemotherapy and radiotherapy often cause anorexia, nausea, vomiting and mucositis, which may make eating difficult for several weeks. Nutritional support may be indicated when there is severe malnutrition (i.e. >10% weight loss of ideal body weight) or illness-reducing food intake that is likely to persist for more than 5 days.

The two major principles of nutritional support need to be taken into consideration:

1. If the gut is functioning, use it.
2. Parenteral nutrition (PN) is rarely useful if used for less than 5 days.

Types of nutritional support include:

- normal diet
- nutritional supplements taken orally (e.g. high-energy/high-protein drinks)
- enteral nutrition given via a fine-bore nasogastric feeding tube/PEG/jejunostomy tube
- parenteral nutrition.

(See also Ch. 19.)

Fatigue

The physical effects of fatigue and loss of physical performance during chemotherapy and radiotherapy have been reported in the literature as affecting up to 70% of patients[32,33] and up to 30% of patients report a loss of energy for years following completion of treatment.[32,34] The physical effects of fatigue and loss of physical performance following HSCT in particular have also been reported in the literature. Most post-transplant quality of life studies[35–38] include the effects of fatigue on daily living, and one study[39] found that females reported significantly more fatigue than males or the normal population. Another study reported that 40% of patients need up to a year for full recovery of physical functioning, and loss of stamina prevents about 30% of patients from going back to work during the first 2 years after stem cell transplant.[40] Some patients never regain their pre-transplant energy levels and learn to adjust, making life choices such as changes in career or leisure activities.

Increasingly, transplant centres are looking at and setting up rehabilitation programmes.

(See also Ch. 34.)

Psychological needs

Patients undergoing HSCT have tremendous psychosocial pressures that may be physical, emotional or financial in nature. They are embarking on a life-threatening treatment modality, which includes being administered potentially fatal doses of chemotherapy and/or radiotherapy. Unlike most treatments, HSCT is optimally undertaken when a patient is in remission and therefore well. They are not entering into a treatment regimen to make them feel better from illness but are choosing to make themselves very unwell in order to achieve the long-term goal of remission, which holds no guarantees.

The transplant may be undertaken in a centre some distance from the patient's home. This will make visiting difficult for family and friends, and for some people this means a lengthy separation from other family members. A sense of isolation during and post transplant has been described, whether physical barrier nursing was undertaken or not. The energy required during and after transplantation is considerable. Patients tire of the rigors of treatment, and both they and their families often feel the pressure of not knowing what will happen.

During the transplant process, medical problems are likely to take priority over psychological needs. However, the psychological stresses of transplant for both the patient and family are considerable and should not be trivialised. For many reasons, both families and patients may experience guilt, relief, fear, anger, depression and anxiety. A number of authors[37,42,43] found that a small percentage of transplant recipients continue to experience long-term psychological disabilities 5–6 years later.

Long-term effects

The long-term effects of transplant are multidimensional[34] and result from a combination of:

- the delayed effects of chemotherapy and radiotherapy
- being a cancer survivor
- confronting death and life-threatening illness
- loss of control
- facing an uncertain future disease course.

Some of these problems are discussed below.

Fertility

Chemotherapy and radiotherapy often cause temporary or permanent reproductive difficulties. The extent of these problems depends on the patient's age and sex and on the dosage and duration of treatment. Most patients who receive TBI as part of their conditioning treatment become sterile. However, sexual desire and function usually return to normal after transplantation, although some studies describe long-term problems with intimacy and sexuality.[37,41,42]

Infertility is common among men who are treated with chemotherapy or radiotherapy. For this reason, men are usually encouraged to consider sperm banking before treatment begins if they wish to father children after transplantation.

Menstrual irregularities often develop in women who have received high-dose chemotherapy. Although menstruation may return up to 2 years after transplantation in younger women, patients over the age of 25 years old are likely to go through early menopause. Hormone replacement therapy can help relieve the symptoms of menopause and may be recommended for other medical reasons. Cryopreservation of fertilised or unfertilised eggs before transplant is possible for some women who have not become infertile through induction treatment.

Sterility can be a psychologically distressing side effect and therefore should be addressed by the patient, partner, family and healthcare team before and after transplantation.

(See also Chs 32 and 33.)

Growth

Studies have shown that some children treated with TBI may have impaired growth, particularly when single-dose TBI is given.

(See also 'The late effects of chemotherapy' section in Ch. 35.)

Cataracts

Cataracts may occur 3–6 years after TBI. Roughly three-quarters of patients who receive single-dose TBI develop cataracts. The number is reduced to about 20% in patients who receive fractionated radiation doses or in those who do not receive TBI. Patients who develop cataracts generally need corrective surgery, which often restores normal vision.[26]

Secondary malignancies

Because HSCT has been performed for only a few decades, not all of the long-term effects of the procedure are known. There is some concern that high-dose chemotherapy, irradiation, immunosuppression, stem cell mobilisation or other unknown factors related to the procedure may increase the risk for secondary cancers. Studies have shown that the risk varies considerably depending on the patient's age, general health, menopausal status (for women) and previous history of radiation and may be between 5% and 10%.[26] The dosage and type of drug given also affect the likelihood that a second cancer may develop.

REHABILITATION AND FOLLOW-UP CARE

HSCTs are undertaken in a variety of settings and vary globally according to local practice and legislation such as accreditation:

- inpatients in a specialised transplant unit
- inpatients in a general hospital
- outpatients attending the hospital daily
- in hospital-provided accommodation such as a flat or hotel room
- in the patient's own home with nursing care, blood component therapy and all drug support provided by a specialised transplant community nurse.

Therefore, follow-up care and discharge criteria vary according to local practice and the patient's condition.

Discharge from inpatient care

Patients who are admitted to hospital for transplant will stay in hospital for 1–2 months after HSCT. Hospitalisation time may be reduced when PBSC are used alone rather than with marrow, because engraftment time tends to be faster. The use of haemopoietic growth factors may also shorten the time many patients must spend in the hospital.

Generally, a patient is discharged from the hospital after the neutrophil count is greater than 500 in a standard measure of blood for at least 2 consecutive days. Other considerations are the RBC and platelet counts, the presence or absence of recurrent infections, and the patient's general physical condition. Patients may need frequent platelet and blood transfusions after discharge.

Some patients will need to return to the hospital's outpatient department daily for the first 2 weeks, while others can be seen less frequently. Follow-up visits to the transplant clinic continue every 1–2 weeks for the first several months to ensure that blood counts are normal. Patients are then seen every month for about 6 months. Later, the schedule of check-ups is based on each patient's need. Generally, check-ups are done every 2–6 months. Most follow-up includes

bone marrow aspiration to determine the condition of the marrow.

For allograft recipients, immunosuppression needs careful monitoring to avoid toxicity. Ciclosporin is normally discontinued about 6 months after transplantation. Prophylactic prescription for specific infections is required, including penicillin to prevent pneumococcal sepsis secondary to hyposplenism, aciclovir to prevent reactivation of the herpes simplex virus and zoster virus, and co-trimoxazole or pentamidine to prevent infection with *Pneumocystis carinii*.[26]

Long-term follow-up post HSCT should aim to monitor endocrinology, cardiac function, pulmonary function, bone density, chronic GvHD and the incidence of secondary neoplasm. It should also provide psychological support for patients with ongoing problems and residual effects post transplant and advice in areas such as reimmunisation and fertility.

Vaccination post stem cell transplantation

As the immune system matures following HSCT, immune reactivity during the first month post-graft is extremely low.[43] Cytotoxic and phagocytic white cell function recovers by day 100, but the more specialised functions of T and B lymphocytes may remain impaired for a year or even longer. In patients with chronic GvHD, the immune system remains suppressed for longer. Information on reimmunisation post SCT remains scant, although there are now limited data on the effect of donor age, recipient age, disease and conditioning regimen and the need for immunisation and its efficacy and outcome. Patients who should not be considered eligible for live vaccination after blood or bone marrow transplant are listed in Box 48.1. A recommended immunisation schedule in blood and bone marrow transplant

---

Box 48.1	Patients who should not be considered eligible for live vaccination after blood or bone marrow transplant[43]

All autograft recipients for 2 years
All allograft recipients for 2 years
Patients on immunosuppressive therapy for any reason
Patients suffering from chronic graft versus host disease
Patients suffering from recurrent malignancy after transplantation

Table 48.10   Recommended immunisation schedule in blood and bone marrow transplant recipients excluding those with chronic graft versus host disease[43]

Vaccine	Schedule	Time post BMT	Comments
Diphtheria toxoid	3 doses at monthly intervals	1 year	Very immunogenic, so some centres give only one dose
Haemophilus influenzae (Hib)	2 doses 6 months apart	4 months	In UK only used in under 4's as 'herd' immunity good
Influenza	1 dose annually	6 months	At least for 2 years. In patients with lung problems; vaccinate household contacts
Measles	1 dose	2 years	All children and selected adults
Mumps	1 dose	2 years	All children and selected adults
Pneumococcus	1 dose	2 years	Additional drug prophylaxis may be needed as antibody response is variable
Poliovirus (inactivated)	3 doses at monthly intervals	1 year	
Rubella	1 dose	2 years	Children and potentially fertile females
Tetanus toxoid	3 doses at monthly intervals	1 year	In UK, one dose given only as very immunogenic

BMT, bone marrow transplantation.

recipients excluding those with chronic GvHD is given in Table 48.10.

SURVIVORSHIP ISSUES

Despite all the potential complications, most patients return to an active, working life without continuing treatment. However, the extent to which patients successfully readapt to normal life after HSCT varies as a number of factors, such as prior treatment, demographic and psychological characteristics of the patient, clinical status of the disease and available social support resources,[44] impact in varying degrees.

Many patients need a full year to recover physically and psychologically from transplantation. Relatively minimal attention has been paid towards evaluating and supporting rehabilitation from the potential negative side effects of bone marrow transplant.

Survivorship encompasses not only the ability to function physically but also feelings about self, wholeness and normalcy.

Even after recovery and discharge from the transplant centre, life may not return to 'normal'– the way it was before the illness: medication may be necessary indefinitely, and the patient's lifestyle may have to be changed to help prevent fatigue, avoid infectious diseases and cope with the long-term effects of treatment.

There may be changes in body image to deal with, such as dry eyes, skin changes and sensitivity. Issues of altered sexuality and fertility, and changes in liver and gastrointestinal function may require alterations in diet. Some patients experience changes in their self-image because they have received part of their body from someone else; on the other hand, some people think of their transplantation date as a new 'birthday.'

References

1. Bortin MM, Horowitz MM, Rowlings PA, et al. 1993 Progress report from the International Bone Marrow Transplant Registry. Advisory Committee of the International Bone Marrow Transplant Registry. Bone Marrow Transplant 1993; 12:97–104.

2. Buchsel P, Kapustay P. Blood cell transplantation. Patient Treatment and Support 1995; 2(2):1–14.

3. Urbano-Ispizua A, Schmitz N, de Witte T, et al. Allogeneic and autologous transplantation for haematological diseases, solid tumours and immune disorders: definitions and current practice in Europe in 2003. Bone Marrow Transplant 2002; 29:639–646.

4. Ringden O, Horowitz MM, Gale RP, et al. Outcome after allogeneic BMT for leukaemia in older adults. J Am Med Ass 1993; 270:57–60.

5. Sweetenham JW, Pearce R, Phillip T, et al. High-dose therapy and autologous bone marrow transplantation for intermediate and high grade non-Hodgkin's lymphoma in patients aged 55 years and over, results from European Group for Bone Marrow Transplantation. EBMT Lymphoma Working Party. Bone Marrow Transplant 1994; 14:981–987.

6. Reiter E, Kalhs P, Keil F, et al. Effect of high-dose melphalan and peripheral blood stem cell transplantation on

renal function in patients with multiple myeloma and renal insufficiency: a case report and review of the literature Ann Hematol 1999; 78(4):189–191.

7. Zwaan FE, Hermans J, Barrett AJ, et al. Bone marrow transplantation for acute lymphoblastic leukaemia; a survey of the European Group for Bone Marrow Transplantation (E.G.B.M.T.). Br J Haematol 1984; 58:33–42.

8. Ash RC, Horowitz MM, Gale RP, et al.. Bone marrow transplantation from related donors other than HLA identical siblings; effect of T cell depletion. Bone Marrow Transplant 1991; 7:443–452.

9. Klump TR. Immunohaematologic complications of bone marrow transplantation. Bone Marrow Transplant 1991; 8:159–170.

10. Mehta J, Powles R, Singhal S, et al Transfusion requirements after bone marrow transplantation from HLA identical siblings: effects of donor-recipient ABO incompatability. Bone Marrow Transplant 1996; 18:151–156.

11. Nash RA, Pepe MS, Storb R, et al. Acute graft-versus-host disease: analysis of risk factors after allogeneic marrow transplantation and prophylaxis with cyclosporin and methotrexate. Blood 1992; 80:1838–1845.

12. Gratwohl A, Hermans J, Niederwieser D, et al.. Bone marrow transplantation for chronic myeloid leukaemia: long term results. Chronic Leukaemia Working Party of the European Group for Bone Marrow Transplantation. Bone Marrow Transplant 1993; 12:509–516.

13. Flowers ME, Pepe MS, Longton G, et al. Previous donor pregnancy as a risk factor for acute graft-versus-host disease in patients with aplastic anaemia treated by allogeneic marrow transplantation. Br J Haematol 1990; 74:492–496.

14. Phillips GL. In: Deeg HJ, Klingmann HG, Phillips GL, et al, eds. A guide to blood and bone marrow transplant. 3rd edn. Berlin: Springer; 1999.

15. Apperly J, Gluckman E, Gratwohl A, for the European Group for Blood and Marrow Transplantation. Blood and bone marrow transplantation – the EBMT handbook. Paris: European School of Oncology; 1998.

16. Meisenberg BR, Ferran K, Hollenbach K, et al. Reduced charges and costs associated with outpatient autologous stem cell transplantation. Bone Marrow Transplant 1998; 21(9):927–932.

17. Westermann AM, Holtkamp MM, Linthorst GA, et al. At home management of aplastic phase following high-dose chemotherapy with stem-cell rescue for hematological and non-hematological malignancies. Ann Oncol 1999; 10(5):511–517.

18. Goodman J, Winston D, Greenfield R. A controlled trial of fluconazole to prevent fungal infections in patients undergoing bone marrow transplantation. N Engl J Med 1992; 326:845–851.

19. Slavin MA, Osborne B, Adams R. Efficacy and safety of fluconazole prophylaxis for fungal infections after marrow transplantation – a prospective, randomised, double-blind study. J. Infect Dis 1995; 171:1545–1552.

20. Bodey G, Bueltmann B, Duguid W. Fungal infections in cancer patients: an international autopsy survey. Eur J Clin Microbiol Infect Dis 1992; 11:99–109.

21. Johnson EM, Gilmore MG, Newman J, et al. Preventing fungal infections in immunocompromised patients. Br J Nurs 2000; 9(1):154–164.

22. Dolan S. In: Grundy M, ed. Nursing in haematological malignancy. London: Ballière Tindall/RCN; 2000.

23. Hugh-Jones NC, Wickramsinghe SN. Lecture notes on haematology. 5th edn. Oxford: Blackwells; 1991.

24. Powles R, Stephens M, Kulkarni S, et al. The Royal Marsden Leukaemia and Myeloma Unit Guidelines (unpublished); 2001.

25. Epstein RJ, MacDonald GB, Sale GE, et al. The diagnostic accuracy of the rectal biopsy in acute graft-versus-host disease: a prospective study of 13 patients. Gastroenterology 1980; 78:764–770.

26. Deeg HJ. In: Deeg HJ, Klingmann HG, Phillips GL, et al., eds. A guide to blood and bone marrow transplant. 3rd edn. Berlin: Springer; 1999.

27. Ribaud P, for the European Group for Blood and Marrow Transplantation. Blood and bone marrow transplantation – the EBMT handbook. Paris: European School of Oncology; 1998.

28. Klingmann HG. In: Deeg HJ, Klingmann HG, Phillips GL, et al., eds. A guide to blood and bone marrow transplant. 3rd edn. Berlin: Springer; 1999.

29. Crawford SW. Critical care and respiratory failure. In: Forman S, Blume K, Thomas ED, eds. Bone marrow transplantation. Boston: Blackwell Science; 1994.

30. Miacowski C, Buchsel P. Oncology nursing; assessment and clinical care. St Louis: Mosby; 1999.

31. Lamberts SW, van der Lely AJ, de Herder W, et al. Octreotride. N Engl J Med 1996; 334(4):246–254.

32. Smets EM, Garssen B, Schuster-Uitterhoeve AL, et al. Fatigue in cancer patients. Br J Cancer 1993; 68(2):220–224.

33. Irvine D, Vincent L, Graydon JE, et al. The prevalence and correlates of fatigue in patients receiving treatment with chemotherapy and radiotherapy. A comparison with the fatigue experienced by healthy individuals. Cancer Nurs 1994; 17(5): 367–378.

34. Whedon M, Ferrell BR. Quality of life in adult bone marrow transplant patients: beyond the first year. Semin Oncol Nurs 1994; 10(1):42–57.

35. Saleh US, Brockopp DY. Quality of life one year following bone marrow transplantation: psychometric evaluation of the quality of life in bone marrow transplant survivors tool. Oncol Nurs Forum 2001; 28(9):1457–1464.

36. Zittoun R, Suciu S, Watson M, et al. Quality of life in patients with acute myelogenous leukaemia in prolonged first complete remission after bone marrow transplantation (allogeneic or autologous) or chemotherapy: a cross sectional study of the

EORTC-GIMEMA AML 8A trial. Bone Marrow Transplant 1997; 20:307–315.

37.   Whedon M, Stearns D, Mills LE. Quality of life of long term adult survivors of autologous bone marrow transplantation. Oncol Nurs Forum 1995; 22:10.

38.   Andrykowski MA, Bruehl S, Brady MJ, et al. Physical and psychosocial status of adults one year after bone marrow transplantation: a prospective study. Bone Marrow Transplant 1995; 15:837–844.

39.   Knobel H, Loge JH, Nordoy T, et al. High level of fatigue in lymphoma patients treated with high dose therapy. J Pain Sympt Manag 2000; 19(6):446–456.

40.   Syrjala KL, Chapko MK, Vitaliana PP, et al. Recovery after allogeneic marrow transplantation: a prospective study of predictors of long-term physical and psychosocial functioning. Bone Marrow Transplant 1993; 11:319–327.

41.   Chao NJ, Tierney DK, Bloom JR, et al. Dynamic assessment of quality of life after autologous bone marrow transplantation. Blood 1992; 80:825–830.

42.   Vose JM, Kennedy BC, Bierman PJ, et al. Long term sequelae of autologous bone marrow or peripheral stem cell transplantation for lymphoid malignancies. Cancer 1992; 69:784–789.

43.   Singhal S, Mehta J. In: Barrett J, Treleaven JG, eds. The clinical practice of stem-cell transplantation. Oxford: Isis Medical Media; 1998.

44.   Andrykowski MA, McQuellon RP. In: Barrett J, Treleaven JG, eds. The clinical practice of stem-cell transplantation. Oxford: Isis Medical Media; 1998.

Appendix

Table A1 World Health Organisation toxicity criteria by grade

		0	1	2	3	4
Leukopenia	WBC x 10³	≥4.0	3.0–3.9	2.0–2.9	1.0–1.9	<1.0
	Granulocytes/Bands	≥2.0	1.5–1.9	1.0–1.4	0.5–0.9	<0.5
	Lymphocytes	≥2.0	1.5–1.9	1.0–1.4	0.5–0.9	<0.5
Thrombocytopenia	Plt x 10³	WNL	75.0–normal	50.0–74.9	25.0–49.9	<25.0
Anaemia	Hgb	WNL	10.0–normal	8.0–10.0	6.5–7.9	<6.5
Haemorrhage (clinical)		none	mild, no transfusion	gross, 1–2 units transfusion/episode	gross, 3–4 units transfusion/episode	massive, >4 units transfusion/episode
*Infection		none	mild, no active Rx	moderate, localized infection requires active Rx	severe, systemic infection requires active Rx, specify site	life-threatening, sepsis, specify site

- Fever felt to be caused by drug allergy should be coded as allergy
- Fever due to infection is coded under infection only

		0	1	2	3	4
Fever in absence of infection		none	37.1–38.0°C 98.7–100.4°F	38.1–40.0°C 100.5–104.0°F	>40.0°C (>104.0°F) for less than 24 hours	>40.0°C (104.0°F) for >24 hours or fever with hypotension
GU	Creatinine	WNL	<1.5 × N	1.5–3.0 × N	3.1–6.0 × N	>6.0 × N
	Proteinuria	No change	1+ or <0.3g% or <3g/l	3–10g/l 2–3+ or 0.3–1.0g% or	4+ or >1.0g% or >10g/l	nephrotic syndrome
	Haematuria	neg	micro only	gross, no clots	gross + clots	requires transfusion
	*BUN	<1.5 × N	1.5–2.5 × N	2.6–5 × N	5.1–10 × N	>10 × N

- Urinary tract infection should be coded under infection, not GU
- Haematuria resulting from thrombocytopenia should be coded under hemorrhage, not GU

		0	1	2	3	4
GI	Nausea	none	able to eat reasonable intake	intake significantly decreased but can eat	no significant intake	
	Vomiting	none	1 episode in 24 hours	2–5 episodes in 24 hours	6–10 episodes in 24 hours	>10 episodes in 24 hours or requiring parenteral support
	Diarrhoea	none	increase of 2–3 stools/day over pre-Rx	increase of 4–6 stools/day, or nocturnal stools, or moderate cramping	increase of 7–9 stools/day or incontinence, or severe cramping	increase of ≥10 stools/day or grossly bloody diarrhoea, or need for parenteral support
	Stomatitis	none	painless ulcers, erythema, or mild soreness	painful erythema, oedema, or ulcers, but can eat	painful erythema, oedema or ulcers, and cannot eat	requires parenteral or enteral support

Liver	Bilirubin	WNL		<1.5 × N	1.5–3.0 × N	>3.0 × N
	Transaminase (SGOT, SGPT)	WNL	≤2.5 × N	2.6–5.0 × N	5.1–20.0 × N	>20.0 × N
	Alk Phos or 5'-nucleotidase	WNL	≤2.5 × N	2.6–5.0 × N	5.1–20.0 × N	>20.0 × N
	Liver – clinical	no change from baseline			precoma	hepatic coma
	• Viral hepatitis should be coded as infection rather than liver toxicity					
Pulmonary		none or no change	asymptomatic, with abnormality in PFTs	dyspnoea on significant exertion	dyspnoea at normal level of activity	dyspnoea at rest
	• Pneumonia is considered infection and not graded as pulmonary toxicity unless felt to be resultant from pulmonary changes directly					
Cardiac	Cardiac dysrhythmias	none	asymptomatic transient, requiring no therapy	recurrent or persistent, no therapy required	requires treatment	requires monitoring, or hypotension or ventricular tachycardia or fibrillation
	Cardiac function	none	asymptomatic, decline of resting ejection by less than 20% of baseline value	asymptomatic, decline of fraction resting ejection fraction by more than 20% of baseline value	mild CHF, responsive to therapy	severe or refractory CHF
	Cardiac – ischaemia	none	non-specific T-wave flattening	asymptomatic, ST and T wave changes suggesting ischaemia	angina without evidence for infarction	acute myocardial infarction
	Cardiac – pericardial	none	asymptomatic effusion, no intervention required	pericarditis (rub, chest pain, ECG changes)	symptomatic effusion; drainage required	tamponade; drainage urgently required

Continued

Table A1 World Health Organisation toxicity criteria by grade—cont'd

	0	1	2	3	4
Blood pressure					
Hypertension	none or no change	asymptomatic, transient increase by >20 mmHg (D) or to >150/100 if previously WNL. No treatment required	recurrent or persistent increase by >20 mmHg (D) or to >150/100 if previously WNL. No treatment required	requires therapy	hypertensive crisis
Hypotension	none or no changes	therapy (including transient requiring no orthostatic hypotension)	or other therapy but not requires fluid replacement hospitalization	hospitalization; resolves requires therapy and within 48 hours of stopping the agent	hospitalization for >48 hours requires therapy and hours after stopping the agent
Skin	none or no change	scattered macular or papular eruption or erythema that is asymptomatic	scattered macular or papular eruption or erythema with pruritus or other associated symptoms	generalized symptomatic macular, papular or vesicular eruption	exfoliative dermatitis or ulcerating dermatitis
Allergy	none	transient rash, drug fever <38°C, 100.4°F	urticaria, drug fever >38°C, 100.4°F, mild bronchospasm	serum sickness, bronchospasm, requires parenteral meds	anaphylaxis
*Phlebitis					
Local	none	arm pain	thrombophlebitis, leg pain and swelling with inflammation or phlebitis	hospitalization ulceration	embolus plastic surgery indicated
Alopecia	no loss	mild hair loss	pronounced or total hair loss		
Weight gain/loss	<5.0%	5.0–9.9%	10.0–19.9%	>20%	

Neurological

	0	1	2	3	4
Sensory					
Neuro – sensory	none or no change	mild paraesthesias; loss of deep tendon reflexes	mild or moderate objective sensory loss; moderate paraesthesias	severe objective sensory loss or parenthesias that interfere with function	
Neuro – vision	none or no change			symptomatic subtotal loss of vision	blindness
Neuro – hearing	none or no change	asymptomatic, hearing loss on audiometry only	tinnitus	hearing loss interfering with function but correctable with hearing aid	deafness, not correctable
Motor					
Motor neuro	change none or no	objective findings subjective weakness; no	without significant mild objective weakness impairment of function	impairment of function objective weakness with	paralysis
Neuro – constipation	none or no change	mild	moderate	severe	ileus >96 hours
Psychological					
Neuro – mood	no change	mild anxiety or depression	moderate anxiety or depression	severe anxiety or depression	suicidal ideation
Clinical					
Neuro – cortical	none	mild somnolence or agitation	moderate somnolence or agitation	severe somnolence, agitation, confusion, disorientation or hallucinations	coma, seizures, toxic psychosis
Neuro – cerebellar	none	slight incoordination, dysdiadochokinesia	intention tremor, dysmetria, slurred speech, nystagmus	locomotor ataxia	cerebellar necrosis
Neuro – headache	none	mild	moderate or severe but transient	unrelenting and severe	
Metabolic:					
Hyperglycaemia	<116	116–160	161–250	251–500	>500 or ketoacidosis
Hypoglycaemia	>64	55–64	40–54	30–39	<30
Amylase	WNL	<1.5 × N	1.5–2.0 × N	2.1–5.0 × N	>5.1 × N
Hypercalcaemia	<10.6	10.6–11.5	11.6–12.5	12.6–13.5	13.5
Hypocalcaemia	>8.4	8.4–7.8	7.7–7.0	6.9–6.1	6.0
Hypomagnesaemia	>1.4	1.4–1.2	1.1–0.9	0.8–0.6	0.5
Coagulation:					
Fibrinogen	WNL	0.99–0.75 × N	0.74–0.50 × N	0.49–0.25 × N	#0.24 × N
Prothrombin time	WNL	1.01–1.25 × N	1.26–1.50 × N	1.51–2.00 × N	>2.00 × N
Partial thromboplastin time	WNL	1.01–1.66 × N	1.67–2.33 × N	2.34–3.00 × N	>3.00 × N

*Denotes ECOG specific criteria.

Table A2   Karnovsky scale

100	Able to work. Normal; no complaints; no evidence of disease
90	Able to work. Able to carry on normal activity; minor symptoms
80	Able to work. Normal activity with effort; some symptoms
70	Independent; not able to work. Cares for self; unable to carry on normal activity
60	Disabled; dependent. Requires occasional assistance; cares for most needs
50	Moderately disabled; dependent. Requires considerable assistance and frequent care
40	Severely disabled; dependent. Requires special care and assistance
30	Severely disabled. Hospitalised, death not imminent
20	Very sick. Active supportive treatment needed
10	Moribund. Fatal processes are rapidly progressing

Source: reproduced with permission from Karnofsky DA, Abelmann WH, Craver LF, Burchenal. The use of nitrogen mustards in the palliative treatment of cancer. Cancer 1948; 1:634–656.

Table A3   ECOG performance status

Grade	ECOG
0	Fully active, able to carry on all pre-disease performance without restriction
1	Restricted in physically strenuous activity but ambulatory and able to carry out work of a light or sedentary nature, e.g. light house work, office work
2	Ambulatory and capable of all self-care but unable to carry out any work activities. Up and about more than 50% of waking hours
3	Capable of only limited self-care, confined to bed or chair more than 50% of waking hours
4	Completely disabled. Cannot carry on any self-care. Totally confined to bed or chair
5	Dead

Source: reproduced with permission from Oken MM, Creech RH, Tormey DC, et al. Toxicity and response criteria of the Eastern Cooperative Oncology Group. Am J Clin Oncol 1982; 5:649–655.

Glossary

5-HIAA (5-hydroxyindole acetic acid) – metabolite of serotonin that is excreted in the urine. Elevations in 5-hydroxyindole acetic acid can indicate carcinoid tumour.

ablative – a treatment regime consisting of very high doses of chemotherapy and/or radiotherapy which effectively eradicates haemopoietic cell production in the bone marrow.

adjuvant – treatment given following the initial primary treatment with the intention of improving response.

adverse events – are occasions on which patients are unexpectedly harmed in some way by the treatment rather than by the disease.

adverse healthcare events – are defined as 'an event or omission arising during clinical care and causing physical or psychological injury to a patient'.[1]

agranulocytes – leucocytes that do not have specialised membrane- bound cytoplasmic granules.

alkylation – direct interaction with DNA by chemotherapy.

allogeneic transplant – in allogeneic transplant, another individual, related or not, provides the HSC for the transplant.

alopecia – partial or total loss of hair.

alveolar soft-part sarcoma – tumour of connective tissue enclosing aggregates of large round or polygonal cells; occurs in subcutaneous and fibromuscular tissues.

anaemia – is a disturbance in erythrokinetics that results in a haemoglobin concentration below the expected normal for the age and sex of the patient.[2]

anaphylaxis – occurs when drug binds to IgE antibodies located on the mast cell surface (*anaphylactic reaction*) or triggers the enzymatic cascade of plasma proteins known as the complement system, releasing the biologically active anaphylatoxins C3a and C5a (*anaphylactoid reaction*). In the more common anaphylactic reaction, the drug may cross-react with pre-existing IgE antibodies or bind avidly to specific IgE antibodies produced following previous exposure to the drug.

angiosarcoma – cancer originating in the blood vessels.

anorexia – decreased or lost appetite for food.

anthracycline – type of chemotherapy that disrupts DNA, e.g. doxorubicin or daunorubicin.

antimetabolite – type of anticancer drugs comprising analogues of natural compounds required for DNA or RNA synthesis.

apoptosis – intrinsic mechanism of programmed cell death whereby aged, damaged or unnecessary cells are removed.

Askin's tumour – a characteristic PNET arising in the thorax.

asthenia – weakness.

ataxia – irregular or uncoordinated muscular activity.

AUC – Area under the curve, a measure of total exposure to a drug over time.

autograft – graft of tissues taken and grafted to the same individual. In stem cell transplantation used when the patient is the source of stem cells.

autologous transplant – the patient acts as his own source of HSC.

azoospermia – absent/low levels of sperm.

BCL – oncogenes divided into those that protect the cell from apoptosis (BCL2 itself, BCL-XL and BCL-W) and those that possess a pro-apoptotic function (BAX, BAD, BAK, BID).

bcr (breakpoint cluster region) – a region on chromosome 22 that is involved in the Philadelphia translocation.

benign – non-metastatic growth where the disease is limited within a well-defined capsule and removal is usually curative.

biochemotherapy – combination of chemotherapy and biotherapy (e.g. interferon or interleukin) with standard chemotherapy agent.

blast crisis – chronic myelogenous leukaemia progression to an acute phase with an increased number of immature white blood cells in the circulating blood.

blebbing – protrusion from the surface.

blood return – gentle aspiration and visualisation of blood into a syringe to confirm vein patency.

bolus – usually administration of an IV drug by injection from a syringe.

bone marrow blasts – immature cell with the potential to proliferate into mature blood cells. Increased numbers of blast cells are seen in leukaemia.

botryoid – resembling a bunch of grapes with rounded protuberances.

Breslow thickness – indication of vertical invasion into the subcutaneous tissues for melanoma, used as a prognostic indicator.

bullous – raised area filled with fluid.

canaliculi – in the liver channels between hepatocytes that carry bile to the bile duct. Also used to name channels in the bone.

cancer – state where a variety of normal cell regulatory processes controlling fundamental cell behaviour such as proliferation, death and motility are upset.

cancer cachexia – characterised by progressive weight loss, anorexia, muscle wasting and weakness. It is usually but not always accompanied by anorexia. Cachexia differs from starvation in that individuals fail to adapt to a decrease in intake by reducing metabolic rate and trying to conserve muscle mass.

cannula – a flexible tube containing a needle (stylet), which may be inserted into a blood vessel.[3]

carcinogenic – causing cancer.

cardioprotective – protecting the heart from damage.

cardiotoxicity – causing damage to the heart.

caspases – cysteine proteases that are activated specifically in apoptotic cells and cleave substrate proteins after aspartic acid residues.

catheter-related bloodstream infection – isolation of the same organism from a semiquantitative or quantitative culture of a catheter segment and from the blood (preferably from a peripheral vein) of a patient with clinical symptoms of a bloodstream infection and no other apparent source of infection.

CD8 antigens – members of the immunoglobulin supergene family that are associative recognition elements in major histocompatibility complex class I-restricted interactions.

cell cycle – process where the DNA is duplicated and the cell divides.

cell cycle mediated resistance – a chemotherapy drug is rendered less effective because of accumulation of cells into a phase of the cell cycle in which it is less active, through the action of other drugs given earlier in the combination.

cell kill hypothesis – tumours are best treated when they are small in volume and that treatment must continue until the last cell is killed.

central pontine myelinolysis – noninflammatory demyelination of the central basis pontis.

central venous catheter – catheter that is threaded through the internal jugular, antecubital or subclavian vein, usually with the tip resting in the superior vena cava or right atrium.[3]

cerebellar ataxia – loss of muscle coordination due to cerebral damage.

checkpoints – periods in the cell cycle where checks are made before progressing to the next phase of the cycle: e.g. at the R/START point within G_1 and at the G_2/M border.

chemical phlebitis – inflammation of the vein due to chemical irritation, e.g. from chemotherapy or electrolyte solutions.

chemokines – class of pro-inflammatory cytokines that have the ability to attract and activate leucocytes.

chromosomal translocation – a segment of chromosome is moved from one section of the chromosome to another position or chromosome.

class I tumour – responsive to chemotherapy; cures probable.

class II tumour – responsive to chemotherapy; not often curative but significant palliation.

class III tumour – generally resistant to chemotherapy; drugs not affecting survival.

clinical governance – 'the framework within which healthcare organisations are accountable for continuously improving the quality of their services and safeguarding high standards of care by creating an environment in which excellence in clinical care will flourish.'[4]

clinical stage (CS) – refers to the stage of disease based on physical examination and imaging technique (lymphoma).

CMV (cytomegalovirus) – widespread Herpetoviridae group viral infection. Can be opportunistic in the immunocompromised host. Patients who have been exposed to the virus will remain cytomegalovirus IgG positive.

collagen – a large protein with a high tensile strength found in connective tissue, skin, bone, cartilage and ligaments.

colonised catheter – growth of >15 colony-forming units (semiquantitative cultures) or $>10^3$ (quantitative culture) from the proximal or distal catheter segment in the absence of accompanying clinical symptoms.

combination chemotherapy – principles are that the drugs should all be active as single agents, possess differing mechanisms of action and have minimally overlapping toxicities.

compartment – group of separate muscles which are grouped and enclosed within a fascial membrane.

confluent – rash that runs together to form a patch.

constipation – delayed movement of intestinal content through the bowel; associated with a dry stool, which may be difficult to pass.[5]

controls assurance – 'a holistic concept based on best governance practice. It is a process designed to provide evidence that NHS organisations are doing their "reasonable best" to manage themselves so as to meet their objectives and protect patients, staff, the public and other stakeholders against risks of all kinds.'[6]

crisis state – characterised by massive cell death, end-to-end fusion of chromosomes and the occasional emergence of a variant cell that is termed immortalised and can multiply without limit.

cyclin-dependent kinases (CDKs) – protein family that regulate progression through the cell cycle and through checkpoints.

cytokine – a number of regulatory proteins that are released by cells of the immune system and act as messengers between cells in the generation of an immune response.

cytoplasmic protein kinases – enzymes which add phosphate groups to specific amino acids on substrate proteins.

cytostatic – suppresses cell growth and multiplication.

de novo (new) – often applied to biochemical pathways where metabolites are newly biosynthesised.

diarrhoea – has been defined 'as an abnormal increase in the quantity, frequency and fluid content of stool and associated with urgency perianal discomfort and incontinence'.[7]

direct bolus injection – dose of medication injected all at once intravenously.[3]

DNA (deoxyribonucleic acid) – genetic material contained within a cell's nucleus.

DNA mismatch repair (MMR) – corrects for base mismatches in DNA.

donor lymphocyte infusions (DLI) – DLI refers to any situation where lymphocytes from a previous donor of haematopoietic stem cells are given to the same recipient with the intention to shift the balance between donor and recipient haematopoiesis towards donor type.

drug resistance – considered to result from the high spontaneous mutation rate of cancer cells (i.e. genetic instability). May be caused by 'pharmacological' factors where insufficient drug reaches the cellular target or some change in the target has occurred or through 'post-target' mechanisms where, although the drug has reached the target, the tumour cells are not killed.

dysphagia – difficulty in swallowing, especially solid food.

dysphasia – inability to speak or think in words or inability to understand spoken or written words.

dysuria – difficulty in passing urine.

endocytosis – process where the cell engulfs a drop of the extracellular fluid by forming a vesicle with part of the cell membrane.

endogenous infection – infections caused by micro-organisms that patients carry on their own bodies (normal bacterial flora).

endoprosthesis – internal prosthetic device.

epithelium – covering layer of internal and external surfaces of the body, including the lining of vessels and other small cavities.

erythema – flushing of the skin due to dilatation of capillaries in the dermis.

eschar – devitalised tissue that is hard, black/brown in colour and leathery in appearance and forms after thermal or chemical burns. It is composed of serous exudate, dead dermal cells, leucocytes and several extracellular components, including collagen, fibrinogen and elastin.

exit site infection – erythema, tenderness, induration or purulence within 2 cm of the skin at the exit site of the catheter.

exocytosis – the release of intracellular fluid into the extracellular space.

exogenous infection – infections acquired in hospital from other people, either patients or staff.

extravasate – to leak into the tissues.

extravasation – the leakage and spread of fluid from vessels into the surrounding tissues.

extrinsic contamination – organisms introduced into the intravenous equipment during use.

fatigue – 'subjective, unpleasant symptom which incorporates total body feelings ranging from tiredness to exhaustion creating an unrelenting overall condition which interferes with individuals' ability to function to their normal capacity'.[8]

fibroblast – cells that produce collagen, elastic fibres and ground substance.

flap – area of tissue with a functioning blood supply that is dissected away from underlying structures and transferred from one anatomical site to another.

flare reaction – redness, blotchiness, and may result in the formation of small wheals, having a similar appearance to a nettle rash.

functional compartmental resection – excision of involved muscles, but with preservation of at least one functional muscle in the group.

fungating wound – the extension of a malignant tumour into the structures of the skin producing a raised or ulcerating necrotic lesion.

G_1 phase – where cells are preparing to synthesise DNA but where synthesis of RNA and protein occurs.

gastrointestinal stromal tumours (GIST) – rare non-epithelial malignant tumours of the GI tract.

Gompertzian function – as the size of a tumour increases, its rate of growth slows.

graft versus host disease (GvHD) – complication of bone marrow transplantation. The donated marrow initiates an immune reaction against the recipient's own tissues.

granulocytes – white blood cells with specialised membrane-bound cytoplasmic granules.

ground substance – mixture of fibrin, fibronectin and proteoglycans that fills the space between the collagen fibres and in which various cells are imbedded during wound healing.

growth factors – substances produced by cells that stimulate cell growth.

haemangiopericytoma – type of tumour formed from connective tissue cells and originating from capillaries.

haematopoiesis – the production of blood cells.

haematopoietic stem cell transplant (HSCT) – HSCT refers to any procedure transplanting the haematopoietic cell population into a recipient (the patient), with the intent to repopulate or replace the haematopoietic system totally or partially for transient or permanent periods of time.

haemostasis – the first phase of wound healing where the coagulation cascade is initiated and a blood clot, composed of platelets, fibrin and red blood cells, is formed to seal the wound.

hapten – small molecule which can act like an antigen and combine with an antibody, but is incapable by itself of causing an antibody response.

hazard ratio – statistical likelihood of death or recurrence.

healthcare associated infection (nosocomial infection) – infections that are neither present nor incubating when a patient enters hospital but are acquired during a hospital stay.

hemiparesis – paralysis of one side of the body.

heterogeneity – different type or characteristics.

HLA – human leucocyte antigen – proteins that activate the body's immune system to respond to foreign organisms.

homogeneously staining regions (HSRs) – chromosomes normally show banding when stained. An HSR appears uniform and contains multiple copies of a single gene.

homonymous hemianopia – blindness in the corresponding (right or left) field of vision of each eye.

human cancer models – tissue culture continuous cell lines and human tumours grown as xenografts on immune-suppressed or deficient mice.

human leukocyte antigen (HLA) – HLA or major histocompatability complex (MHC) is the polymorphic gene cluster on chromosome 6 that codes for cell surface proteins involved in tissue recognition.

hydrocephalus – accumulation of cerebrospinal fluid within the skull and dilatation of the cerebral ventricles, most often occurring secondarily to obstruction of the cerebrospinal fluid pathways.

hyperostosis – enlargement or overgrowth of bone.

IAP (inhibitors of apoptosis) – proteins which antagonise the action of caspase 3.

iatrogenic menopause – naturally occurring menopause.

immunocompromised – group of patients with impairment of either or both natural and specific immunity to infection, due to disease (i.e. cancer) or treatment (i.e. radiotherapy, steroids).

immunophenotyping – classification of the immune system cells based on structural and functional differences.

immunosuppressive – drug that suppresses the immune system, thereby reducing the body's resistance to infection or foreign proteins.

implanted vascular access device – consists of a portal attached to a silicone catheter; they are implanted subcutaneously, usually on the chest wall or in the antecubital area, and require access by a needle.

induration – abnormal hardening of tissue as a reaction to inflammation or neoplastic infiltration.

infiltration – infiltration is the inadvertent administration of a non-vesicant drug out of the venous system into the surrounding tissues.[9]

inter-strand cross-links – cross-links on different DNA strands.

interval debulking surgery – plan where the incomplete initial resection is followed by chemotherapy and then further surgery and chemotherapy.

intra-strand crosslinks – involving cross-links on the same strand of DNA.

intrinsic contamination – organisms introduced into the intravenous equipment prior to use.

invasive breast cancer – presence of malignant breast cells that have breached the basement membrane.

irritant drug – can cause local sensitivity and if it infiltrates can cause local inflammation and discomfort but no long-term damage.

karyotypic abnormality – abnormality in the number, form or structure of chromosomes; some are associated with leukaemia subtypes.

lagophthalmos – condition where the eye cannot be completely closed.

Li Fraumeni syndrome – inherited family trait carrying an increased risk of certain types of cancers among family members.

liposarcoma – type of sarcoma arising from lipoblastic cells.

locally advanced (breast cancer) – presentation of a primary cancer that is unsuitable for primary surgery due to either large size and/or involvement with other body structures.

macrophage – phagocytic cell present in connective tissue and several body organs.

maculopapular rash – consisting of spots and raised lumps on the skin.

major histocompatability complex (MHC) – the polymorphic gene cluster on chromosome 6 that codes for cell surface proteins involved in tissue recognition.

malignant – where the disease invades surrounding tissue and spreads around the body.

matched unrelated transplant (MUD) – an unrelated volunteer donor who is HLA matched provides the HSC.

mechanical phlebitis – irritation to the intima of the vein by mechanical means.

Medical Devices Agency (MDA) – executive agency of the Department of Health UK to ensure that all medical devices and equipment meet the appropriate standards of safety, quality and performance, and comply with the relevant European directives.

mesenchymal – tissues relating to the middle layer of the early embryo. Develops into the musculoskeletal, connective tissue, blood, vascular and urinogenital systems and some glands.

metastases – spread or recurrence of secondary tumours at distant sites, including bone, liver, lung or soft tissue.

midline catheter – a peripheral device inserted into an antecubital vein, where the tip is advanced along the vein of the upper arm up to 20 cm, but is not extended past the axilla.

mitomycin C – a prodrug that requires activation by enzymatic reduction to produce a molecule that forms cross-links on DNA.

morbidity – reduction in health or symptoms of disease.

morphology – study of the structure of animal or man.

mortality – death rate.

MRPs – organic ion transporters that are able to transport a wide variety of substances out of cells.

mucositis – an inflammatory reaction of the gastrointestinal, respiratory or genitourinary mucosa, the most common sites being the oral cavity and oesophagus.

murine – mouse.

mutagenic – causing genetic mutation.

myalgia – muscular pain.

myelodysplasia – abnormal change in the bone marrow cells.

myelosuppression – reduction in the bone marrow production of blood cells.

nadir count – in chemotherapy it is the blood's lowest level of the number of blood cells after chemotherapy-induced bone marrow suppression.

necrosis – changes in the cell that show it has died and is being broken down by enzymes.

neo-adjuvant – prior to surgery.

neurofibromatosis – hereditary disorder characterised by brown and white spots on the skin and a tendency to develop nerve tumours.

neurotoxicity – (chemotherapy-induced) result of direct or indirect damage to the central nervous system (CNS), peripheral nervous system or any combination of these.

neutrophil – type of white blood cell capable of phagocytosis that are drawn to areas of inflammation.

non-tunnelled central venous catheter – enters through the skin directly into a central vein.

nosocomial infection – infections that are neither present nor incubating when a patient enters hospital but are acquired during a hospital stay.

nucleotide excision repair (NER) – complex interaction of at least 20 proteins to recognise and excise damaged DNA, then synthesise new DNA to fill the resulting gap and reseal.

odds ratio – statistical likelihood of recurrence.

odynophagia – pain on swallowing.

oesophagitis – inflammation of the oesophageal mucosa.

oncogenes – act in a dominant manner and may be viewed as cell cycle accelerators.

opportunistic infections – infections caused by organisms that do not normally cause infections in persons with normal immune responses.

oral mucositis – inflammation of the lining of the oral cavity; also known as stomatitis.

osteoblasts – develop from fibroblasts and produce bone tissue.

p53 – protein that plays a fundamental role in normal cell cycle progression and apoptosis but which is inactivated by a variety of means in the vast majority of tumours. Its function is to bind to particular DNA sequences, leading to the activation of adjacent genes, such as those involved in cell cycle arrest.

Paget's disease – type of ductal carcinoma, associated with eczema-like changes of the nipple.

pancytopenia – reduction of all blood cells after chemotherapy.

parenchyma – the functional rather than the structural elements of an organ.

peripheral cannula – a flexible tube containing a needle (stylet), which may be inserted into a blood vessel.[3]

peripherally inserted central catheter (PICC) – a catheter which is inserted via the antecubital veins in the arm and is advanced into the central veins, with the tip located in the lower third superior vena cava (SVC).[10–12]

phagocytosis – engulfment and digestion of foreign particles, including bacteria, by a cell.

phase I clinical trials – phase I clinical trials are the first use of an investigational drug in humans.

phase II clinical trials – a phase II clinical trial is designed to determine the anticancer activity of an investigational drug against specific types of tumours.

phase III clinical trials – a phase III trial aims to establish the usefulness of the investigational drug in the treatment of the specified cancer through large randomised controlled trials (RCTs) comparing the new treatment with the current standard treatment.

phase IV clinical trials – the phase IV trial seeks to monitor adverse effects of a new drug after it has been approved for marketing.

phlebitis – inflammation of a vein, in some cases with pain and erythema.

phosphatase – enzymes opposite in effect to kinases in that they remove phosphate groups, generally leading to inactivation.

phosphorylation – creation of a new phosphate-derived product from an organic molecule.

pleomorphic – having different forms at each stage of the life cycle.

Plummer–Vinson syndrome (Patterson–Kelly syndrome) – a syndrome with a number of characteristics that include increased incidence of oesophageal carcinoma.

pluripotent stem cell disease – where the patient may lack any normal stem cells.

point mutations – single amino acid changes in specific positions of the gene.

primary cachexia – cachexia without a mechanical or functional aetiology.

prodrug – a compound that is converted in the body into its active form.

proptosis – abnormal bulging of the eyeball.

randomised controlled trial – a clinical trial that involves at least one test treatment and one control treatment, where the treatments to be administered are selected by a random process.

relative resistance – drug interaction that leads to decreased cytotoxicity (antagonism).

rete – network or plexus or resembling a network, particularly blood vessels or nerves.

retroperitoneal – the back of the abdominal space.

rhabdomyosarcomas – thought to arise from primitive mesenchymal cells with the capacity for rhabdomyoblastic development.

S phase – cell cycle phase where there is a doubling of the DNA content.

sarcomas – malignant neoplasms derived from mesenchymal connective tissue.

scalp hypothermia – application of cold to the scalp in an effort to reduce hair loss from some types of chemotherapy.

sclerosant – injectable irritant used to produce blood vessel occlusion.

second gap (G$_2$) phase – where the cell is preparing for cell division.

secondary cachexia – food intake is diminished as a result of treatment side effects.

senescence – state of being old.

sentinel node – first lymph node(s) to receive drainage from a cancer-containing area of the breast.

Sertoli cells – testis cells that produce sperm.

single arm study – there is no randomisation and all eligible patients receive the investigational drug at the same dose.

skin-tunnelled catheter ('Hickman' catheter) – a catheter that lies in a subcutaneous tunnel with the exit site midway from the anterior chest wall and the tip lying at the junction of the SVC and right atrium or within the SVC or upper right atrium.[13]

slough – devitalised tissue that is soft, moist and often stringy in consistency. It is usually yellow, white and/or grey in colour and has a similar composition to eschar but with a larger number of leucocytes present.

spermatogenesis – manufacture of sperm in the seminiferous tubules.

stage – main determinant of prognosis in cancer; staging takes into account tumour size, nodal involvement, presence of metastases and histological grade.

stem cell – the most primitive cells in the bone marrow from which all types of blood cell can develop.

steroidogenesis – production of androgens, including testosterone.

stomatitis – inflammation of the lining of the oral cavity.

superior vena cava – second largest vein of the body, returning deoxygenated blood from the upper half of the body to the right atrium.[3]

syngeneic transplant – an identical twin of the patient acts as the source for HSC.

telomeres – repetitive DNA sequences (TTAGGG in humans) and associated proteins present at the ends of chromosomes.

teratogenic – causing abnormality in development (of the fetus).

thrombocytopenia – low platelet count.

thrombophlebitis – vein inflammation associated with thrombus formation.

topoisomerase I & II – enzymes important in maintaining DNA topology and in DNA replication and recombination, as they introduce transient double- or single-stranded DNA breaks followed by strand passage and rejoining.

transcription factors – bind to specific DNA sequences and activate the transcription of genes.

tubulin – tubulin is localised in the centrosome of the cell and is involved in nucleation of microtubule assembly during the cell cycle.

tumour suppressors – act as cell cycle retarders.

tunnel infection – erythema and tenderness in the tissue over the catheter and >2 cm from the exit site.

vascular access devices (VADs) – a VAD is inserted either into a vein or an artery, via the peripheral or central vessels, to provide for either diagnostic or therapeutic purposes.[14]

venous spasm – pain along the vein caused by local irritation usually by drugs[15] or temperature.

vesicant – an irritant drug that has the potential to cause blistering, severe tissue damage and even necrosis if extravasated and usually requires some form of management.

wide excision margins – surgical removal of the whole tumour in one piece with a margin of normal tissue surrounding it.

winged infusion device – or 'butterfly', is a steel needle with a short section of tubing attached which can be used to give bolus injections intravenously.

xerostomia is a subjective feeling of mouth dryness.

References

1. Department of Health. An organisation with a memory. Report of an Expert Group on Learning from Adverse Events in the NHS. London: The Stationary Office; 2000.

2. Groeger JS. Critical care of the cancer patient. St Louis: Mosby Year Book; 1991:8–92.

3. Mosby's pocket dictionary of nursing, medicine and professions allied to medicine, 1995 UK edition. Anderson KN, Anderson LE, eds. London: Mosby; 1995.

4. NHS Health Service Circular. Clinical governance – quality in the new NHS. SC 1999/065. London: Department of Health; 1999.

5. Winney J. Constipation. Nurs Stand 1998; 13(11):49–56.

6. NHS Health Service Circular. Governance in the new NHS: controls assurance statements, 1999/2000 – risk management and organisational controls. HSC 1999/123. London: Department of Health; 1999.

7. Cope DG. Management of chemotherapy induced diarrhoea and constipation. Nurs Clin N Am 2001; 36(4):695–707, vi.

8. Ream E, Richardson A. Fatigue in patients with cancer and chronic obstructive airways disease: a phenomenological enquiry. Int J Nurs Stud 1997; 34(1):44–53.

9. Oncology Nursing Society. Cancer chemotherapy guidelines and recommendations for practice. Pittsburgh: Oncology Nursing Press, 1999.

10. Hadaway LC. Developing an intraactive intravenous education and training program. J Intraven Nurs 1999; 22(2):87–93.

11. Goodwin M, Carlson I. The peripherally inserted catheter: a retrospective look at 3 years of insertions, J Intraven Nursing 1993; 16(2):92–103.

12. Gabriel J. Long term venous access. In: Dougherty L, Lamb J, eds. Intravenous therapy in nursing practice 1999, Edinburgh: Churchill Livingstone; 1999.

13. Davidson T, Al Mufti, R. Hickman central venous catheters in cancer patients. Cancer Topics 1997; 10(8):10–14.

14. Dougherty L, Lister S. The Royal Marsden manual of clinical nursing procedures. 6th edn. Oxford: Blackwell Science, 2004.

15. Weinstein SM. Antineoplastic therapy. In: Plumer's principles and practice of IV therapy. 7th edn. Philadelphia: JB Lippincott; 2000.

Index

Notes

Page numbers suffixed by 't' indicate material in tables: page numbers suffixed by 'f' indicate material in figures: page numbers suffixed by 'b' indicate material in boxes

To save space in the index, the following abbreviations have been used:

ALL - acute lymphoblastic leukaemia
AML - acute myeloid leukaemia
CLL - chronic lymphocytic leukaemia
CML - chronic myeloid leukaemia
5-FU - 5-fluorouracil

GvHD - graft-versus-host disease
NHL - non-Hodgkin's lymphoma
NSCLC - non-small cell lung cancer
SCT - stem cell transplantation
vs. indicates a differential diagnosis or comparison.

Journals of related interest

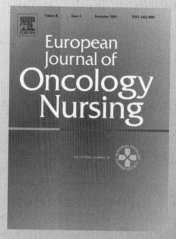

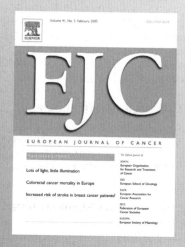

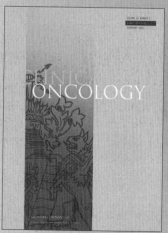

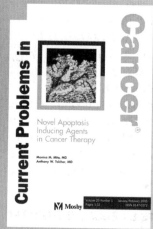

You can order these, or any other Elsevier title (Churchill Livingstone, Saunders, Mosby, Baillière Tindall, Butterworth-Heinemann), from your local bookshop, or, in case of difficulty, direct from us on:

EUROPE, MIDDLE EAST & AFRICA
Tel: +31 20 485 3757
www.elsevierhealth.com/journals

ASIA & AUSTRALIA
Tel: +65 6349 0222
www.elsevierhealth.com/journals

CANADA
Tel: +1 866 276 5533
www.elsevier.ca

USA
Tel: +1 877 839 7126
www.elsevierhealth.com/journals

ELSEVIER